The Biological Effects of Glutamic Acid and Its Derivatives

Developments in Molecular and Cellular Biochemistry

V. A. NAJJAR, *series editor*

Volume 1

MARTINUS NIJHOFF/DR W. JUNK PUBLISHERS   THE HAGUE/BOSTON/LONDON   1981

The Biological Effects of Glutamic Acid and Its Derivatives

Edited by
V. A. NAJJAR

Reprinted from
Molecular and Cellular Biochemistry, Vols. 38 and 39, 1981

MARTINUS NIJHOFF/DR W. JUNK PUBLISHERS   THE HAGUE/BOSTON/LONDON   1981

Distributors:

for the United States and Canada

Kluwer Boston, Inc.
190 Old Derby Street
Hingham, MA 02043
USA

for all other countries

Kluwer Academic Publishers Group
Distribution Center
P.O. Box 322
3300 AH Dordrecht
The Netherlands

Library of Congress Cataloging in Publication Data
Main entry under title:

The Biological effects of glutamic acid and its
    derivatives.

    (Developments in molecular and cellular
biochemistry ; v. 1)
    "Reprinted from Molecular and cellular bio-
chemistry, vols. 38 and 39, 1981."
    1. Glutamic acid--Physiological effect--Ad-
dresses, essays, lectures. I. Najjar, V. A.
(Victor A.), 1914-   . II. Molecular and
cellular biochemistry. III. Series.
QP562.G5B56 1981   599.01'9245   81-20731
                                        AACR2

ISBN-13: 978-94-009-8029-7   e-ISBN-13: 978-94-009-8027-3
DOI: 10.1007/978-94-009-8027-3

Introduction to 'Developments in molecular and cellular biochemistry'

Molecular and Cellular Biochemistry is an international journal that covers a wide range of biophysical, biochemical and cellular research. This type of coverage is intended to acquaint the reader with the several parameters of biological research that are relevant to various fields of interest. Unlike highly specialized journals, it does not bring into focus a particular field of investigation on a monthly basis. Accordingly, it has been decided to supplement its present wide scope by periodic presentations of a restricted area of research in the form of book-length volumes. These volumes will also be published in hard covers as a book series entitled, *Developments in Molecular and Cellular Biochemistry*. Each volume will focus on an active topic of interest which will be covered in depth. It will encompass a series of contributions that deal exclusively with one single well-defined subject.

The present volume, *The Biological Effects of Glutamate and Its Derivatives,* is the first one in the book series. The second volume will deal extensively with *Immunologically Active Peptides*.

It is the editor's hope that *Molecular and Cellular Biochemistry* will fulfill its intended role of service to the international community of biological scientists.

The biological effects of glutamic acid and its derivatives

During the past decade, there has been much active research into the effects of glutamic acid and its derivatives on several target organs, particularly the nervous system. It is also involved in the γ-glutamyl cycle through the activity of the enzyme γ-glutamyl transpeptidase. Equally important are the poly-γ-glutamyl derivatives of folic acid. These have been scattered in many scientific journals, some in basic science journals and others in technical publications. In view of this and the rapid advances in this area during the past decade, it was deemed advisable to bring together many of these investigations into one single publication. This has been done under the auspices of *Molecular and Cellular Biochemistry,* an international journal, and has now been published as Volume 1 of 'Developments in Molecular and Cellular Biochemistry'.

Victor A. Najjar, Editor in chief

Contents

Hippocampal glutamate receptors

Michel Baudry and Gary Lynch
Dept. of Psychobiology, University of California, Irvine, CA 92717, U.S.A.

Summary

For years, the hippocampus has been the privileged domain of anatomists and electrophysiologists for investigating various neurobiological processes. The present review deals with recent work which shows that this structure is also well suited to study the role of glutamate as a neurotransmitter and more particularly the characteristics of glutamate receptors and their possible involvement in hippocampal function. After a brief description of the main anatomical features of the hippocampus, we attempt a critical evaluation of the electrophysiological studies of hippocampal glutamate receptors. We then describe the properties of Na-independent ^{3}H-glutamate binding sites in hippocampal membranes, and discuss the possibility that these binding sites are related to postsynaptic glutamate receptors. Finally we show that these binding sites are extremely labile and that hippocampal membranes possess various mechanisms which regulate their number. In particular we develop the idea that the calcium-stimulation of ^{3}H-glutamate binding in hippocampal membranes may be the mechanism by which electrical activity regulates the number of glutamate receptors at hippocampal synapses and thus induces long-lasting changes in synaptic transmission.

Introduction

Because of its relatively simple anatomical organization, the hippocampus has become increasingly popular as a model for the study of basic neurobiological processes. The cell bodies of hippocampal neurones form two densely packed and widely separated layers while the dendrites are arranged in parallel arrays stretching for considerable distances from the somata. The major extrinsic and intrinsic fiber projections travel in well defined layers oriented at right angles to the axis of the dendrites. Thus a given lamina of the hippocampus consists, for the most part, of dendritic segments from one cell type and synapses generated by one or two afferents, a situation which vastly simplifies the problem of analyzing well-defined inputs and their targets.

While most of the work exploiting these properties has involved anatomical or physiological questions, neurochemists have begun using the hippocampus for the study of transmitters and their receptors. The possibility that acidic amino acids are used as transmitter in excitatory synapses·in the central nervous system (CNS) has come under particularly intense investigation (1–5). The hippocampus proves to have effective systems for the uptake and release of glutamate (6) and there is evidence which indicates that glutamate or a related compound is released during synaptic transmission (7). The hippocampus also possesses high affinity binding sites for glutamate (8) and one category of these possesses certain characteristics which render it a reasonable candidate for a post-synaptic receptor (9). It is this subject which forms the topic of the present paper. In the following sections we will review physiological and biochemical studies of glutamate receptors in hippocampus and attempt

Molecular and Cellular Biochemistry 38, 5–18 (1981).   0300–8177/81/0381–0005/$ 2.80.

to relate these to each other and to the possible role of amino acids as transmitters. We shall also summarize recent evidence that the number of glutamate binding sites in hippocampal membranes is regulated by calcium-sensitive enzymes and consider the possibility that this form of receptor 'plasticity' is related to certain rather extraordinary physiological properties of hippocampal synapses. Before beginning the discussion of binding sites, it is appropriate that we first outline the various pathways within hippocampus which have been used in physiological and biochemical studies.

Anatomy of the hippocampus

Fig. 1 illustrates the major pathways and subdivisions of hippocampal formation. The dentate gyrus is composed of a 'C' shaped row of granule cell bodies, the dendrites of which generate a homogeneous, essentially cell-free molecular layer. This dendritic field is innervated by afferents from the entorhinal cortex ('perforant path') and ipsilateral ('associational' projections) and contralateral ('commissural' projections) hippocampus proper.

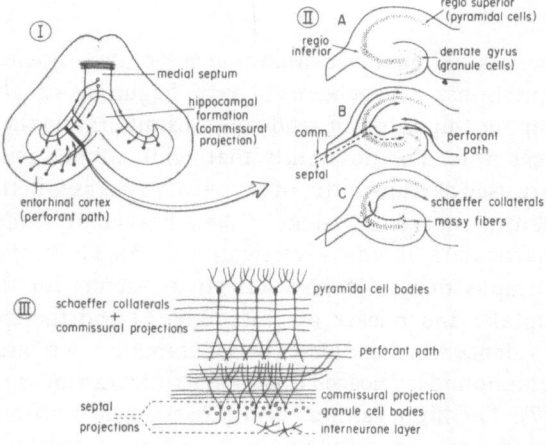

Fig. 1. Schematic illustration of major subdivisions and pathways of the hippocampus. The drawing at the top left is a horizontal view of the forebrain and illustrates the relative positions of hippocampus, entorhinal cortex and the septum (I). Three successive sections through the hippocampus are shown on the right; these indicate the subdivison (dentate gyrus, regio inferior, and regio superior) extrinsic and intrinsic pathways of the structure (II). At the bottom is shown a picture of the cell types of the regio superior and dentate gyrus including the distribution of key inputs (III).

These inputs are strictly segregated with the perforant path innervating the outer 3/4 of the molecular layer while the pyramidal cell projections share the inner portions of the dendritic trees (see ref. (10) for a review). The septum sends a cholinergic projection to the dentate gyrus but it is not yet clear if this terminates on the granule cells directly or instead is targeted for a population of interneurones (see ref. (11) for a review). The granule cell bodies are densely innervated by a group of subjacent basket cells; there is good evidence that these cells use GABA as their transmitter (12).

The granule cell axons, the mossy fibers, collect together on the inner face of the 'C' formed by the dentate gyrus and travel together as a bundle across the proximal dendrites of the pyramidal cells of the nearby regio inferior of the hippocampus proper. These fibers generate enormous boutons which are unusual in that they contain high concentrations of zinc and in all probability, enkephalin (13). The remaining portions of the pyramidal cell dendrites are innervated by the pyramidal cells of the ipsilateral and contralateral hippocampus as well as by the entorhinal cortex. The regio inferior pyramidal cells produce a dense bilateral projection to the apical dendrites of the regio superior pyramidal cells; this is the so-called Schaeffer-commissural projection and has been the subject of many neurophysiological studies.

Neurophysiological studies of amino acid receptors in hippocampus

Effects of various amino acids on cell physiology

A variety of neurophysiological techniques have been used to study amino acid receptors in hippocampus and in general the data accord well with those obtained for other structures. Attempts have also been made to determine if these receptors are used by several of the synaptic systems in hippocampus and, while certainly not conclusive, the results have been encouraging.

When applied by iontophoresis, glutamate and aspartate both cause a marked increase in the firing rates of hippocampal pyramidal and granule cells (14, 15). These effects are produced by application to the dendritic trees as well as to the cell bodies, occur with extremely short latencies, and can be elicited by simply removing the 'holding' current on the glutamate electrode (15). The excitatory action of both amino acids is completely suppressed by iontophoretic application of glutamic acid diethyl ester (GDEE) in the regio superior; however, this drug has no effect on aspartate in the dentate gyrus (16). GDEE appears to have no effect on cell firing changes produced by acetylcholine in dentate gyrus (16, 17) and hippocampus proper (15). Segal (18) has measured the effects of pressure application of amino acids to the dendrites on the membrane potential and conductance of the CAI pyramidal cell body and reports that glutamate produces a marked depolarization of the pyramidal cells followed by a long lasting hyperpolarization. He also found evidence for an inhibitory interneurone which appears to have an extremely rapid response to glutamate. Somewhat surprisingly, D-glutamate proved to have about the same potency as the L-isomer. Quisqualic and D,L-homocysteic acids were about 25 times more potent than glutamate while kainic acid was the most powerful amino acid tested, being some 100 times as effective as glutamate. However, kainic acid had a slower onset time than did glutamic acid and its effects persisted for a much longer period than did glutamate, suggesting that the two amino acids may be operating in a qualitatively different fashion. The effects of glutamate were blocked by D-glutamylglycine (DGG), 2-amino-5 phosphonovaleric acid (2APV) and GDEE, in that order of efficiency.

Effects of amino acid antagonists on synaptic physiology

There have been several recent attempts to block synaptic potentials in hippocampus with antagonists of the excitatory amino acids. Two of the better controlled studies have employed iontophor-etic application of these drugs to the granule cells of the dentate gyrus. Wheal & Miller (17) report that GDEE, at concentrations which block iontophor-etically applied glutamate, inhibits cell discharges elicited by stimulation of the perforant path but not by stimulation of the medial septum. Atropine, which blocks ACh but not glutamate-induced excitation of the granule cells, suppresses cell discharges elicited by stimulation of the medial septum but not those caused by perforant path activation. Hicks & McLennan (16) found that iontophoretically applied GDEE blocked cell discharge elicited by glutamate but not those recorded in response to aspartate or its analogue N-methyl-DL-aspartate (NMDA) (as noted above, however, GDEE has not been reported to block aspartate in the *regio superior*). D-a-aminoadipate (D-α-AA) produced a converse set of results: it blocked the aspartate response without influencing the response of the granule cells to glutamate. GDEE inhibited the discharge of the granule cells to perforant path but not commissural stimulation while D-α-AA produced the opposite pattern of results in 7 cells (Table 1).

Taken together these results make a reasonable case for the following conclusions: 1) a 'glutamate' receptor is used in the perforant path synapses but not in the connections arising from the commissural projections; 2) an 'aspartate' (or NMDA preferring) receptor is involved in transmission across the commissural but not perforant path synapses. It bears emphasizing that the physiological measures used in these studies, namely spike discharges, are both physically and temporally removed from the transmission process: the experiments measure the effects of the drugs on the responses of the granule cells to EPSP's but not the effects of the drugs on the EPSP's themselves. The selectivity of drug action (e.g., GDEE blocks one

Table 1. The effect of three drugs applied by iontophoresis on the granule cell discharges elicited by putative transmitters or electrical stimulation of dentate gyrus afferents (see text for abbreviations).

	Glutamate	Aspartate	Acetylcholine	Perforant path	Comm. project	Medial septum
GDEE[a,b]	block	no effect	no effect	block	no effect	no effect
D-α-AA[a]	no effect	block	not tested	no effect	block	not tested
atropine[b]	no effect	not tested	block	no effect	not tested	block

[a] Based on Hicks & McLennan (16).
[b] Based on Wheal & Miller (17).

input but not another) tends to rule out generalized effects on the electronic properties of the granule cells; however, the afferents used are located at different levels of the dendritic trees and the possibility that they are differentially influenced by manipulations of the physiological properties of the primary dendrites and somata of the granule cells cannot be excluded. Hicks & McLennan (16) also report that D-α-AA causes an increase in the background firing rate of the granule cells. Since the increased firing is blocked by the GABA antagonist bicuilline, they assume that the effect is due to the actions of α-AA on a group of aspartate-driven inhibiting interneurones. While this is a reasonable interpretation, it must be noted that bicuculline has been shown to have multiple effects on hippocampal neurones (19) and therefore its actions in this pivotal control experiment cannot be assumed with certainty to be due to an antagonism of GABA. Furthermore, removal of tonic inhibition by α-AA would have been expected to produce an enhanced response by the granule cells to both glutamate and perforant path stimulation and this apparently did not occur.

Local application of antagonists via pressure injection has also been used to study the effects of antagonists on synaptic transmission in hippocampus. Segal (18) found that D-glutamylglycine (DGG). 2-amino-5-phosphonovaleric acid (2APV), and GDEE infusion into the apical dendrites of the regio superior pyramidal cells blocked EPSP's (recorded intracellularly) produced by stimulation of the Schaeffer-commissural inputs to these regions. However, he does not describe controls for potential non-specific effects of the drugs and accordingly these data must be considered as preliminary in nature.

Electrophysiological studies using the in vitro hippocampal slice

The *in vitro* slice method affords the opportunity to perfuse the hippocampus with drugs at known concentrations, as well as to identify their locus of action. While these features should be of great value in assessing the possible role of amino acid receptors in synaptic transmission, the pharmacological results thus far obtained with the slice have not been conclusive. Aminophosphonobutyric acid (APB) has been reported to block the synaptic field potentials generated by stimulation of the perforant path in the dentate gyrus (20) and by the Schaeffer-commissural fibers in the regio superior (20, 21). Interestingly, GDEE was found to be ineffective with bath applications although, as noted above, it does block responses when applied by pressure to the dendritic fields of regio superior or by ionto-phoresis to the cell bodies of the granule neurones (see Table 1).

While suggestive, these experiments do not satis-factorily establish that the observed actions of the drugs are due to post-synaptic receptor blockade. The concentrations of APB used in the above studies cause an increased discharge of the pyra-midal cells (20) and are close to levels which produce pronounced physiological disturbances in slices. White *et al.* (20) argue that the increase in the frequency of cell firing produced by APB is due to the reduction of activity of inhibitory interneurones (via a suppression of amino acid innervation of these cells) but the effect could as well be due to a partial depolarization of the neurones. It has been reported that APB does not reduce antidromic potentials or fiber volleys in the slice (20); however, it is not clear if these extracellular measures are sufficiently sensitive to detect the small degree of depolarization needed to reduce release and post-synaptic excitatory potentials. It should be em-phasized that relatively small drops in the mem-brane potential of nerve terminals have been shown to cause substantial decrements in transmitter release. In light of this, it is imperative that the sensitivity of controls for depolarization and non-specific effects etc. be carefully calibrated in phar-macological experiments using slices and to date this has not been done.

In summary, several lines of evidence point to the conclusion that hippocampus contains a full com-plement of acidic amino acid receptors. Further-more, while individual experiments are not entirely satisfactory, the body of data suggests that these receptors are involved in synaptic transmission. There are points of confusion which require atten-tion; chief among these is that GDEE blocks synaptic responses when applied by iontophoresis but appears relatively ineffective when perfused through slices.

Biochemical studies of hippocampal glutamate receptors

In addition to the physiological measures described above, receptors can also be analyzed using biochemical events associated with the interaction between them and their transmitters. In many cases this event can be the stimulation of an enzymatic activity linked to the receptor (e.g. β-adrenergic receptor and adenylate cyclase) (22). While excitatory amino acids induce an increased level of cyclic GMP in cerebellar slices (23), with a pharmacology relatively similar to that of the electrophysiological receptors (24), there have been no attempts to use this approach in hippocampal slices. Another biochemical approach to the study of receptors consists in measuring changes in ionic fluxes elicited by the transmitter, as exemplified in studies of the acetylcholine receptors (25). A recent study (26) showed that glutamate modifies sodium fluxes in striatal slices, but this procedure has not yet been applied to the identification of hippocampal glutamate receptors. The most popular technique for studying receptors in the past decade has been to measure the binding of an appropriate ligand to purified membranes. While simple and direct, these procedures suffer from the drawback that they do not provide any guarantee that the binding sites are part of a physiologically active receptor. Therefore, binding studies typically incorporate efforts to establish if the sites under study possess various properties which *a priori* would be expected of a 'true' receptor (27). Several of these anticipated properties are: 1) an affinity in the concentration range over which the ligand is known to produce physiological effects, 2) saturability, 3) reversibility, 4) a regional and subcellular localization consistent with those of its action, 5) a relative binding affinity of analogues which correlates with their physiological effects. Several groups have used some or all of these criteria in attempts to identify glutamate receptors in a number of preparations (27–34). Although kainic acid was initially thought to label glutamate receptors (35), more recent studies have clearly shown that it binds to a site separate from the glutamate receptors (36, 37). In the absence of specific agonists or antagonists, the ligand which has been generally used is glutamate itself, which raises the problem of distinguishing presynaptic uptake and postsynaptic receptor sites. In the case of GABA, the binding to uptake sites requires sodium and this feature has been used to distinguish between these 2 categories of sites (38). Although Roberts (28) reported the existence in cortical membranes of what appeared to be Na-independent and Na-dependent sites for glutamate, a later study on cerebellar membranes (32) did not substantiate this point. On the other hand, Vincent & McGeer (39), using rat striatal membranes, showed that binding of glutamate in the presence of sodium was labeling sites likely associated with high-affinity uptake. Given that the data on this crucial point were not in complete agreement, it was necessary to begin the analysis of glutamate binding sites in hippocampus with an analysis of the effects of monovalent cations.

Effects of monovalent cations on hippocampal ^3H-glutamate binding

When the effects of a wide range of concentrations were tested, it was found that sodium exerts a remarkable biphasic effect on ^3H-glutamate binding to hippocampal membranes (Fig. 2) (9). Very low concentrations of sodium (0.1 to 5 mM) induce a dose-dependent inhibition of the binding with an IC_{50} of about 0.75 mM and a maximum inhibition (at 2.5 mM) of 80%. Concentrations of sodium higher than 10 mM cause a dose-dependent stimulation of the binding with an

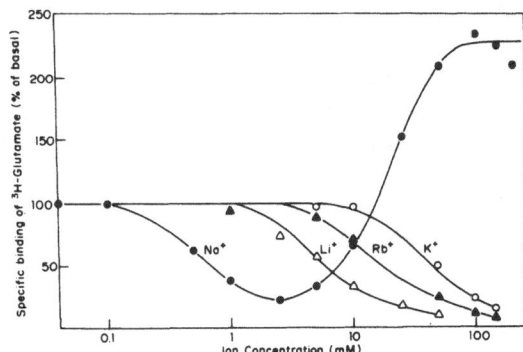

Fig. 2. Effects of monovalent cations on ^3H-glutamate binding to rat hippocampal membranes. Rat hippocampal membranes were prepared and immediately assayed for ^3H-glutamate binding as described in Baudry & Lynch (9,59), in the presence of the various cations. Results represent specific binding of ^3H-glutamate determined by the amount of binding displaced by 0.1 mM cold glutamate and are expressed as percent of the binding measured in the absence of sodium. Mean of three different experiments. Data from Baudry & Lynch (9,40).

EC_{50} of about 25 mM and a maximum stimulation of about 250%. The inhibitory effect of the sodium ion is shared by several monovalent cations (Fig. 2), with lithium, caesium, and potassium exhibiting an IC_{50} of 6.5 mM, 20 mM and 55 mM, respectively (40). This order of potency suggests that the inhibitory effect is relatively selective for sodium since there is a 10-fold difference in IC_{50} between sodium and lithium and almost a 100 fold difference between sodium and potassium. This pattern of results is most easily explained by the existence of two glutamate binding sites in hippocampus, one of which ('Na-independent') is inhibited by sodium and one of which ('Na-dependent') requires the cation. As will be developed below, pharmacological experiments provide strong support for this hypothesis.

A similar biphasic effect of sodium is also found in cerebellar membranes although, possibly due to a different balance of the Na-independent and the Na-dependent binding sites in this structure compared to hippocampus, high concentrations of sodium still produce a net inhibitory effect; this probably explains the apparently contradictory results of Roberts (28) and Foster & Roberts (32).

When the binding of various concentrations of ^3H-glutamate was measured in the presence of various monovalent cation concentrations, it was found that the maximum number of binding sites was decreased without any obvious changes in the apparent affinity of glutamate for the receptors excluding a direct competition effect of sodium on the binding (40). In addition, recent studies showed that treatment of membranes with the detergent Triton X-100 suppresses the inhibitory effect of low sodium concentrations on ^3H-glutamate binding, suggesting that the inhibitory effect of the cation does not involve a direct action on the binding site (Baudry *et al.*, submitted). Neurophysiological studies have indicated that the glutamate receptor is likely to be linked to a sodium conductance channel (41) and by analogy with other neurotransmitter receptors (for example GABA with chloride (42) and glycine with chloride (43)) it is possible that the sodium-induced decrease in binding reflects some interaction between the sodium channel and the glutamate receptors. Conceivably the inhibitory effect is due to a feed-back regulatory mechanism in which opening and subsequent interactions of the channel with sodium ions result in an inhibition of the association of glutamate to its recognition site.

Kinetic and pharmacological properties of ^3H-glutamate binding

When the association of ^3H-glutamate to hippocampal membranes was studied in the absence of sodium, the binding occurred rapidly and equilibrium was reached within about 15 min. (9). The second-order association constant (K_1) was estimated to be 0.57 μM^{-1} min^{-1}. Equilibrium was achieved more rapidly for the Na-dependent binding (less than 5 minutes) and the second-order association constant was found to be 1.18 μM^{-1} min^{-1}. The dissociation of ^3H-glutamate bound to hippocampal membranes induced by adding an excess of gold glutamate was extremely rapid at 30 °C; the time for half-dissociation of the Na-independent binding was about 1 minute corresponding to a dissociation rate constant (K_{-1}) of 0.65 min^{-1}, whereas the corresponding values for the Na-dependent binding were 0.5 min and 1.3 min^{-1}. The ratio of K_{-1} to K_1 gives an estimate of the equilibrium dissociation constant Kd which according to the above data would be about 1 μM for both the Na-independent and the Na-dependent sites.

^3H-Glutamate binding to hippocampal membranes in the absence or presence of sodium is saturable and Scatchard analysis revealed a homogeneous population of binding sites in the range of glutamate concentrations studied (50 nM to 10 μM). The Na-independent binding exhibited a Kd of about 500 nM and a maximum number of sites of 6.5 pmol/mg protein, whereas the Na-dependent binding exhibited a Kd of 2500 μM and a maximum number of sites of 75 pmol/mg protein (9). These numbers provide an explanation for the two to three fold increase in binding elicited by high sodium concentration observed at a ^3H-glutamate concentration of 100 nM. In both cases the Hill coefficient was not significantly different from unity indicating the absence of apparent cooperativity of the binding of glutamate to the two sites.

Thus the equilibrium dissociation constants estimated from saturation kinetics or association and dissociation kinetics, are in reasonably good agreement, although the very rapid dissociation rate of the binding may be responsible for imprecise values of the dissociation rate constants. It should be noted that the above-described studies used a filtration method, and there are theoretical considerations (44) which indicate that this technique should not measure such relatively low affinity binding sites. However, because the association rates are relatively slow as compared to an association reaction governed solely on free diffusion, the filter method appears to give a reasonably accurate estimate of the binding properties. In the case of the Na-dependent binding the slow association rate probably reflects glutamate binding to a sodium receptor complex as has been suggested from uptake studies (45). The slow association rate for the Na-independent binding might reflect some conformational changes taking place at the receptor level.

As stressed previously, the pharmacological properties of the physiological receptors in hippocampus are still poorly characterized in part due to uncertainty about efficacy and specificity of the various agonists and antagonists. Nevertheless we attempted to measure the ability of several putative agonists and antagonists to compete with ³H-glutamate binding in the absence or presence of sodium. In the absence of sodium, ³H-glutamate binding exhibited some degree of stereoselectivity: the L-isomers of glutamate or aspartate were 10–20 times more potent in inhibiting the binding than

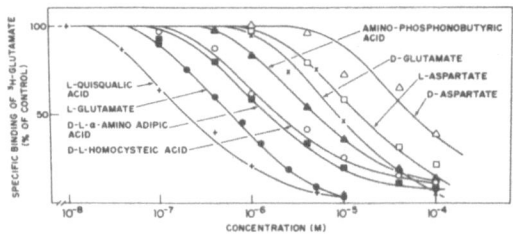

Fig. 3 Inhibition of Na-independent ³H-glutamate binding by various analogs. Concentration-response curves for various analogs were obtained for ³H-glutamate binding to rat hippocampal membranes at a ³H-glutamate concentration of 100 nM. Results are expressed as percent binding measured in the absence of any analogs and are means of three experiments.

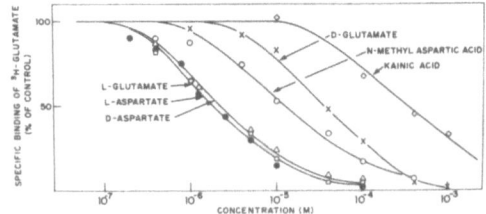

Fig. 4. Inhibition of Na-dependent ³H-glutamate binding by various analogs Same legend as in Fig. 3 except that the binding was conducted in the presence of 150 mM sodium chloride.

were the D-isomers, while glutamate was 10 times more effective than was aspartate (Fig. 3). Several excitatory amino acids, among which L-quisqualic, L-ibotenic and DL-homocysteic acids, were very potent inhibitors of glutamate binding, with K_1 values of 0.12, 1.2 and 2 μM respectively. Although all these compounds have powerful excitatory effects on neurones, only the physiological actions of quisqualic acid have been linked to a glutamate receptor (41). Kainic acid and N-methyl-D,L-aspartic acid (NMDA) were totally devoid of inhibitory effect on Na-independent binding whereas they produce a concentration-dependent inhibition of the Na-dependent binding (Fig. 4); this correlates well with their inhibitory effect towards the high-affinity uptake (8). Among the putative antagonists, D-α-aminoadipate (αAA) and α-aminophosphonobutyric acid (APB) proved to be strong inhibitors of Na-independent ³H-glutamate binding, but had no significant effect on the Na-dependent ³H-glutamate binding. On the other hand, glutamate diethylester (GDEE) was a very poor inhibitor of the Na-independent ³H-glutamate binding, requiring very high concentrations to induce partial blockade. A very similar pharmacological profile has been reported for the Na-independent ³H-glutamate binding in cerebellar membranes by Foster & Roberts (32). This pattern of results does not accord well with the findings of studies using iontophoretic application of drugs. As described above GDEE is a rather specific antagonist of glutamate-induced excitation of neurones while D-α-AA has little effect in this regard – this is the reverse of their effects on Na-independent glutamate binding. Perhaps the simplest explanation is that multiple sites exist and the Na-independent binding site is distinct from that involved in mediating the effects of iontophoretically applied glutamate. If this were to prove to be the case, the question of which site, if either, is associated with synaptic receptors would assume paramount importance. It bears repeating in this context that GDEE proved to be a very poor blocker of synaptic potentials in hippocampus when applied by perfusion, although it has been reported to be effective when administered by iontophoresis. It is also possible that the artificial environment in which binding assays are conducted distorts their properties such that aberrant pharmacological profiles emerge – the potent effects of various cations on glutamate binding may prove pertinent to this point. These issues will be considered further in a later section.

Localization and ontogeny of ³H-glutamate binding sites

The number of Na-dependent binding sites exhibits a marked regional difference which correlates with the regional distribution of high-affinity uptake sites (Fig. 5), while the Na-independent binding sites show little variation in numbers across brain areas (9). This absence of regional variation is not totally surprising since glutamate is able to excite most neurones in the CNS, suggesting a widespread distribution of glutamate receptors, which is also in agreement with the proposed role of

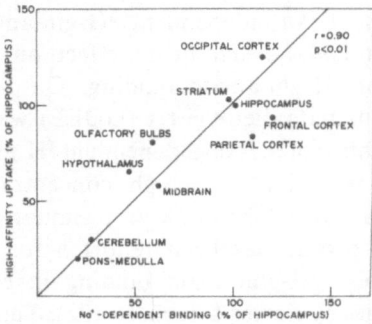

Fig. 5. Correlation between the regional distribution of Na-dependent ³H-glutamate binding and high-affinity uptake. Data are from Baudry & Lynch (9) and are expressed as percent of the values found in the hippocampus. Mean of 4 different experiments.

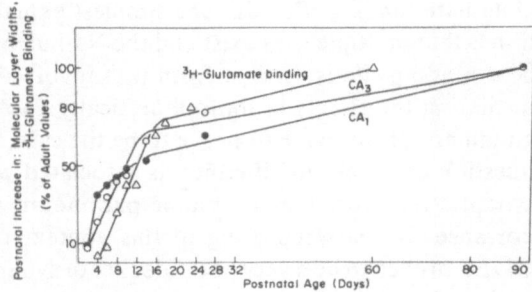

Fig. 6. Postnatal increase in Na-independent ³H-glutamate binding in rat hippocampal membranes and widths of CA₁ and CA₃ molecular layers. The data for the ³H-glutamate binding are from Baudry *et al.* (47) and those for the changes in the widths of CA₁ and CA₃ molecular layers have been generously provided by Dr R. Loy. They are expressed as percentage of the adult values.

glutamate as an excitatory neurotransmitter of a large number of anatomical pathways (46).

More interesting is the developmental pattern of the Na-independent binding sites in hippocampus. The amount of binding sites, expressed as pmol/hippocampus, increases 40 times between the posnatal day (PND) 4 and adult. The binding sites are added at a very fast rate between PND 6 and 18 and at a slower pace thereafter (47). This time-course is very similar to that of synapse addition in the hippocampal formation (48). Hippocampal pyramidal cells undergo their final division before birth and during the first two postnatal weeks they extend dendrites and establish synaptic contacts with their afferent connections (49). This is reflected by an increase in the size of the dendritic trees of the pyramidal cells (50) and thus in the width of the molecular layers of regio superior and regio inferior (Fig. 6); in fact the addition of ³H-glutamate binding sites seems to parallel very closely the increase in molecular layer widths. The analysis of the changes in the dentate gyrus is complicated by the fact that granule cells continue to be added after birth (51); however as is the case with the pyramidal cell fields, the dentate gyrus is invaded by its major afferents during the first two postnatal weeks.

When expressed in terms of density of sites, i.e., pmol/mg protein, glutamate binding exhibits a very different developmental pattern. The density of sites increases 3 fold between PND 4 and PND 9 when it reaches a maximum, and then slowly decreases to reach adult values at PND 23. The simplest interpretation is that following PND 9, proteins are added faster than are ³H-glutamate binding sites. In this regard it is noteworthy that astroglial cells invade the hippocampus at the beginning of the second postnatal week. Myelination does not start before the second or third postnatal week and therefore the reduction in density of binding sites possibly reflects glial cell maturation and myelination. These data offer strong evidence that the Na-independent ³H-glutamate binding sites are not associated with glial cells or myelin but, rather, are associated with some element of the synaptic complexes. A recent study on the development of the Na-independent ³H-glutamate binding sites in rat cerebellar membranes reached a similar conclusion (33).

Subcellular localization of the Na-independent ³H-glutamate binding sites also indicated that these sites are associated with synapses, since they were highly enriched in synaptic plasma membranes and in synaptic junctions (52), whereas only small amounts of binding were associated with myelin or mitochondria (32).

Are the Na-independent glutamate binding sites glutamate receptors?

A reasonable case can be made for the conclusion that the Na-dependent ^{3}H-glutamate binding sites are related to the high-affinity uptake of glutamate; their regional distribution, pharmacological profiles, and even their dependency on sodium, all resemble the properties of the high-affinity glutamate uptake process. Certain characteristics of the Na-independent sites suggest that these may be post-synaptic receptors but the evidence is not yet compelling. Lesions of hippocampal afferents do not cause a reduction in sodium-independent binding (unpublished observation), suggesting that these sites are either on target dendrites or glial cells and the developmental studies cited above tend to rule out the latter location. Furthermore, subcellular fractionation studies suggest that the sites are enriched in synaptic junctions. With regard to the criteria outlined earlier, the binding is saturable, reversible and has a regional and subcellular distribution which is consonant with what would be expected of a physiological receptor. Further evaluation of the relationship between the Na-independent sites and synaptic receptors will require additional evidence on two issues. First, it would be most helpful if an estimate could be made of the concentration range over which glutamate acts physiologically; this information could indicate whether or not the Na-independent site possess an appropriate Kd for glutamate. Experiments using slices or dissociated cells could conceivably provide data on this issue although the possibility of extrajunctional excitatory receptors with higher affinities than synaptic receptors as well as the very effective uptake systems found in neurones might well generate misleading conclusions. Second, and of more immediate interest, further work is needed on the pharmacology of both physiologically effective receptors and glutamate binding sites and the relationship of these sites to synaptic transmission. As discussed, there are enough discrepancies between the pharmacologies of the Na-independent

site and iontophoretically applied glutamate to raise the possibility that two distinct sites are studied by these techniques. However, only the dentate gyrus has received detailed investigation using the iontophoretic approach and there are suggestions in the literature that drugs may operate somewhat differently elsewhere in hippocampus (for example, GDEE does not block aspartate in the dentate gyrus but is does in the regio superior). Furthermore, the effects of iontophoretic application of drugs on synaptic potentials does not agree well with the results of experiments using perfusion. These areas of confusion indicate that additional pharmacologial studies, perhaps combining techniques as well as using a broader range of analogues, will be needed before it will be possible to determine if the Na-independent site possesses the appropriate pharmacological profile for a physiologically effective glutamate receptor, to say nothing of a true post-synaptic receptor.

Possible involvement of glutamate receptors in hippocampal physiological plasticity

The hippocampus exhibits a remarkable degree of anatomical and physiological 'plasticity'. Very brief trains of high frequency stimulation produce an increase in synaptic efficiency which persists for weeks or even longer (long-term potentiation: 'LTP') (53,54). Neurophysiological studies have provided evidence that the LTP effect is due to a change in the synaptic connections ((55) for a review), thereby raising the possibility that post-synaptic receptors undergo some form of modification following high frequency activity. These findings, coupled with the development of a convenient and sensitive assay for a possible glutamate receptor, prompted us to investigate first, the possibility that hippocampal ^{3}H-glutamate binding sites are modifiable and second, the role, if any, receptor plasticity might play in the long-term potentiation effect. For two reasons, we began our studies with an analysis of the effects of calcium on ^{3}H-glutamate binding: a) experiments using a variety of systems have shown that calcium exerts profound effects on membrane organization, including surface receptors (see (56) for a review) and b) ion manipulation experiments using *in vitro* hippocampal slices suggest that the LTP effect is quite sensitive to calcium levels (57) as well as to drugs which block the binding of calcium to calmodulin (58).

Effect of calcium on ^{3}H-glutamate binding and a possible mechanism for the regulation of binding sites

Whereas monovalent cations induce a marked inhibition of the Na-independent ^{3}H-glutamate binding to hippocampal membranes, several divalent cations produce a strong stimulation of this binding. Calcium, manganese and strontium increase the binding two to three fold with apparent EC_{50}'s of 30, 300 and 400 M respectively (Fig. 7). Magnesium also increases the binding by about 20% at 5 mM, whereas cobalt and barium are ineffective up to 10 mM and inhibit ^{3}H-glutamate binding at higher concentrations (40). Scatchard analysis of ^{3}H-glutamate binding in the presence of calcium indicates that calcium increases the maximum number of binding sites without changing their apparent affinity for glutamate. Moreover this stimulatory effect of calcium on the number of glutamate receptors is partially irreversible; when hippocampal membranes are preincubated with calcium and then washed to eliminate the cations, these membranes still exhibit a higher number of binding sites than control, untreated membranes.

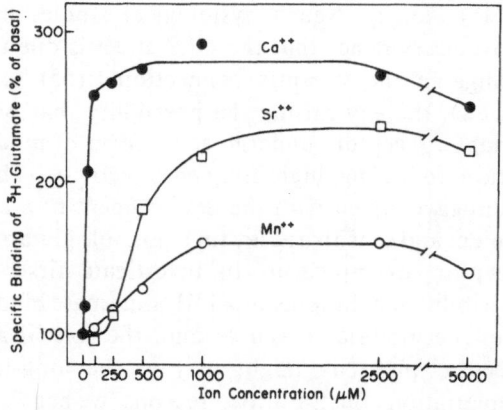

Fig. 7. Effect of various divalent cations on Na-independent ^{3}H-glutamate binding. Hippocampal membranes were prepared as described in Baudry & Lynch (9) except that 2.5 mM EGTA was included in all the solutions during the preparation. After washing the EGTA, ^{3}H-glutamate binding was assayed in the presence of various divalent cations (chloride salts). Results are expressed as percentage of the binding measured in the absence of added cations and are means of 3-6 experiments.

This suggests that the effect of calcium is indirect and requires the participation of an unknown number of intermediate steps. This is also indicated by several other lines of evidence: a) neonatal hippocampal membranes do not exhibit the stimulatory effect of calcium on ^{3}H-glutamate binding until PND 10 (47). Thus glutamate binding sites appear before the onset of the calcium effect; b) Calcium ions do not stimulate ^{3}H-glutamate binding at temperatures below 15–20 °C (Baudry *et al.,* submitted); c) treatment of membranes with Triton X-100 at concentrations which only slightly reduce ^{3}H-glutamate binding, totally suppresses the effect of calcium on the binding (Baudry *et al.,* submitted); d) calcium ions at concentrations as high as 250 μM do not stimulate ^{3}H-glutamate binding in cerebellar membranes, whereas the effect is maximal in hippocampal, striatal or cortical membranes at these concentrations (59).

Pharmacological studies have provided important clues as to the possible cellular and molecular mechanisms which might be involved in the stimulatory effect of calcium on ^{3}H-glutamate binding (59). Thus it appears that reducing or alkylating agents as well as variety of proteinase inhibitors decrease both basal and calcium stimulated ^{3}H-glutamate binding (59); moreover some of these agents namely, N-ethyl maleimide (NEM) and leupeptin, a tripeptide generally considered as a specific inhibitor of thiol proteases (60), do not affect basal ^{3}H-glutamate binding but totally suppress the increase in binding sites produced by calcium (61, 62). This suggests that calcium exerts its actions by stimulating a membrane-bound calcium-sensitive proteinase. This hypothesis is strengthened by the fact that two exogenous proteinases, trypsin and chymotrypsin, induce an increased number of ^{3}H-glutamate binding sites in hippocampal membranes (59). Previous studies have shown that nervous tissue contains calcium and temperature-sensitive thiol proteinases (63–65) but these require concentrations of calcium a hundred times higher than that required to stimulate ^{3}H-glutamate binding. However, recent studies provided evidence that hippocampal and cortical synaptic membranes contain calcium-dependent, leupeptin-sensitive, proteolytic activity, with an apparent affinity for calcium of about 30 μM (61). The substrate of this calcium-dependent proteinase appears to be a high-molecular weight doublet protein (Mr above 200 000) which has been found in purified postsynaptic densities preparations (66), and which may belong in the category of actin-binding proteins. This would agree well with what is known of the substrates of soluble calcium activated proteinases in brain and other tissues (65).

Taken together these data indicate that the calcium stimulation of ^{3}H-glutamate binding could be due to the calcium-induced activation of a membrane-bound proteinase; the subsequent proteolysis of its substrate protein might reveal binding sites which were inaccessible, possibly through a local change in membrane organization.

Long-term potentiation and changes in ^{3}H-glutamate binding sites

The regulatory mechanism described above has several characteristics which make it an obvious candidate for the substrate of the long-term potentiation effect (Table 2). First, the effect of calcium on glutamate binding is partially irreversible, which is consonant with the fact that LTP induction is dependent on calcium and is virtually irreversible. Second, during postnatal development, LTP cannot be elicited before postnatal day 10 in the regio superior (47,68) and this is close to the age at which the calcium stimulation effect appears. Third, cerebellar membranes do not exhibit this effect of calcium and it does not appear that LTP is found in cerebellum.

These arguments led us to test for the effects of brief bursts of high frequency stimulation on ^{3}H-glutamate binding in hippocampus. In a first set of experiments we found that hippocampal slices accumulated more ^{3}H-glutamate following stimulation than control, unstimulated slices; this increased accumulation was restricted to the stimulated terminal field and was still present 30 min after the stimulating train (69). No changes in GABA or

tyrosine accumulation could be detected under these conditions. Moreover, membranes prepared from stimulated slices exhibited an increased number of glutamate binding sites, without changes in affinity for glutamate, as compared to membranes prepared from control, unstimulated slices (69).

In a second set of experiments we used a 'minislice' preparation which uses only the regio superior subfield; in this preparation the great majority of the synapses originate from the regio inferior pyramidal cells and through the use of multiple stimulating electrodes it is possible to activate very large numbers of these. Despite its very small size, the minislice exhibits physiological responses which are not greatly different from those recorded from hippocampus *in vivo*. Our preliminary data with this preparation confirms the earlier finding that high frequency stimulation causes a marked increase in ^{3}H-glutamate binding.

A molecular model for long-term potentation

Taken together, the above data can be integrated in the following multiple-stage molecular model (70, 71):

1) High-frequency stimulation results in an influx of calcium in the postsynaptic dendrites (72, 73).

2) This influx of calcium results, directly or indirectly through the eventual participation of mitochondria (71), in a transitory increase in cytoplasmic free calcium. Although this point is still controversial, it is not unlikely that calcium concentration, which in the resting state is in the order of 0.1 μM, can increase two or more orders of magnitude to reach concentrations as high as 10 or 100 μM, at least locally.

3) This, in turn, activates the postulated membrane-bound calcium-dependent proteinase, causing the proteolysis of some membrane-associated components such as neurofilaments or actin-bin-

Table 2. Correlation between the characteristics of LTP and the effect of calcium on ^{3}H-glutamate binding.

Characteristics of LTP	Calcium effect on ^{3}H-glutamate binding
Increased synaptic transmission	Increased number of ^{3}H-glutamate binding sites
Depends on external Ca^{++} (57)	Effect of Ca^{++} partly irreversible (40)
Ca^{++} can be substituted by Sr^{++} (67)	Mimicked by Sr^{++} and Mn^{++} (Fig. 7)
Absent before PND 10 (47,68)	Absent before PND 10 (47)
Never been reported in cerebellum	Absent in cerebellar membranes (49)

16

ding proteins. (It has been shown that most of the substrates of neutral calcium-activated proteinases from different tissues share the ability to bind actin (65).)

It is then reasonable to propose that the breakdown of this substrate causes changes in membrane organization such that glutamate receptors, which were otherwise inaccessible, become exposed to the ligand. This would provide an increase in synaptic transmission which would last as long as the life of these new receptors. The question of the half-life of neurotransmitter receptors is still unresolved, but it is interesting to note that in their theory of selective stabilization of synapses, Changeux & Danchin (74) postulate that synaptic receptors, once aggregated, remain for the entire life of the synapse. If this were to hold true for central synapses, the increase in glutamate receptors possibly occuring after LTP would persist infinitely. This model also has the potential to account for the structural changes which have been shown to accompany LTP (75). Neurofilaments are thought to perform important muscle-like contractile functions in cells such as cell shape maintenance (76). Thus if the calcium-dependent proteinase acts on such a category of protein, it would be possible that the same mechanism which triggers the change in receptor numbers also triggers the change in the shape of synaptic contacts.

Prospects

The results described above do not provide a clear description of the postsynaptic glutamate receptor(s). Electrophysiological studies, although still in a preliminary stage, have provided evidence for the existence of at least three different receptors for excitatory amino acids: one preferentially stimulated by glutamate and sensitive to GDEE, a second responding preferentially to N-methyl-D,L-aspartic acid and sensitive to D-α-aminoadipic acid and finally a separate receptor for kainic acid. Whether these receptors are junctional or extrajunctional is an open question – GDEE, for instance, does not antagonize synaptic responses, when perfused through hippocampal slices. The availability of a new generation of antagonists as well as the development of the hippocampal slice preparation should allow a better understanding and description of the various receptors. Bioche-

mical studies have mainly focussed on the characterization of ^{3}H-glutamate binding sites in hippocampal membranes. They clearly demonstrated that the Na-dependent high-affinity ^{3}H-glutamate binding site corresponds to a high-affinity uptake site, whereas a population of Na-independent high-affinity binding sites have several properties of a physiological postsynaptic receptor. The pharmacology of these binding sites presents some puzzling features and does not correlate well with that of the receptors defined by the electrophysiologists. Here again, the study of new antagonists in various ionic conditions should shed some light on the complexity of these binding sites and hopefully reconcile biochemical and physiological studies.

However, one of the most exciting results of the biochemical approach has been the demonstration that the Na-independent binding sites are remarkably labile and can be regulated in a number of ways. Thus a 'down' regulation is exerted by sodium ions and might represent a negative feedback mechanism due to the link between glutamate recognition site and sodium conductance channels. The physiological signification of this phenomenon is not clear at the moment but is an obvious theme for future investigation. Conversely, an 'up' regulation is exerted by calcium ions, which in very low concentration (micromolar range) produce partially irreversible increase in receptor numbers. A detailed and testable molecular model has been proposed to explain the stimulatory effect of calcium which may be in fact related to a more general mechanism of regulation of cell surface receptors. Moreover the relationships of such a molecular mechanism with some forms of synaptic plasticity have been explored using the hippocampal slice preparation. More precisely, we proposed that the calcium stimulation of glutamate receptors could be the basis for the long-term potentiation of synaptic transmission which occurs in hippocampus following electrical repetitive stimulation. The predictions of such a model may provide new avenues of research for the pharmacology of learning and memory.

Acknowledgements

We wish to acknowledge the constant help and support of Elizabeth Smith and Denise Arst who participated in some of the experiments described above. We also are very grateful to Karen Zfaty for her devoted secretarial assistance.

These studies were supported by research grants NIMH MH19793-09, NSF BNS 76-17370-04 and NSF AG00538-4.

References

1. Fonnum, F., Ed., 1978. Amino Acids as Chemical Transmitters, Plenum Press, New York.
2. Usherwood, P. N. R., 1978. Advances in Comp. Physiol. and Biochem. 1: 227–309.
3. Johnson, J. L., 1978. Prog. in Neurobiol. 10: 155–202.
4. Roberts, P. J., Storm-Mathisen, J. & Johnston, G., Eds., 1980. Glutamate as a Transmitter, John Wiley Press, New York.
5. DiChiara, G. & Gessa, G. L., Eds., 1980. Glutamate as a Neurotransmitter, Raven Press, New York.
6. Nadler, J. V., Vaca, K. V., White, W. F., Lynch, G. S. & Cotman, C. W., 1976. Nature 260: 538–540.
7. Wieraszko, A. & Lynch, G., 1979. Brain Res. 160: 372–376.
8. Baudry, M. & Lynch, G., 1979. Europ. J. Pharmacol. 57: 283–285.
9. Baudry, M. & Lynch, G., 1981. J. Neurochem. 36: 811–820.
10. Lynch, G. & Cotman, C. W., 1975. In: The Hippocampus (Isaacson, R. & Pribram, K., eds.), Vol. 1, pp. 123–155, Plenum Publishing Co., New York.
11. Lynch, G., Rose, G. & Gall, C., 1978. In: Functions of the Septohippocampal System, Ciba Foundation Symposium, Vol. 58, pp. 5–24, Elsevier, North-Holland.
12. Storm-Mathisen, J., 1972. Brain Res. 40: 215–235.
13. Gall, C., Brecha, N., Chang, T. & Karten, H., 1981. J. Comp. Neurol., in press.
14. Biscoe, T. J. & Straughan, D., 1966. J. Physiol. 183: 341–359.
15. Spencer, H. J., Gribkoff, V. U., Cotman, C. M & Lynch, G., 1976. Brain Res. 105: 471–481.
16. Hicks, T. P. & McLennan, H., 1979. Can. J. Physiol. Pharmacol. 57: 973–978.
17. Wheal, H. V. & Miller, J. J., 1980. Brain Res. 182: 145–155.
18. Segal, M., 1980. In Glutamate as a Neurotransmitter (DiChiara, G. & Gessa, G. L., eds.) pp. 217–226 Raven Press, New York.
19. Curtis, D. R., Duggan, A. W., Felix, D., Johnston, G. A. R. & McLennan, H., 1971. Brain Res. 33: 57–73.
20. White, W. F., Nadler, J. V. & Cotman, C. W., 1979. Brain Res. 164: 177–194.
21. Dunwiddie, T. V., Madison, D. & Lynch, G. S., 1978. Brain Res. 150: 413–417.
22. Limbird, L. E. & Lefkowitz, R. J., 1976. Molec. Pharmacol. 12: 559–567.
23. Ferrendelli, J. A., Chang, M. M. & Kinscherf, D. A., 1974. J. Neurochem. 22: 535–540.
24. Garthwaite, J. & Balazs, R., 1980 in Glutamate as a Neurotransmitter (DiChiara, G. & Gessa, G. L., eds.) pp. 317–326, Raven Press, New York.
25. Kasai, M. & Changeux, J. P., 1971. J. Memb. Biol. 6: 1–16.
26. Luini, A., Goldberg, D. & Teichberg, V. I., 1980. Abstract Society for Neuroscience, v. 10, p. 189.
27. Hollenberg, M. D. & Cuatrecasas, P., 1979 in The Receptors (O'Brien, R. D., ed.) vol. 1, pp. 193–213.
28. Roberts, P. J., 1976. Nature 252: 399–401.
29. Michaelis, E. K., 1975. Biochem. Biophys. Res. Comm. 65: 1004–1012.
30. Michaelis, E. K., Michaelis, M. L. & Boyarsky, L. L., 1974. Biochim. Biophys. Acta 367: 338–348.
31. De Robertis, E. & Fiszer De Plazas, S., 1976. J. Neurochem. 26: 1237–1243.
32. Foster, A. C. & Roberts, P. J., 1978. J. Neurochem. 31: 1467–1477.
33. De Barry, J., Vincendon, G. & Gombos, G., 1980. FEBS Letters 109: 175–179.
34. Biziere, K., Thompson, H. & Coyle, J. T., 1980. Brain Res. 183: 421–433.
35. Simon, J. P., Contrera, J. F. & Kuhar, M. J., 1976. J. Neurochem. 26: 141–147.
36. Schwarcz, R. Scholz, D. & Coyle, J. T., 1978. Neuropharmacology 17: 147–151.
37. Coyle, J. T., Zaczek, R., Slevin, J. & Collins, J., 1980 in Glutamate as a Neurotransmitter (DiChiara, G. & Gessa, G. L., eds.) pp. 337–346, Raven Press, New York.
38. Enna, S. J. & Snyder, W. H., 1977. Mol. Pharmacol. 13: 442–453.
39. Vincent, S. R. & McGeer, E., 1980. Brain Res. 184: 99–108.
40. Baudry, M. & Lynch, G., 1979. Nature 282: 748–750.
41. Anderson, C. R., Cull-Candy S. G. & Miledi, R., 1976. Nature 261: 151–153.
42. Mohler, H. & Okada, T., 1978. Mol. Pharmacol. 14: 256–265.
43. Young, A. B. & Snyder, S. H., 1974. Proc. Nat. Acad. Sci. (USA) 71: 4002–4005.
44. O'Brien, R. D., 1979 in The Receptors (O'Brien, R. D., ed.), vol. 1, pp. 311–333, Plenum Press, New York.
45. Wheeler, D. D., 1979. J. Neurochem. 33: 883–894.
46. Fonnum, F., Lund-Karlsen, R., Malthe-Sorensen, D., Skrede, K. K. & Walaas, I., 1979. Prog. Brain Res. 51: 167–191.
47. Baudry, M., Arst, D., Oliver, M. & Lynch, G., 1981. Developmental Brain Res. 1: 37–48.
48. Gall, C., McWilliams, R. & Lynch, G., 1980. J. Comp. Neur., 193: 1047–1062.
49. Loy, R., Lynch, G. & Cotman, C., 1977. Brain Res. 121: 229–243.
50. Loy, R., 1980. Anat. and Embryol. 159: 257–275.
51. Schlessinger, A. R., Cowan, W. M. & Gottlieb, D. I., 1975. J. Comp. Neurol. 159: 149–176.
52. Cotman, C. W., Foster, A. & Lanthorn, T., 1980 in Glutamate as a Neurotransmitter (DiChiara, G. & Gessa, G. L., eds.) pp. 1–27, Raven Press, New York.
53. Bliss, T. V. P. & Lomo, T., 1973. J. Physiol. (Lond.) 232: 331–356.
54. Bliss, T. V. P. & Gardner-Medwin, A. T., 1973. J. Physiol. (Lond.) 232: 357–374.
55. Lynch, G., Gall, C. & Dunwiddie, T., 1973. In: Progress in Brain Research (Corner, M. A., ed.) pp. 113–128, Elsevier Scientific Publishing Co., Amsterdam.
56. Nicolson, G. L., 1979. Curr. Top. Dev. Biol. 13: 305–338.
57. Dunwiddie, T. V. & Lynch, G. S., 1978. J. Physiol. (Lond.) 276: 353–367.

18

58. Finn, R., Browning, M. & Lynch, G., 1980. Neuroscience Letters 19: 103–108.
59. Baudry, M. & Lynch, G., 1980. Proc. Nat. Acad. Sci. (USA) 77: 2298–2302.
60. Toyo-Oka, T., Shimizu, T. & Masaki, T., 1978. Biochem. Biophys. Res. Commun. 82: 484–491.
61. Vargas, F., Greenbaum, L. & Costa, E., 1980. Neuropharmacology 19: 791–794.
62. Baudry, M., Bundman, M., Smith, E. & Lynch, G., 1981. Science, in press.
63. Gilbert, D. S., Newby, B. J. & Anderton, B. H., 1975. Nature 256: 586–589.
64. Schlaepfer, W. W. & Hasler, M. B., 1979. Brain Res. 168: 299–309.
65. Pant, H. C. & Gainer, H., 1980. J. Neurobiol. 11: 1–12.
66. Cohen, R. S., Blomberg, F., Berins, K. & Siekevitz, P., 1977. J. Cell Biol. 74: 181–191.
67. Wigstrom, H. & Swann, J. W., 1980. Brain Res. 194: 181–191.
68. Harris, K. M., Teyler, T. M. & Cruce, W. L. R., 1980. Abstracts Society for Neuroscience vol. 10, p. 86.
69. Baudry, M., Oliver, M., Creager, R., Wierszko, A. & Lynch, G., 1980. Life Sci. 27: 325–330.
70. Baudry, M. & Lynch, G., 1980. Exp. Neurol. 68: 202–204.
71. Lynch, G. & Baudry, M., 1981. Proceedings of the Meeting 'Brain Synaptic Plasticity' Philadelphia, October 1980.
72. Hotson, J. R., Prince, D. A. & Schwartzkroin, P. A., 1979. J. Neurophysiol. 42: 889–895.
73. Wong, R. K. S., Prince, D. A. & Basbaum, A. I., 1979. Proc. Nat. Acad. Sci. (USA) 76: 986–990.
74. Changeux, J. P. & Danchin, A., 1976. Nature 264: 705–712.
75. Lee, K., Schottler, F., Oliver, M. & Lynch, G., 1980. J. Neurophysiol. 44: 247–258.
76. Edelman, G. M., 1976. Science 192: 218–226.

Received January 14, 1981.

Enzymatic synthesis and function of folylpolyglutamates

John J. McGuire and Joseph R. Bertino
Dept. of Pharmacology Yale University School of Medicine New Haven, CT 06510, U.S.A.

Summary

Derivatives of folic acid occur in nature predominantly as poly (γ-glutamyl) derivatives containing 2–8 glutamate residues. The data regarding the function of these derivatives, and their biosynthesis by eucaryotic and procaryotic folylpolyglutamate synthetases, is reviewed.

The most universal functions of folylpolyglutamates appear to be (a) as the actual cofactors in vivo for folate dependent enzymes, (b) as inhibitors of folate dependent enzymes for which they are not substrates, and (c) to increase retention of folates after they are transported into cells as monoglutamates. Folylpolyglutamates also have numerous specialized functions in specific organisms, e.g. as structural components of some coliphage, and as allosteric regulators in *Neurospora crassa*.

A single enzyme appears responsible for synthesis of all polyglutamate derivatives, regardless of length. With the recent introduction of sensitive assays this folylpolyglutamate synthetase has begun to be characterized. Although procaryotic and eucaryotic synthetases have many dissimilar properties, both types catalyze the ATP-dependent addition of L-glutamate to the γ-carboxyl of the glutamate present in the folate. Both types also require a monovalent cation and a relatively high pH. The most significant differences between the two types are in their folate substrate specificity and the product lengths derived from various folates.

The mechanism of the bacterial enzyme has been studied and an acyl phosphate intermediate is indicated.

List of abbreviations

The term folate is used to refer to the general class of compounds derived from folic acid. The symbols (ℓ) and (d) denote the natural and unnatural diastereoisomers of folates, respectively, which are the result of the assymetric center introduced at C-6 during reduction, and do not indicate optical rotation. All folates contain L-glutamate unless otherwise indicated. The abbreviations used are: PteGlu, pteroylglutamic acid, folic acid; H_2PteGlu, 7, 8-dihydrofolic acid; H_4PteGlu, 5, 6, 7, 8-tetrahydrofolic acid; 5-HCO-, 10-HCO-, 5, 10-CH_2-, and 5-CH_3-H_4PteGlu, 5-formyl-, 10-formyl-, 5, 10-methylene-, and 5-methyltetrahydrofolic acid, respectively; H_2Pte, dihydropteroic acid; poly (γ-glutamyl) derivatives of all forms are indicated by a following subscript n, where n is the total number of glutamates, e.g., PteGlu$_2$ is PteGlu-γ- Glu; CHO, Chinese Hamster Ovary; FPGS, folylpolyglutamate synthetase; HPLC, high pressure liquid chromatography; DHFR, dihydrofolate reductase; SHMT, serine hydroxymethyltransferase; AICAR, 5-amino-4-imidazole carboxamide ribonucleotide.

Introduction

A. Structure and function of folates

The folates (Fig. 1) are a family of vitamins that

Molecular and Cellular Biochemistry 38, 19–48 (1981).   0300–8177/81/0381–0019/$ 6.20.

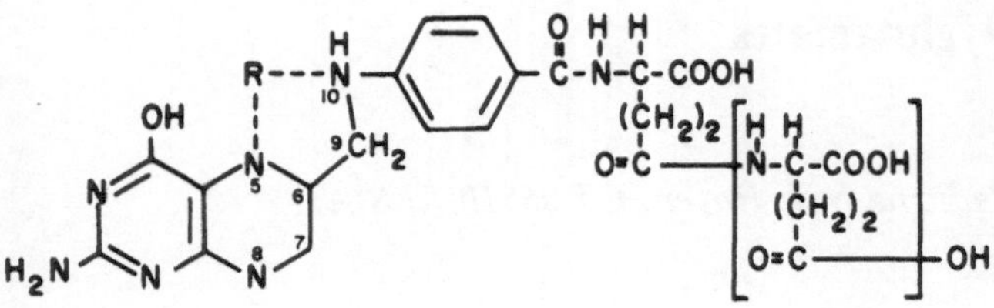

SUBSTITUENT (R)	POSITION
-CH₃	5
-CH₂-	5 and 10
=CH- (methenyl)	5 and 10
-HCO	5 or 10
-CH = NH (formimino)	5

Fig. 1. Structure of tetrahydrofolate and its one-carbon derivatives. Folates consist of a heterocyclic pteridine moiety (including C-9), p-aminobenzoic acid (pABA), and L-glutamic acid. The compound containing only the pteridine and pABA is pteroic acid, and so all folates can be described as derivatives of pteroylglutamate (PteGlu). The pyrazine portion of the pteridine can exist in fully oxidized, 7, 8-dihydro-, or 5, 6, 7, 8-tetrahydro (shown) states. In biological systems, one-carbon substituents are attached only to tetrahydrofolate at positions 5, 10, or as bridges between these two positions. The six natural one-carbon units occur at the oxidation level of methanol, formaldehyde, or formate.

serve as coenzymes in a number of reactions. The discovery of folic acid and various folate forms, and the determinations of their chemical structures have been the subject of several reviews (1, 2).

One-carbon units attached to tetrahydrofolate are utilized in the biosynthesis of a variety of cellular components, including purines, thymidine, and amino acids, and in the initiation of protein synthesis in bacteria and eucaryotic mitochondria (Fig. 2). The one-carbon units are generally derived from glucose (through the serine pathway), but also may be obtained from degradative and scavenging pathways. The different one-carbon units are all interconvertible (Fig. 2) with the exception of 5-CH₃-H₄PteGlu whose synthesis is generally thought to be irreversible in vivo (3).

B. Natural occurrence of folates

Investigations on the natural occurrence of folates, up to 1969, have been reviewed by Blakley (2). Later work has been reviewed by Hoffbrand (4), Baugh and Krumdieck (5), Scott and Weir (6), and Covey (7). The latter three reviews are particularly useful because they discuss in detail the problems and inadequacies of present methodology for determining the form of natural folates.

In general, intracellular folates do not contain a single glutamate, but rather a poly(γ-glutamyl) chain is attached (Fig. 1). The length of this chain varies from 2 to 8 total glutamates under normal conditions. However, derivatives containing up to 12 glutamates have been isolated (8a).

There is generally a distribution of lengths centered around a predominant species, the length of which varies with the organism. Thus, *E. coli* contains predominantly pentaglutamates, but significant amounts of tetra- and hexaglutamate are found. Yeast contains predominantly heptaglutamates with lesser amounts of hexa- and octaglutamates (8b). Mammalian cells often contain pentaglutamates as the predominant folate (6). The only known exceptions to this pattern of multiple lengths are the *Clostridia* which contain only triglutamates (9).

C. Scope of this review

Folylpolyglutamates have been recognized as chemical entities almost since the discovery of folic acid. However, until recently little was known about their possible functions and essentially nothing was known about their biosynthesis except through in vivo radiolabelling studies. Interpretation of the results of these in vivo studies is complicated because transport and metabolism of the labeled folate (or precursor) occurs simultaneously with the polyglutamylation reactions. This review will summarize the experimental evidence for proposed functions of folylpolyglutamates and the most recent data on their biosynthesis in cell free systems.

II. Physiological functions of folylpolyglutamates

The observation that all organisms have the capacity to synthesize folylpolyglutamates, including organisms which are unable to biosynthesize folic acid, suggests that folylpolyglutamates are vital to cellular metabolism. However, the exact function of these derivatives has remained obscure.

21

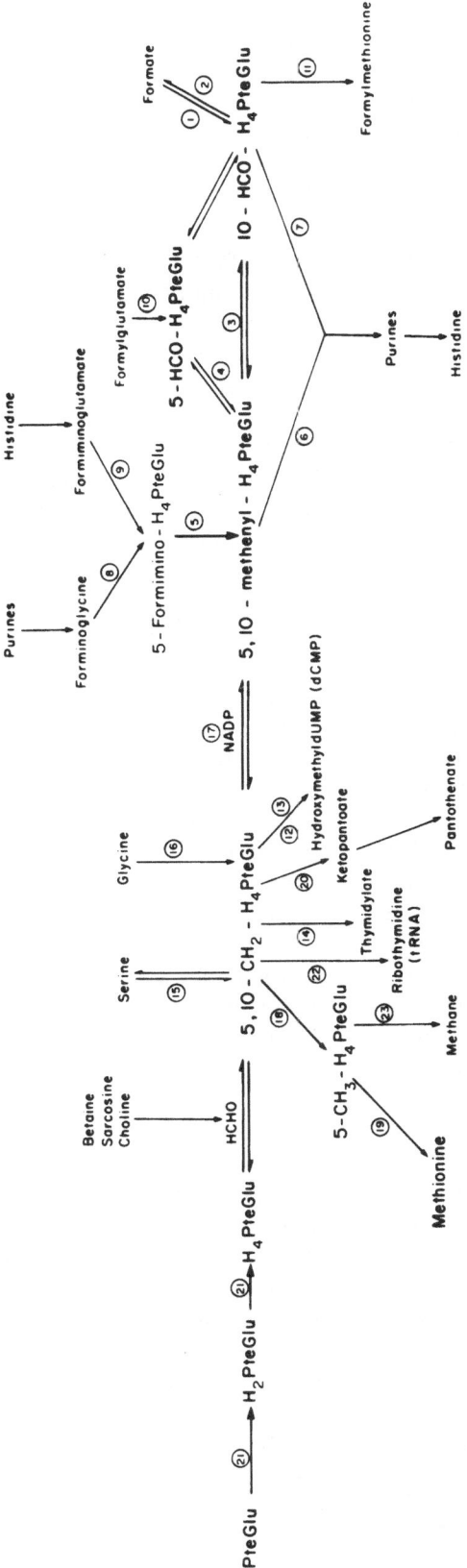

Fig. 2. Biosynthesis and utilization of one carbon units in tetrahydrofolate mediated reactions. (Based on Blakley (2), and Rader and Huennekens (141)). This figure is a composite of folate mediated reactions that occur in procaryotes and eucaryotes. Not all reactions are carried out by any single species. Numbers refer to the following enzymes: 1, 10-formyltetrahydrofolate synthetase; 2, 10-formyltetrahydrofolate deacylase; 3, 5, 10-methenyltetrahydrofolate cyclohydrolase; 4, 5-formyltetrahydrofolate cyclodehydrase; 5, 5-formiminotetrahydrofolate cyclodeaminase; 6, glycinamide ribonucleotide transformylase; 7, 5-amino-4-imidazole carboxamide ribonucleotide (AICAR) transformylase 8, formiminoglycine formiminotransferase; 9, formiminoglutamate formiminotransferase; 10, N-formylglutamate transformylase; 11, methionyl-tNRA transformylase; 12, deoxycytidylate hydroxymethyltransferase; 13, deoxyuridylate hydroxymethyltransferase; 14, thymidylate synthetase; 15, serine hydroxymethyltransferase; 16, enzyme system responsible for oxidative decarboxylation of glycine; 17, 5, 10-methylenetetrahydrofolate dehydrogenase; 18, 5, 10-methylenetetrahydrofolate reductase; 19, methionine synthetase; 20, Ketopantoate hydroxymethyltransferase (58); 21, dihydrofolate reductase; 22, folate-dependent ribothymidyl synthase (70); 23, enzyme system responsible for methanogenesis.)

Some experimental evidence exists indicating that folylpolyglutamates are storage forms of the vitamin, are active as co-factors and inhibitors in one-carbon metabolism, and because of their polyanionic nature are retained intracellularly. Besides these general functions, folylpolyglutamates have been shown to be required for a variety of more specialized functions and postulated to be involved in others.

A. Folylpolyglutamates as storage forms of folate

Folylpolyglutamates were first detected because folate extracted from yeast would not serve as a growth factor for folate requiring bacteria unless it was treated with extracts of a variety of organisms (10). This suggested that the folate in yeast was in a form different from folic acid. Isolation and analysis of this yeast folate revealed its structure to be folic acid with six additional molecules of glutamic acid in peptide linkage (11). The linkages were later unequivocally demonstrated to be all γ-linkages (12, 13). Extracts which made this folylpolyglutamate available as a bacterial growth factor were shown to contain an enzyme – pteroylpolyglutamate hydrolase – which removed the γ-peptide chain (14).

Folylpolyglutamates and pteroylpolyglutamate hydrolase were found to be ubiquitous, and since only the hydrolyzed forms were active bacterial growth factors, and the monoglutamates were active in newly discovered folate dependent enzyme reactions, it was widely assumed that the folylpolyglutamates were merely storage forms of the vitamin. It is now known that the requirement for hydrolysis of folylpolyglutamates before bacterial utilization resulted from ineffective transport of these forms by the bacteria rather than their not being utilized as coenzymes. Gawthorne and Smith (15) proposed that their finding of 75–99% of liver folate as polyglutamates was consistent with a storage function, although it is equally consistent with their being metabolically active. A preliminary communication (16) noted that, while normal rat liver contained predominantly pentaglutamates, proliferating liver (following partial hepatectomy) contained shorter polyglutamates. This suggested that the shorter forms were required for DNA synthesis (i.e., were metabolically active) and thus implied that larger forms were for storage. How-ever, Lavoie et al. (17) found no such difference in the proportion of longer polyglutamates in normal and regenerating rat liver. Neither did they find it in other proliferating versus quiescent cells. No difference was detected in proliferating and non-proliferating human fibroblasts (18). Moran et al. (19) demonstrated that L1210 cells contained only folylpolyglumates whether grown on optimal folate or a suboptimal concentration which allowed 88% of the optimal growth rate. If polyglutamates were storage forms, a relative increase in the monoglutamate content would be expected in the latter case.

Despite this evidence that folylpolyglutamates are not solely storage forms, there are suggestions that a degree of storage might occur. Under culture conditions which permitted biosynthesis of folic acid in an amount twenty to thirty-fold greater than that required for maximum cell growth, *Diplococcus pneumoniae* still converted >85% of the intracellular folate into polyglutamates (20). The studies (19) showing the presence of only folylpolyglutamates in L1210 cells grown on optimal and suboptimal folate also demonstrated that folate deprived cells (0.76 pmol intracellular folate/10^6 cells) grew at 88% the rate of folate sufficient cells (5.6 pmol/10^6 cells). Thus a sevenfold decrease in the folate pool, with no apparent change in the relative distribution within the pool, caused only a 12% decrease in growth rate. In these examples, normally growing cells had a folate pool, as folylpolyglutamates, which was in excess of the growth requirement. This suggests cells retained metabolically inactive folates or used the expanded folate pool at a reduced flux rate per molecule. Either of these alternatives would fit a broad definition of storage. Another relevant observation is that many reduced folates, but not 5-CH_3-H_4PteGlu, inhibit bovine liver dihydrofolate reductase, and thus feedback inhibit their own synthesis (21). The lack of inhibition by 5-CH_3-H_4Pte-Glu is consistent with its synthesis, at least partially, as a storage derivative. The role of polyglutamates in this system has not been investigated.

B. Folylpolyglutamates as substrates for folate dependent reactions

The evidence that folylpolyglutamates serve as co-factors in folate dependent reactions (Figure 2) is drawn almost exclusively from in vitro studies using isolated enzymes, and folylpolyglutamates synthesized chemically and enzymatically (Table 1).

1. Dihydrofolate reductase (DHFR). Kinetics with polyglutamate substrates have been investigated with both bacterial and mammalian DHFR enzymes. The DHFR of *Streptococcus faecalis R* is one of the few enzymes showing a substantial increase in K_m for a polyglutamate (22). Since this was an early study, it is possible that the $H_2PteGlu_3$ substrate was impure. The *Lactobacillus casei* DHFR (23) reduced saturating levels (50 μM) of $H_2PteGlu_n$ (n = 1, 3, 6) at the same rate indicating identical V_{max}. The earliest studies on mammalian DHFR all compared $H_2PteGlu$ only with $H_2PteGlu_3$ since $PteGlu_3$ was provided by the Lederle group (12). The calf thymus (24, 25) and sheep liver (26) enzymes exhibited a small decrease in K_m and a small increase in V_{max} values for the triglutamate compared to the monoglutamate. The L1210 enzyme (27) also exhibited a slightly increased (30%) V_{max} with $H_2PteGlu_3$ as the substrate as compared to $H_2PteGlu$. A more extensive study of this DHFR and several others from human sources with $H_2PteGlu_n$ (n = 1, 3, 5, 7) as substrates was performed by Coward et al. (28). Their results (Table 1) also indicated either equivalent K_m and V_{max} values for all chain lengths or the K_m values were slightly decreased and the V_{max} increased with increasing chain length. A similar pattern of changes was observed with all these DHFR when $PteGlu_n$ (n = 1, 3, 5, 7) were tested except the respective K_m values were 10-fold higher than the $H_2PteGlu_n$ substrates (28). DHFR from a methotrexate resistant line of human KB cells also showed only slight differences in kinetic parameters between the mono- and pentaglutamate dihydro derivatives (29). The data with the pentaglutamate derivative may be of importance because mammalian cells generally contain predominantly folylpentaglutamates (6).

2. Serine hydroxymethyltransferase (SHMT). SHMT was the first folate dependent reaction (other than pteroylpolyglutamate hydrolase) demonstrated to use folylpolyglutamate substrates. The conversion of serine to glycine by co-factor depleted extracts of *Clostridium* HF required factors present in boiled extracts of *Clostridium cylindros-porum* (30). These factors were shown to be polyglutamate derivatives of different folates, and they were responsible for the observed activity because no monoglutamates were detectable (31). This enzyme probably only prefers polyglutamates since some monoglutamates were active at substrate levels. A similar activity occurs in extracts of *Pseudomonas* AM1 since the maximum rate of serine synthesis was achieved at a level of triglutamate only 10% that of the monoglutamate (32). The purified SHMT of *Clostridium cylindrosporum* (Table 1) showed a small decrease in K_m value as the chain length increases to the triglutamate (33). No data are available on the relative V_{max}. The enzymes from *Bacillus subtilis* (34) *Bacillus megaterium* (35), *Candida utilis* (a yeast) (35), and *Coprinus lagopus* (a basidiomycete fungus (35) utilized mono- and triglutamate substrates about equally well. The rabbit liver SHMT (36) displayed a K_m for the triglutamate which was half that of the monoglutamate, but the V_{max} were similar. The heptaglutamate was active with this enzyme in the same concentration range as the other substrates but insufficient amount was available for an accurate determination of K_m and V_{max}.

3. Methylenetetrahydrofolate reductase. Substantial reductions in K_m values were observed with increasing polyglutamate chain length for all methylenetetrahydrofolate reductases (Table 1) indicating they were more efficient substrates. The K_m for the *Lactobacillus casei* enzyme decreased as the chain length increased reaching a nine-fold reduction at the heptaglutamate (37). The V_{max} was unaffected. The reductase of *Bacillus subtilis* apparently had the same V_{max} with the mono- and triglutamates but no data are available on the relative K_m values (34). The rat liver enzyme displayed a sevenfold decrease in K_m, but a fivefold decrease in V_{max}, for the penta- compared to the monoglutamate (Table 1) (38). The result is probably a marginal advantage for the polyglutamate form. Pentaglutamate activity with the rat liver reductase was competitively inhibited by the monoglutamate and its K_i was similar to its K_m as a substrate indicating that both substrates were utilized by the same enzyme. Effects of polyglutamate length on activity of this enzyme were most evident with the pig liver reductase (39). The V_{max} values remained relatively constant for all lengths between

Table 1. Folylpolyglutamates as substrates for folate dependent reactions.

Enzyme	Source	Substrate (concentration)[a]	Ref[b]	K_m (n=1)	V_{max}[2] (n=1)	K_m (n=2)	V_{max}[2] (n=2)	K_m (n=3)	V_{max}[2] (n=3)	K_m (n=4)	V_{max}[2] (n=4)	K_m (n=5)	V_{max}[2] (n=5)	K_m (n=6)	V_{max}[2] (n=6)	K_m (n=7)	V_{max}[2] (n=7)
Dihydrofolate Reductase (EC 1.5.1.3)	Streptococcus faecalis R.	$H_2PteGlu_n$ (μM)	a	4	1			40									
	Sheep Liver	$H_2PteGlu_n$ (μM)	b	1.2	1			0.83	1.27			0.8	2.12			1.3	2.61
	Calf Thymus	$H_2PteGlu_n$ (μM)	c	100	1			62	1.15			120	1.97			21	1.18
	Calf Thymus	$H_2PteGlu_n$ (μM)	d	1.4	1			1.2	0.89								
	L1210	$PteGlu_n$ (μM)	e	20	1			81	3.8			1.3	0.51			1.3	0.54
	Human Erythrocytes	$H_2PteGlu_n$ (μM)	e	5.9	1			4.2	0.71								
	Human AML	$PteGlu_n$ (μM)	e	47	1			52	3.33			28	1.33			28	0.94
	Human AML	$H_2PteGlu_n$ (μM)	e	3.6	1			10	2.43			1.5	0.93			0.6	1.08
	Human ALL	$PteGlu_n$ (μM)	e	74	1			33	0.93			49	1.47			39	1.0
	Human ALL	$H_2PteGlu_n$ (μM)	e	3.5	1			1.8	0.93			9.3	1.99			36	0.8
	Human KB/MTX	$PteGlu_n$ (μM)	e	73	1			18	2.5			16	1.04				
	Human KB/MTX	$H_2PteGlu_n$ (μM)	f	0.67	1							0.58	0.92				0.5
Serine Hydroxy-methyltransferase (EC 2.1.2.1)	Clostridium cylindrosporum	(l)-$H_4PteGlu_n$ (μM)	g	19	1			12									
Methylenetetra-hydrofolate Reductase (EC 1.1.1.68)	Rabbit Liver	(dl)-$H_4PteGlu_n$ (μM)	h	180	1			83	1								
	Lactobacillus casei	(l)-5-CH_3-$H_4PteGlu_n$ (μM)	i	9.5	1			4.8	0.90			1.8	0.85			1.1	0.82
	Rat Liver	(dl)-5-CH_3-$H_4PteGlu_n$ (μM)	j	45	1							6	0.19				
	Pig Liver	(l)-5,10-CH_2-$H_4PteGlu_n$ (μM)	k	7.1	1.0	5.2	1.76	1.7	1.71	0.62	1.73	0.26	0.64	0.10	0.68	0.51	0.68
Methionine Synthetase (B₁₂ independent) (EC 2.1.1.14)	Escherichia coli	(dl)-$H_4PteGlu_n$ (μM)	l		0			25	1								
	Escherichia coli	(dl)-$H_4PteGlu_n$ (μM)	m		0			8	1								
	Escherichia coli	(l)-5-CH_3-$H_4PteGlu_n$ (μM)	n		0			2.4	1								
	Lactobacillus casei	(l)-5-CH_3-$H_4PteGlu_n$ (μM)	o	40	1							0.34	4.5				
	Neurospora crassa	(dl)-5-CH_3-$H_4PteGlu_n$ (μM)	p		0	0.96	1	0.82	1								
	Saccharomyces cerevisiae	(dl)-5-CH_3,CH_3-$H_4PteGlu_n$ (μM)	p		0	0.43	1	0.38	1								
Methionine Synthetase (B₁₂ dependent) (EC 2.1.1.13)	Escherichia coli	(dl)-$H_4PteGlu_n$ (μM)	l	150	1												
	Escherichia coli	(dl)-$H_4PteGlu_n$ (μM)	m	180	1												
Methylenetetra-hydrofolate Dehydrogenase (EC 1.5.1.5)	Rat Liver	(dl)-$H_2PteGlu_n$ (μM)	j	25	1			24	1.24			8	0.63				
	Bovine Brain	(dl)-$H_2PteGlu_n$ (μM)	q	73	1			8.8	0.9			28	1.74			22	1.91
	Clostridium cylindrosporum	(l)-5,10-CH_2-$H_4PteGlu_n$ (μM)	r	26	1												
	Calf Thymus	(dl)-$H_2PteGlu_n$ (μM)	s	25	1			6.8	0.81			3.0	1.04				
	Pig Liver	(l)-5,10-CH_2-$H_4PteGlu_n$ (μM)	t						0.83							2.7	0.80

Table 1 (Continued)

Enzyme (EC)	Source	Substrate	Ref	Values
Formyltetrahydrofolate Synthetase (EC 6.3.4.3)	Clostridium cylindrosporum	(l)-H$_4$PteGlu$_n$	u	0.29, 1, 0.025, 1, 1
	Pigeon Liver	(l)-10-HCO-H$_4$PteGlu$_n$ (μM)	v	10, 1, 0.12, 1, 0.12, .62
	Sheep Liver	(dl)-H$_4$PteGlu$_n$	w	1
	Sheep Liver	(dl)-H$_4$PteGlu$_n$ (μM)	x,y	4.6, 1, 110, 0.16, 1, 0.16, 1.6
	Rat Liver	(dl)-H$_4$PteGlu$_n$ (μM)	z	400, 1, 0.06, 6, 6
	Bovine Liver	(dl)-H$_4$PteGlu$_n$ (μM)	z	100, 1, 10, 10, 1.9
	Pig Liver	(l)-H$_4$PteGlu$_n$ (μM)	t	89, 1, 2.0, 0.98, 0.37
	Pig Liver	(l)-H$_4$PteGlu$_n$ (μM)		61, 1, 25, 1.25, 25, 1.25
Thymidylate Synthetase (EC 2.1.1.45)	Lactobacillus casei	(l)-H$_4$PteGlu$_n$ (μM)	aa	2.2, 2.2, 2.2, 2.2
	Lactobacillus casei	(l)-H$_4$PteGlu$_n$ (μM)	bb	15
	Human	(dl)-H$_4$PteGlu$_n$ (μM)	cc	30, 2, 2
AICAR transformylase (EC 2.1.2.3)	Chicken Liver	(dl)-10-HCO-H$_4$PteGlu$_n$ (μM)	dd	674, .11, 0.16, 1.0, 0.13, 1.8, 0.10
Ketopantoate Hydroxymethyltransferase	Escherichia coli	(dl)-H$_4$PteGlu$_n$ (μM)	ee	180, 1, 100, 100, 1, 200, 1
Formimino-glutamate Formiminotransferase (EC 2.1.2.5)	Pig liver	(l)-H$_4$PteGlu$_n$ (μM)	t	48, 1, 31, 0.87, 3.5, 0.96, 4.6
Formimino-glycine Formiminotransferase (EC 2.1.2.4)	Clostridium cylindrosporum	(l)-H$_4$PteGlu$_n$ (μM)	ff	24, 1, 14, 1.40, 1.40
Formimino-tetrahydrofolate Cyclodeaminase (EC 4.3.1.4)	Clostridium cylindrosporum	(l)-formimino-H$_4$PteGlu$_n$ (μM)	gg	31, 1, 29, 3.3

1. a) Blakley and McDougall (22). b) Morales and Greenberg (26). c) Nath and Greenberg (24). c) Coward et al, (28). d) Greenberg et al (25). L1210/MTX is a subline of mouse L1210 leukemia cells which is resistant to methotrexate. Human erythrocytes were isolated from a patient with polycythemia vera. Human acute myelocytic leukemia blasts were isolated from a patient. The spleen of a human patient with acute lymphatic leukemia was obtained shortly after death. f) Domin et al. (29). A methotrexate resistant line of human KB cells. g) Uyeda and Rabinowitz (33). h) Blakley (36). i) Shane and Stokstad (37). j) Cheng et al. (38). k) Matthews and Baugh (39). l) Guest and Jones (40a). m) Jones et al. (42). n) Whitfield et al. (43). o) Shane and Stokstad (37). p) Burton et al. (44). q) Coward et al. (49). r) Uyeda and Rabinowitz (56). s) Yeh and Greenberg (52). t) MacKenzie and Baugh (53). u) Himes and Rabinowitz (56). v) Curthoys and Rabinowitz (57). w) Jaenicke and Brode (59a). x) Brode and Jaenicke (59b). y) Jaenicke and Brode (59c) z) Lewis et al. (23). bb) Kisliuk et al. (60). aa) Himes et al. (61). cc) Dolnick and Cheng (63). dd) Baggott and Krumdieck (64). ee) Powers and Snell (58). ff) Rabinowitz and Himes (66). gg) Uyeda and Rabinowitz (67).

2. Relative V$_{max}$.

3. Units of concentration following substrate (in parenthesis) are the units of the K$_m$ value for the particular substrate.

26

the mono- and heptaglutamate, but the K_m values decreased with each additional glutamate until the hexaglutamate (Table 1). The total decrease in K_m was seventyfold.

4. Methionine synthetase. The activity of folyl-polyglutamates as substrates for methionine synthetase was first investigated in *E. coli*. This organism has two methionine synthetases; the most important difference between the two is that one requires vitamin B_{12} while the other does not (40a, b). The B_{12} dependent enzyme used both mono- and triglutamate derivatives (41) while the B_{12} independent synthetase used only the triglutamate (40a, 42, 43). With the B_{12} independent enzyme the diglutamate has been reported to be as active as the triglutamate (44) and inactive (41), and the heptaglutamate was active (42). Although the exact length required is in doubt, this methionine synthetase is polyglutamate specific and is the only well documented example of such an enzyme.

The vitamin B_{12} independent methionine synthetases of *Candida utilis* (35), *Caprinus lagopus* (35), *Aerobacter aerogenes* (45), *Salmonella typhimurium* (46), *Bacillus subtilis* (34), and rat liver mitochondria (47) all required a triglutamate for activity. *Lactobacillus casei* has a B_{12} independent enzyme (37) which utilized both mono- and pentaglutamate $5\text{-}CH_3\text{-}H_4PteGlu_n$ derivatives, but the pentaglutamate was about 500 times more effective (Table 1). Higher plants (e.g., green beans, spinach, and barley sprouts) contained an enzyme similar to that of *L. casei.* (48).

There is a single example (in *Bacillus megaterium*) of a B_{12} dependent methionine synthetase which exhibited a requirement for a polyglutamate substrate (35).

The cytoplasm of mammalian cells contains only a B_{12} dependent methionine synthetase (49). An early study of this enzyme from pig liver (50) demonstrated that the mono- and triglutamates were used almost equally well. Rat liver methionine synthetase (38) exhibited Michaelis-Menten kinetics with $5\text{-}CH_3H_4PteGlu_n$ (n = 1, 5). The pentaglutamate had a lower V_{max} but its affinity was three times greater than the monoglutamate (Table 1). The bovine brain enzyme (49), exhibited similar kinetics, and independent of their length, displayed a greater affinity for polyglutamate substrates. (Table 1). The V_{max} was increased with poly-

glutamates, and thus the polyglutamates were very efficient substrates. With both the rat liver and bovine brain enzymes $5\text{-}CH_3H_4PteGlu$ competitively inhibited the substrate activity with the polyglutamates indicating both species bind to the same active site.

5. Methylenetetrahydrofolate dehydrogenase (Table 1). Methylenetetrahydrofolate dehydrogenase from *Clostridium cylindrosporum* (51) exhibited a threefold decrease in K_m and little change in V_{max} as chain length increased from mono- to triglutamate. Similar results, as far as V_{max}, were obtained with calf thymus enzyme (52). The most complete study was done on the pig liver enzyme (53) which is part of a trifunctional folate protein in eucaryotes (54, 55). Using $(\ell)\text{-}5,10\text{-}CH_2\text{-}H_4PteGlu_n$ (n = 1, 3, 5, 7) the V_{max} was again insensitive to chain length. The K_m, however decreased with increasing length until the pentaglutamate (Table 1). The penta- and heptaglutamate behaved similarly.

6. Formyltetrahydrofolate synthetase. The clostridial formyltetrahydrofolate synthetase has been particularly well characterized with regard to polyglutamate specificity. The K_m for $H_4PteGlu_3$ in the forward reaction was tenfold lower than for $H_4PteGlu$ (56) while the K_m for $10\text{-}HCO\text{-}H_4PteGlu_3$ in the back reaction was 100-fold lower than for the monoglutamate (57). There was little effect of glutamate chain length on V_{max} in either direction. This enzyme used all $H_2PteGlu_n$ up to n = 7 as substrates (58). The pigeon liver enzyme used saturating levels of mono-, tri-, and heptaglutamate derivatives at the same rate (59a). Although the diglutamate value was clearly anomalous, perhaps from an impure $PteGlu_2$ starting material, the general trend for the sheep liver synthetase was to decrease K_m sharply and increase V_{max} as the chain length increased (59b, c). Both the rat and bovine liver synthetases showed dramatic declines in K_m as the chain length extended to the pentaglutamate (60). Similarly large decreases were noted with the pig liver enzyme up to the triglutamate (53). The penta- and heptaglutamate substrates showed such strong substrate inhibition that kinetic data could not be obtained.

7. Thymidylate synthetase. E. coli thymidylate

synthetase utilized mono- and triglutamate substrates (27). The *Lactobacillus casei* enzyme displayed the same preference for a polyglutamate (lower K_m, higher V_{max}) regardless of its length (23, 61). This polyglutamate preference was also noted in folate substrate binding studies (62). In studies on a human thymidylate synthetase 5, 10-CH_2-$H_4PteGlu_5$ had a sixteenfold lower K_m and a two fold higher V_{max} than the monoglutamate (63).

8. AICAR transformylase. The activity of the chicken liver enzyme was strikingly affected by folylpolyglutamate substrates (64). The K_m for its monoglutamate substrate was very high, and at physiological concentrations of this substrate (1–2 μM) the monoglutamate would be inactive. Triglutamate and longer polyglutamates had K_m values which were three- to six-hundredfold lower than the monoglutamate while their V_{max} were decreased six to tenfold. The K_m values for the polyglutamates were very near the intracellular substrate concentration and thus they would be readily utilized.

9. Ketopantoate hydroxymethyltransferase. Ketopantoate hydroxymethyltransferase, an enzyme of the pantothenic acid biosynthetic pathway, displayed a preference for polyglutamates (58). The V_{max} for all lengths were equivalent but derivatives between tri- and hexaglutamate had K_m values half those of the mono-, di-, and heptaglutamates (Table 1).

10. Formiminoglutamate formiminotransferase. The one-carbon fragment of formiminoglutamate, an intermediate in histidine degradation, enters the one-carbon pool by transfer of the formimino group to $H_4PteGlu_n$. In mammals, at least, this formiminotransferase activity is part of a bifunctional folate enzyme which also contains formiminotetrahydrofolate cyclodeaminase activity (65). The pig liver formiminotransferase showed a decided preference for pentaglutamate and longer polyglutamates (53). Their V_{max} were about the same as the monoglutamate; but their K_m values were tenfold lower.

11. Formiminoglycine formiminotransferase. During purine degradation in clostridial species, formiminoglycine is formed. It is metabolized in a manner analogous to formiminoglutamate (66). $H_4PteGlu_3$ had a 40% higher V_{max} and a K_m value about half that observed with the monoglutamate in the formiminotransferase reaction (66).

12. Formiminotetrahydrofolate cyclodeaminase. Formiminotetrahydrofolate formed either from formiminoglutamate or formiminoglycine is converted to 5, 10-methenyltetrahydrofolate by formiminotetrahydrofolate cyclodeaminase. The clostridial enzyme (67) again showed a preference for the tri- over the monoglutamate. The two derivatives had equal K_m values, but the V_{max} of the triglutamate was over threefold higher. The pig liver enzyme could not be tested directly for substrate activity with 5-formimino-$H_4PteGlu_n$, but inhibition studies with $PteGlu_n$ (n = 1, 3, 5, 7) suggested a strong preference for polyglutamates, particularly those of pentaglutamate length (53).

13. Correlation of in vitro activity and the predominant folylpolyglutamate form in vivo. If folylpolyglutamates are the preferred substrates for folate dependent enzymes in vivo, a correlation might exist between the predominant intracellular folylpolyglutamate length and the optimal length determined with isolated enzymes. Baggott and Krumdieck (64) have pointed out that in determining the optimal length of polyglutamates, the V_{max}/K_m values are what must be compared. An increased ratio indicates a more efficient substrate. In most instances good agreement exists between the optimal length determined in this manner and the published value for the predominant length of the source in question. Agreement is noted with the enzymes and folates of pig liver (6) *E. coli* (58), L1210 cells (19) and *L. casei* (6). A particularly good example of this correlation is *Clostridium cylindrosporum*. This organism contains only pteroyltriglutamates (9, 66) and each of the five clostridial enzymes investigated (Table 1) functioned more efficiently with a triglutamate substrate than with the corresponding monoglutamate. The kinetic data on the clostridial enzymes also illustrate the varied effects that polyglutamates can have on substrate activity. Since K_m and V_{max} are independent parameters which can increase, decrease, or remain unchanged, there are nine possible combinations of effects that polyglutamates could have. Three combinations (e.g., K_m decreases, V_{max} increases) lead unambiguously to higher V_{max}/K_m ratios, two combinations (e.g., K_m increases, V_{max} increases) give either higher or lower V_{max}/K_m ratio depending on the magnitude of each change, three combinations (e.g., K_m increases, V_{max} decreases) lead unambiguously to lower V_{max}/K_m ratios, and one combination (K_m and V_{max} both unchanged) leads to an unchanged ratio. Four different combinations, all leading to more favorable substrate activity by the triglutamate, were observed with these five clostridial enzymes. All other enzymes for which complete data are available (Table 1) have either unchanged or increased V_{max}/K_m for polyglutamate as compared to monoglutamate substrates. The only exception is when $PteGlu_n$ are used as substrates for mammalian DHFR, but these are not physiological substrates for the mammalian enzyme.

14. 'Channeling'. Organisms can increase their metabolic efficiency through the use of multienzyme complexes and multifunctional proteins (68). Multifunctional proteins consist of a single type of polypeptide chain, but they have multiple catalytic or binding functions (69). Such proteins have unique catalytic properties (68) including: (a) each activity in the protein can be coordinately regulated by a single effector, (b) if sequential enzymes in a pathway are involved, 'channeling' or compartmentalization of intermediates can occur so such intermediates never appear free in solution. An intermediate could be transferred directly between active sites, confined to a non-mixing solvent layer on the enzyme surface, or be physically trapped by the protein structure. In any case, the intermediate does not equilibrate with bulk solvent. This 'channeling' may allow not only more rapid establishment of the steady state, it may also effect the actual conditions at the steady state, (c) inherent properties of the protein which could lead to lower K_m values and/or a higher V_{max} for a reaction relative to the same activity not in a multifunctional protein.

Two multifunctional proteins have been identified in mammalian folate metabolism. The sequential activities 10-HCO-H_4PteGlu synthetase, 5, 10-methenyl-H_4PteGlu cyclohydrolase, and 5, 10-CH_2-H_4PteGlu dehydrogenase are located in a single protein species in pig (54) and sheep (55) livers. These combined activities have been called C_1-THF synthase (THF = H_4PteGlu) (70). The sequential activities of formiminoglutamate formiminotransferase and 5-formimino-H_4PteGlu cyclodeaminase (called here, combined formimino activities) are also associated with a single protein species (65).

Investigations as to whether these multifunctional proteins display unusual kinetic properties (specifically, channeling of intermediates) with mono- and polyglutamate substrates have been performed. With monoglutamate, H_4PteGlu, the combined formimino activities did not retain the intermediate (5-formimino-H_4PteGlu), and it was detectable in the solvent (53). When H_4PteGlu$_3$ was the substrate some intermediate appeared in the solvent. Part was channeled directly through the second reaction. With H_4PteGlu$_5$, channeling through the second reaction was complete and no free intermediate was detectable. The authors speculated that this channeling was kinetically advantageous moreover, it did not allow accumulation of a labile intermediate which has no known function in folate metabolism. With the C_1-THF synthase partial channeling of the monoglutamate through the dehydrogenase/cyclohydrolase steps was observed (71). Polyglutamate substrates up to heptaglutamate showed approximately the same degree of partial channeling (53). The authors noted that this incomplete channeling was vital because free 5, 10-methenyl-H_4PteGlu$_n$ is required for de novo purine biosynthesis. These examples demonstrate that channeling does occur in mammalian folate metabolism and polyglutamate forms of folates can contribute substantially to the channeling.

An unanswered question of great importance is how the K_m and V_{max} values obtained for the separate activities of these proteins compare to the values when the combined activities act in concert. Is an intermediate added to an in vitro assay actually utilized in exactly the same manner as the intermediate generated in situ? If not, the kinetic constants obtained for individual activities of multifunctional proteins must be interpreted with caution.

15. Summary. These studies demonstrate that folylpolyglutamates are substrates for many if not all folate dependent enzymes. No monoglutamate specific enzyme has been identified, although there are enzymes which will use only polyglutamates. In nearly every case, a polyglutamate is as good a substrate as the monoglutamate and in many cases it is better, having either a lower K_m, a higher V_{max}, or both. As emphasized by Baggott and Krumdieck (64) the ratio V_{max}/K_m is a better way to analyze the relative effectiveness of these substrates. This ratio is generally the same or higher with polyglutamate substrates and often the highest ratio is achieved with the length of polyglutamate which predominates in the organism used as the enzyme source. These observations in vitro are consistent with folylpolyglutamates serving as the preferred cofactors for one-carbon transfer in vivo. In addition, there is suggestive evidence from in vivo studies that folylpolyglutamates allow more efficient growth of organisms (37, 72).

The preference shown in vitro for folylpolyglutamates does not mean that monoglutamate forms are not utilized as such in vivo. The evidence clearly indicates that $5\text{-}CH_3\text{-}H_4PteGlu$ is transported into cells and the one carbon unit is rapidly utilized (73). However, cellular metabolism cannot be supported entirely by even reduced folate monoglutamates. Wild type CHO cells grew optimally on restrictive medium with 10 ng/ml of $5\text{-}HCO\text{-}H_4PteGlu$, while a mutant capable of $5\text{-}HCO\text{-}H_4PteGlu$ transport and only lacking any ability to make folylpolyglutamates, was unable to grow on the same medium even if 100 μg/ml (10^4 increase) $5\text{-}HCO\text{-}H_4PteGlu$ was included (74). These results and the lack of significant levels of intracellular monoglutamates indicate that folylpolyglutamates are quantitatively the most important co-factors and are, in fact, essential for cellular one-carbon metabolism.

The mechanisms by which polyglutamates are better utilized as substrates are varied. The polyglutamate chain is often used only for increased binding as evidenced by a decreased K_m with no difference in V_{max} (39, 57). In those reactions where either both the K_m and V_{max} are changed or just the V_{max} is changed, the polyglutamate chain must also influence the active site, perhaps by inducing a conformational change. Folylpolyglutamates can also influence activity by being channeled preferentially through multifunctional proteins.

C. Folylpolyglutamates as inhibitors of folate dependent reactions

A number of folate dependent enzymes are inhibited by monoglutamate or polyglutamate forms of folates which are not substrates of the reaction (Table 2). The concentration at which significant inhibition occurs is often within the physiological range, especially for the polyglutamates. This has led to the hypothesis that folate metabolism could be regulated, in part, by the relative amounts of the substrates and these inhibitors.

1. Dihydrofolate reductase. A folylpolyglutamate inhibitor of mouse leukemia (L1210) cell and *E. coli* dihydrofolate reductases was isolated from *E. coli* and identified as $10\text{-}HCO\text{-}PteGlu_5$ (75). This identification was based on its characteristic spectrum and quantitative amino acid analysis. This pentaglutamate compound was seven times more inhibitory for the leukemic enzyme than the corresponding monoglutamate, and was inhibitory at physiological concentrations. Interestingly, the *E. coli* reductase was over fourthousandfold less sensitive to this natural inhibitor than the leukemic enzyme, and the inhibitory effect was independent of chain length.

2. Methylenetetrahydrofolate reductase. An extremely detailed study of inhibition of pig liver methylenetetrahydrofolate reductase by $H_2PteGlu_n$ (n = 1-6) has been performed (39). The dihydro derivatives were all competitive inhibitors with respect to 5, $10\text{-}CH_2\text{-}H_4PteGlu_1$. The K_i for $H_2PteGlu$ was the same whether the mono- or triglutamate substrate was present suggesting the K_i values obtained with the dihydropolyglutamates with the monoglutamate substrate may be valid against the polyglutamates as well. Inhibition increased with polyglutamate length up to hexaglutamate, which was 500-fold more inhibitory than the monoglutamate. Since the K_i of the hexaglutamate (13 nM) is well within the physiological range of $H_2PteGlu_n$ concentration, this inhibition may be important in vivo. A linear relationship was noted between the -log K_i and number of glutamates, indicating that each additional glutamate (up to six) caused an identical increase in apparent binding energy (39).

3. Methionine synthetase. The B_{12} independent methionine synthetase of *E. coli*, which absolutely required $5\text{-}CH_3\text{-}H_4PteGlu_3$ (see above) as a sub-

Table 2. Folylpolyglutamates as inhibitors of folate dependent reactions.

Enzyme	Source	Ref[1]	Substrate	Inhibitor	Value (concentration)	n=1	n=2	n=3	n=4	n=5	n=6	n=7
Dihydrofolate Reductase (EC 1.5.1.3)	Escherichia coli	a	$H_2PteGlu_1$	$10\text{-}HCO\text{-}PteGlu_n$	$I_{50}(mM)$	0.096				0.066		
	L1210/MTX	a	$H_2PteGlu_1$	$10\text{-}HCO\text{-}PteGlu_n$	$I_{50}(\mu M)$	0.1				0.015		
Methylenetetra-hydrofolate Reductase (EC 1.1.1.68)	Pig Liver	b	$5,10\text{-}CH_2\text{-}H_4PteGlu_1$	$H_2PteGlu_n$	$K_i(\mu M)$	6.5	1.7	0.7	0.2	0.04	0.013	0.065
	Pig Liver		$5,10\text{-}CH_2\text{-}H_4PteGlu_3$	$H_2PteGlu_n$	$K_i(\mu M)$	6.5						
5,10-methenyl-tetrahydrofolate Cyclohydrolase (EC 3.5.4.9)	Pig Liver	c	$5,10\text{-}methenyl\text{-}H_4PteGlu_1$	$PteGlu_n$	$I_{50}(\mu M)$	195		60		18		18
Thymidylate Synthetase	T2 Phage	d	$5,10\text{-}CH_2\text{-}H_4PteGlu$	$PteGlu_n$	$I_{50}(\mu M)$	70	8	8	8	8	9	10
	T2 Phage	e	$5,10\text{-}CH_2\text{-}H_4PteGlu$	$PteGlu_n$	$I_{50}(\mu M)$	>60					0.6	
	T2 Phage	e	$5,10\text{-}CH_2\text{-}H_4PteGlu$	$PteGlu_n$	$I_{50}(\mu M)$						>10	
	Escherichia coli	d	$5,10\text{-}CH_2\text{-}H_4PteGlu$	$PteGlu_n$	$I_{50}(\mu M)$	180	11	5	4	4	5	4
	Escherichia coli	e	$5,10\text{-}CH_2\text{-}H_4PteGlu$	$PteGlu_n$	$I_{50}(\mu M)$						>60	
	Escherichia coli	e	$5,10\text{-}CH_2\text{-}H_4PteGlu$	$PteGlu_n$	$I_{50}(\mu M)$						7	
	Escherichia coli	a	$5,10\text{-}CH_2\text{-}H_4PteGlu$	$PteGlu_n$	$I_{50}(\mu M)$						0.1	
	Escherichia coli	a	$5,10\text{-}CH_2\text{-}H_4PteGlu$	$5\text{-}HCO\text{-}H_4PteGlu_n$	$I_{50}(\mu M)$	200	20	3	3	2	1	0.7
	Lactobacillus casei	d	$5,10\text{-}CH_2\text{-}H_4PteGlu$	$PteGlu_n$	$I_{50}(\mu M)$	150	30	0.8	0.4	0.4	0.6	
	Lactobacillus casei	a	$5,10\text{-}CH_2\text{-}H_4PteGlu$	$PteGlu_n$	$I_{50}(\mu M)$						0.9	
	Lactobacillus casei	f	$5,10\text{-}CH_2\text{-}H_4PteGlu$	$H_2PteGlu_n$	$I_{50}(\mu M)$	300	20	3.2			3.2	
	Lactobacillus casei	a	$5,10\text{-}CH_2\text{-}H_4PteGlu$	$5\text{-}HCO\text{-}H_4PteGlu_n$	$I_{50}(\mu M)$					1	1.7	
	Human	g	$5,10\text{-}CH_2\text{-}H_4PteGlu$	$PteGlu_n$	$K_i(\mu M)$	40		3		2		
	Human	g	$5,10\text{-}CH_2\text{-}H_4PteGlu_3$	$H_2PteGlu_n$	$K_i(\mu M)$						6	
Formiminotetra-hydrofolate Cyclodeaminase	Pig Liver	c	$5\text{-}formimino\text{-}H_4PteGlu_1$	$PteGlu_n$	$I_{50}(\mu M)$	70		13		1.0		2.3

1. a) Friedkin et al. (75). b) Matthews and Baugh (39). Values for n=2, 3, 4, and 5 have been estimated from a figure. c) MacKenzie and Baugh (53). d) Kisliuk et al. (77). e) Maley et al. (78). f) Kisliuk et al. (23). g) Dolnick and Cheng (63). The first set of values in each case is in the absence of $MgCl_2$, the second value is in the presence of 50 mM $MgCl_2$.

strate, was weakly inhibited by PteGlu$_3$ (43). At 6 and 140 μM 5-CH$_3$-H$_4$PteGlu$_3$ the I$_{50}$ values for PteGlu$_3$ were about 1 and 3 mM, respectively. These concentrations of PteGlu$_3$ are so high as to be without physiological significance.

4. 5, 10-methenyltetrahydrofolate cyclohydrolase. Pig liver 5, 10-methenyltetrahydrofolate cyclohydrolase is one activity of a trifunctional protein in folate metabolism. The other two activites, formyltetrahydrofolate synthetase and 5, 10-methylenetetrahydrofolate dehydrogenase, use polyglutamate substrates more effectively than monoglutamates (Table 1). Since the polyglutamate substrates for the cyclohydrolase were not available, its preference for polyglutamates was indirectly determined by testing the inhibitory potency of the series PteGlu$_n$ (n = 1, 3, 5, 7) (53). The assumption was made that the relative inhibitory potency of these polyglutamates would parallel the polyglutamate substrate activity, although the absolute values would be different. Inhibition increased with chain length (Table 2) until PteGlu$_5$, which was ten-fold more inhibitory than PteGlu, and thus the cyclohydrolase displayed preferential binding of polyglutamate inhibitors, and probably also of polyglutamate substrates. The dehydrogenase and cyclohydrolase activities of this trifunctional protein both show their maximum effect with a pentaglutamate derivative (53). Unfortunately, substrate activity of the synthetase with pentaglutamates could not be tested.

5. Thymidylate synthetase. Inhibition of thymidylate synthetase by folylpolyglutamates has been of special interest since the description by Friedkin et al (76) of a potent, naturally occurring folylpolyglutamate inhibitor. This inhibitor was isolated and identified as 5-HCO-H$_4$PteGlu$_5$ (75). Using a series of synthetic 5-HCO-H$_4$PteGlu$_n$ (n = 1-6), inhibition was shown to increase twohundredfold as the chain length increased. The natural inhibitor had the same potency as synthetic 5-HCO-H$_4$PteGlu$_5$, and they were both hundredfold more inhibitory than 5-HCO-H$_4$PteGlu. This natural inhibitor was an even more potent inhibitor of *L. casei* thymidylate synthetase (75) than it was of the *E. coli* enzyme.

Other folylpolyglutamates have also been tested as thymidylate synthetase inhibitors. The enzymes of T2 phage and *E. coli* (77, 78) as well as *L. casei* (77) and human sources (63) have I$_{50}$ values for polyglutamate forms of PteGlu which are nine to two hundred and fiftyfold less than for the monoglutamate. Significantly, the polyglutamates of H$_2$PteGlu – one product of the thymidylate synthetase reaction – are very potent inhibitors of the reaction catalyzed by the *L. casei* (23) and human enzymes (63). Kisliuk et al. (23) suggested that this product inhibition occurs at a low enough concentration as to be physiologically significant. Inhibition by folylpolyglutamates is not just a function of the polyglutamate moiety because p-aminobenzoylhexaglutamate and hexaglutamate do not inhibit this reaction at concentrations 10^4 above the I$_{50}$ level of PteGlu$_6$ (23).

6. Formiminotetrahydrofolate cyclodeaminase. Formiminotetrahydrofolate cyclodeaminase is part of a bifunctional protein in pig liver (65). Its polyglutamate substrates were unavailable for testing and thus its preference for polyglutamates was determined indirectly by its inhibition by PteGlu$_n$ (n = 1, 3, 5, 7) (53). A seventyfold increase in inhibition was observed for the most inhibitory compound, the pentaglutamate, compared to the monoglutamate. This indicates a preference for polyglutamates, particularly pentaglutamates, which is similar to results for substrate activity for the second activity present, formiminoglutamate formiminotransferase (Table 1).

7. Other possible sites of inhibition. Other folate dependent enzymes are known to be potently inhibited by non-substrate, monoglutamate folates. Rabbit liver serine hydroxymethyltransferase is inhibited by both 5-CH$_3$- and 5-HCO-H$_4$PteGlu (79). Dihydrofolate reductase and 5, 10-methenyltetrahydrofolate cyclohydrolase from bovine liver are each inhibited by a number of folate monoglutamates, but particularly 5, 10-CH$_2$-H$_4$PteGlu (21). If polyglutamates of these forms are more potent inhibitors, as suggested by Table 2, some would be effective inhibitors in the physiological concentration range. Inhibition by the various polyglutamyl folates could mean that the intermediates in folate metabolism are intimately involved in its regulation.

8. Physiological significance. In many instances

inhibition was observed with $PteGlu_n$ (n>1); forms which do not occur intracellularly under normal conditions. This inhibition, therefore, can be of little direct in vivo significance, and none has been claimed in these studies. The real usefulness of these results is that they may give us a notion of the relative increase in binding to be expected from polyglutamylation. This is particularly important in cases (53) where the actual polyglutamate substrates are difficult to synthesize and test. Inhibition by $PteGlu_n$ might usefully serve as a quick, first test of an enzyme's response to polyglutamyl derivatives. More information on $PteGlu_n$ inhibition of enzymes whose polyglutamate substrate specificity is established (Table 1) would be necessary to establish the validity of this test.

Instances where both the folylpolyglutamate form and the concentration at which it inhibits are physiological have led to various proposals that the relative levels of polyglutamate substrates and inhibitors could regulate folate enzymes, and hence folate metabolism (23, 39, 80). Inhibition of thymidylate synthetase by $H_2PteGlu_n$ (23, 63), a product of the reaction, would prevent depletion of the reduced folate pool if $H_2PteGlu_n$ were not being reduced at a sufficiently rapid rate. Matthews and Baugh (39) have proposed that mammalian 5, 10-CH_2-$H_4PteGlu$ reductase might also be regulated by $H_2PteGlu_n$. In mammalian cells 5, 10-CH_2-$H_4PteGlu$ can be used for either methionine (through the reductase) or thymidylate biosynthesis (Fig. 2). When DNA synthesis occurs and the demand for thymidylate is high, the rapid flux through thymidylate synthetase might cause a rise in the levels of $H_2PteGlu_n$ which would inhibit 5, 10-CH_2-$H_4PteGlu$ reductase and free more 5, 10-CH_2-$H_4PteGlu$ for thymidylate biosynthesis. Presumably thymidylate synthetase itself would not be inhibited by a small rise in $H_2PteGlu_n$ (above) because its K_i is much higher. Bertino and Hillcoat (81) have pointed out the difficulty of specifically inhibiting an enzyme in such a system of close interaction and interconverting forms, but regulatory mechanisms of this type occur in other complex enzyme systems, such as glycolysis, so such a system may be possible in folate metabolism.

D. Folylpolyglutamates as forms required for intracellular retention of folate

Since cells only transport folates which are smaller than those that predominate within that cell type, and the highly anionic nature of folylpolyglutamates limits their ability to diffuse through membranes, polyglutamylation may serve to trap or retain folates intracellularly. Since *Diplococcus pneumoniae* was able to concentrate folate, relative to the medium, and it was all as polyglutamates, it was suggested there might be a relation between the concentrative ability and polyglutamylation (20). Buehring et al. (82) noted that intracellular folates of *L. casei* had longer chains than folates in the medium, although both were polyglutamates. This suggested that shorter polyglutamates were preferentially released and thus polyglutamylation aided retention. Further experiments with *L. casei* (72, 83) demonstrated that both the affinity and maximum velocity of transport decreased with increasing polyglutamate chain length. Assuming influx and efflux occurred by the same mechanism, the degree of retention would be directly related to chain length. These same experiments showed that [^{3}H]folic acid would efflux from *L. casei* after short term incubation where no metabolism occurred. At longer incubation times, as polyglutamates were formed, the efflux rate dropped drastically, even though the intracellular folate concentration was the same as in short term. The little folate material that did efflux was determined to be a diglutamate. This again suggests that longer polyglutamates were preferentially retained. *Corynebacterium sp.* growth medium contained a higher proportion of triglutamates than were found intracellularly, where tetraglutamates predominated, suggesting preferential retention of longer derivatives (84). Preferential transport of shorter derivatives was evident in studies (85) where the cytotoxicity for *S. faecalis* of methotrexate (a folate analog) and its polyglutamates was examined. As the chain length increased to heptaglutamate there was a 10^4fold decrease in cytotoxicity, and presumably a similar decline in transport. Mammalian cells share this property of reduced permeability to polyglutamates. Monoglutamates are readily transported into and efflux from mammalian cells (86, 87). However, Hoffbrand et al. (88) demonstrated that $PteGlu_3$ entered human marrow cells and lymphocytes less than 5% as well as PteGlu. Decreased permeability of hepatoma cells to polyglutamates was suggested (89) because once polyglutamates of methotrexate were formed, efflux of methotrexate was extremely slow even though the total intracellular methotrexate concentration was hundredfold above the protein bound fraction.

The most convincing evidence that folylpolyglutamates are involved in retention of folates is derived from work on two mutant CHO cell lines: AUX B1, which is auxotrophic for glycine, adenosine, and thymidine, and AUX B3, which is auxotrophic only for glycine and adenosine. Complementation analysis and reversion frequency data showed that these mutants contained a single recessive mutation in the same gene (74). Since the compounds required for growth all use folate dependent pathways (Fig. 2), a single central block in folate metabolism was postulated. The transport rate of folates and the levels of a number of folate dependent enzymes were all identical in the wild type and mutants, however the mutants were found to be unable to concentrate [³H]folate to the same extent as wild type cells. AUX B1 and AUX B3 had [³H]folate pools 10 and 40%, respectively, that of wild type cells under the same growth conditions. The pools were not only smaller, but also qualitatively different from wild type in that (a) 96 and 85% of the intracellular [³H]folate of AUX B1 and AUX B3, respectively, could efflux after long term incubation in [³H]folate, while little efflux occurred from wild type cells, and (b) chromatography of intracellular folates showed that wild type cells contained predominantly pentaglutamates while AUX B1 contained only monoglutamates and AUX B3 contained mono-, di-, and possibly some triglutamates. The data suggested that a single defect in the biosynthesis of folylpolyglutamates caused the multiple auxotrophy in these mutant cells. Further, the decreased folate pools and extensive folate efflux found in the mutants must be the result of this inability to synthesize polyglutamates and thus polyglutamate forms must aid in the retention of folates (74).

The defective synthesis of folylpolyglutamates in these lines was traced to a lack of folylpolyglutamate synthetase (FPGS) in AUX B1 and a defective FPGS in AUX B3 (90). It was also demonstrated that spontaneous revertants of the mutants simultaneously regained FPGS activity and a proportionally increased capacity to retain folates, further supporting the retention hypothesis (90).

Although the evidence clearly supports retention by cells of polyglutamates, the degree of retention is a function of both the polyglutamate length and the cell type. In L1210 cells, which contain predominantly pentaglutamates (19) transport of the form of methotrexate containing one additional glutamate [MTX(G$_1$)] had a fifteen-fold higher K$_t$ than methotrexate with an equivalent V$_{max}$ (consistent with retention). However, the efflux rate of both derivatives was the same (91). This argues that (a) efflux kinetics might not always be readily predicted by influx kinetics, and (b) this diglutamate, and perhaps those of natural folates, are not retained any better than the monoglutamate. Permeability of mammalian cells to folyldiglutamates is suggested by the results with AUX B3 which synthesizes di- and possibly triglutamates. Both its lower folate pool and high amount of efflux indicate that the diglutamate is not retained well. The triglutamate may have less ability to cross membranes, since it is transported by human marrow cells only 1–5% as well as the monoglutamate (88). However, as noted above, this influx data may not give a true representation of efflux. In bacteria similar results are obtained as for example where diglutamates escape from *L. casei* (83), and tri- and tetraglutamates escape from *Corynebacterium sp.* (84).

The data on the predominent length that occur in natural sources (6) and the limited data on influx and efflux of polyglutamates suggest that cells have evolved polyglutamate biosynthetic machinery that will synthesize lengths just longer than any which will pass the cellular membrane by either active transport or diffusion. In mammalian cells triglutamate will barely pass the membrane and these cells have pentaglutamates as the predominent lengths. In *L. casei* derivatives up to heptaglutamate enter the cell (92a) although the K$_m$ for influx increases dramatically and the V$_{max}$ decreases as the chain length extends (83). *L. casei* contains predominantly octaglutamates (82). Only diglutamates or shorter derivatives enter *S. faecalis* (92b) and its intracellular folates are mostly tetraglutamates (82). Cells can thus retain the levels of folates necessary for cellular growth while avoiding wasteful synthesis of excessively long polyglutamates.

E. Miscellaneous functions of folylpolyglutamates

1. T-even bacteriophage assembly. Synthesis of the

tail section of T-even bacteriophage specifically requires six molecules of $H_2PteGlu_6$ which is bound in the tail baseplate (93). This folate does not appear to be active as a cofactor, but apparently is only structural. The polyglutamate chain may provide a flexible linkage between the baseplate and the tail fibers. Synthesis of this folate is a phage, not host, function and is probably catalyzed by a phage protein using the host folate pool as its substrate. This structural role is very specific for the hexaglutamate in that neither penta- nor hepta-glutamates could be substituted, and conjugase treatment of the folate led to inactivation of the phage.

2. Effects on other enzymes. Folylpolyglutamates are implicated in the activities of two additional enzymes, although their role is unclear. Using radiolabeled folate, a folate binding protein was identified in rat liver mitochondria (94). The binding protein was partially purified, and the bound folate was identified as a single folate species, $H_4PteGlu_5$ (95). Recently (96), the homogeneous protein was shown also to contain riboflavin, and to catalyze sarcosine dehydrogenase and dimethylglycine dehydrogenase activities. One product of these reactions is formaldehyde, and the $H_4PteGlu_5$ was postulated (96) to act as a formaldehyde 'trap' because formaldehyde will react non-enzymatically with $H_4PteGlu_n$ to form 5, 10-CH_2-$H_4PteGlu_n$ (97). It is also possible that formaldehyde transfer is mediated by the enzyme. If it is enzyme mediated the fact that protein, as isolated, contains only $H_4PteGlu_5$ suggests this polyglutamate is the cofactor in vivo. This would be the only example where the in vivo cofactor has been positively identified (excluding the *Clostridia* which contain only triglutamates).

The second enzyme with which folylpolyglutamates are reported to interact is uroporphyrinogen I synthetase, an enzyme of heme biosynthesis. During studies of lead toxicity, it was noted that the enzyme from hemolysates was inhibited by 0.1 mM $PbCl_2$, but the hepatic enzyme was unaffected (98). A dialyzable factor was isolated from liver which would protect against $PbCl_2$ inhibition (99). This factor had fluorescence and UV spectra similar to pteridines, and the factor antagonized [³H]PteGlu binding to a specific folate binding protein, but none of the common monoglutamates had the

protective effect. Hydrolysis of the factor with chicken pancreas pteroylpolyglutamate hydrolase, which yields a pteroyldiglutamate end product, inactivated the factor (99) suggesting it was larger than a diglutamate. $PteGlu_3$ did not protect against $PbCl_2$ inhibition, while $PteGlu_6$ was effective. The isolated factor, however, was estimated to be protective at much lower concentrations than $PteGlu_6$, so it was assumed the protective factor must be a reduced/substituted polyglutamate. The natural factor also stimulated purified uroporphyrinogen I synthetase activity by threefold. A factor with similar properties of activation was separated from the enzyme during purification (100), but it is not clear whether this activator and the dialyzable factor are identical. The mechanism of the protection/activation is unknown, but it is not simple chelation (99). The finding (discussed in reference 100) that a one-carbon transfer may be involved in this synthetase reaction may give a clue to the function of the folate. Regardless of its function, the protection/activation role clearly requires a folylpolyglutamate.

3. Enzyme stabilization. Folylpolyglutamates may be important in regulating cellular levels of folate dependent enzymes through substrate (or inhibitor) stabilization. Bertino and Hillcoat (81) have pointed out that the levels of folate dependent enzymes could be regulated even if they were not subject to induction or repression. Binding of a folate ligand could stabilize the enzyme against intracellular degradation and turnover, thus leading to an increased intracellular concentration. Dihydrofolate reductase levels can be increased in vivo by such a mechanism (81). Since polyglutamate substrates and inhibitors generally have higher affinities for folate enzymes than monoglutamates (Table 1 and 2), folylpolyglutamates could be more effective stabilizing agents.

This principle has been elegantly demonstrated in vitro with *L. casei* thymidylate synthetase (101). *L. casei* thymidylate synthetase is inactivated by several proteases. Neither $PteGlu_1$ nor $PteGlu_2$ effected the rate of inactivation, while $PteGlu_3$ gave partial protection. $PteGlu_4$ through $PteGlu_7$ offered the greatest protection. The simultaneous presence of $PteGlu_n$ and dUMP, the nucleotide substrate for the enzyme, offered greater protection which again increased with chain length. dUMP and PteGlu$_5$ gave virtually complete protection against inactivation. These results indicate that binding of folylpolyglutamates could significantly alter the turnover rate of a folate dependent enzyme in vivo, and the extent of the effect depends on the length of polyglutamate. Polyglutamate substrates and inhibitors could both serve this function.

4. Allosteric effectors. Folylpolyglutamates may serve as allosteric effectors of non-folate reactions. Cystathionine γ-synthase of *Neurospora crassa* catalyzes the formation of cystathionine, the immediate precursor of homocysteine. Homocysteine is transmethylated with 5-CH$_3$-H$_4$PteGlu$_n$ to form methionine. 5-CH$_3$-H$_4$PteGlu$_n$ antagonize the feedback inhibition of cystathionine γ-synthase by S-adenosylmethionine, and serve as specific, essential activators of the synthase (102). Both of these functions were increasingly effective as the chain length increased. This activation also operates in vivo because a mutant which lacks methylenetetrahydrofolate reductase activity, and thus cannot synthesize 5-CH$_3$-H$_4$PteGlu$_n$, also lacks cystathionine γ-synthase activity in vitro unless extracts are supplemented with 5-CH-$_3$H$_4$PteGlu$_n$ (102). The preference for polyglutamate forms is also evident in vivo as mutants which can synthesize 5-CH$_3$-H$_4$PteGlu$_1$, but are deficient in FPGS activity and thus unable to make longer forms, also cannot synthesize cystathionine (102). The authors postulated that this would allow synthesis of methyl acceptor (homocysteine) only if adequate supplies of methyl donor (5-CH$_3$-H$_4$PteGlu$_n$) was present, and thus would allow regulation of methionine biosynthesis.

5. Effects on enzyme kinetic constants. Folylpolyglutamates may affect the kinetics of a reaction in ways other than those previously mentioned. For several reactions the kinetic constants for other substrates are altered in the presence of a folylpolyglutamate substrate. For example, the K_m for formate of the formyltetrahydrofolate synthetases of rat and bovine liver are decreased 6 and 70 fold, respectively, in the presence of a pentaglutamate substrate (60).

In two other examples – human thymidylate synthetase (63) and pig liver methylenetetrahydrofolate reductase (39) – the K_m values of the second substrate are significantly increased. Subtle chan-

ges in enzyme mechanism and mode of inhibition may also appear when polyglutamates are used instead of monoglutamates (39, 77).

III. Enzymatic synthesis of folylpolyglutamates in cell free systems

A. Introduction

Folylpoly-γ-glutamates, as discussed above, are generally the only forms of folate found intracellularly. Since the chain length of these intracellular polyglutamates always exceeds the longest form that can be transported efficiently, it follows that all cells must have their own enzyme system, folylpolyglutamate synthetase (FPGS), for synthesis of polyglutamates. As briefly described above the synthesis of folylpolyglutamates has been in-

Table 3. Specific activity of folylpolyglutamate synthetase in crude extracts of different sources.

Source	Substrate	Specific activity[a]
Escherichia coli[b]	10-HCO-H$_4$PteGlu	18 600
Corynebacterium sp.[c]	H$_4$PteGlu	10 000
Neurospora crassa[d]	H$_4$PteGlu	6 530
Mouse liver[e]		~60
Rat liver[f]	H$_4$PteGlu	320
Rabbit liver[g]	H$_4$PteGlu	183
Sheep liver[h]	H$_4$PteGlu	50
Chinese hamster ovary[g]	H$_4$PteGlu	107
Chinese hamster ovary (AUX B1)[g]	H$_4$PteGlu	0–3
Chinese hamster ovary (AUX B2)[g]	H$_4$PteGlu	78
Chinese hamster ovary (AUX B3)[g]	H$_4$PteGlu	17
Chinese hamster lung (V-79)[g]	H$_4$PteGlu	131
Chinese hamster lung (V-79 ght-1)[g]	H$_4$PteGlu	1–3

a) Defined as pmol folylpolyglutamate product synthesized/ h/mg protein. b) Masurekar and Brown (110). c) Shane (103). Value presented is at saturating glutamate. Under standard assay conditions value is 4 900. d) Ritari et al. (108). e) Moran and Colman (129). f) McGuire et al. (107). g) Taylor and Hanna (90). AUX B1 and ght-1 are mutants auxotrophic for glycine, adenosine (hypoxanthine), and thymidine. AUX B2 is auxotrophic for glycine. AUX B3 is auxotrophic for glycine and adenosine. h) Gawthorne and Smith (15).

vestigated in vivo and much useful information has been obtained. However, study of the FPGS in cell free systems has been slow and difficult because (a) the FPGS is present in relatively low amounts in all sources examined (Table 3), including species, such as *Corynebacterium sp.* (103) which overproduce folylpolyglutamates, (b) the FPGS is an extremely unstable protein (103) (McGuire, et al., unpublished work), and (c) simple assays have only recently been developed (90, 104).

Although all sources have low absolute amounts of activity, procaryotes have 50–100 times more activity than higher eucaryotes (Table 3). This difference in FPGS activity contrasts with the folate polyglutamate pools observed for these two classes which are the same order of magnitude (64, 103, 105). In addition, characterization of the FPGS partially purified from procaryotes and eucaryotes reveals several significant differences (see below). Whether these differences are related to differences in the function of this enzyme and/or its products in procaryotes and eucaryotes remains to be determined.

The number of enzymes involved in the synthesis of folylpolyglutamates by a given organism has been investigated in several cases. The maximum number of enzymes would be required if either one enzyme were responsible for synthesis of all polyglutamate lengths of each particular folate form, or if all folyldiglutamates were synthesized by one enzyme, all triglutamates by a second, etc., or if each enzyme added only one glutamate to one folate form. A single enzyme could be reponsible if it either made all lengths of all folates, or if it made polyglutamates of one or more folates and relied on the dynamics of intracellular folate metabolism to supply the proper intermediate(s).

The most convincing evidence on this point has been obtained for Chinese Hamster Ovary (CHO) cells where a single enzyme is indicated by the genetic studies of McBurney and Whitmore (74) and the elegant biochemical studies of Taylor and Hanna (90, 106). From wild-type CHO cultures, which synthesize pteroylpentaglutamates, McBurney and Whitmore (74) isolated a cell line following mutagenesis which was unable to synthesize folylpolyglutamates. The reversion frequency of the mutant was consistent with a single genetic lesion as the cause of the defective synthesis. Taylor and Hanna (90) demonstrated that crude extracts and

twentyfivefold purified FPGS from wild-type CHO cells could both synthesize diglutamate and higher lengths of $H_4PteGlu$, and the purified FPGS could make polyglutamates of a number of different folate derivatives. Extracts of the mutant cell line simultaneously lost the ability to make the diglutamate of any folate, and the ability to convert $H_4PteGlu_2$ or $H_4PteGlu_3$ to longer polyglutamates. This loss was not the result of the presence of a nondialyzable inhibitor, the presence of a very active conjugase, or repression of the FPGS under the permissive conditions required to grow the mutant. Extracts of spontaneous revertants of the mutant simultaneously regained the ability to synthesize all diglutamates, and greater lengths of $H_4PteGlu$. Finally (106), it was demonstrated that the revertant cells contained an FPGS with altered properties suggesting that the original mutation was in the FPGS structural gene rather than a regulatory gene. The evidence accumulated is consistent with a single FPGS being responsible for synthesis of all folylpolyglutamates in CHO cells, at least to the pentaglutamate state.

Circumstantial evidence from several other sources also bears on this point. The finding (107) that a partially purified rat liver FPGS can synthesize pentaglutamate derivatives, the predominant length in rat liver, from monoglutamates, and the observation that all folate monoglutamates have similar pH optima for activity, is consistent with rat liver also containing a single FPGS. In *Corynebacterium sp.* (103) the relative activities of crude extracts and a seventhousandfold purified FPGS with mono- and polyglutamyl substrates are nearly identical suggesting that this organism also possesses a single enzyme. *Neurospora crassa* (108, 109) was reported to have a diglutamate synthetase and a separate enzyme which synthesized higher polyglutamates. This assignment was based on the partial separation of the two activities by ammonium sulfate fractionation, and on the observation that extracts of two purportedly non-allelic mutants had one activity but not the other. Recent evidence (reference 103, footnote 2) that the two activities in *Neurospora* are not separable by ammonium sulfate fractionation contradicts these findings and suggests again that a single enzyme is responsible. More than one enzyme may be present in *Escherichia coli* (110) because the isolated FPGS only synthesized diglutamates of its preferred substrate,

10-HCO-H$_4$PteGlu, while *E. coli* contains predominantly pentaglutamate derivatives (58). This observation is ambiguous, however, because synthesis of longer polyglutamates by crude extracts could not be detected either, indicating perhaps that the reaction conditions (i.e., pH, type or concentration of folate) were not optimal. In that regard, the original description of the crude *E. coli* FPGS (111) demonstrated synthesis of di- and triglutamates from H$_4$PteGlu, a poorer substrate. H$_4$PteGlu$_2$ was itself a substrate. Thus a single enzyme from *E. coli* may utilize 10-HCO-H$_4$PteGlu to form diglutamates and then utilize H$_4$PteGlu$_2$ (or other diglutamate folates) produced in the course of metabolism to form longer polyglutamates.

The tissue distribution of mammalian FPGS has recently been investigated. The tissue distribution was determined in rat using assay conditions optimal for the rat liver FPGS (104). The highest specific activity was found in the liver, a tissue containing predominantly pteroylpentaglutamates (112–114) and the highest amount of total folate (105). FPGS activity was detectable in spleen, stomach, lung, small intestine, and brain, but not in heart or kidney. Heart, and other muscle tissue, contains only very low levels of folates (105) and hence would not require high synthetase activity. The lack of activity by folylpolyglutamate-rich kidney may have two explanations, besides the kidney FPGS having optimal assay conditions different than liver. Kidney contains high levels of a folate binding protein (115) which might deplete H$_4$PteGlu in the assay (6). Second, kidney contains very high levels of pteroylpolyglutamate hydrolase which could degrade products as they were synthesized (2).

The subcellular localization of the mammalian liver FPGS has been determined. In rat liver (104) the highest specific activity and the largest per cent of total activity (75%) was found in the cytosol. Other subfractions had less total activity in the order: nuclear > mitochondrial/lysosomal ≃ microsomal. The specific activity of all these fractions was about the same. The high activity of the nuclear fraction is most likely the result of its contamination with whole cells and the occlusion of considerable amounts of cytosol in this low speed pellet. In sheep liver (15) the subcellular distribution was similar except the microsomal fraction had a much higher specific activity than the mitochondrial. The distribution of FPGS activity paralleled the subcellular distribution of folylpolyglutamates as determined by microbiological assay (15, 116).

The FPGS activity of the mitochondrial fraction is of interest because mitochondria contain folylpolyglutamates (15) and must have their own FPGS, since it is unlikely that polyglutamates are transported into this organelle. Simple explanations for the low specific activity of FPGS in this fraction are: incomplete disruption of mitochondria before assay, disruption caused a partial inactivation of the FPGS, high levels of contaminating pteroylpolyglutamate hydrolase from the lysosomes known to sediment with mitochondria (116) and reaction conditions which were not optimal for the mitochondrial FPGS. A more subtle explanation may lie in the general observation that many aspects of mitochondrial metabolism are more similar to procaryotic than eucaryotic metabolism (117), a relationship which suggests that mitochondria arose as bacterial endosymbionts of primitive eucaryotes. Since many catalytic properties of bacterial FPGS are different from those of the mammalian enzyme, particularly the extremely strict folate substrate specificity of the bacterial enzymes, it is conceivable that more activity would be detected in mitochondria if assay conditions optimal for the bacterial enzymes were used.

The gene for human FPGS has recently been assigned to chromosome 9 by Taylor et al. (118) through somatic cell genetics techniques. Human lymphocytes were fused with a mutant CHO cell line lacking FPGS, and hybrids were isolated in medium selective for the FPGS$^+$ phenotype. Isozyme and cytogenetic analysis allowed the assignment of the structural gene for human FPGS to chromosome 9. In addition, hybrids were shown to contain the human gene product rather than a revertant CHO FPGS.

B. Assays for folylpolyglutamate synthetase activity

The lack of a simple, rapid, sensitive assay for FPGS activity has been the major obstacle to study of this enzyme in cell free systems. FPGS was first detected in extracts of *Escherichia coli* (111) using electrophoretic separation of reactants and products, and identification by bioautography. The sheep liver FPGS was assayed by separating labeled pteroylmonoglutamates from their polyglutamate products by gel sieving chromatography (15). These assays were extremely time consuming and difficult to scale up for large numbers of samples; thus they were impractical for use in enzyme purification. FPGS activity has also been assayed by using labeled glutamate and a charcoal adsorption assay (110, 119). After incubation, labeled glutamate ligated to unlabeled folates is separated from free glutamate by adsorbing the aromatic folate on charcoal, removing free glutamate by washing, and eluting the polyglutamate product from the charcoal with ethanolic ammonia. This assay is both simple and easy to perform in large numbers, and has proven useful for the study of sources containing higher levels of FPGS (e.g., *E. coli* and *N. crassa*). It is not useful for sources with low activity because the blank value (counts as product in the absence of either folate or enzyme) is high, and elution from charcoal has been found to be non-quantitative by many workers. Another assay (120) also measures incorporation of labeled glutamate into unlabeled folates, but at the end of the incubation the folates are cleaved by Zn/HCl treatment to a family of labeled p-aminobenzoyl-polyglutamates which are then converted to azo dye derivatives. The azo derivatives are easily separated from free glutamate by adsorption chromatography. This simple method gives extremely low blanks, and thus high sensitivity, and is easily performed on large numbers of samples. However, it has recently been shown (121, 122) that many folate derivatives are not cleaved by the Zn/HCl treatment and are thus not quantifiable. The assay is thus satisfactory for use in assaying activity with a limited number of substrates. A sensitive, rapid assay with a slightly higher blank value, but which can quantitate FPGS activity with any natural folate or analog as substrate, has been independently developed in two laboratories (90, 104).

This assay depends on the separation on DEAE-cellulose minicolumns of labeled glutamate – which is incorporated into folylpolyglutamates from free glutamate. Separation of folylpolyglutamates from unincorporated [3H] glutamate in these assays is not trivial. All FPGS have K_m values for L-glutamate which are much higher than the apparent K_m for the best folate substrate. Thus, under assay conditions with saturating glutamate and folate, the glutamate concentration is typically millimolar while the folate is in the low micromolar range. Activity in crude extracts, particularly of mammalian tissues, is low (Table 3). For example, rat liver crude extracts can synthesize only 150 pmol of polyglutamate under conditions of linearity with respect to time and enzyme concentration. This represents 1.7% conversion of the initial folate monoglutamate, but only 0.015% of the labeled glutamate is incorporated. Any assay method must, therefore, be able to separate labeled folylpoly-glutamate from a seventhousandfold excess of free labeled glutamate.

FPGS activity determinations in crude extracts must be carefully controlled to avoid artifacts caused by the presence of other enzymes. For example, glutamyl tRNA synthetase activity could be measured with labeled glutamate and endogenous tRNA[Glu] by either the charcoal adsorption or DEAE-cellulose assays. The product of the glutamate dehydrogenase reaction, α-Ketoglutarate, binds to DEAE-cellulose under standard washing conditions and thus would be counted as product (McGuire et al., unpublished work). The increased apparent activity can easily be corrected by controls lacking folate. Factors leading to artifactually low activity are sometimes more difficult to circumvent. The effects of contamination by folate binding proteins and pteroylpolyglutamate hydrolase were discussed above. Metabolism of the folate substrate to another form would be particularly troublesome in sources where FPGS substrate specificity is strict. An important source of error is the high levels of adenosine triphosphatase activity in many crude extracts (McGuire et al., unpublished work) which rapidly lead to rate limiting ATP concentrations. This problem can be alleviated by use of an ATP regenerating system, short incubation times, and higher initial levels of ATP. High levels of ATP (10 mM) do not inhibit either the rat liver (107) or mouse leukemia L5178Y FPGS (McGuire et al., unpublished work). The ultimate proof for folylpolyglutamate synthesis in crude extracts must come from folate product identification. This can be done by double radio-label studies, pteroylpolyglutamate hydrolase sensitivity, isolation of products and showing they promote growth of appropriate folate requiring bacteria, or co-chromatography of the products (or their p-aminobenzoylpolyglutamate derivatives) with authentic standards.

Using these assays a few FPGS have been partially purified. One, the FPGS of *Corynebacterium sp.* (103) has been purified seventhousand-fold to 95% purity. These enzymes have been used in characterization studies the results of which are discussed below.

C. Molecular properties

Since only one FPGS has been purified to near homogeneity there is little data on physical properties except for molecular weights. Using calibrated gel seiving columns the M_r determined are: *E. coli* (110) 42 000, *Corynebacterium sp.* (103) 51 000 and rat liver (107), 69 000.

D. Catalytic properties

1. Kinetic constants. The kinetic constants for ATP, L-glutamate, and folate substrates have been determined in several instances (Table 4). In addition, crude sheep liver FPGS required 5–10 mM L-glutamate for saturation so its K_m is probably near that of rat liver (15). The K_m values are generally unremarkable except for an indication that the bacterial enzymes have significantly lower K_m's than the liver enzyme for both ATP and L-glutamate.

Determination of the K_m for ATP with FPGS must be made with extreme care. The actual substrate of the reaction is Mg-ATP and free ATP acts as an inhibitor (103). Thus, the ratio of Mg^{+2} to ATP^{+4} in the reaction mixture has a pronounced effect on activity. The absolute requirement of the rat liver enzyme for Mg^{+2} is also consistent with Mg-ATP as the true substrate (107). When the ratio of Mg^{+2} to ATP is such that free ATP is present at equilibrium, the activity of rat liver FPGS is inhibited relative to the same ATP level where all the ATP is present as the Mg^{+2} chelate, which indicates that free ATP is inhibitory in this case also (McGuire et al., unpublished work). A further anomaly was noted in the kinetics at low Mg-ATP concentrations with the rat liver enzyme. Activity was non-linear with respect to time at low (but not high) Mg-ATP concentrations, and this non-linearity was not the result of enzyme inactivation, limiting substrate, or product inhibition (107). If linearity with respect to time is not rigorously maintained, the kinetics appear sigmoidal and the observed K_m value is larger than the true value.

2. Effect of pH and temperature. All FPGS display high pH optima when tested with their preferred substrate (Table 5). The pH optima of rat liver FPGS with a variety of folate monoglutamates are also high and identical (107). The low or non-existent activity of all these enzymes near or below pH 7 may explain why some workers have been unable to detect activity (74). Unfortunately, it is not possible to directly compare the pH values of Table 5 because the temperature during the pH measurement is generally not stated and many workers list the pH of the buffer stock solution rather than the actual pH of the assay. The assay pH may be as much as one pH unit different from the nominal value as a result of dilution, temperature effects, and mixing with other assay components (McGuire et al., unpublished work). The buffer species generally has little or no effect on activity at the optimal pH (15, 90, 103, 107). Tris-HCl, triethanolamine-HCl, diethanolamine-HCl,

Table 4. Kinetic constants of folylpolyglutamate synthetases.

Source	Km value of substrate				
	L-glutamate	ATP	H₄PteGlu	10-HCO-H₄PteGlu	5, 10-CH₂-H₄PteGlu
	mM	μM	μM	μM	μM
Escherichia coli[a]	0.18	N.D.[a]	10	2	10
Corynebacterium sp.[b]	0.16	18	2.1	N.D.[b]	N.D.[b]
Rat liver[c]	0.65	≅70	N.D.[c]	N.D.[c]	N.D.[c]

a) Masurekar and Brown (110). Km for ATP not determined (N.D.) but saturation was achieved at 0.2 mM ATP (1 mM MgCl₂). b) Shane (128). N.D. = not determined. c) McGuire et al. (107). N.D. = not determined. Complex kinetics with folate substrates make determination of K_m values impossible (see section on Folate products).

Table 5. pH dependence of folylpolyglutamate synthetase activity.

Source	pH		
	Maximum activity	½ Maximum activity	Inactive
Escherichia coli[a]	9.0– 9.8	8.2; 10.4	<7.0
Corynebacterium sp[b]	10	8.5[f]	<7.0[f]
Rat liver[c]	8.2– 8.6	7.7; 9	
Sheep liver[d]	8.4	7.8; 9[f]	
Chinese hamster ovary[e]	8.5–10.2	8.0[f]	<7.5[f]

a) Masurekar and Brown (110). b) Shane (103). c) McGuire et al. (107). Values are pH in the assay mixture at 37 °C. d) Gawthorne and Smith (15). e) Taylor and Hanna (90). f) Values estimated from figure in appropriate reference.

ethanolamine-HCl, Tris-glycine, imidazole, and Na-glycine all gave similar activity. Phosphate buffer was inhibitory (103) presumably because of product inhibition. Borate buffer was also inhibitory probably because its complexation with the vicinal diol of ATP lowers the effective ATP concentration. This latter hypothesis could be tested by replacing ATP with dATP which is also a substrate (90, 103, 107) but which cannot form these complexes.

The optimum temperature for assaying FPGS activity has been determined as 50° for *E. coli*[110] and 37–41.5° for rat liver (107). Rat liver FPGS activity is less at 22° and is almost undetectable at 50° or 0°. The CHO synthetase (90) also inactive at 0°. Other sources have only been assayed at 37 °C.

3. Activation by monovalent cations. Synthetases commonly require a monovalent cation for activity (123, 124). This cation may be required at the catalytic site (124) or to promote a specific conformational change required for catalysis (123) or for the structural integrity of the protein (125). Monovalent cation requirements are often one of two types: K^+, NH_4^+, and Rb^+ activate while Na^+ and Li^+ are ineffective, or Na^+ and Li^+ are active and the K^+ group is ineffective (123).

The FPGS all absolutely require a monovalent cation for activity and are of the K^+ activated type. The greatest extent of activation was achieved with K^+ but Rb^+ and NH_4^+ were also activators (Table 6) while Li^+, Na^+, and Cs^+ were ineffective at any concentration. The FPGS of *N. crassa* (126) is reported to have an absolute requirement for K^+ but no details are available. Only the CHO synthetase appears to lack this requirement (90); the FPGS in crude extracts is stimulated a maximum of 15% at 30 mM K^+. This may be misleading, however, because the crude rat liver synthetase is also not dependent on exogenous K^+ while the

Table 6. Monovalent cation activation of folylpolyglutamate synthetase.

Source	K^+		NH_4^+		Rb^+	
	Conc.[a]	Activity[b]	Conc.[a]	Activity[b]	Conc.[a]	Activity[b]
	mM		mM		mM	
Escherichia coli[d]	200	1	50	0.5	300	0.6
Corynebacterium sp.[e]	200	1	200	0.4	N.D.[c]	
Rat liver[f]	20	1	10	0.8	50	0.7
Sheep liver[g]	120	1	N.D.[c]		N.D.[c]	

a) Concentration of ion as chloride salt giving optimal activity. b) Activity as per cent relative to K^+. c) N.D. = not determined. d) Masurekar and Brown (110). e) Shane (103). f) McGuire et al. (107). g) Gawthorne and Smith (15).

purified enzyme shows absolute dependence (107). Thus, there is either enough K^+ in this tissue to fulfill the requirement or other factors in crude extracts can substitute effectively.

4. Effect of divalent cations. All FPGS require Mg^{+2} because the Mg-ATP chelate is the true substrate of the reaction (see section above). The *E. coli* FPGS will utilize Mn^{+2} but not Ca^{+2} as a replacement (110). The *Corynebacterium sp.* FPGS will not use Co^{+2} or Mn^{+2} as the divalent cation (103). Effectiveness of divalent cations other than Mg^{+2} has not been evaluated with the rat liver enzyme because under standard assay conditions other ions (including Mn^{+2}, Ca^{+2}, Co^{+2}, and Zn^{+2}) formed unidentified complexes and precipitated (McGuire et al., unpublished work). This occurred rapidly in most cases, but with Mn^{+2} precipitation was slow. Using other buffer species in assays did not prevent precipitation.

5. Other effectors. FPGS activity was reported to be slightly increased in the livers of vitamin B_{12} deficient sheep (127), but no increase was detected when CHO cells were cultured in medium lacking B_{12} (90), and addition of various B_{12} forms to assays did not stimulate CHO FPGS activity (90). Intravenous injections of L-methionine slightly lowered FPGS activity in sheep liver (127). This effect is probably indirect because L-methionine neither activates nor inhibits the partially purified rat liver FPGS (McGuire et al., unpublished work). Coenzyme A stimulated the FPGS of *N. crassa* but was non-essential (126). Neither coenzyme A nor acetyl coenzyme A, however, had any effect on the *Corynebacterium sp.* synthase (103). The stimulation observed with coenzyme A with the *N. crassa* synthetase might result from the reducing ability of the coenzyme A sulfhydryl group. Both reduced folates (2) and the FPGS (107) are labile if inadequate levels of reducing agents are present.

6. Substrate specificity and inhibitors. a. ATP. All FPGS absolutely require a nucleoside triphosphate for activity and ATP or dATP generally give highest activity. The products of ATP utilization in this reaction are ADP and P_i (103, 110, 128). The *E. coli* enzyme will utilize GTP and dATP at 20% and 45%, respectively, the rate of ATP, while TTP, CTP, UTP, XTP, ITP and ADP are inactive (110).

The *Corynebacterium sp.* synthetase utilizes ATP, dATP, and UTP (in order of effectiveness) and CTP, GTP, and TTP are essentially inactive (103). The sheep liver enzyme utilizes ATP but not GTP (15). The CHO enzyme utilizes dATP 1.5 times more effectively than ATP which is more effective than GTP. ADP, CTP, UTP, and TTP were inactive (90). The rat liver FPGS will use ATP, dATP, GTP, and dGTP but not UTP, TTP, ADP, or AMP (107). Of the ATP analogs which were not substrates, a few were inhibitors. Both ADP and AMP were inhibitory for the *Corynebacterium sp.* (103) and mouse liver (129) synthetases. The β,γ-methylene analog of ATP was a very potent inhibitor of the *Corynebacterium sp.* FPGS (103).

It had been noted earlier (107) that FPGS were purine nucleoside triphosphate specific but the data on the *Corynebacterium sp.* enzyme conflicts with this. Data from more sources are required before deciding whether *Corynebacterium sp.* is an exception to this generalization.

b. Glutamate. All FPGS display absolute specificity for L-glutamate as a variety of analogs are neither substrates nor inhibitors (Table 7). In-

Table 7. Glutamate analogs inactive as substrates and inhibitors of folylpolyglutamate synthetase.

Compound	Reference[1]
D-glutamate	a, b, d, e
L-glutamine	a, b, c, e
L-aspartate	a, b, d, e
L- or DL-aminoadipate	a, b, e
DL-aminopimelate	b
glutarate	b
2-hydroxyglutarate	b
2-oxoglutarate	b
L-α-aminobutyrate	b
L-γ-aminobutyrate	b
L-methionine sulfoximine	b, e
L-methionine	b, f
L-lysine	b
glycine	b, e
N-acetylglutamate	b
N-methylglutamate	f
glutathione	c, e
p-aminobenzoate	a, e
γ-L-glutamyl-L-glutamate	a, c, e

[1] a) *Escherichia coli:* Masurekar and Brown (110). b) *Corynebacterium sp.:* Shane (103). c) Sheep liver: Gawthorne and Smith (15). d) Chinese Hamster Ovary cells: Taylor and Hanna (90). e) Rat liver: McGuire et al. (107). f) Rat liver: McGuire et al., unpublished observation.

activity of D-glutamate demonstrates the stereo-specificity of the enzyme while the ineffectiveness of L-aspartate, L-α-aminoadipate, and L-α-amino-pimelate (containing one less, one more, and two more methylene carbons, respectively, than glutamic acid) demonstrates the strict size specificity of the glutamate binding site. Common amino acids, a peptide containing a γ-glutamyl linkage (glutathione; γ-Glu-Cys-Gly), as well as other structural analogs of glutamate also do not bind to the enzyme. The lack of binding by N-acetylglutamate is striking because its structure closely resembles the amide linkage of the folylpolyglutamate products.

It was first observed that the *E. coli* synthetase (111) would not use pre-formed γ-glutamyl peptides as substrates for folylpolyglutamate synthesis. No products were detected with either γ-glutamyl-glutamate or γ-glutamyl-γ-glutamylglutamate, and H$_2$Pte or H$_4$PteGlu as the substrate. The generality of this observation (Table 7) suggests that glutamates are always added stepwise. This suggestion has been confirmed recently in a study of the kinetic mechanism of the *Corynebacterium sp.* synthetase (128) (see below). It would be of interest to determine the effect of γ-glutamylglutamate on the FPGS of *Diplococcus pneumoniae* because it has been suggested, on the basis of in vivo experiments, that it makes peptides and incorporates them into folates (20).

In two cases weak inhibition by glutamate analogs was noted. The rat liver FPGS (107) was inhibited slightly by high concentrations of 2-oxoglutarate (α-Ketoglutarate), and L-glutamate-γ-methylester was a poor inhibitor of the *Corynebacterium sp.* synthetase with fourteenfold less affinity than L-glutamate (103). Considering the high inhibitor concentrations required and the low degree of inhibition it is conceivable that in both cases contaminating L-glutamate was responsible for the decreased labeled glutamate incorporation.

c. Folate substrates. The folate substrate specificity of FPGS is dependent on the source of the enzyme (Table 8). The *E. coli* synthetase will utilize only three naturally occurring monoglutamyl folates (110). The 10-HCO-H$_4$PteGlu derivative (K$_m$ = 2 μM) is the preferred substrate suggesting that it may be the physiologically important substrate for addition of the first glutamate. In the physiological range of folate concentrations (10 μM), the highly

purified *Corynebacterium sp.* synthetase utilizes only H$_2$Pte, H$_4$PteGlu, and 5, 10-CH$_2$-H$_4$PteGlu (103). Other natural folates are essentially inactive, although in some instances this is merely the result of a very low affinity for the enzyme (Table 8). The possibility that dihydrofolate synthetase and FPGS are two activities of the same protein in this bacterium is suggested by their seventhousandfold co-purification in constant ratio (103). *Neurospora crassa* FPGS has been reported to utilize only tetrahydrofolates as substrates (126). Three reduced folate monoglutamates show significant activity with the sheep liver (15) and CHO (90) synthetases indicating that the higher eucaryotic enzymes have broader folate substrate specificity. The CHO enzyme also utilizes H$_4$PteGlu$_2$ and H$_4$PteGlu$_3$ but not PteGlu and thus was classified as specific for reduced folates. However, substrate activity of PteGlu was tested in the absence of reducing agents, and it is known that at least one mammalian enzyme, the rat liver FPGS (107), is unstable in the absence of reducing agents. Brody (120) found that the specificity of the rat enzyme was broader because PteGlu and reduced folates were substrates. The significance of this brief report is unclear since the assay used primarily measures the newly discovered enzymes tetrahydrofolate: amino acid ligase and folate diglutamate: amino acid transpeptidase, and their activity could be mistaken as FPGS (130). Partially purified rat liver enzyme does, however, possess very broad folate specificity (107). In the physiological range of folate concentrations, every folate serves as a substrate although several, including 5-CH$_3$-H$_4$PteGlu, have low activity. The early observation (131) that 5-CH$_3$-H$_4$PteGlu was not a substrate for rat liver crude FPGS is undoubtedly the result of its low relative activity which would not be detectable in crude extracts. The high activity of H$_4$PteGlu and 10-HCO-H$_4$PteGlu with the rat liver enzyme at the lowest concentration (5 μM) suggests these derivatives may serve as the physiological substrates for the first reaction. It has been briefly reported (129) that at physiological concentrations (1 μM) a mouse liver preparation exhibited broad specificity as follows: H$_2$PteGlu>H$_4$PteGlu, 5-HCO-H$_4$Pte-Glu>PteGlu$_3$>>PteGlu.

7. Folate products. Detailed product analysis has been performed in a limited number of cases. The *E.*

Table 8. Folate substrate specificity of folylpolyglutamate synthetase.

Source	Substrate conc. (μM)	Relative activity of substrate[a]							
		H_2Pte	PteGlu	$H_2PteGlu$	$H_4PteGlu$	$5\text{-}CH_3\text{-}H_4PteGlu$	$5\text{-}HCO\text{-}H_4PteGlu$	$5,10\text{-}CH_2\text{-}H_4PteGlu$	$10\text{-}HCO\text{-}H_4PteGlu$
Escherichia coli[b]	150	0	0.02 (70 μM)	0	0.14	0	0	0.23	1
Corynebacterium sp.[c]	10	.48	.002	.07	1	0.02	0.006	0.67	0.04
	100	.15	.002	.16	1	0.08	0.03	1.32	0.17
	1000	.16	.006	.13	1	0.71	0.37	1.16	0.73
Neurospora crassa[d]			0	0	1	0			0
Rat Liver[e]			0.33		1	0			1
Rat Liver[f]	5		0.16	0.56	1	0.19	0.18	0.68	0.88
Rat Liver[g]	35		0.47	0.84	1	0.48	0.27	0.64	0.54
Sheep Liver[h]	1.2				1	0.51	0.40		
Chinese Hamster	20				1	0.16	0.45		
Ovary[i]	100		0.03		1				

a) Relative activity is defined as the ratio of FPGS activity to the activity of the preferred substrate of that particular FPGS. b) Masurekar and Brown (110). c) Shane (103). d) Sakami et al. (126). e) Spronk (131). f) Brody (120). g) McGuire et al. (107). h) Gawthorne and Smith (15). i) Taylor and Hanna (90).

44

coli FPGS is only capable of diglutamate synthesis with its preferred substrate, 10-HCO-H$_4$PteGlu (110). The product was identified by its spectral characteristics on isolation, by its growth promoting ability for *L. casei,* and double radiolabel experiments. Earlier studies indicated that with H$_4$PteGlu (a poorer substrate) both di- and triglutamate products could be obtained (111). The *Corynebacterium sp.* synthetase (103) formed only diglutamate products from its monoglutamate substrates (at 100 μM; see Table 8), except for 5, 10-CH$_2$-H$_4$PteGlu with which the triglutamate form was just detectable. A single glutamate was added to these substrates because their respective di- and triglutamate derivatives were very poor substrates, again with the exception of the methylene derivatives (103). (dℓ)-5, 10-methylene-H$_4$PteGlu$_2$ had up to 15% of the activity found with H$_4$PteGlu and derivatives as long as tetraglutamate, the predominant intracellular length of *Corynebacterium sp.* folates (84) were sometimes detected (103). 5, 10-methylene-H$_4$PteGlu$_3$ was also utilized, albeit extremely poorly, and the product was identified as the tetraglutamate. Thus, with both bacterial enzymes, only a single glutamate was readily added to the monoglutamate substrates. Synthesis of the longer derivatives which predominate in these species (58, 84) was extremely slow relative to the diglutamate. This rate was deemed rapid enough, however, to account for the in vivo rate of folylpolyglutamate biosynthesis (103). The mammalian enzymes are able to synthesize longer polyglutamates quite readily with H$_4$PteGlu as the substrate. The CHO synthetase (90) converted H$_4$PteGlu to di-, tri-, and tetraglutamate forms as determined by double radiolabel of the products, and co-chromatography with standards. The partially purified rat liver FPGS (107) synthesized polyglutamates of H$_4$PteGlu up to the pentaglutamate, the predominant length of folylpolyglutamate in rat liver (112–114). The identification of these products as folylpolyglutamates was based on their HPLC behavior compared to standards, double radiolabel studies, conjugase sensitivity, and amino acid analysis of labeled product. It was first observed with the CHO synthetase (90) that synthesis of longer derivatives was promoted as the initial H$_4$PteGlu concentration was decreased. An identical effect on product formation from H$_4$PteGlu by the partially purified

rat liver synthetase was investigated in detail (107). It was concluded that average product length was inversely dependent on the initial monoglutamate concentration, and that longer polyglutamates could be synthesized in higher absolute amounts at low monoglutamate concentration even though total product formation was lower. This inverse relationship is observed with some other (e.g., 10-HCO-H$_4$PteGlu), but not all folates (e.g., PteGlu) (132). No such effect is seen with the highly purified *Corynebacterium sp.* FPGS as the same products are synthesized from H$_4$PteGlu and 5, 10-CH$_2$-H$_4$PteGlu regardless of their initial concentration (133).

This effect could make mammalian folate metabolism more efficient in vivo in that rapid synthesis of longer polyglutamates would occur under conditions of folate deficiency when their special qualities of increased retention and efficiency of one-carbon transfer would be particularly advantageous. This effect may also correlate with the observations made in vivo (82, 134), including in rat liver (105), that low extracellular folate concentration led to accumulation of longer polyglutamates in cells, while high folate concentration led to shorter polyglutamates.

8. Stereospecificity for folate substrates. Chemical or electrochemical reduction of PteGlu to H$_4$PteGlu introduces an asymmetric center at C-6 and produces two diastereoisomers (2). Chemical methods for preparing one-carbon derivatives from this H$_4$PteGlu also yield both diastereoisomers. For nearly all folate enzymes where stereospecificity has been examined, only one isomer is utilized and it is the same one as occurs naturally. One exception to this rigid stereospecificity is the glycineamide ribonucleotide transformylase of chicken liver (135) which used the unnatural isomer of 5, 10-methenyl-H$_4$PteGlu at 0.8% the rate of the natural isomer. The transport of reduced folates also may not be stereospecific (72, 136), but this question has not been completely answered (137). Although generally not substrates, the unnatural isomer or its polyglutamate form may inhibit a folate dependent reaction (23, 138). Direct studies with the *E. coli* FPGS (110) showed only the natural isomer of 10-HCO-H$_4$PteGlu was a substrate and the unnatural isomer was a weak competitive inhibitor. Indirect, in vivo evidence suggests that the FPGS of

L. casei is not stereospecific, however (139). It has been directly demonstrated that the rat liver FPGS is not stereospecific for $H_4PteGlu$, and probably also not with 10-HCO- or 5-CH_3-$H_4PteGlu$ (107). The two purified diastereoisomers of $H_4PteGlu$ have about the same affinity for the rat liver FPGS, and the apparent V_{max} of the unnatural isomer is 50% that of the natural, indicating it is a good substrate. The substrate activity of the unnatural isomer was demonstrated not to be the results of a racemization producing the natural isomer (107). The lack of stereospecificity of the mammalian enzyme is perhaps not surprising considering its relative lack of specificity with respect to the pteridine portion of the molecule (see Table 8 and 9).

9. Folate analogs as substrates and inhibitors. Limited testing of folate analogs has been performed with nearly all FPGS described, however extensive testing to determine the structural requirements for activity has been performed with only two synthetases (Table 9). The *E. coli* FPGS (110) is quite strict in its specificity for a fully reduced, formylated derivative as neither 10-HCO-$H_2PteGlu$ or 10-CH_3-$H_4PteGlu$ are substrates. The 4-hydroxy substituent is non-essential, the 4-amino analog of 10-HCO-$H_4PteGlu$ (10-HCO-H_4-aminopterin) is active, but the 4-amino group itself is insufficient (aminopterin is inactive). The activity of 11-HCO-H_4homofolate, an analog with an extra methylene group between C-9 and N-10, indicates some flexibility in the active site as long as all other determinants are present. On the basis of its broad folate specificity (Table 8) and its lack of stereospecificity, the rat liver FPGS (107) might be expected to utilize as substrates a wide variety of folate analogs (Table 9). The substrate activity of aminopterin and methotrexate indicate the 4-hydroxy group can be replaced by an amino group without loss of activity (this substituent actually increases activity). The N-10 position can accommodate the unnatural methyl group without effect since 10-CH_3-PteGlu and methotrexate are as active as the corresponding unmethylated compounds. Replacement of the N-5 and N-8 by carbons also give an active substrate, 5, 8-dideazafolate (140). Finally, 5-CH_3-H_4homofolate is a substrate indicating, again, the lack of specificity of the folate binding site.

Folate analogs not utilized as substrates were tested as potential inhibitors of the rat liver FPGS (107). Neither the analog of methotrexate containing aspartate nor the analog of folic acid

Table 9. Substrate activity of folate analogs for folylpolyglutamate synthetase.

Analog	FPGS				
	E. coli[a]	*Coryn. sp.*[b]	*N. crassa*[c]	Rat Liver[d]	CHO[e]
Pte-D-Glu				−	
10-HCO-Pte	−				
10-HCO-H_4Pte	−				
10-HCO-$H_2PteGlu$	−				
10-CH_3-PteGlu	−			+	
10-CH_3-$H_4PteGlu$	−				
H_4-homofolate			−		+
11-HCO-H_4homofolate	+				
5-CH_3-H_4homofolate				+	
Aminopterin (2, 4-diamino-PteGlu)	−	+		+	
10-HCO-H_4aminopterin	+				
Methotrexate (2, 4-diamino-10-CH_3-PteGlu)		−		+	
2, 4-diamino-10-CH_3-PteAsp				−	
5, 8-dideazafolate				+	

a) Masurekar and Brown (110). b) Shane (103). c) Sakami et al. (126). d) McGuire et al. (107). e) Taylor and Hanna (90).

containing D-glutamate were inhibitory. Thus in contrast to the lack of pteridine specificity, the binding specificity for the terminal glutamate appears absolute.

E. Mechanism of the reaction

The mechanism of the FPGS reaction has been investigated only with the *Corynebacterium sp.* synthetase (128). With this enzyme it was possible to examine a single step of the reaction, that is the conversion of $H_4PteGlu$ to the diglutamate. Initial velocity, product inhibition, and competitive inhibition studies indicated an ordered ter ter mechanism with substrates binding in the order: Mg-ATP, $H_4PteGlu$, L-glutamate, and products released in the order: ADP, $H_4PteGlu_2$, and P_i. An important implication of this mechanism is that the folate must leave the active site after each glutamate is added. Thus, sequential addition of glutamate to bound folate is not possible.

Acknowledgements

The authors wish to thank Dr. James K. Coward, Department of Chemistry, Rensselaer Polytechnic Institute, Troy, New York for his comments on this manuscript. The invaluable assistance of Patricia M. Kerley in preparing this review is gratefully acknowledged.

Support for the preparation of this review was provided by National Cancer Institute Research Grant CA08010 and by Postdoctoral Traineeship 5-T32-CA09085 (to John J. McGuire). Joseph R. Bertino is an American Cancer Society Professor of Medicine and Pharmacology.

References

1. Stokstad, E. L. R., 1979. Fed. Proc. 38: 2696–2698.
2. Blakley, R. L., 1969. Frontiers of Biology Eds. Neuberger, A. & Tatum, E. L. Vol. 13, North-Holland, Amsterdam.
3. Kutzbach, C. & Stokstad, E. L. R., 1971. Biochim. Biophys. Acta 250: 459–477.
4. Hoffbrand, A. V., 1975. Prog. in Hematology 9: 85–105.
5. Baugh, C. M. & Krumdieck, C. L., 1971. Ann. N. Y. Acad. Sci. 186: 7–28.
6. Scott, J. M. & Weir, D. G., 1976. Clinics in Hematology 5: 547–568.
7. Covey, J. M., 1980. Life Sciences 26: 665–678.
8 a. Nakamura, K. & Kozloff, L. M., 1978. Biochim. Biophys. Acta, 540: 313–319.
8. b. Bassett, R., Weir, D. G. & Scott, J., 1976. J. Gen. Microbiol. 93: 169–172.
9. Curthoys, N. P., Scott, J. M. & Rabinowitz, J. C., 1972. J. Biol. Chem. 247: 1959–1964.
10. Binkley, S. B., Bird, O. D., Bloom, E. S., Brown, R. A., Calkins, D. G., Campbell, C. J., Emmett, A. D., Pfiffner, J. J., 1944. Science 100: 36–37.
11. Pfiffner, J. J., Calkins, D. G., Bloom, E. S. & O'Dell, B. L., 1946. J. Am. Chem. Soc. 68: 1392.
12. Boothe, J. H., Semb, J., Waller, C. W., Angier, R. B., Mowat, J. H., Hutchings, B. L., Stokstad, E. L. R. & SubbaRow, Y., 1949. J. Am. Chem. Soc. 71: 2304–2308.
13. Semb, J., Boothe, J. H., Angier, R. B., Waller, C. W., Mowat, J. H., Hutchings, B. L. & SubbaRow, Y., 1949. J. Am. Chem. Soc. 71: 2310–2315.
14. Bird, O. D., Binkley, S. B., Bloom, E. S., Emmett, A. D. & Pfiffner, J. J., 1945. J. Biol. Chem. 157: 413–414.
15. Gawthorne, J. M. & Smith, R. M., 1973. Biochem. J. 136: 295–301.
16. Whitehead, V. M., 1973. Clin. Res. 21: 571.
17. Lavoie, A., Tripp, E., Parsa, K. & Hoffbrand, A. V., 1975. Clin. Sci. Mol. Med. 48: 67–73.
18. Hoffman, R. M. & Erbe, R. W., 1974. J. Cell Biology 63: 141a.
19. Moran, R. G., Werkheiser, W. C. & Zakrzewski, S. F., 1976. J. Biol. Chem. 251: 3569–3575.
20. Sirotnak, F. M., Donati, G. J. & Hutchison, D. J., 1963. J. Bacteriol. 85: 658–665.
21. Rowe, P. B. & Lewis, G. P., 1973. Biochemistry 12: 1962–1968.
22. Blakley, R. L. & McDougall, B. M., 1961. J. Biol. Chem. 236: 1163–1167.
23. Kisliuk, R. L., Gaumont, Y. & Baugh, C. M., 1974. J. Biol. Chem. 249: 4100–4103.
24. Nath. R. & Greenberg, D. M., 1962. Biochemistry 1: 435–441.
25. Greenberg, D. M., Tam, B.-D., Jenny, E. & Payes, B., 1966. Biochim. Biophys. Acta 122: 423–435.
26. Morales, D. R. & Greenberg, D. M., 1964. Biochim. Biophys. Acta 85: 360–376.
27. Plante, L. T., Crawford, E. J. & Friedkin, M., 1967. J. Biol. Chem. 242: 1466–1476.
28. Coward, J. K., Parameswaran, K. N., Cashmore, A. R. & Bertino, J. R., 1974. Biochemistry 13: 3899–3903.
29. Domin, B. A., Cheng, Y.-C. & Hakala, M. T., 1979. Chemistry & Biology of Pterdinies Eds. Kisliuk, R. L. & Brown, G. M., Elsevier-North Holland, New York, pp. 395–399.
30. Wright, B. E. & Stadtman, T. C., 1956. J. Biol. Chem. 219: 863–871.
31. Wright, B. E., 1956. J. Biol. Chem. 219: 873–883.
32. Large, P. J. & Quayle, J. R., 1963. Biochem. J. 87: 386–396.
33. Uyeda, K. & Rabinowitz, J. C., 1968. Arch. Biochem. Biophys. 123: 271–278.
34. Salem, A. R., Pattison, J. R. & Foster, M. A., 1972. Biochem. J. 126: 993–1004.
35. Salem, A. R. & Foster, M. A., 1972. Biochem. J. 127: 845–853.

36. Blakley, R. L., 1957. Biochem. J. 65: 342–348.

37. Shane, B. & Stokstad, E. L. R., 1977. J. Gen. Microbiol. 103: 261–270.

38. Cheng, F. W., Shane, B., Stokstad, E. L. R., 1975. Can. J. Biochem. 53: 1020–1027.

39. Matthews, R. G. & Baugh, C. M., 1980. Biochemistry 19: 2040–2045.

40. a. Guest, J. R. & Jones, K. M., 1960. Biochem. J. 75: 12p–13p.

40. b. Whitfield, C. D. & Weissbach, H., 1968. Biochem. Biophys. Res. Commun. 33: 996–1003.

41. Guest, J. R., Friedman, S., Dilworth, M. J. & Woods, D. D., 1964. Ann. N.Y. Acad. Sci. 112: 774–790.

42. Jones, K. M., Guest, J. R. & Woods, D. D., 1961. Biochem. J. 79: 566–574.

43. Whitfield, C. D., Steers, E. J., Jr. & Weissbach, H., 1970. J. Biol. Chem. 245: 390–401.

44. Burton, E., Selhub, J. & Sakami, W., 1969. Biochem. J. 111: 793–795.

45. Morningstar, J. F., Jr. & Kisliuk, R. L., 1965. J. Gen. Microbiol. 39: 43–51.

46. Cauthen, S. E., Foster, M. A. & Woods, D. D., 1966. Biochem. J. 98: 630–635.

47. Wang, F. K., Koch, J. & Stokstad, E. L. R., 1967. Biochemische Z. 346: 458–466.

48. Burton, E. G. & Sakami, W., 1969. Biochem. Biophys. Res. Commun. 36: 228–234.

49. Coward, J. K., Chello, P. L., Cashmore, A. R., Parameswaran, K. N., DeAngelis, L. M. & Bertino, J. R., 1975. Biochemistry 14: 1548–1552.

50. Loughlin, R. E., Elford, H. L. & Buchanan, J. M., 1964. J. Biol. Chem. 239: 2888–2895.

51. Uyeda, K. & Rabinowitz, J. C., 1967. J. Biol. Chem. 242: 4378–4385.

52. Yeh, Y.-C. & Greenberg, D. M., 1965. Biochim. Biophys. Acta 105: 279–291.

53. MacKenzie, R. E. & Baugh, C. M., 1980. Biochim. Biophys. Acta 611: 187–195.

54. MacKenzie, R. E., 1973. Biochem. Biophys. Res. Commun. 53: 1088–1095.

55. Paukert, J. L., Straus, L. D. & Rabinowitz, J. C., 1976. J. Biol. Chem. 251: 5104–5111.

56. Himes, R. H. & Rabinowitz, J. C., 1962. J. Biol. Chem. 237: 2903–2914.

57. Curthoys, N. P. & Rabinowitz, J. C., 1972. J. Biol. Chem. 247: 1965–1971.

58. Powers, S. G. & Snell, E. E., 1976. J. Biol. Chem. 251: 3876–3793.

59. a. Jaenicke, L. & Brode, E., 1961. Biochemisches Z. 334: 108–132.

59. b. Brode, E. & Jaenicke, L., 1961. Biochemisches Z. 334: 328–341.

59. c. Jaenicke, L. & Brode, E., 1961. Biochemisches Z. 334: 342–356.

60. Lewis, G. P., Salem, M. E. & Rowe, P. B., 1979. Chemistry and Biology of Pteridines Eds. Kisliuk, R. L. & Brown, G. M., Elsevier-North Holland, New York, pp. 441–442.

61. Kisliuk, R. L., Gaumont, Y., Baugh, C. M., Galivan, J., Maley, F. & Maley, G. F., 1978. Fed. Proc. 37: 1427.

62. Galivan, J. H., Maley, F. & Baugh, C. M., 1976. Biochem. Biophys. Res. Commun. 71: 527–534.

63. Dolnick, B. J. & Cheng, Y.-C., 1978. J. Biol. Chem. 253: 3563–3567.

64. Baggott, J. E. & Krumdieck, C. L., 1979. Biochemistry 18: 1036–1041.

65. Slavik, K., Zizkovsky, V., Slavikova, V. & Fort, P., 1974. Biochem. Biophys. Res. Commun. 59: 1173–1184.

66. Rabinowitz, J. C. & Himes, R. H., 1960. Fed. Proc. 19: 963–970.

67. Uyeda, K. & Rabinowitz, J. C., 1967. J. Biol. Chem. 242: 24–31.

68. Gaertner, F. H., 1978. Trends Biochem. Sci. (March): 63–65.

69. Kirschner, K. & Bisswanger, H., 1976. Annu. Rev. Biochem. 45: 143–166.

70. Delk, A. S., Nagle, D. P., Jr. & Rabinowitz, J. C., 1980. J. Biol. Chem. 255: 4387–4390.

71. Cohen, L. & MacKenzie, R. E., 1978. Biochim. Biophys. Acta 522: 311–317.

72. Shane, B. & Stokstad, E. L. R., 1976. J. Biol. Chem. 251: 3405–3410.

73. Nixon, P. F., Slutsky, G., Nahas, A. & Bertino, J. R., 1973. J. Biol. Chem. 248: 5932–5936.

74. McBurney, M. W. & Whitmore, G. F., 1974. Cell 2: 173–182.

75. Friedkin, M., Plante, L. T., Crawford, E. J. & Crumm, M., 1975. J. Biol. Chem. 250: 5614–5621.

76. Friedkin, M., Crawford, E. J., Donovan, E. & Pastore, E. J., 1962. J. Biol. Chem. 237: 3811–3814.

77. Kisliuk, R. L., Gaumont, Y., Baugh, C. M., Galivan, J., Maley, G. F. & Maley, F., 1979. Chemistry and Biology of Pteridines (Kisliuk, R. L. & Brown, G. M., eds.) Elsevier North Holland, New York, pp. 431–435.

78. Maley, G. F. & Maley, F. & Baugh, C. M., 1979. J. Biol. Chem. 254: 7485–7487.

79. Schirch, L. & Ropp, M., 1967. Biochemistry 6: 253–257.

80. Krumdieck, C. L., Cornwell, P. E., Thompson, R. W. & White, W. E., Jr., 1977. Folic Acid. Biochemistry and Physiology in Relation to the Human Nutrition Requirement. National Academy of Sciences, Washington, D.C., pp. 25–42.

81. Bertino, J. R. & Hillcoat, B. L., 1968. Adv. Enz. Regulation 6: 335–349.

82. Buehring, K. U., Tamura, T. & Stokstad, E. L. R., 1974. J. Biol. Chem. 249: 1081–1089.

83. Shane, B. & Stokstad, E. L. R., 1975. J. Biol. Chem. 250: 2243–2253.

84. Shane, B., 1980. J. Biol. Chem. 255: 5649–5654.

85. Nair, M. G. & Baugh, C. M., 1973. Biochemistry 12: 3923–3927.

86. Nahas, A., Nixon, P. F. & Bertino, J. R., 1972. Cancer Res. 32: 1416–1421.

87. Goldman, I. D., 1971. Ann. N.Y. Acad. Sci. 186: 400–422.

88. Hoffbrand, A. V., Tripp, E., Houlihan, C. M. & Scott, J. M., 1973. Blood 42: 141–146.

89. Galivan, J., 1979. Cancer Res. 39: 735–743.

90. Taylor, R. T. & Hanna, M. L., 1977. Arch. Biochem. Biophys. 181: 331–344.

91. Sirotnak, F. M., Chello, P. L., Piper, J. R. & Montgomery, J. A., 1978. Biochem. Pharm. 27: 1821–1825.

92. a. Tamura, T., Shin, Y.-S., Williams, M. A. & Stokstad, E. L. R., 1972. Anal. Biochem. 49: 517–521.

48

92. b. Baugh, C. M., Stevens, J. C. & Krumdieck, C. L., 1970. Biochim. Biophys. Acta 212: 116–125.
93. Kozloff, L. M., 1980. BioSystems 12: 239–247.
94. Zamierowski, M. M. & Wagner, C., 1977. J. Biol. Chem. 252: 933–938.
95. Wittwer, A. J. & Wagner, C., 1979. Fed. Proc. 38: 393.
96. Wittwer, A. J. & Wagner, C., 1980. Proc. Natl. Acad. Sci. USA 77: 4484–4488.
97. Kallen, R. G. & Jencks, W. P., 1966. J. Biol. Chem. 241: 5851–5863.
98. Piper, W. N. & Tephly, T. R., 1974. Life Sciences 14: 873–876.
99. Piper, W. N. & Van Lier, R. B. L., 1977. Mol. Pharm. 13: 1126–1135.
100. Piper, W. N., Van Lier, R. B. L. & Hardwicke, D. M., 1979. In: Chemistry and Biology of Pteridines (Kisliuk, R. L. & Brown, G. M., eds.) Elsevier-North Holland, New York, pp. 329–334.
101. Galivan, J., Maley, F. & Baugh, C. M., 1977. Arch. Biochem. Biophys. 184: 346–354.
102. Selhub, J., Savin, M. A., Sakami, W. & Flavin, M., 1971. Proc. Nat. Acad. Sci. USA 68: 312–314.
103. Shane, B., 1980. J. Biol. Chem. 255: 5655–5662.
104. McGuire, J. J., Kitamoto, Y., Hsieh, P., Coward, J. K. & Bertino, J. R., 1979. In: Chemistry and Biology of Pteridines (Kisliuk, R. L. & Brown, G. M., eds.) Elsevier-North Holland, New York, pp. 471–476.
105. Richardson, R. E., Healy, M. J. & Nixon, P. F., 1979. Biochim. Biophys. Acta 585: 128–133.
106. Taylor, R. T. & Hanna, M. L., 1979. Arch. Biochem. Biophys. 197: 36–43.
107. McGuire, J. J., Hsieh, P., Coward, J. K. & Bertino, J. R., 1980. J. Biol. Chem. 255: 5776–5788.
108. Ritari, S. J., Sakami, W., Black, C. W. & Rzepka, J., 1973. Neurospora Newsletter 20: 26–27.
109. Ritari, S. J., Sakami, W. & Black, C. W., 1973. Neurospora Newsletter 20: 27.
110. Masurekar, M. & Brown, G. M., 1975. Biochemistry 11: 2424–2430.
111. Griffin, M. J. & Brown, G. M., 1964. J. Biol. Chem. 239: 310–316.
112. Shin, Y.-S., Williams, M. A. & Stokstad, E. L. R., 1972. Biochem. Biophys. Res. Commun. 47: 35–43.
113. Houlihan, C. M. & Scott, J. M., 1972. Biochem. Biophys. Res. Commun. 48: 1675–1681.
114. Leslie, G. I. & Baugh, C. M., 1974. Biochemistry 13: 4957–4961.
115. Kamen, B. A. & Caston, J. D., 1975. J. Biol. Chem. 250: 2203–2205.
116. Shin, Y.-S., Chan, C., Vidal, A. J., Brody, T. & Stokstad, E. L. R., 1976. Biochim. Biophys. Acta 444: 794–801.
117. Fridovich, I., 1974. Life Sciences 14: 819–826.
118. Taylor, R. T., Hanna, M. L., Jones, C. & Kao, F.-T., 1980. Fed. Proc. 39: 655.
119. Ritari, S. J., Sakami, W., Black, C. W. & Rzepka, J., 1975. Anal. Biochem. 63: 118–129.
120. Brody, T., 1976. Federation Proc. 35: 1344.
121. Lewis, G. P. & Rowe, P. B., 1979. Anal. Biochem. 93: 91–97.
122. Baugh, C. M., Braverman, E. B., Nair, M. G., Horne, D. W., Briggs, W. T. & Wagner, C., 1979. Anal. Biochem. 92: 366–369.
123. Evans, H. J. & Sorger, G. J., 1966. Annu. Rev. Plant Physiol. 17: 47–76.
124. Suelter, C. H., 1970. Science 168: 789–795.
125. Himes, R. H. & Harmony, J. A. K., 1973. CRC Crit. Rev. Biochem. 1: 501–535.
126. Sakami, W., Ritari, S. J., Black, C. W. & Rzepka, J., 1973. Fed. Proc. 32: 471.
127. Gawthorne, J. M. & Smith, R. M., 1974. Biochem. J. 142: 119–126.
128. Shane, B., 1980. J. Biol. Chem. 255: 5663–5667.
129. Moran, R. G. & Colman, P. D., 1980. Proc. Am. Assoc. Cancer Res. 21: 25.
130. Brody, T. & Stokstad, E. L. R., 1979. In: Folic Acid in Neurology, Psychiatry, and Internal Medicine (Botez, M. I. & Reynolds, E. H., eds.) Raven Press, New York, pp. 55–62.
131. Spronk, A. M., 1973. Fed. Proc. 32: 471.
132. McGuire, J. J., Hsieh, P., Coward, J. K. & Bertino, J. R., 1980. Fed. Proc. 39: 1699.
133. Shane, B., Brody, T. & Stokstad, E. L. R., 1979. In: Chemistry and Biology of Pteridines (Kisliuk, R. L. & Brown, G. M., eds.) Elsevier-North Holland, New York, pp. 341–346.
134. Bassett, R., Weir, D. & Scott, J., 1976. Biochem. Soc. Trans. 4: 500–502.
135. Caperelli, C. A., Benkovic, P. A., Chettur, G. & Benkovic, S. J., 1980. J. Biol. Chem. 255: 1885–1890.
136. White, J. C., Bailey, B. D. & Goldman, I. D., 1978. J. Biol. Chem. 253: 242–245.
137. Sirotnak, F. M., Chello, P. L., Moccio, D. M., Kisliuk, R. L., Compebine, G., Gaumont, Y. & Montgomery, J. A., 1979. Biochem. Pharm. 28: 2993–2997.
138. Scott, V. F. & Donaldson, K. O., 1964. Biochem. Biophys. Res. Commun. 14: 523–526.
139. Shane, B. & Stokstad, E. L. R., 1977. J. Gen. Microbiol. 103: 249–259.
140. Acharya, S. P. & Hynes, J. B., 1975. J. Heterocycl. Chem. 12: 1283–1286.
141. Rader, J. I. & Huennekens, F. M., 1973. In: The Enzymes (Boyer, P. D., ed.) 3rd edition, v. 9, pp. 197–223.

Revision received December 29, 1980.

δ-Aminolaevulinic acid and amino acid neurotransmitters

M. J. W. Brennan and R. C. Cantrill

Brain Research Group, Dept. of Medical Biochemistry, School of Pathology, University of the Witwatersrand Medical School and South African Institute for Medical Research, Johannesburg 2001, South Africa

Summary

The effects of the porphyrin precursor δ-aminolaevulinic acid (ALA) on γ-aminobutyric acid (GABA) and L-glutamate transmitter systems was investigated in rat brain. It was found that ALA inhibited GABA and glutamate uptake and stimulated basal efflux of the amino acids in purified nerve endings. These effects were evident only at relatively high concentrations of ALA (at least 100 μM). Such concentrations probably do not occur in the nervous systems of patients suffering from acute porphyria. In addition, it was found that ALA inhibited the stimulated release of GABA from nerve endings probably by acting as an agonist at GABA autoreceptors. This effect was found at very low concentrations of ALA (1 μM). It is therefore likely that the neuropsychiatric manifestations of the acute porphyric attack are attributable, to some extent, to reduced GABA release at central synapses.

Introduction

The hereditary hepatic porphyrias, namely acute intermittent porphyria (AIP), porphyria variegata (PV) and hereditary coproporphyria (HC), are a group of diseases involving overproduction of porphyrins, porphyrin precursors or both. In the last 30 years, great advances have been made in understanding the mechanisms of porphyrin synthesis and their control; this has resulted in a good understanding of the genetic defects underlying these diseases (1–4). Acute attacks of the hepatic porphyrias are, however, characteristically accompanied by neuropsychiatric symptoms and signs. These are well documented and large series of case histories have been reported for AIP (5,6), PV (7,8) and HC (9,10). In decreasing order of frequency, there may be motor neuropathy, confusion, psychiatric manifestations, hyperexcitability and epileptic-type seizures. Psychiatric manifestations include depression, anxiety, insomnia and an organic brain syndrome. The aetiology of the neural dysfunction in the acute attack is unknown; several mechanisms have, however, been suggested at a neurochemical level.

1) Neurotoxicity of porphyrin precursors: Excretion of the porphyrin precursors δ-aminolaevulinic acid (ALA) and porphobilinogen (PBG) is increased during acute porphyric attacks. In fact, this is the only gross biochemical abnormality common to all three hereditary hepatic porphyrias. It is possible that these precursors gain access to the nervous system and exert direct neurotoxic effects. Several observations suggest that such an explanation might be plausible. There is good evidence, from the case reports of many patients in acute porphyric episodes, that the onset of neurological symptoms is accompanied by raised excretion of ALA and PBG (11) and there is a rough correlation between the level of precursor excretion and the clinical severity of the attack (12). ALA and PBG can be detected in the cerebrospinal fluid (CSF), where they are not normally present, of patients during acute attacks of porphyria (13,14) and ALA can

Molecular and Cellular Biochemistry 38, 49–58 (1981).   0300-8177/81/0381-0049/$ 2.00.

pass the blood-brain barrier of rats and mice at plasma concentrations known to occur in the acute porphyric attack (15–17). In addition, brain tissue concentrations of ALA remain elevated after blood concentrations have returned to normal (17). Becker *et al.* (18) have shown that brain slices can concentrate ALA through an energy dependent process, and consequently brain tissue levels of ALA might exceed CSF levels. Finally, all effective treatments of the acute attack, high carbohydrate diet (19,20), intravenous haematin infusion (13,21–25) or propranolol administration (26), suppress porphyrin precursor production in these patients and decreased precursor excretion almost always accompanies or precedes clinical improvement (8).

Early studies on the possible neurotoxicity of porphyrin precursors conducted *in vivo* or on isolated organs have been subject to some controversy. Several of these investigations have suggested that ALA is pharmacologically inert (27–30). However, these studies can now be criticised on a number of points. In the experiments on isolated organs, very low levels of porphyrin precursors were tested against limited physiological parameters (27,28). The *in vivo* experiments (29,30) were conducted over a relatively short period of time, the levels of ALA were not measured in the plasma, and neither the uptake into the nervous system nor the rate of clearance by the kidneys was taken into account. In other studies conducted *in vivo,* evidence for neurotoxic effects has been reported. Experiments in which the porphyrinogenic drug allylisopropylacetamide was administered to rats, resulting in increased excretion of ALA, have shown effects such as deep sleep (31), weakness and ataxia involving the hind limbs (32), increased susceptibility to isonicotinyl hydrazide-induced convulsions (33) and acute flaccid paresis in pantothenate deficient rats (34). In addition, recent work in which ALA was administered chronically and acutely to rats and mice (15) or injected directly into the central nervous systems of rats (35) has demonstrated convincing behavioural effects including convulsions.

In addition to these behavioural effects, the mechanism of which is unknown, ALA has been shown to have a wide variety of pharmacological actions *in vitro*. Thus, ALA inhibits transmitter release at the neuromuscular junction (36,37), inhibits ventral and dorsal root responses and depresses dorsal root potentials in the frog spinal cord (38), and depolarises frog muscle fibres (39). These findings might be explicable on the basis of a nonspecific metabolic action of ALA such as inhibition of the $(Na^+ + K^+)$-ATPase (40).

2) Defect in neural haem biosynthesis: The metabolic defects in the hereditary hepatic porphyrias have been demonstrated in tissues other than the liver including erythrocytes (41–43), fibroblasts (44–46), and amniotic cells (44). It is therefore quite possible that defects exist in all tissues, including neurons. This hypothesis is supported by the observation of significant peripheral neuropathy in latent hereditary hepatic porphyria patients, some of whom have never had an acute attack (47). Since very little is known about haem biosynthesis in the central and peripheral nervous systems, the consequences of a postulated defect in the synthetic pathways are largely speculative. The concept of a latent genetic defect in neural tissue is, perhaps, better invoked as an explanation for the degenerative changes seen in the nervous system of the porhyric *post mortem* than as a mechanism for the reversible neuropsychiatric manifestations of the acute attack.

3) Defect in hepatic haemoprotein function: It is conceivable that defective haemoprotein function in the liver could relate to nervous system injury. The precise mechanism of this interaction is ill-defined and the evidence for it tenuous. A major portion of hepatic haem is utilised for the maintenance of microsomal cytochromes (22). The finding that porphyric patients in acute attack show impaired metabolism of salicylamide (48) and antipyrine (49) suggests that there may be a cytochrome P_{450} deficiency in the liver with failure of its oxidising function. The significance of these observations in the aetiology of the neural dysfunction in the acute attack is obscure. In addition, many drugs, such as the barbiturates, induce hepatic cytochrome P_{450} and are also powerful inducers of acute episodes in porphyric patients (50).

4) Toxic metabolites of porphyrin precursors: Patients in acute attacks of porphyria excrete increased amounts of a monopyrrolic compound indistinguishable from kryptopyrrole (2,4-dimethyl-3-ethylpyrrole) (51,52). Kryptopyrrole is structurally related to ALA and PBG although it is not necessarily a metabolite of either. It has been reported in the urine of patients with various types

of psychosis (53,54), although the identification of the compound in these studies is suspect (55). Kryptopyrrole has also been reported to cause increased excretion of porphyrins in experimental animals (52). It is therefore possible that any neurotoxic effects of kryptopyrrole are mediated via an increase in ALA or PBG concentrations in the plasma.

Other metabolites of porphyrin precursors (such as 5-oxo-2-hydroxyPBG) have been detected in experimental animals (56); it is not known whether these are neurotoxic or whether they are excreted by patients in the acute attack.

5) Unrelated mechanisms: The neuropsychiatric manifestations of the acute attack of porphyria might be related only indirectly to the enzymatic defect in haem biosynthesis. Thus it is possible that critical metabolites are depleted or that neurotoxic substances, unrelated to haem precursors, accumulate in acute porphyria. Abnormalities in the metabolism of zinc, pyridoxine, vitamin E and glycine have been postulated (57). Thus far, these cannot be related to the pathophysiology of acute porphyria.

ALA is an omega amino acid with a 5 carbon chain similar in structure to the inhibitory transmitter γ-aminobutyric acid (GABA) and the excitatory amino acid L-glutamate (Fig. 1). It is therefore possible that the neuropsychiatric symptomatology of the acute porphyric attack results from the interaction of ALA with GABAergic or glutamatergic systems in the brain. The work described here represents a systematic investigation of the effects of ALA on the uptake, release and receptor binding of these important amino acid neurotransmitters.

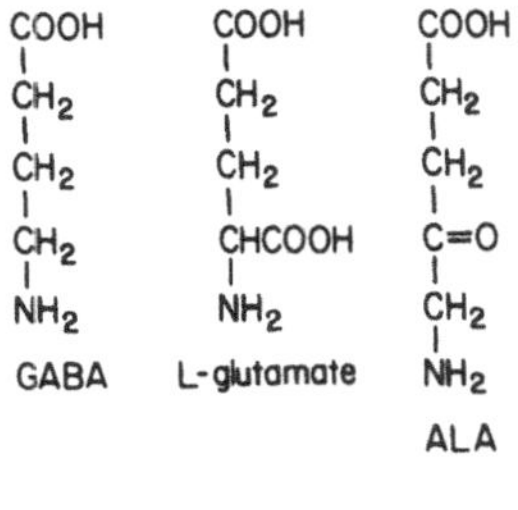

Fig. 1. Structural analogues of GABA and L-glutamate. ALA is an omega amino acid with a 5 carbon chain similar in structure to GABA and glutamate.

Materials and methods

ALA, unlabelled GABA and L-glutamate were supplied by the Sigma Chemical Company, St. Louis, MO. All other chemicals were of Analar reagent grade purchased from commercial sources.

Fresh synaptosomes prepared from the cerebral cortices of adult Wistar rats were resuspended in 0.32 M glucose to give a protein concentration of about 5 mg/ml and diluted 1:10 with ice-cold incubation medium (final concentrations: 128 mM NaCl; 5 mM KCl; 2.7 mM CaCl$_2$; 1.2 mM MgSO$_4$; 10 mM Tris-HCl buffer at pH 7.35). In experiments involving GABA, 0.1 mM aminooxyacetic acid was added to the buffer to prevent GABA catabolism. One ml aliquots of the suspension were preincubated at 37 °C for 15 min in a water bath in an air atmosphere.

Uptake of amino acids by synaptosomes

2,3-^{3}H-GABA, specific activity 54 Ci/mmol; L-U-^{14}C-glutamate, specific activity 290 mCi/mmol; 4-^{14}C-ALA, specific activity 54 mCi/mmol were purchased from the Radiochemical Centre, Amersham. The ^{3}H-GABA was diluted with unlabelled GABA to give a specific activity of 10 Ci/mmol; ^{14}C-glutamate and ^{14}C-ALA were used at the specific activities quoted above. Following the 15 min preincubation, a small volume (1% of the final volume) of a solution containing a known concentration of radiolabelled amino acid was added to the incubation tubes to give a concentration in the tube of 0.5 μM. Addition of unlabelled amino acid gave a final concentration in the range 0.5–50 μM. In experiments examining the effect of ALA on transmitter uptake, ALA was added to the incubation medium and the synaptosomes preincubated in the presence of ALA. Incubation was continued for a further 10 minutes after the addition of the label. Uptake was terminated by rapid filtration through Millipore filters (0.45 μm pore) and the filters washed with 3 ml of medium at 37 °C. Control experiments to account for radioactivity non-specific bound to the filters were carried out. Filters were solubilised in 10 ml of Aquagel I liquid scintillant (Chemlab) and counted in a Packard Tricarb spectrometer at 37% efficiency.

Release of preloaded transmitters

Release of label from the synaptosomes was monitored using a superfusion system previously described (58–60). One ml aliquots of synaptosome suspension preloaded in the presence of 0.5 μM labelled transmitter were layered on Millipore filters (0.45 μm pore) resting on filter supports constituting the bottoms of four parallel superfusion chambers (61) and thermostatically maintained at 37 °C. The chambers were connected to a multichannel peristaltic pump, the excess medium drawn off at maximum flow rate, and the filters washed with 10 ml of control medium (concentrations as described above) containing 30 mM glucose. The flow rate was adjusted to 0.5 ml/min and 1 min fractions collected directly into scintillation counting vials. Superfusion was continued for 10 min to establish a baseline rate of transmitter efflux; the control medium was then exchanged for the test medium and superfusion continued for a further 15 min. Aquagel I, 5 ml, was added to each vial and the radioactivity of the vials counted. Radioactivity remaining on the filters was counted in the same way. Stimulation of transmitter release was calculated as the percentage increase in efflux over the baseline unstimulated level.

GABA receptor binding

The sodium-independent binding of ^{3}H-GABA to rat cortical membranes was studied at 4 °C by the method of Enna & Snyder (62). Adult Wistar rats were decapitated and the cortices rapidly homogenised in 15 volumes of ice-cold 0.32 M sucrose. The homogenate was centrifuged at 1000 g for 10 min, the pellet discarded, and the supernatant centrifuged at 20 000 g for 20 min. A suspension of the crude mitochondrial pellet in distilled water was dispersed with a Brinkmann Polytron PT-10 (setting 6) for 30 s and centrifuged at 8000 g for 20 min. The supernatant fluid was collected, and the pellet, a bilayer with a soft, buffy coat, was rinsed carefully with the supernatant fluid to collect the upper layer. This suspension was centrifuged at 48 000 g for 20 min, and washed once in distilled water. The membranes were stored at –20 °C for at least 18 h. For the GABA binding assay, frozen pellets were resuspended in water, maintained at 25 °C for 20 min, and centrifuged at 48 000 g for 10

min. Aliquots of these membranes (0.8–1.2 mg protein) were incubated in quadruplicate at 4 °C for 5 min in 2 ml of 0.05 M Tris-citrate buffer (pH 7.1) containing ^{3}H-GABA (specific activity 54 Ci/mmol, Amersham) alone or in the presence of 1 mM unlabelled GABA or ALA at various concentrations. After incubation, the tubes were centrifuged at 48 000 g for 10 min, the fluid decanted, and the pellets rinsed superficially with two 5 ml aliquots of ice-cold distilled water. Bound radioactivity was extracted into 1.5 ml Protosol (New England Nuclear), 10 ml Aquagel I added, and radioactivity counted. Total specific ^{3}HGABA binding was obtained by subtracting from the total bound radioactivity the amount not displaced by 1 mM unlabelled GABA. In some experiments membranes were separated from the incubation medium by filtration through Whatman GF/C glass fiber filters. Filters were washed with two 3 ml aliquots of buffer, disintegrated by vigorous shaking in 10 ml Aquagel I, and counted for radioactivity. This latter procedure was adopted in an attempt to select for high affinity GABA binding sites in the membrane preparation.

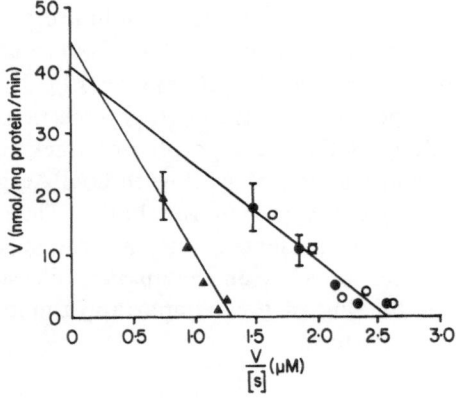

Fig. 2. Kinetic analysis of the uptake of labelled GABA into rat cerebral synaptosomes. The uptake was measured as described in Materials and methods after a 10 minute incubation with varying concentrations of ^{3}H-GABA. In experiments examining the effect of ALA on the uptake of ^{3}H-GABA, synaptosomes were preincubated in the presence of ALA for 15 min before addition of 0.5 μM ^{3}H-GABA. In this Eadie-Hofstee plot, the uptake rate (v) is plotted as a function of the uptake rate over the GABA concentration (v/s). Each point is the mean of at least 8 experiments, and the lines represent the best fit to the data by the method of least squares. Standard error bars are shown where these are greater than the size of the points.

Key: ●—●, control medium; ○—○, 0.15 mM ALA; ▲—▲, 0.75 mM ALA.

Experimental and discussion

Kinetics of ³H-GABA uptake and effect of ALA

The uptake of GABA into the synaptosome fraction was measured over a range of concentrations from 0.5–50 μM. There is considerable disparity in the values of the apparent Km for high

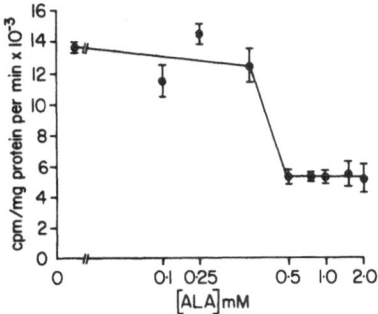

Fig. 3. Effect of eight increasing concentrations of ALA on ³H-GABA uptake into the synaptosome fraction of rat cerebral cortex. Uptake was measured as described in Materials and methods following preincubation in the presence of ALA. The points are means ± S.E.M. of 4 independent experiments.

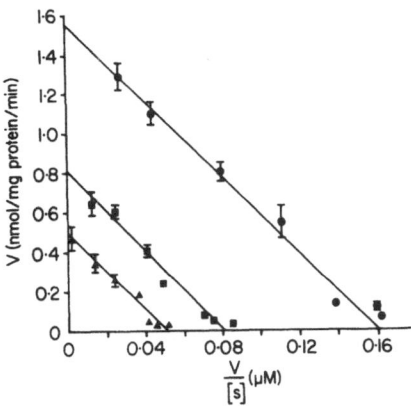

Fig. 4. Kinetic analysis of the uptake of labelled L-glutamate into rat cerebral synaptosomes. The uptake was measured using a rapid Millipore filtration technique after 10 minutes incubation with varying concentrations of ¹⁴C-glutamate. In experiments examining the effect of ALA on uptake of ¹⁴C-glutamate, synaptosomes were preincubated in the presence of ALA for 15 min before addition of 0.5 μM ¹⁴C-glutamate. In this Eadie-Hofstee plot, the uptake rate (v) is plotted as a function of the uptake rate over the glutamate concentration (v/s). Each point is the mean of at least 8 experiments, and the lines represent the best fit to the data by the method of least squares. Standard error bars are shown where these are greater than the size of the points.
Key: ●—●, control medium; ■—■, 0.15 mM ALA; ▲—▲, 0.75 mM ALA.

affinity GABA uptake reported for various GABA transport systems. Values reported for transport in rat cerebral cortex slices and cerebral homogenates are 24 μM and 19 μM respectively (63), those for transport in rat brain synaptosomes include 0.42 μM (64), 4 μM (65), 19 μM (66) and 3.9 μM (67). The apparent Km of 16.5 μM calculated from the data shown in the Eadie-Hofstee plot (Fig. 2) is thus within the range of reported values for the synaptosomal high affinity GABA transport mechanism.

Preincubation of synaptosomes in the presence of low concentrations of ALA (0.05–0.25 mM) had no appreciable effect on ³H-GABA uptake (Fig. 3). Concentrations in the range of 0.5–2.0 mM, however, markedly inhibited ³H-GABA accumulation by the nerve endings. The inhibition was maximal at 0.5 mM (63%) and a further increase in ALA concentration up to 2 mM was unable to effect greater inhibition. A double reciprocal plot of the data shown in Fig. 2 (68) indicated that, at an ALA concentration of 0.75 mM, the inhibition was of a linear competitive mode. The Eadie-Hofstee plot (Fig. 2) showed near competitive inhibition and yielded a Ki for ALA of 467.5 μM.

Kinetics of ¹⁴C-glutamate uptake and effect of ALA

Accumulation of glutamate by the synaptosomes was measured over a concentration range of 0.5–50 μM. An apparent Km of 9.8 μM was

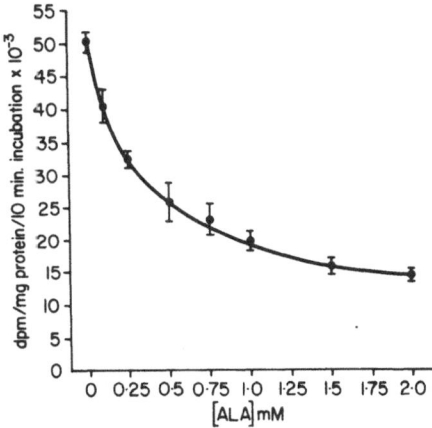

Fig. 5. Effect of seven increasing concentrations of ALA on ¹⁴C-glutamate uptake into the synaptosome fraction of rat cerebral cortex. Uptake was measured as described in Materials and methods following preincubation in the presence of ALA. The points are means ± S.E.M. of 4 independent experiments.

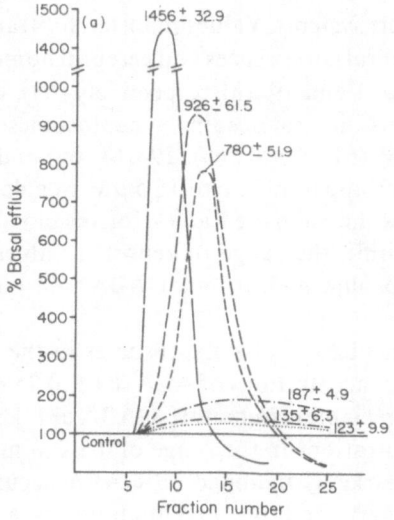

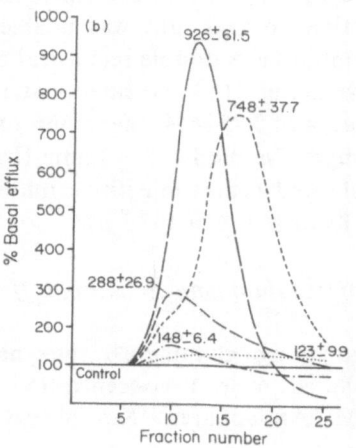

Fig. 6a-b. A plot of percentage change in efflux of ³H-GABA from preloaded synaptosomes (baseline efflux = 100%) against fraction number. The arrow represents the changeover from control medium to the test medium containing in a: —, control; ---, 0.75 mM ALA; · · ·, 0.1 mM ALA; — —, 1.0 mM ALA; -·-·, 0.25 mM ALA; - - -, 5.0 mM ALA; —·—·, 0.5 mM ALA; and in b: —, control; ---, 55 mM K⁺; . . ., 0.1 mM ALA; ·-△-, 0.1 mM ALA and 55 mM K⁺; — —, 1.0 mM ALA; - -, 1.0 mM ALA and 55 mM K⁺. The first few fractions were very variable in each case and are not shown. Each curve is an average of 3 experiments, and the figures are the maximum stimulation (mean ± S.E.M. of 3 experiments) elicited by the test medium. Superfusion rate was 0.5 ml/min and 1 min fractions were collected. The curve passes through every experimental point; however, these have not been shown for reasons of clarity.

calculated from the data shown in the Eadie-Hofstee plot (Fig. 4). There is, again, some disparity in the Km values reported for glutamate transport in various nerve tissue preparations. Levi & Raiteri (69) obtained only a low affinity component (Km = 0.4 mM) for uptake into brain slices from adult rats, but observed a high affinity uptake process (Km = 31 μM) in 'mini-slices' or prisms. A Km value of 20 μM has been reported for glutamate uptake into rat brain cortex slices (70) and one of 29.8 μM for uptake into the crude synaptosome fraction rat cortex (71).

The effect of ALA on ¹⁴C-glutamate accumulation was examined over a range of concentrations up to 2.0 mM (Fig. 5). Preincubation of synaptosomes in the presence of ALA markedly inhibited subsequent uptake of ¹⁴C-glutamate, and the inhibition was maximal at an ALA concentration of 2.0 mM. Kinetic analysis (Fig. 4) showed that the inhibition was of a noncompetitive type. There is a discrepancy in the values of the inhibition constant calculated from the data of Fig. 4. At an ALA concentration of 0.15 mM, a Ki of 170 μM was obtained, while at an ALA concentration of 0.75 mM a value of 350 μM was calculated. The reasons for this difference are not clear.

Stimulation of basal ³H-GABA efflux by ALA: effect of ALA on K⁺-induced release: High concentrations of ALA (0.75–5.0 mM) in the superfusion medium produced very marked stimulation of ³H-GABA efflux (Fig. 6a). The maximum stimulation of GABA efflux obtained by homoexchange with unlabelled GABA is 705 ± 60% (mean ± S.E.M. of 3 experiments) at a concentration of 1 mM GABA (58). Thus the stimulation produced by ALA is greater than can be accounted for by an exchange mechanism.

Membrane depolarisation induced by 55 mM K⁺ in the superfusion medium stimulated ³H-GABA release by about 200% (Fig. 6b). ALA reduced this K⁺-stimulated release of GABA in a dose-dependent fashion (Fig. 7). The reduction was significant at an ALA concentration of 1 μM, and, at a concentration of 100 μM, 75% of the stimulated release was abolished. The concentration of ALA which inhibited 50% of the K⁺-stimulated release was approximately 10 μM. In all cases the reduction was prevented by the GABA receptor antagonists bicuculline or picrotoxin (1 μM) (Table 1). ALA at 1 μM or 10 μM exhibited no effects on the

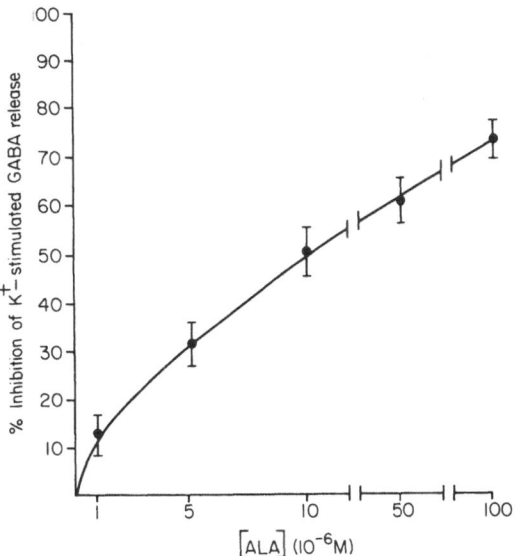

Fig. 7. A dose-response curve for the inhibition of K$^+$-induced GABA release by ALA. The horizontal axis gives concentration of ALA ($\times 10^{-6}$ M) on a logarithmic scale. Represented on the vertical axis is the % inhibition of K$^+$-stimulated (55 mM) GABA release. Each point is the mean % inhibition ± S.E.M. (n = 4). The curve is the best fit to the data by the method of least squares (r^2 = 0.97).

Table 1. Drug effect on the K$^+$-stimulated release of GABA from preloaded synaptosomes.

Drug present	Induced release (% increase over baseline control)	Mean drug effect on induced release
55 mM K$^+$ alone (6)	188 ± 26.9*	
10^{-4} M ALA alone (4)	23 ± 9.9	
55 mM K$^+$ + 10^{-4} M ALA (4)	48 ± 6.4**	−74.5%
55 mM K$^+$ + 10^{-4} M ALA + 10^{-6} M bicuculline (4)	191 ± 13.2	+1.6%
55 mM K$^+$ + 10^{-5} M ALA (4)	92 ± 13.5**	−51.1%
55 mM K$^+$ + 10^{-5} M ALA + 10^{-6} M picrotoxin (4)	187 ± 10.2	−0.5%
55 mM K$^+$ + 10^{-6} M ALA (4)	163 ± 7.5***	−13.0%
55 mM K$^+$ + 10^{-6} M ALA + 10^{-6} M bicuculline (4)	197 ± 13.1	+4.8%

Experiments were carried out as described in Materials and methods. The values in parentheses indicate the number of times the experimental conditions in the first column were repeated. Baseline efflux was calculated as % total tissue stores released per fraction (0.57 ± 0.068%, n = 7). The second column refers to the % increase in efflux over this control baseline level; in each case the mean ± S.E.M. is given. Statistical significance was calculated using the two-sided Student t-test. The third column represents the average drug-induced change compared with the release caused by 55 mM K$^+$ alone. ALA at concentrations $<10^{-4}$ M had no effect on the basal release of radioactivity from the synaptosomes. Bicuculline and picrotoxin alone (10^{-6} M or 10^{-5} M) did not facilitate the release of GABA, presumably because the flow of superfusion fluid removed any GABA as it was released. In the absence of negative feedback effects to antagonise, the GABA antagonists had no effect on release.

* Substitution of Mg$^+$ for Ca$^+$ in the medium did not significantly affect basal release of radioactivity, although 76 ± 2.2% (n = 4) of the K$^+$ (55 mM)-induced release was Ca^{2+} dependent.
** P < 0.001, significant difference from 55 mM K$^+$ alone.
*** P < 0.05, significant difference from 55 mM K$^+$ alone.

basal release of GABA. Neither bicuculline nor picrotoxin alone (1 μM or 10 μM) modified the basal release of radioactivity from the nerve endings.

Recently there has been strong evidence that the release of GABA is subject to negative feedback control through presynaptic receptors on GABA-ergic terminals (72–75). The demonstration that ALA reduces the stimulated release of GABA and that the reduction is prevented by specific receptor antagonists suggests that ALA is an agonist at GABA autoreceptors. Indeed, it seems to be a fairly potent agonist, inhibiting 50% of the stimulated release at a concentration of 10 μM.

Stimulation of basal ^{14}C-glutamate efflux by ALA

High concentrations of ALA (0.75–5.0 mM) produced significant stimulation of ^{14}C-glutamate efflux from preloaded synaptosomes (Fig. 8). No stimulation of efflux was obtained at ALA concentrations of 0.5 mM or lower.

Membrane depolarisation with 55 mM K$^+$ stimulated glutamate release by 105 ± 4% (n = 3) (Fig. 8). ALA at concentrations up to 1 mM did not significantly affect the stimulated release of glutamate. This contrasts with the reduction in K$^+$-stimulated release of GABA produced by low concentrations of ALA.

Uptake of ^{14}C-ALA by synaptosomes

Synaptosomes were incubated in the presence of a range of concentrations of ^{14}C-ALA (0.5–50 μM) for a range of time periods (10–30 min). There was no detectable accumulation of radioactivity by the synaptosomes when compared to control experiments accounting for nonspecific binding to the Millipore filters. There is evidence that ALA can be

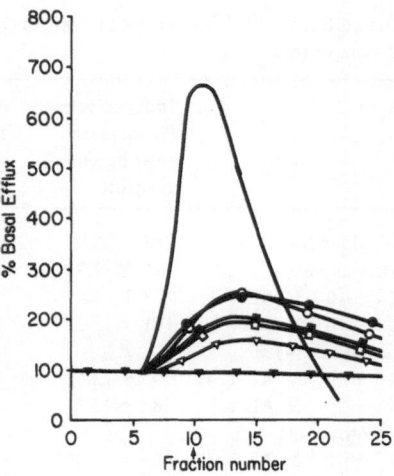

Fig. 8. Stimulation of ¹⁴C-glutamate efflux from preloaded synaptosomes. Shown is the percentage change in efflux (baseline efflux = 100%) against fraction number. The arrow represents the changeover from control medium to the test medium containing: v—v, control medium; v—v, 0.75 mM ALA; ●—●, 1.0 mM ALA; —, 5.0 mM ALA; ■—■, 55 mM K⁺; □—□, 55 mM K⁺ and 0.1 mM ALA; O—O, 55 mM K⁺ and 1.0 mM ALA. The first few fractions were very variable in each case and are not shown. Each curve is an average of 3 superfusion experiments. Variation between individual curves was less than 10% of the mean.

concentrated by brain slices through an energy dependent process (18). Such uptake is probably into a compartment other than the nerve ending.

Effect of ALA on GABA receptor binding

Using the standard GABA receptor binding technique of Enna & Snyder (62), ALA displaced ³H-GABA from its high affinity receptor site with an inhibition constant of about 300 μM. This value does not correlate with the IC₅₀ of 10 μM for ALA in reducing stimulated GABA release. It is therefore possible that ALA binds selectively to the autoreceptors which do not constitute a significant proportion of the sites labelled using the standard centrifugation technique.

Using a filtration technique a single class of GABA receptors having a very high affinity was uncovered. The Ki for ALA in displacing binding to these receptors was 7.5 μM. This correlates well with the potency of ALA in inhibiting GABA release. It is therefore possible that ALA is a selective agonist at the autoreceptors and that these can be assayed by a modification in the binding procedure.

ALA has been shown to inhibit the $(Na^+ + K^+)$-ATPase isolated from red blood cells and from rabbit brain (40). Inhibition of the synaptosomal $(Na^+ + K^+)$-ATPase by 100 μM ouabain produces approximately 100% stimulation of GABA efflux (76); consequently it is not possible that the large stimulation of efflux of GABA and glutamate elicited by ALA is due solely to inhibition of the APTase. Considering the nonspecific action of ALA on the basal efflux of GABA and glutamate, it is likely that this effect is mediated by some as yet undefined toxic action of the compound. Inhibition of the ATPase is known to reduce the ion linked uptake of a number of neurotransmitters. It is therefore possible that this action explains the inhibition of GABA and glutamate transport caused by ALA.

The effects of ALA on uptake and basal efflux of the amino acid transmitters is evident only at relatively high concentrations of ALA. It is very unlikely that such concentrations are reached in the brain during the acute porphyric attack (35). Nevertheless, it has been demonstrated that ALA can penetrate the blood-brain barrier of the rat at plasma concentrations known to occur in AIP and appear in the CSF in micromolar concentrations (16). In addition, CSF levels of 16–20 μM have been recorded in patients during acute attacks characterised by hyperexcitability and convulsions (14). Our findings strongly support a direct mechanism whereby ALA acts to inhibit GABA release from inhibitory nerve endings. This effect is evident *in vitro* at concentrations as low as and lower than those already recorded in the central nervous system during acute porphyric episodes.

Acknowledgement

This work was supported in part by grants from the South African Medical Research Council and the Atomic Energy Board of South Africa.

References

1. Bloomer, J. R., 1976. Gastroenterology 71: 689–701.
2. Elder, G. H., Gray, C. H. & Nicholson, D. C., 1972. J. Clin. Pathol. 25: 1013–1033.
3. Pimstone, N., 1975. Mod. Trends Gastroenterology 5: 375–381.

4. Tschudy, D. P., Valsamis, M. & Magnussen, C. R., 1975. Ann. Intern. Med. 83: 851–864.

5. Goldberg, A., 1959. Q. J. Med. 28: 183–209.

6. Stein, J. A. & Tschudy, D. P., 1970. Medicine 49: 1–16.

7. Dean, G., 1971. The Porphyrias; A story of inheritance and environment, Pitman, London.

8. Eales, L., 1963. S. Afr. J. Lab. Clin. Med. 9: 151–162.

9. Goldberg, A., Rimington, C. & Lockhead, A., 1967. Lancet i: 623–636.

10. McIntyre, N., Pearson, A. J. G., Allan, D. J., Craske, S., West, G. M. I., Moore, M. R., Beattie, A. D., Paxton, J. & Goldberg, A., 1971. Lancet i: 560–564.

11. Becker, D. M., 1972. PhD thesis, University of the Witwatersrand, Johannesburg.

12. Ackner, B., Cooper, J. E., Gray, C. H., Kelley, M. & Nicholson, D. C., 1961. Lancet i: 1256–1260.

13. Bonkowsky, H. L., Tschudy, D. P., Collins, A., Doherty, J., Bossenmaier, I., Cardinal, R. & Watson, C. J., 1971. Proc. Natl. Acad. Sci. U.S.A. 68: 2725–2729.

14. Sweeney, V. P., Pathak, M. A. & Asbury, A. K., 1970. Brain 93: 369–380.

15. McGillion, F. B., Moore, M. R. & Goldberg, A., 1973. Scot. Med. J. 18: 133.

16. McGillion, F. B., Thompson, G. G., Moore, M. R. & Goldberg, A., 1974. Biochem. Pharmacol. 23: 472–474.

17. McGillion, F. B., Thompson, G. G. & Goldberg, A., 1975. Biochem. Pharmacol. 24: 299–301.

18. Becker, D. M., Kramer, S. & Viljoen, J. D., 1974. J. Neurochem. 23: 1019–1023.

19. Welland, F. H., Hellman, E. S., Gaddis, E. M., Collins, A., Hunter, G. W. & Tschudy, D. P., 1964. Metabolism 13: 232–250.

20. Bonkowsky, H. L., Magnussen, C. R., Collins, A. R., Doherty, J. M., Hess, R. A. & Tschudy, D. P., 1976. Metabolism 25: 405–414.

21. Watson, C. J., Dhar, G. J., Bossenmaier, I., Cardinal, R. & Petryka, Z. J., 1973. Ann. Intern. Med. 79: 80–83.

22. Watson, C. J., 1975. New Engl. J. Med. 293: 605–607.

23. Dhar, G. J., Bossenmaier, I., Petryka, Z. J., Cardinal, R. & Watson, C. J., 1975. Ann. Intern. Med. 83: 20–30.

24. Petersen, A., Bossenmaier, I., Cardinal, R. & Watson, C. J., 1976. J. Am. Med. Ass. 235: 520–522.

25. Watson, C. J., Pierach, C. A., Bossenmaier, I. & Cardinal, R., 1977. Proc. Natl. Acad. Sci. U.S.A. 74: 2118–2120.

26. Blum, I. & Atsmon, A., 1976. S. Afr. Med. J. 50: 898–899.

27. Goldberg, A., Paton, W. D. M. & Thompson, J. W., 1954. Br. J. Pharmacol. 9: 91–94.

28. Jarrett, A., Rimington, C. & Willoughby, D. A., 1956. Lancet i: 125–127.

29. Marcus, R. J., Wetterberg, L. Yuwiler, A. & Winters, W. D., 1970. Electroencephalogr. Clin. Neurophysiol. 29: 602–607.

30. Shanley, B. C., Taljaard, J. J. F., Deppe, W. M. & Joubert, S. M., 1972. S. Afr. Med. J. 46: 84.

31. Biempica, L., Kosower, V. & Novikoff, A., 1967. Lab. Invest. 17: 171–189.

32. Yuwiler, A., Wetterberg, L. & Geller, E., 1970. Biochem. Pharmacol. 19: 189–195.

33. Kosower, N. & Rock, R. A., 1968. Nature 217: 565–567.

34. DeMatteis, F. & Rimington, C., 1962. Lancet i: 1332–1334.

35. Shanley, B. C., Neethling, A. C., Percy, V. A. & Carstens, H., 1975. S. Afr. Med. J. 49: 576–580.

36. Feldman, D. S., Levere, R. D. & Lieberman, J. S., 1968. J. Clin. Invest. 47: 33A.

37. Feldman, D. S., Levere, R. D., Lieberman, J. S., Cardinal, R. A. & Watson, C. J., 1971. Proc. Natl. Acad. Sci. U.S.A. 68: 383–386.

38. Loots, J. M., Becker, D. M., Meyer, B. J., Goldstuck, N. & Kramer, S., 1975. J. Neural Transm. 36: 71–81.

39. Becker, D. M., Goldstuck, N. & Kramer, S., 1975. S. Afr. Med. J. 49: 1790–1792.

40. Becker, D. M., Viljoen, J. D. & Kramer, S., 1971. Biochim. Biophys. Acta 225: 26–34.

41. Strand, L. J., Meyer, U. A., Felsher, B. F., Redeker, A. G. & Marver, H. S., 1972. J. Clin. Invest. 51: 2530–2536.

42. Sassa, S., Granick, S., Bickers, D. R., Bradlow, H. L. & Kappas, A., 1974. Proc. Natl. Acad. Sci. U.S.A. 71: 732–736.

43. Magnussen, C. R., Levine, J. B., Doherty, J. M., Cheeseman, J. O. & Tschudy, D. P., 1974. Blood 44: 857–868.

44. Sassa, S., Solish, G., Levere, R. D. & Kappas, A., 1975. J. Exp. Med. 142: 722–731.

45. Bonkowsky, H. L., Tschudy, D. P., Weinbach, E. C., Ebert, P. S. & Doherty, J. M., J. Lab. Clin. Med. 85: 93–102.

46. Bickers, D. R., Keogh, L., Rifkind, A. B., Harber, L. C. & Kappas, A., 1977. J. Invest. Derm. 68: 5–9.

47. Mustajoki, P. & Seppalainen, A. M., 1975. Br. Med. J. 2: 310–312.

48. Song, C. S., Bonkowsky, H. L. & Tschudy, D. P., 1974. Clin. Pharmac. Ther. 15: 431–435.

49. Anderson, K. E., Alvares, A. P., Sassa, S. & Kappas, A., 1976. Clin. Pharmac. Ther. 19: 47–54.

50. Meyer, U. A., 1976. Progress in liver diseases (Popper, H. and Schaffner, F., eds.), pp. 280–293, Grune & Stratton, New York.

51. Irvine, D. G. & Wetterberg, L., 1972. Lancet ii: 1201.

52. Brodie, M. J., Graham, D. J. M., Thompson, G. G., Moore, M. R. & Goldberg, A., 1976. Clin. Sci. Molec. Med. 50: 431–434.

53. Irvine, D. G., Bayne, W. & Miyashita, H., 1969. Nature 224: 811–813.

54. Sohler, A., Beck, R. & Noval, J. J., 1970. Nature 228: 1318–1320.

55. Jacobson, S. J., Rapport, H. & Ellman, G. L., 1975. Biol. Psychiat. 10: 91–93.

56. Frydman, R. B., Tomaro, M. L., Frydman, B. & Wanschelbaum, A., 1975. FEBS Lett. 51: 206–210.

57. Meyer, U. A. & Schmid, R., 1974. Brain dysfunction in metabolic disorders (Plum, F., ed.) Res. Publ. Assoc. Nerv. Ment. Dis. 53: 211–223, Raven Press, New York.

58. Brennan, M. J. W. & Cantrill, R. C., 1978. J. Neurochem. 31: 1339–1341.

59. Brennan, M. J. W. & Cantrill, R. C., 1979. J. Neurochem. 32: 1781–1786.

60. Brennan. M. J. W. & Cantrill, R. C., 1979. J. Neurochem. 33: 721–725.

61. Cantrill, R. C. & Brennan, M. J. W., 1980. Experientia 36: 141–142.

62. Enna, S. J. & Snyder, S. H., 1975. Brain Res. 100: 81–97.

63. Iversen, L. L. & Johnston, G. A. R., 1971. J. Neurochem. 18: 1939–1950.

58

64. Henn, F. & Hamberger, A., 1971. Proc. Natl. Acad. Sci. U.S.A. 68: 2686–2690.
65. Martin, D. L., 1973. J. Neurochem. 21: 345–356.
66. Somoza, E., Pugnaire, M. P., Munoz, L. M., Portal, C. G., Ibanez, A. E. & DeFeudis, F. V., 1977. J. Neurochem. 28: 1197–2000.
67. Hitzemann, R. J. & Loh, H. H., 1978. J. Neurochem. 30: 471–477.
68. Brennan, M. J. W. & Cantrill, R. C., 1979. S. Afr. J. Sci. 75: 126–129.
69. Levi, G. & Raiteri, M., 1973. Life Sci. 12: 81–88.
70. Balcar, V. J. & Johnston, G. A. R., 1972. J. Neurobiol. 3: 295–301.

71. Takagaki, G., 1978. J. Neurochem. 30: 47–56.
72. Snodgrass, S. R., 1978. Nature 273: 392–394.
73. Mitchell, P. R. & Martin, I. L., 1978. Nature 274: 904–905.
74. Brennan, M. J. W., Cantrill, R. C. & Epstein, H., 1979. 4th Natl. Congr. S. Afr. Biochem. Soc. 102.
75. Brennan, M. J. W. & Cantrill, R. C., 1979. Nature 280: 514–515.
76. Raiteri, M., Federico, R., Coletti, A. & Levi, G., 1975. J. Neurochem. 24: 1243–1250.

Reprint requests to M. J. W. Brennan.

Received August 6, 1980.

γ-Glutamylamine cyclotransferase

An enzyme involved in the catabolism of ε-(γ-glutamyl)lysine and other γ-glutamylamines

Mary Lynn Fink and J. E. Folk
Laboratory of Biochemistry, National Institute of Dental Research, National Institutes of Health, Bethesda, MD 20205, U.S.A.

Summary

γ-Glutamylamine cyclotransferase, an enzyme found in a number of animal tissues and cells, catalyzes the conversion of ε-(L-γ-glutamyl)-L-lysine to free lysine and 5-oxo-L-proline as well as the release of free amines and the formation of 5-oxo-L-proline from a variety of other L-γ-glutamylamines. Among its substrates are both the mono- and di-γ-glutamyl derivatives of putrescine, spermidine and spermine, and a derivative of ε-(L-γ-glutamyl)-L-lysine in which both the α-amino group and the carboxyl group of the lysine moiety are blocked. The enzyme does not act on most γ-glutamyl-α-amino acids, nor is it active toward the ε-lysyl derivatives of L-aspartic acid or D-glutamic acid. Derivatives of ε-(L-γ-glutamyl)-L-lysine in which the α-amino or the α-carboxyl function of the glutamyl moiety is blocked also do not serve as substrates. The specificity of γ-glutamylamine cyclotransferase is in accordance with the proposal that it functions biologically in the latter stages of the catabolism of products of the action of transglutaminases. Some suggestions as to the manner in which γ-glutamylamine cyclotransferase serves this function are made based on present knowledge of protein degradation.

I. Introduction

γ-Glutamylamine cyclotransferase catalyzes the release of free amines from γ-L-glutamylamines with the concomitant cyclization of the glutamic acid moiety to 5-oxo-L-proline (synonyms: pyroglutamic acid, 5-pyrrolidone-2-carboxylic acid) in accordance with the following reaction:

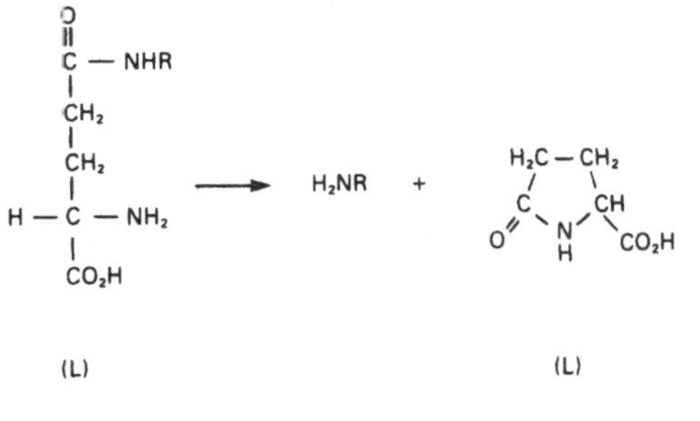

The recent discovery of this enzyme (1) was a consequence of our ongoing interest in the metabolic fate of ε-(γ-glutamyl)lysine crosslinks and of other protein-bound γ-glutamylamine products of transglutaminase action. Stimulus was supplied by the known resistence of the crosslink to digestion by proteases (2, 3) together with reports that the isopeptide, ε-(γ-glutamyl)lysine, can sustain the growth of rats and chicks on lysine-deficient diets (4, 5). These reports suggested the presence of an activity capable of releasing lysine from ε-(γ-glutamyl)lysine and a search for the enzyme responsible for the disassembly of this dipeptide was undertaken. The finding of the widely distributed enzyme, γ-glutamylamine cyclotransferase, which catalyzes not only the breakdown of ε-(γ-glutamyl)lysine, but that of a variety of other γ-glutamylamines provides evidence for a catabolic pathway for products of the transglutaminase reaction.

Molecular and Cellular Biochemistry 38, 59–67 (1981).   0300–8177/81/0381–0059/$ 1.80.

II. The ε-(γ-glutamyl)lysine crosslink and polypeptide γ-glutamylamine conjugates: products of the transglutaminase reaction

Covalent crosslinking through ε-(γ-glutamyl)lysine bonds is essential to the functional or structural integrity of a number of mammalian proteins (for review, see ref. 6). Among these are fibrin, coagulated seminal vesicular proteins and various keratins. Identification of the isopeptide, ε-(γ-glutamyl)lysine, after exhaustive proteolytic digestion of various tissues, cells and whole organisms provides evidence for crosslinking, albeit in many cases the proteins involved have not been identified (7–11). Similar evidence for γ-glutamylpolyamine conjugates in both cells and extracellular fluid has been obtained (12).

ε-(γ-Glutamyl)lysine crosslinks and other monosubstituted γ-amides of peptide-bound glutamic acid are formed by the catalytic action of members of a widely distributed group of enzymes called transglutaminases. Several reviews covering the properties and distribution of the various enzymes have appeared (6, 13, 14). The transglutaminase reaction (reaction 2) occurs by way of a Ca^{2+}-

$$-GLU-\overset{\displaystyle\ulcorner NH_2}{} \quad + \quad H_2NR \quad \longrightarrow \quad -GLU-\overset{\displaystyle\ulcorner NHR}{} \quad + \quad NH_3 \qquad (2)$$

dependent acyl transfer mechanism in which carboxamide groups of peptide-bound glutamine residues serve as acyl donors and in which amino groups in a wide variety of primary amines can act as acyl acceptors. Included are many alkyl amines such as methylamine and ethylamine (15–17) aromatic amines such as phenethylamine (15) diamines (15, 18) the polyamines, spermine and spermidine (12, 15, 18) and the biogenic amine, histamine (15). The fluorescent amine, monodansylcadaverine (N-(5-aminopentyl)-5-dimethylaminoaphthalene-1-sulfonamide) is an especially sensitive acceptor substrate for transglutaminases and possesses the additional property of being easily detectable (19). Several amino acid esters and amides serve as acceptor substrates (15, 20); free amino acids do not (15). The product of amine incorporation in each case is a peptide-bound γ-glutamylamine (-Glu-NHR in reaction 2). Participation of ε-amino groups of peptide-bound lysine

residues as acyl acceptors, leads to formation of ε-(γ-glutamyl)lysine crosslinks (reaction 3). Cross-

$$-GLU-\overset{\displaystyle\ulcorner NH_2}{} \quad + \quad -LYS- \quad \longrightarrow \quad \overset{\displaystyle -LYS-}{\underset{\displaystyle -GLU-}{\displaystyle |}} \quad + \quad NH_3 \qquad (3)$$

linking can also occur as a result of diamine or polyamine incorporation (reaction 4) (12, 18). In

$$2-GLU-\overset{\displaystyle\ulcorner NH_2}{} \quad + \quad H_2N-R-NH_2 \quad \longrightarrow \quad -GLU-\overset{\displaystyle\ulcorner NH-R-NH\urcorner}{}-GLU- \quad (4)$$
$$+ \ 2NH_3$$

this type of crosslinking the amine forms a bridge between two peptide-bound glutamine residues.

Systematic studies carried out to examine the amine specificity of transglutaminases reveal a preference of the enzyme for amines possessing a methylene chain equal in length to that of the sidechain of a lysine residue (21). Evidence for an extended amine binding site and a stereopreference for L-lysine has been obtained by the use of lysine peptide derivatives (21, 22)[a].

In contrast to the broad specificity of transglutaminases toward acceptor substrates, these enzymes act solely on peptide-bound glutamine residues; peptide-bound asparagine residues do not serve as substrates (20, 26, 27).

III. γ-Glutamylamine cyclotransferase

A. Discovery and isolation

Despite an accumulation of information on the production and distribution of ε-(γ-glutamyl)lysine crosslinks and protein-bound γ-glutamylamines, there has been little attention directed toward the

---

[a] Only the un-ionized forms of amines are reactive as acceptor substrates for transglutaminases (15, 23). When one estimates the proportion of various amines in reactive form at physiological pH levels and temperature it becomes evident that a considerably larger fraction of the primary amino groups of polyamines are in a reactive form than are the ε-amino groups of lysine residues (e.g., spermine, pK_a 7.92 and 8.81 at 37°[24]; lysine ε-amino group, $pK_a \sim 10.6$[25]). Thus, the concentration dependency of the reactive forms of amines as substrates for transglutaminases must be taken into account when considering the relative effectiveness of biological amines as substrates.

metabolic fate of these products of transglutamine-ase action. We have recently described an enzyme that we believe is involved in the catabolism of these crosslinks and γ-glutamylamine bonds (1). This enzyme, γ-glutamylamine cyclotransferase, acts on γ-glutamylamines to form free amines; lysine is a product of its action on the isopeptide, ε-(γ-glutamyl)lysine. The occurrence of this enzyme in a number of mammalian tissues serves to explain the observation that ε-(γ-glutamyl-)lysine can replace lysine in the diet of test animals (4, 5) and that lysine is released from this isopeptide as a result of its incubation with homogenates of various tissues (28, 29).

The kidney is the richest source of γ-glutamyl-amine cyclotransferase in the rabbit. Enzymic activity is found both in kidney cortex and medulla. Partial purification of the enzyme from rabbit kidney homogenates is accomplished by a procedure involving ion-exchange chromatography, salt fractionation, and size-exclusion chromatography.

Procedures employed for assay of γ-glutamyl-amine cyclotransferase activity include measurement of lysine released from ε-(γ-glutamyl)lysine and determination of monodansylcadaverine formed from γ-glutamylmonodansylcadaverine. Lysine is conveniently measured by reverse phase high pressure liquid chromatography after reaction with the fluorescent reagent, 2-methoxy-2,4-diphenyl-3-(2H)furanone[b] (30, 31) or by ion exchange chromatography on a short column coupled with on-stream reaction with o-phthalaldehyde. Monodansylcadaverine is detected by thin layer chromatography. Quantitative determinations are carried out after column separation on polyamide.

B. The enzymic reaction

Lysine was the only product detected, when ε-(γ-glutamyl)lysine was incubated with purified γ-glutamylamine cyclotransferase and portions of the reaction mixture were examined by conventional amino acid analysis. If, however, the reaction was allowed to go to completion and the products were hydrolyzed with acid prior to analysis, glutamic acid was also detected and was found in equimolar amounts with lysine. The undetected product was isolated and shown to be 5-oxo-L-proline. Since neither glutamic acid nor glutamine was converted to 5-oxoproline upon incubation with γ-glutamyl-amine cyclotransferase, it was concluded that the enzyme reaction does not proceed through hydrolysis, but rather by way of an internal cyclic transfer which produces 5-oxoproline while releasing lysine, as depicted in reaction 1.

C. Substrate specificity

The compounds that have been tested as substrates for γ-glutamylamine cyclotransferase are listed in Table 1. The activity toward each of the compounds is tabulated relative to the activity of the enzyme toward ε-(L-γ-glutamyl)-L-lysine (compound 1).

The requirement for the γ-glutamyl moiety is suggested by the failure of ε-formyl-L-lysine (compound 2) and ε-acetyl-L-lysine (compound 3) to function as substrates. The importance of this portion in substrates is evidenced by the lack of activity toward analogs of ε-(γ-glutamyl)lysine, such as ε-(β-aspartyl)lysine, ε-(β-aminoglutaryl)-lysine, and ε-(glutaryl)lysine, (compounds 4 through 6, respectively), that are unable to form the 5-membered pyrrolidone ring through intramolecular cyclization. The stereospecific requirement of the enzyme for the L-γ-glutamyl portion of the substrate is apparent from its failure to act on ε-(γ-D-glutamyl)-L-lysine (compound 7). That ε-(γ-L-glutamyl)-D-lysine (compound 8) is an efficient substrate demonstrates a lack of stereospecificity toward the lysine moiety of the dipeptide. Compounds in which the α-carboxyl group of the glutamic acid residue is in peptide linkage (compounds 9–11) are not substrates. A compound in which the α-amino group of the glutamic acid moiety is blocked by acetylation, (compound 12), is also not a substrate. It seems probable, therefore, that both the α-carboxyl and α-amino functions in the γ-glutamyl portion of a compound must be free in order for it to serve as a substrate.

[b] 2-Methoxy-2,4-diphenyl-3(2H)-furanone is obtained as a racemic mixture. Reaction of this reagent with L-lysine to give the *bis* substituted amino acid should result in the formation of four stereoisomers. Three non-equivalent peaks were obtained when samples of this fluorescent derivative of L-lysine were chromatographed on a microbondapak C_{18} column with methanol and 10 mM ammonium bicarbonate in equal volumes as eluant. The ratios of areas of these peaks were the same in all analyses and thus measurement of the area of any one peak could be used for quantitation.

Table 1. Substrate specificity of γ-glutamylamine cyclotransferase[a].

No.	Compound	Relative activity
1.	ε-(L-γ-glutamyl)-L-lysine	100
2.	ε-Formyl-L-lysine	<1
3.	ε-Acetyl-L-lysine	<1
4.	ε-(L-β-aspartyl)-L-lysine	<1
5.	ε-(D,L-β-aminoglutaryl)-L-lysine	<1
6.	ε-(glutaryl)-L-lysine	<1
7.	ε-(D-γ-glutamyl)-L-lysine	<1
8.	ε-(L-γ-glutamyl)-D-lysine	170
9.	α-Acetyl-ε-[γ-(L-glutamylglycine)]-L-lysine methyl ester	<1
10.	α-Acetyl-ε-[γ-(L-glutamyl-L-valine ethyl ester)]-L-lysine methyl ester	<1
11.	N-[γ-(L-glutamylglycylglycylglycine)]-isobutylamine	<1
12.	α-Acetyl-ε-(N-acetyl-L-γ-glutamyl)-L-lysine methyl ester	<1
13.	α-Acetyl-ε-(L-γ-glutamyl)-L-lysine methyl ester	115
14.	L-γ-glutamylmethylamine	15
15.	L-γ-glutamylethylamine	30
16.	L-γ-glutamylisopropylamine	35
17.	L-γ-glutamyl-n-butylamine	95
18.	L-γ-glutamylisobutylamine	85
19.	L-γ-glutamyldansylcadaverine	40
20.	L-glutamine	_[b]
21.	α-(L-γ-glutamyl)-L-lysine	<1
22.	L-γ-glutamyl-L-methionine	<1
23.	L-γ-glutamyl-L-glutamine	<1
24.	L-γ-glutamylglycine	4
25.	L-γ-glutamylglycyl-β-alanine	<1
26.	L-γ-glutamyl-β-alanine	65
27.	L-γ-glutamyl-β-alanylglycine	56
28.	L-γ-glutamyl-D,L-β-aminoisobutyric acid	48
29.	L-γ-glutamyl-D,L-β-amino-n-butyric acid	15
30.	L-γ-glutamylputrescine	95
31.	N^1,N^4-bis-(L-γ-glutamyl)putrescine	+[c]
32.	N^1 and N^8-(L-γ-glutamyl)spermidines	34
33.	N^1,N^8-bis-(L-γ-glutamyl)spermidine	+[c]
34.	N^1-(L-γ-glutamyl)spermine	81
35.	N^1,N^{12}-bis-(L-γ-glutamyl)spermine	+[c]
36.	L-γ-glutamylhistamine	15

[a] Reactions were carried out in phosphate buffer at pH 7.5 using 3.33 mM compound except compounds 32–35; these were tested at 1 mM.

[b] Activity was determined by monitoring glutamine concentration; no decrease in glutamine concentration was observed.

[c] Product formation was rapid. Rates were not measured since more than one amine product was formed. The γ-glutamylamine products are also substrates.

Analogs of ε-(L-γ-glutamyl)L-lysine in which the L-lysine portion is replaced by D-lysine (compound 8) or by α-N-acetyl-L-lysine methyl ester (compound 13) are excellent substrates. Indeed, most L-γ-glutamylamines (compound 14–18) are substrates, with some important exceptions. Glutamine (compound 20) is not a substrate, nor is α-(L-γ-glutamyl)-L-lysine (compound 21). None of the γ-glutamyl-α-amino acids tested (compounds 22 and 23) were found to be substrates, with the exception of γ-glutamylglycine (compound 24), for which the enzyme displays a very weak activity. It is interesting in this respect that γ-glutamylglycyl-β-alanine (compound 25) is not a substrate. It is quite likely that other γ-glutamyl peptides do not function as substrates. Displacement of the carboxyl group to the β-position, as in γ-L-glutamyl-β-alanine (compound 26), γ-L-glutamyl-β-alanylglycine (compound 27), and the γ-glutamyl-β-aminobutyric acid derivatives (compounds 28 and 29) restores substrate properties. Both mono- and di- γ-glutamyl derivatives of the diamine, putrescine, (compounds 30 and 31), and the polyamines, spermidine and spermine (compounds 32–35), are substrates. In addition to its action on γ-glutamyl derivatives of the naturally occurring polyamines, γ-glutamylamine cyclotransferase also catalyzes release of the biogenic amine, histamine from γ-glutamylhistamine (compound 36).

Although the data of Table 1 show a broad specificity of γ-glutamylamine cyclotransferase toward the amine portion of substrates, there are pronounced variations in the effectiveness of the various γ-glutamylamines as substrates. These differences certainly reflect influences of amine structure on interactions between substrate and enzyme.

D. Properties and distribution

γ-Glutamylamine cyclotransferase has been purified approximately 200-fold from kidney homogenates. The best preparations, however, are not homogenous as evidenced by the finding of multiple bands after polyacrylamide gel electrophoresis in sodium dodecyl sulfate. The exclusion chromatographic properties of the enzyme are consistent with an apparent molecular weight of less than 25 000.

At saturating levels of ε-(L-γ-glutamyl)-L-lysine the most highly purified enzyme preparations catalyze the release of 32 μmoles of lysine per hr per mg protein at pH 7.4 and 30°. The $K_{m(app)}$ with this substrate was estimated to be 0.23 ± 0.1 mM. γ-Glutamylamine cyclotransferase exhibits a broad pH optimum between 6.8 and 8.5. The enzyme is inactive at pH 4.

The effects of a number of reagents on γ-glutamylamine cyclotransferase activity are summarized in Table 2. Compounds that inhibit serine proteases, i.e., diisopropylphosphorofluoridate and phenylmethylsulfonylfluoride, do not inhibit the cyclotransferase. The use of these compounds has supplied evidence that during incubation in some tissues and cell extracts the cyclotransferase in inactivated proteolytically. Pronounced losses in enzymic activity occur when the enzyme is treated with 4-hydroxymercuribenzoic acid or 5,5′ dithio-bis(2-nitrobenzoic acid). However, other reagents known to modify protein -SH groups, e.g., iodo-acetamide, N-ethylmaleimide and cysteamine, are without substantial effect on activity.

Table 2. Effect of some reagents on γ-glutamylamine cyclotransferase activity toward the substrate, ε-(L-γ-glutamyl)-L-lysine.

Reagent	Concentration	Relative activity
None		100
Iodoacetic acid	2.5 mM	94
Iodoacetamide	2.5 mM	96
Glutathione	2.5 mM	82
Dithiothreitol	2.5 mM	73
N-Ethylmaleimide	2.5 mM	92
Cysteamine	2.5 mM	96
4-Hydroxymercuribenzoic acid	0.5 mM	12
5,5′-Dithio-bis-(2-nitro-benzoic acid)	1.0 mM	12
EDTA	2.5 mM	76
Phenylmethylsulfonylfluoride	1.0 mM	100
Diisopropylphosphorofluoridate	1.0 mM	100

Several analogs and derivatives of ε-(L-γ-glutamyl)-L-lysine were tested as potential inhibitors of γ-glutamylamine cyclotransferase. The results given in Table 3 show that of those compounds tested, ε-(D-γ-glutamyl)-L-lysine is the most effective inhibitor.

γ-Glutamylamine cyclotransferase is widely distributed in rabbit tissues and cells. Although the highest concentrations are found in kidney, there are substantial amounts in pancreas and testes. Heart, spleen and skin contain low levels of activity. Measurable amounts of cyclotransferase activity are found in peritoneal neutrophils, in reticulocytes, and in white and red blood cells, but not in blood plamsa. Human peripheral lymphocytes were found to contain the enzyme, as were those lines of human lung fibroblasts and Chinese hamster ovary cells tested.

E. Relationship to other enzymes involved in glutamate metabolism

5-Oxo-L-prolinase, an enzyme widely distributed in mammalian tissues, catalyzes the conversion of 5-oxo-L-proline to L-glutamate (32–34) (Reaction 5). This enzyme is thought to link the reactions

Table 3. Inhibition of γ-glutamylamine cyclotransferase by analogs of ε-(L-γ-glutamyl)-L-lysine.

Inhibitor	Inhibitor concentration	Substrate [ε-(L-γ-glutamyl)-L-Lysine] concentration	Relative activity
None			100
ε-(D,L-β-aminoglutaryl)-L-lysine	5.0 mM	0.75 mM	70
ε-Glutaryl-L-lysine	2.5 mM	2.5 mM	68
	2.5 mM	0.25 mM	36
N-acetyl-ε-(N-acetyl-L-γ-glutamyl)-L-lysine methyl ester	5.0 mM	0.5 mM	60
N-acetyl-ε-(L-γ-glutamyl-α-ethyl ester)-L-lysine methyl ester	5.0 mM	0.5 mM	75
ε-(D-γ-glutamyl)-L-lysine	2.5 mM	2.5 mM	50
	2.5 mM	0.25 mM	5

involved in the utilization of glutathione with those that lead to its synthesis (32, 34). Thus, 5-oxoproline is a metabolite of glutathione; that is, it is product of the action of γ-glutamyl*amino acid* cyclotransferase[c] on γ-glutamylamino acids (Reaction 6) which are formed in turn from glutathione

through transpeptidation with amino acids (for review, see ref. 37). Although γ-glutamyl*amine* cyclotransferase which is described in detail here and γ-glutamyl*amino acid* cyclotransferase are separate enzymes with distinctly different specificities (compare reactions 1 and 6), each of these enzymes catalyzes the production of 5-oxo-L-proline, the substrate for 5-oxo-L-prolinase. It is probable, therefore, that glutamate is an eventual metabolite of ε-(γ-glutamyl)lysine and other γ-glutamylamines.

γ-Glutamylputrescine occurs as the free γ-glutamylamine in rat and bovine brain and its production from putrescine in rat brain has been demonstrated (38)[d]. Another free γ-glutamylamine, γ-

glutamylhistamine, is produced as a major metabolite of histamine in the ganglia of a marine mollusk (41). Labeling studies indicate that the γ-glutamyl portion of this compound originates from free glutamate. Although little is known concerning either the biological role of these γ-glutamylamines or the enzymic mechanisms for their production *in vivo*, it has been shown that γ-glutamyl transpeptidase is capable of catalyzing their formation *in vitro* (38, 39, 40). Thus, it is possible that the biological production of certain free γ-glutamylamines occurs by means other than through the degradation of transglutaminase products, i.e., by a mechanism other than that of enzymic breakdown of protein-amine conjugates[e] (Sections II and IV). Radiolabeled γ-glutamylputrescine (38) and γ-glutamylhistamine (40) formed upon intraventricular injection of the respective labeled amine into rat brain are rapidly degraded indicating their efficient metabolism. Since γ-glutamylputrescine and γ-glutamylhistamine serve as substrates for γ-glutamylamine cyclotransferase *in vitro* (Table 1) and since this enzyme occurs in brain (1), it is likely that γ-glutamylamine cyclotransferase is indeed the enzyme responsible for turnover of these free γ-glutamylamines.

IV. Considerations on the role of γ-glutamylamine cyclotransferase in the catabolism of transglutaminase products

Observed changes in cellular levels of transglutaminase activity have provided bases for speculation on the involvement of the transglutaminases in diverse cellular functions and processes (for review, see ref. 14). Consistent with the widespread occurrence of these enzymes in cells is recent evidence for ε-(γ-glutamyl)lysine bonds in a variety of normal

---

[c] For clarity, the enzyme designated γ-glutamyl cyclotransferase (γ-L-glutamyl-L-amino acid γ-glutamyltransferase (cyclizing) EC 2.3. 2.4) (35, 36) is referred to here as γ-glutamylamino acid cyclotransferase.

[d] The formation of γ-glutamyl derivatives of several biogenic amines including those of tyramine, noradrenaline, dopamine, serotonin, and histamine has been demonstrated by injection of the radioactive amines into rat brain (39, 40). It is not known whether these γ-glutamyl compounds exist normally in brain since the experiments were carried out under conditions very different from physiological ones; i.e., with the use of intraventricular injections of large doses of amines and, in most cases, after blockade of the normal metabolic route by administration of monoamine oxidase inhibitor. It is interesting with regard to the possible metabolism of these γ-glutamylamines that their degradation was attributed to the action of brain γ-glutamyl *amino acid* cyclotransferase (39). This conclusion was based on experiments conducted with enzyme partially purified from rat brain. Enzyme purified from rat kidney showed no activity toward the γ-glutamylamines.

[e] Putrescine-protein conjugates have been isolated from both human amniotic fluid (42) and from human blood plasma (43). Although an involvement of transglutaminases in their formation is suggested, no information is as yet available as to the mode of amine attachment. The finding of labeled γ-glutamylputrescine in proteolytic digests of the protein fraction prepared from human blood lymphocytes that had been incubated with [³H]putrescine is strong evidence for transglutaminase-catalyzed incorporation of putrescine (12). The putrescine-protein conjugates from this source have not, however, been isolated or identified.

cells, both prokaryotic and eukaryotic (9). The finding of very low concentrations of this isopeptide bond in all cells examined, however, has prompted the suggestion that the ϵ-(γ-glutamyl)lysine bond serves a normal function in most cells that is more specialized than simply that of maintaining gross forms of protein structure and limiting degrees of extensibility (9). The occurrence of protein-bound γ-glutamylputrescine and γ-glutamylspermidine in normal human peripheral blood lymphocytes supplies evidence for transglutaminase-catalyzed incorporation of these amines in cells. The low concentrations of γ-glutamylamines in lymphocytes and the fact that they occur as *mono*-γ-glutamyl derivatives indicates that they do not have a crosslinking role and is further support for the suggestion that cellular transglutaminases have a specialized function.

We have considered the possibility that the production of ϵ-(γ-glutamyl)lysine crosslinked proteins or other protein-amine conjugates constitutes one or more steps in certain vital cellular processes. In those cases where the ϵ-(γ-glutamyl)lysine crosslink is not a fundamental structural feature, its disassembly, as well as the disassembly of other protein γ-glutamyl bonds, would occur as a normal part of the intracellular turnover of transglutaminase-modified proteins. There is no indication that γ-glutamyl bonds in protein are cleaved without prior degradation of the modified proteins; it seems unlikely that cleavage of these bonds occurs through the reverse action of transglutaminases because this reaction is slow and inefficient (20, 44). It is possible that transglutaminase-modified proteins in cells are degraded in such a manner that substrates for γ-glutamylamine cyclotransferase are rapidly and preferentially formed. This seems reasonable in light of evidence for very rapid and efficient breakdown of protein to the amino acid level by cellular systems (for reviews, see refs. 45–47). This idea becomes especially attractive in view of the fact that proteins with abnormal structures are degraded especially rapidly within cells, (46, 47) and when one considers the possibility that the aberrations induced by transglutaminase-modification may signal this type of breakdown. Certain other types of post-translational covalent protein modifications, e.g., phosphorylation (47) and glycosylation (48), have also been considered as possible steps in protein degradation.

We have conducted preliminary experiments to test for the products of breakdown of a transglutaminase-modified protein in cell-free preparations from rabbit reticulocytes. Incubation in this system of a succinylated derivative of casein into which [^{14}C]methylamine had been incorporated by transglutaminase action led to the rapid production of trichloroacetic acid soluble labeled products. Samples of the acid soluble material from digests in which between 50% and 75% of the labeled protein had become acid soluble were analyzed, and essentially all of the radioactivity was found in two components – γ-glutamylmethylamine and methylamine. This finding is in accordance with the presence of measurable levels of γ-glutamylamine cyclotransferase in rabbit reticulocyte extracts (Section IIID).

Two extracellular events are known to occur as consequences of transglutaminase catalysis. These are the crosslinking of the fibrin clot during hemostasis (for review, see ref. 6), and the production of the vaginal plug by postejaculatory crosslinking of proteins in rodent seminal plasma (for review, see ref. 14). There is evidence that during the course of the covalent polymerization of fibrin in normal blood plasma, both cold-insoluble globulin (fibronectin) (49) and α_2-plasmin inhibitor (50) are attached to fibrin through ϵ-(γ-glutamyl)lysine bonds. The finding that polyamines are incorporated through γ-glutamyl linkage into a number of proteins of rat seminal plasma during clotting (12) adds another dimension to extracellular transglutaminase products. The question arises as to the biological mechanism for disposal of ϵ-(γ-glutamyl)lysine bonds and γ-glutamylamines that occur in the proteins of body fluids. It is possible that transglutaminase modified-extracellular proteins and protein complexes, like unmodified protein and a spectrum of other soluble and particulate materials are internalized by phagocytic cells, transported to cell lysosomes, and there degraded. Support for this suggestion is evidence of a specific receptor-mediated endocytotic mechanism for internalization of soluble crosslinked fibrin-fibrinogen complexes (51). It is doubtful that disassembly of ϵ-(γ-glutamyl)lysine and other γ-glutamylamines by γ-glutamylamine cyclotransferase occurs within lysosomes. Intralysosomal pH varies between 4.5 and 5.5 (52) – well outside of the broad optimum for activity of the amine cyclotransferase.

It is believed that intralysosomal hydrolysis of proteins, in general, gives rise to amino acids which cross the lysosomal membrane and enter the cytosol (53). The permeability of secondary lysosomes of mouse peritoneal macrophages to a number of dipeptides (54) raises the possibility that ϵ-(γ-glutamyl)lysine and other γ-glutamylamines are also capable of crossing the lysosomal membrane. Whether γ-glutamylamines are formed within lysosomes as a consequence of hydrolysis of transglutaminase-modified extracellular proteins and, if so, whether their γ-glutamylamine cyclotransferase-catalyzed conversion to 5-oxoproline and free amines occurs in an extralysosomal fashion are topics under consideration.

Acknowledgements

We thank Dr Alton Meister for advice and encouragement, and for the samples of L-γ-glutamyl-D,L-β-aminoisobutyric acid and L-γ-glutamyl-D,-L-β-amino-n-butyric acid. We also express our appreciation to Dr Stanley Stein, Hoffman-LaRoche, for the gift of 2-methoxy-2,4-diphenyl-3-(2H)-furanone and his helpful suggestions on its use in the determination of lysine.

References

1. Fink, M. L., Chung, S. I. & Folk, J. E., 1980. Proc. Natl. Acad. Sci. USA 77: 4564–4568.
2. Matacíc, S. & Loewy, A. G., 1968. Biochem. Biophys. Res. Commun. 30: 356–362.
3. Pisano, J. J., Finlayson, J. S. & Peyton, M. P., 1968. Science 160: 892–893.
4. Mauron, J., 1970. J. Int. Vitaminol. 40: 209–227.
5. Waibel, P. E. & Carpenter, K. J., 1972. Br. J. Nutr. 27: 509–515.
6. Folk, J. E. & Finlayson, J. S., 1977. Adv. Pro. Chem. 31: 1–133.
7. Rice, R. H. & Green, H., 1979. Cell 18: 681.
8. Hanigan, H. & Goldsmith, L. A., 1978. Biochim. Biophys. Acta 522: 589–601.
9. Matacíc, S. S. & Loewy, A. G., 1979. Biochim. Biophys. Acta 576: 263–268.
10. Buxman, M. M. & Wuepper, K. D., 1978. J. Histochem. and Cytochem. 26: 340–348.
11. Birckbichler, P. J., Carter, H. A., Orr, G. R., Conway, E. & Patterson, M. K., Jr., 1978. Biochem. Biophys. Res. Comm. 14: 232–237.
12. Folk, J. E., Park, M. H., Chung, S. I., Schrode, J., Lester, E. P. & Cooper, H. L., 1980. J. Biol. Chem. 255: 3695–3700.
13. Folk, J. E. & Chung, S. I., 1973. Adv. Enzymol. 38: 109–191.
14. Folk, J. E., 1980. Ann. Rev. Biochem. 49: 517–531.
15. Clarke, D. D., Mycek, M. J., Neidle, A. & Waelsh, H., 1959. Arch. Biochem. Biophys. 79: 338–354.
16. Lorand, L. & Ong, H. H., 1966. Biochemistry 5: 1747–1753.
17. Pincus, J. H. & Waelsh, H., 1968. Arch. Biochem. Biophys. 126: 44–52.
18. Schrode, J. & Folk, J. E., 1978. J. Biol. Chem. 253: 4837–4840.
19. Lorand, L., Rule, N. G., Ong, H. H., Furlanetto, R., Jacobsen, A., Dawney, J., Oner, N. & Bruner-Lorand, J., 1968. Biochemistry 7: 1214–1223.
20. Chung, S. I., Shrager, R. I. & Folk, J. E., 1970. J. Biol. Chem. 245: 6424–6435.
21. Gross, M., Whetzel, N. K. & Folk, J. E., 1977. J. Biol. Chem. 252: 3752–3759.
22. Schrode, J. & Folk, J. E., 1979. J. Biol. Chem. 254: 653–661.
23. Folk, J. E. & Cole, P. W., 1966. Biochim. Biophys. Acta 122: 244–264.
24. Hirschman, S. Z., Lang, M. & Felsenfeld, G., 1967. Biopolymers 5: 227–233.
25. Jenks, W. P. & Regenstein, J., 1970. In: Handbook of Biochem. Ed. H. A. Sober, 2nd ed., The Chemical Rubber Co., Cleveland, pp. J187–J226.
26 Neidle, A., Mycek, M. J., Clarke, D. D. & Waelsh, H., 1958. Arch. Biochem. Biophys. 77: 227.
27. Neidle, A. & Acs, G., 1961. Fed. Proc. 20: 234.
28. Raczynski, G., Snochowski, M. & Buraczewski, S., 1975. Br. J. Nutr. 34: 291–296.
29. Finot, P.-A., Mottu, F., Bujard, E. & Mauron, J., 1978. Adv. in. Exp. Med. Biol. 105: 549–570.
30. Weigele, M., DeBernardo, S., Leimgruber, W., Clieland, R. & Grunberg, E., 1973. Biochem. Biophys. Res. Commun. 54: 899–906.
31. Udenfriend, S. & Stein, S., 1977. In: Peptides: Proceedings of the Fifth American Peptide Symposium. Eds. M. Goodman and J. Meienhofer, Wiley and Sons, pp. 14–26.
32. Van Der Werf, P., Orlowski, M. & Meister, A., 1971. Proc. Natl. Acad. Sci. USA 68: 2982–2985.
33. Van Der Werf, P., Griffith, O. & Meister, A., 1975. J. Biol. Chem. 250: 6686–6692.
34. Van Der Werf, P., Stephani, R. A., Orlowski, M. & Meister, A., 1973. Proc. Natl. Acad. Sci. USA 70: 759–761.
35. Orlowski, M., Richman, P. G. & Meister, A., 1969. Biochemistry 8: 1048–1055.
36. Orlowski, M. & Meister, A., 1973. J. Biol. Chem. 248: 2836–2844.
37. Orlowski, M. & Meister, A., 1971. In: The Enzymes Ed. P. D. Boyer, 3rd edn., Academic Press Inc., New York, pp. 123–151.
38. Nakajima, T., Kakimoto, Y., Tsuji, M. & Konishi, H., 1976. J. Neurochem. 26: 115–118.
39. Tsuji, M., Matsuoka, Y. & Nakajima, T., 1977. J. Neurochem. 29: 633–638.
40. Konishi, H. & Kakimoto, Y., 1976. J. Neurochem. 27: 1461–1463.
41. Weinrich, D., 1979. J. Neurochem. 32: 363–369.
42. Seale, T. W., Chan, W.-Y., Shulka, J. B. & Rennert, O. M., 1979. Clin. Chim. Acta 95: 461–472.

43. Seale, T. W., Chan, W.-Y., Shulka, J. B. & Rennert, O. M., 1979. Arch. Biochem. Biophys. 198: 164–174.

44. Folk, J. E., 1969. J. Biol. Chem. 244: 3707–3713.

45. Segal, H. L. & Doyle, D. J., (eds.), 1978. Protein Turnover and Lysosome Function, Academic Press, New York.

46. Goldberg, A. L. & Dice, J. L., Jr., 1974. Ann. Rev. Biochem. 43: 835–869.

47. Goldberg, A. L. & St. John, A. C., 1976. Ann. Rev. Biochem. 45: 747–803.

48. Kalish, F., Chovick, N. & Dice, J. F., 1979. J. Biol. Chem. 254: 4475–4481.

49. Mosher, D. F., 1976. J. Biol. Chem. 251: 1639–1645.

50. Sakata, Y. & Aoki, N., 1980. J. Clin. Invest. 65: 290–297.

51. Sherman, L. A. & Lee, J., 1977. J. Exp. Med. 145: 76–85.

52. Ohkuma, S. & Poole, B., 1978. Proc. Natl. Acad. Sci. USA 75: 3327–3331.

53. Cohn, Z. A., 1975. In: Proteases and Biological Control, Eds. E. Reich, D. B. Rifkin & E. Shaw, Cold Spring Harbor Laboratory, pp. 483–493.

54. Ehrenreich, B. A. & Cohn, Z. A., 1969. J. Exp. Med. 129: 227–243.

Received August 5, 1980.

GABA and the enteric nervous system

A neurotransmitter function?

K. R. Jessen

MRC Neuroimmunology Project, Dept. of Zoology, University College London, Gower Street, London WC1E 6BT, Great Britain

Summary

GABA and GABA-related properties in the enteric nervous system of the gastrointestinal tract, the third and most complex division of the vertebrate autonomic nervous system, have been the subject of relatively few studies. This chapter aims at being a comprehensive review of these investigations.

With respect to GABA the enteric nervous system shows in some respects similarities with, and in others, notable differences from other parts of the peripheral nervous system.

Like the cell bodies of other autonomic and sensory neurons, the cell bodies of enteric neurons possess bicuculline and picrotoxin sensitive GABA receptors, the activation of which leads to depolarization, probably mediated by increase in Cl^- conductance. Further, in common with other peripheral glia, the cell membrane of the enteric glial cells appears to contain β-alanine sensitive high affinity transport sites by which they can accumulate exogenous GABA.

However, the present evidence, although not completely conclusive, suggests that unlike other parts of the peripheral nervous system, the enteric ganglia may contain a population of GABA-ergic neurons; in vertebrates such neurons have hitherto been thought to be present in the brain and spinal cord only. At present the most important single strand of evidence for this notion is the demonstration of a population of enteric neurons possessing high affinity transport sites for GABA, while it is supported by studies of GAD and GABA content, the effects of GABA receptor blockade on gut motility and GABA release.

Introduction

Some twenty years ago, Hobbiger (1) speculated, on the basis of pharmacological studies, that GABA, then recently discovered as a constituent of nervous tissue, might have a role in neurotransmission in the enteric nervous system of the vertebrate gut. Subsequent work, however, soon focussed on GABA in relation to the vertebrate central nervous system, partly because early measurements of endogenous GABA levels failed to detect GABA in peripheral nervous tissue, suggesting that in vertebrates GABA was only present in the brain and spinal cord. It has since become accepted that in vertebrates GABA serves as a neurotransmitter in the central nervous system only, while it is recognized that several GABA-related properties such as GABA receptors (Matthews & Roberts), (2) de Groat (3), Bowery & Brown (4), high affinity glial uptake of GABA (Young et al. (5), Schon & Kelly (6, 7), the GABA synthesizing enzyme GAD and endogenous GABA (Beart et al. (8), Kanazawa et al. (9), Osborne et al. (10), Bertilson et al. (11)) are in fact widespread in the vertebrate peripheral nervous system, where they do not, however, seem to be related to the presence of GABA ergic neurons or conventional GABA-mediated synaptic transmission (for reviews see Iversen & Kelly (12), Roberts et al. (13), Nistri & Constanti (14)).

Recently several lines of evidence have emerged,

Molecular and Cellular Biochemistry 38, 69–76 (1981). 0300-8177/81/0381-0069/$ 1.60.

70

which indicate that this view may need re-evaluation since they suggest that the enteric nervous system may indeed contain a population of GABA ergic neurons. The enteric nervous system constitutes the third division of the autonomic nervous system, the other two being the sympathetic and parasympathetic divisions (Langley (15), Gabella (16), Wood (17), Furness & Costa (18)). In addition to efferent neurons innervating intestinal muscle, blood vessels and glands, it contains both sensory neurons and interneurons. It is now believed that this complex system employs a number of different neurotransmitters in addition to acetylcholine and noradrenaline, the classical neurotransmitters of the vertebrate periphery. Thus GABA is the latest member in a group of putative enteric neurotransmitters, which at present consists of purine nucleotides, 5-HT or a 5-HT like substance and several peptides including vasoactive intestinal polypeptide (VIP), substance-P and enkephalin (for reviews see Burnstock & Hökfelt (19), Furness & Costa (18)).

2. GABA and the enteric nervous system

In the first study of GABA actions in the gut, Hobbiger (1) found that the effects of GABA on isolated small intestine from guinea pigs, rabbits and rats were complex and species dependent. In the guinea pig where the GABA effects were most pronounced, it caused contraction and(or) relaxation of the ileum, the contraction being abolished by atropine, a blocker of cholinergic neuromuscular transmission in the gut. GABA also acted to a limited extent as an antagonist of acetylcholine, nicotine and histamine. Furthermore, GABA at a concentration of 10^{-5} M prevented the propagation of peristaltic waves, initiated by increasing the intraluminal pressure in a segment of the guinea pig ileum *in vitro*. These results led Hobbiger to speculate that GABA 'might be concerned in the activity of intestinal muscles *in vivo*'. In a subsequent paper, dealing with the antagonism by GABA to the actions of 5-HT and nicotine on the guinea pig ileum, Hobbiger (20) concluded that the GABA effects 'appear to be the result of an action of GABA on those neuronal structures which are involved in the transmission of impulses generated by both the stimulant drugs' (i.e. 5-HT and nico-

tine). The anti-acetylcholine and anti-nicotine effects of GABA, as well as its potent anti-5-HT action on the guinea pig ileum were confirmed by Florey & McLennan (21). Similar results were obtained by Inouyne, *et al.* (22) who in addition confirmed Hobbiger's observation that at a concentration of 10^{-4} M, GABA blocked peristalsis in the guinea pig small intestine. They were the first to observe that the effects of GABA on the gut were antagonized by picrotoxin, a drug which later came into widespread use together with bicuculline as GABA antagonists defining the classical GABA receptor (see De Feudis (23)). In agreement with Hobbiger (20) they concluded that GABA acts on 'those neuronal structures which are involved in the transmission of impulses generated by 5-HT and nicotine'.

Significant steps forward in this field were not made until some twenty years later. In a pharmacological study of the guinea pig ileum and colon Krantis *et al.* (24) confirmed the conclusions of earlier workers that GABA receptors seem to be absent from intestinal muscle. They found that the effects of GABA on the contractile state of the guinea pig ileum and distal colon were abolished by tetrodotoxin and that GABA had no detectable effects on nerve free preparations of the guinea pig ileum. For the guinea pig taenia coli, however, there are reports that GABA causes contractions which are not antagonized by atropine and therefore presumably not caused by GABA activation of cholinergic neurons (Rikimaru & Suzuki (25), Ishizawa & Picles (26)). This may indicate direct action of GABA on the smooth muscle of this tissue, although it remains possible that also here GABA acts indirectly by releasing an excitatory neurotransmitter other than acetylcholine.

Krantis *et al.* (24) also concluded that GABA receptors were present on at least two populations of neurons in the enteric nervous system, i.e. the cholinergic neurons that contract intestinal muscle and the intrinsic inhibitory neurons that relax it, thus partly clarifying the complex contraction/-relaxation effects of GABA observed by Hobbiger (1) and Inouye *et al.* (22). Further, they provided evidence that the action of GABA on these receptors was blocked by bicuculline. Direct demonstration of picrotoxin sensitive GABA receptors on enteric neurons was achieved in 1979 by Grafe *et al.* (27). By recording intracellularly from the enteric neurons in the myenteric plexus of the guinea pig ileum following bath-application of GABA, they showed that the drug reversibly depolarized, by up to 20 mV, 33 out of 44 neurons tested. The depolarization was accompanied by an increase in membrane conductance, the threshold concentration for obtaining the effect was between 5×10^{-6} and 10^{-5} M and it was abolished by picrotoxin, confirming the observations by Inouyne et al. (22). Furthermore GABA reduced the amplitude of the fast excitatory post-synaptic potentials which can be evoked in neurons of the myenteric plexus following focal electrical stimulation of fiber tracts in the plexus (Grafe et al. (27) It is not known whether this inhibition is due to a pre- or a post-synaptic action of GABA although the apparent absence of axo-axonic synapses in the myenteric plexus (Gabella (28)) may seem to favour a post-synaptic mechanism. The ionic mechanism of GABA action on enteric neurons appears to be similar to that most commonly thought to operate in other peripheral neurons, i.e. an increase in the Cl^- conductance of the cell membrane. Thus the effects of GABA are reversibly abolished in a Cl^- free solution and the reversal potential of the GABA response is close to the Cl^- equilibrium potential (Dr C. J. Mayer, personal communication). Further, the actions of GABA are blocked by furosemide and piretamide which are considered to block Cl^- channels (Dr A. Krantis, personal communication).

Since it was known that bicuculline and picrotoxine sensitive GABA receptors were present on sympathetic and sensory neurons and that GABA suppressed synaptic transmission through sympathetic ganglia (for refs. see 'Introduction') these results were not surprising. They could be viewed as bringing the enteric neurons into line with other autonomic neurons in possessing GABA receptors which are pharmacologically similar to those of central neurons, but are apparently not concerned with the mediation of synaptic GABA ergic neurotransmission.

In 1979, however, Jessen et al. (29) showed that unlike sympathetic and sensory ganglia, the enteric ganglia contain neurons which possess high affinity transport sites for ^{3}H-GABA. Such uptake sites are pharmacologically and functionally different from GABA receptors (Roberts et al. (13)) and have so far only been found on putative or established GABA ergic neurons (see below). Working on the myenteric plexus of the guinea-pig taenia coli they employed light and electron microscopic auto-radiography to show selective labelling of a small population of neurons following incubation of the tissue in 2×10^{-8} M ^{3}H-GABA for 20 min. This was observed both following incubation of pieces of gut wall containing the plexus and also when tissue culture preparations of the plexus (Jessen et al. (30)) were incubated with the radioactive ligand (Fig. 1). The labelled neurons were always small to medium sized and constituted about 5% or less of the total population of neurons. The labelling was unaffected by β-alanine (10^{-3} M) a selective blocker of nonneuronal GABA transport (Iversen & Kelly (12)) and was greatly reduced or abolished in the presence of cis-1,3-aminocyclohexane carboxylic acid (ACHC), an inhibitor of neuronal GABA transport (Bowery et al. (31)). The presence of neurons in the enteric nervous system that become selectively labelled following incubation in low concentrations of ^{3}H-GABA has been confirmed in the chicken and rat myenteric plexus maintained in tissue culture (Ms M. J. Saffrey, personal communication; Dr K. R. Jessen, unpublished observations) and in the myenteric plexus of the guinea pig small intestine by Krantis (32). Using whole mounts of the myenteric plexus he found that autoradiographic labelling was present not only over scattered neurons inside the ganglia but also in the nerve strands that connect them, as well as in those nerve bundles which run from the plexus into the surrounding musculature. This labelling was almost totally abolished by DABA (10^{-3} M) which preferentially blocks neuronal GABA transport (Iversen & Kelly (12)). Uptake of ^{3}H-GABA into nerve bundles outside the myenteric plexus has also been found in fibers running inside the circular and longitudinal muscle layers of the guinea pig caecum (Dr K. R. Jessen, unpublished observations). The pattern of radioactive labelling observed following incubation with ^{3}H-β-alanine, which is selectively taken up by glial cells (Iversen & Kelly (12)) was quite different, the grains forming a diffuse cover over the plexus. This would be the distribution expected if glial cells were the sites of accumulated radioactivity; this labelling was not affected by DABA (Krantis (32)).

All available evidence concerning the neuronal distribution of high affinity membrane transport

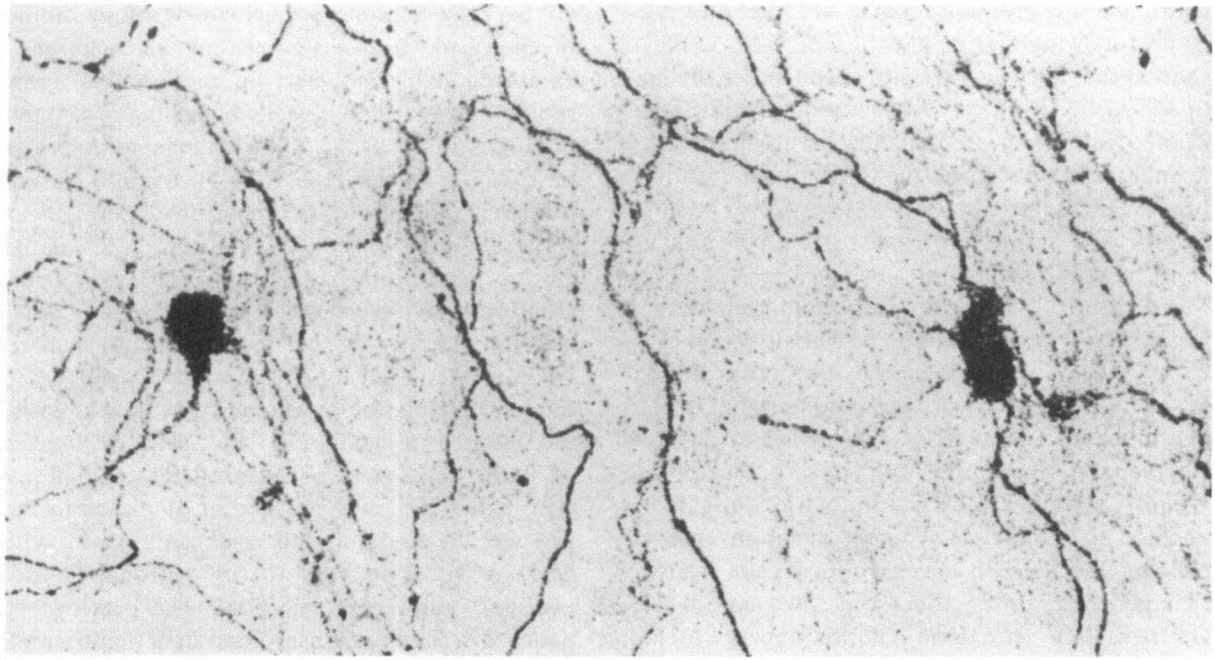

Fig. 1. Autoradiograph showing uptake of ^{3}H-GABA into neurons from enteric ganglia grown in tissue culture. Two neuronal cell bodies and several neuronal processes are heavily labelled with autoradiographic grains, indicating that these cellular elements possess high affinity uptake sites for ^{3}H-GABA. Faint background labelling is due to a limited ^{3}H-GABA uptake into the enteric glial cells which form a flat sheet underlying the neurons. The autoradiograph was prepared following the incubation of explants of the guinea pig myenteric plexus, maintained in culture for 14 days, in 2×10^{-8} M ^{3}H-GABA, 10^{-3} M β-alanine for 20 min at room temperature ($\times$ 440).

sites for GABA suggests that such sites are restricted to those neurons which use GABA as a neurotransmitter, although it remains possible that some GABA-ergic neurons do not share this property (see Iversen & Kelly (12); Roberts *et al.* (13)). This contention has recently received support from the studies of Brandon *et al.* (33) who showed that in the rabbit retina high affinity GABA uptake sites and the localization of GAD, the enzyme that synthesizes GABA from glutamic acid, show an identical pattern of distribution, strongly indicating that both properties reside in the same neurons. Similarly in a study of ^{3}H-GABA uptake into spinal cord neurons in tissue culture Farb *et al.* (34) found that no identifiable cholinergic neurons showed high affinity GABA uptake. Thus the presence of high affinity GABA uptake has been widely used for the identification of GABA-ergic neurons, both following injection of ^{3}H-GABA *in vivo* as well as after *in vitro* incubation of tissue slices or neurons maintained in tissue culture (e.g. Iversen & Bloom (35), Sotelo *et al.* (36), Schon & Iversen (37), Lasher

(38), Brandon *et al.* (33), White *et al.* (39)). The studies on ^{3}H-GABA uptake in the enteric nervous system therefore suggest that, unlike other parts of the vertebrate peripheral nervous system, it contains a population of GABA ergic neurons.

Investigating this possibility further, Jessen *et al.* (29) measured the specific activity of GAD in homogenates of the myenteric plexus, assessed the ability of the isolated, intact plexus to synthesize and accumulate ^{3}H-GABA following incubation with its immediate precursor, ^{3}H-glutamic acid, and measured the levels of endogenous GABA in isolated strips of the taenia coli muscle, containing the myenteric plexus. The results are shown in Table 1. In summary it was found that homogenates of plexus showed significant GAD activity and the intact plexus accumulated about 3.3 times more newly synthesized ^{3}H-GABA than did sympathetic ganglia, where synthesis and accumulation of ^{3}H-GABA presumably takes place in glial cells only (Iversen & kelly (12)), but about half the levels of cerebellar slices which are thought to be rich in

Table 1. GABA content and metabolism in the guinea pig myenteric plexus and other tissues.

	Myenteric plexus	Sympathetic ganglia	Cerebellum	Striated muscle
GAD activity (μmol/0.1 g protein/h)	2.18	NT	NT	NT
Amount of endogenous GABA (n mol/g wet weight)	17.5*	NT	NT	5.7
Accumulated ^{3}H-GABA after synthesis from ^{3}H-glutamic acid (mol/mg protein)	4.0×10^{-13}	9.6×10^{-14}	8.0×10^{-13}	NT
Accumulated ^{3}H-homocarnosine after synthesis from ^{3}H-glutamic acid (mol/mg protein)	2.6×10^{-13}	O	O	NT

NT Not tested

* This value represents the GABA content of the taenia coli muscle containing the myenteric plexus, the plexus itself constituting only a very small fraction of the total tissue mass.

For experimental details see Jessen *et al.* (29) (1979).

GABA ergic neurons (Roberts *et al.* (13)). The plexus also synthesized and accumulated ^{3}H-homocarnosine, a dipeptide of unknown function found in brain. The taenia coli muscle including the myenteric plexus possessed about three times more endogenous GABA than a control specimen of striated muscle. These results are all in agreement with the hypothesis that there is a small population of GABA ergic neurons in the gut, although care is needed in the interpretation of the data since it appears that low levels of GABA and GAD are found in the vertebrate periphery outside GABA ergic neurons (see 'Introduction'). On the other hand the amounts of both GABA and GAD contained in a population of enteric neurons would be severely underestimated in measurements of the kind described here. Endogenous GABA levels were assessed in muscle specimens of which the myenteric plexus only constitutes a very small fraction. Therefore GABA content of a small population of enteric neurons would be greatly diluted. Since autoradiographic labelling of GABA uptake sites is common in nerve fibers outside the myenteric plexus (see above) and no labelled nerve terminals or varicosities are observed within the ganglia of the

guinea pig myenteric plexus of the taenia coli (Ms M. E. Dennison, personal communication) it seems likely that the putative GABA ergic neurons project to targets outside the plexus. All such fibers are however severed in the preparation used to measure GAD activity. These experiments would therefore mainly assess the GAD activity contained in the GABA ergic neuronal cell bodies, which is very low in comparison to the GAD content of nerve terminals of GABA ergic neurons (Barber & Saito (40), Wood *et al.* (41)).

In their study of enteric GABA receptors discussed earlier Krantis *et al.* (24) observed that in the guinea pig distal colon, neither the ascending excitatory nor the descending inhibitory component of the enteric reflex was affected by blockage of GABA receptors by bicuculline or by desensitization of the receptors by prolonged exposure to GABA. Investigating further the possible involvement of GABA in intestinal motility Krantis (42) (1979) found, however, that in the same preparation, both treatments markedly affected the rate of propulsion of faecal pellets along isolated gut segments. While GABA (3×10^{-5} g/ml) and bicuculline (3.7×10^{-5} g/ml) after exposure for 8–10 min completely stopped motility in some preparations, they most commonly reduced the propulsion rate by 45–50%. These effects were readily reversible following removal of the respective drugs and it was suggested that GABA was involved in specific reflex pathways (Krantis (42)).

Krantis has also made a preliminary study of GABA release from the myenteric plexus in which he demonstrated a tetrodotoxin sensitive release of preloaded ^{3}H-GABA from gut preparations upon electrical stimulation or depolarization of the tissue with solutions containing high concentrations of K^+ (Dr A. Krantis, personal communication).

3. Conclusions

The results reviewed above demonstrate that with respect to GABA and GABA-related properties, the enteric nervous system shows in some respects similarities with, and in others, notable differences from other parts of the peripheral nervous system.

Like the cell bodies of other autonomic and sensory neurons, the cell bodies of enteric neurons possess bicuculline and picrotoxin sensitive GABA receptors, the activation of which leads to depolarization, probably mediated by increase in Cl^-conductance. Further, in common with other peripheral glia, the cell membrane of the enteric glial cells appears to contain β-alanine sensitive high affinity transport sites by which they can accumulate exogenous GABA.

However, the present evidence, although not completely conclusive, suggests that unlike other parts of the peripheral nervous system, the enteric ganglia may contain a population of GABA ergic neurons; in vertebrates such neurons have hitherto been thought to be present in the brain and spinal cord only (see Roberts et al. (13)). At present the most important single strand of evidence for this notion is the demonstration of a population of enteric neurons possessing high affinity transport sites for GABA, while it is supported by studies of GAD and GABA content, the effects of GABA receptor blockade on gut motility and GABA release.

It may be tempting to speculate that the function of these putative GABA ergic neurons in the gut must be connected with the enteric neuronal GABA receptors and glial GABA uptake. The presence of these features does, however, not constitute evidence in favour of the hypothesis that there are GABA ergic neurons in the gut, since they are also found in parts of the nervous system where there is no evidence for GABA ergic neurons, such as sympathetic and sensory ganglia. Therefore neuronal GABA receptors and glial GABA uptake do not appear to be specifically related to synaptic GABA ergic neurotransmission. The significance of these properties in the peripheral nervous system remains unclear, although they might be related to hormonal neuromodulatory function of glial-derived GABA in extracellular fluids (see e.g. Iversen & Kelly (12)).

The chemical and morphological complexities of the synaptic interactions involved in the neuronal control of gut movements, secretion and blood flow are only beginning to be understood and it is at this stage difficult to suggest what might be the specific role of a small population of enteric GABA ergic neurons. This is further hampered by the paucity of information about the distribution and projections of these cells in the gut wall as well as our limited knowledge regarding the action of GABA on gut tissue; it has not been investigated, for instance, whether GABA affects intestinal blood supply or secretion. Furthermore, it is difficult to interpret most of the available functional studies of GABA in the gut, i.e. the investigations into the effects of exogenous GABA on intestinal motility (Hobbiger (1, 20), Florey & McLennan (21), Inoyne et al. (12), Krantis et al. (24)) because of the widespread occurrence of neuronal GABA receptors. The observed effects may well be due to GABA action at these extrasynaptic receptors. They would then be comparable to the inhibitory effects of GABA on transmission through sympathetic ganglia and unrelated to specific synaptic GABA ergic transmission (Matthews & Roberts (2), de Groat (3), Bowery & Brown (4). Alternatively it is possible that the effects of exogenous GABA on gut motility do to some extent reflect stimulation of GABA ergic enteric pathways. Because of this difficulty, experiments involving the blockade by GABA antagonists of endogenous GABA activity may be more useful in unravelling the function of enteric GABA ergic synapses. Such studies, although only preliminary, suggest that a GABA ergic link may be specifically involved in some, but not all, intestinal motility reflexes (Krantis (42), Krantis *et al.* (24)).

The enteric GABA neurons appear to send their axons into the axon bundles which lie inside the intestinal muscle coat. Such bundles are characteristic of the innervation of gut muscle, where single nerve fibers are hardly ever found. In these nerves vesicle filled varicosities, which are the presumed transmitter-releasing sites, are found not only in axons lying at the surface of the bundles, facing the muscle, but also in fibers lying well inside the bundles, where they are in close proximity to other nerve fibers (Gabella (28)). It has been suggested that the significance of this arrangement may lie in the opportunity it provides for presynaptic modulation of enteric neuro-muscular transmission (Jessen *et al.* (43)). This might explain the presence of nerve fibers inside these bundles containing putative transmitters which are known not to affect the muscle directly, but do influence the release of other enteric transmitters, as appear to be the case for enkephalin-containing fibers in nerves inside the longitudinal muscle of the guinea pig taenia coli (Coocks & Burnstock (44), Jessen *et al.* (43)). GABA does not appear to have any direct effect on the contractile state of gut musculature, while it has been widely implicated as a presynaptic modulator of transmitter release in the central nervous system, e.g. from substance-P containing terminals in the substantia nigra and from the primary afferent terminals of sensory neurons in the spinal cord (for reviews see Levy (45), Vizi (46)). Since GABA ergic fibers are present within axon bundles in intestinal muscle, it is worth investigating whether the putative GABA ergic neurons in the gut might act by modulating presynaptically the release of neuro-muscular transmitters from intestinal nerves.

References

1. Hobbiger, F., 1958. J. Physiol. 142: 147–164.
2. Matthews, R. J. & Roberts, B. J., 1961. J. Pharmacol. Exptl. Ther. 132: 19–22.
3. de Groat, W., 1970. J. Pharmac. Exptl. Ther. 172: 384–396.
4. Bowery, N. G. & Brown, D. A., 1974. Br. J. Pharmac. 50: 205–218.
5. Young, J. A. C., Brown, D. A., Kelly, J. S. & Schon, F., 1973. Brain Res. 63: 479–486.
6. Schon, F. & Kelly, J. S., 1974. Brain Res. 66: 275–288.
7. Schon, F. & Kelly, J. S., 1974. Brain Res. 66: 289–300.
8. Beart, P. M., Kelly, J. S. & Schon, F., 1974. Biochem. Soc. Trans. 2: 266–268.
9. Kanazawa, I., Iversen, L. L. & Kelly, J. S., 1976. J. Neurochem. 27: 1267–1269.
10. Osborne, N. N., Wu, P. H. & Neuhoff, V., 1974. Brain Res. 74: 175–181.
11. Bertilson, L., Suria, A. & Costa, E., 1976. Nature 260: 540–541.
12. Iversen, L. L. & Kelly, J. S., 1975. Biochem. Pharmacol. 24: 933–938.
13. Roberts, E., Chase, T. N. & Tower, D. B. (eds.), 1976. GABA in Nervous System Function, Raven press, New York.
14. Nistri, A. & Constanti, A., 1979. Prog. Neurobiol. 13: 117–235.
15. Langley, J. N., 1921. The Autonomic Nervous System Part 1. Heffer, London.
16. Gabella, G., 1976. Structure of the Autonomic Nervous System. Chapman & Hall, London.
17. Wood, J. D., 1979. Integrative Functions of the Autonomic Nervous System (Brooks, McC., Koizumi, K. & Sato, A., eds.), pp. 177–193, University of Tokyo Press.
18. Furness, J. B. & Costa, M., 1980. Neurosci. 5: 1–20.
19. Burnstock, G. & Hökfelt, T., 1979. Neurosci. Res. progr. Bull. 17: 379–519.
20. Hobbiger, F., 1958. J. Physiol. 144: 349–360.
21. Florey, E. & McLennan, H., 1959. J. Physiol. 145: 66–76.
22. Inouye, A., Fukuda, M., Tsuchiya, K. & Tsujioka, T., 1960. Jap. J. Physiol. 10: 167–182.
23. De Feudis, F. V., 1977. Progr. Neurobiol. 9: 123–145.
24. Krantis, A., Costa, M., Furness, J. B. & Orbach, J., 1980. Eur. J. Pharmacol. 67: 461–468.
25. Rikimaru, A. & Suzuki, R., 1971. Tohoku J. Exp. Med. 103: 303–310.
26. Ishizawa, M. & Pickles, V. R., 1975. Br. J. Pharmacol. 54: 279P.
27. Graefe, P., Galvan, M. & Mayer, C., 1979. Eur. J. Physiol. 382: R44.
28. Gabella, G., 1979. Intern. Rev. Cytol. 59: 129–193.
29. Jessen, K. R., Mirsky, R., Dennison, M. E. & Burnstock, G., 1979. Nature 281: 71–74.
30. Jessen, K. R., McConnell, J. D., Purves, R. D., Burnstock, G. & Chamley-Campbell, J., 1978. Brain Res. 152: 573–579.
31. Bowery, N. G., Jones, G. P. & Neal, M. J., 1976. Nature 264: 281–284.
32. Krantis, A., 1980. Proc. Austral. Physiol. Pharmacol. Soc. 11: 134P.
33. Brandon, C., Lam, D. M. K. & Wu, J., 1979. Proc. Natl. Acad. Sci. USA 76: 3557–3561.
34. Farb, D. H., Berg, D. K. & Fischbach, G. D., 1979. J. Cell Biol. 80: 651–661.
35. Iversen, L. L. & Bloom, F. E., 1972. Brain Res. 41: 131–143.
36. Sotelo, C., Privat, A. & Drain, M. J., 1972. Brain Res. 45: 302–308.
37. Schon, F. & Iversen, L. L., 1974. Life Sci. 15: 157–175.
38. Lasher, R. S., 1974. Brain Res. 69: 235–254.
39. White, W. F., Snodgrass, S. R. & Dichter, M., 1980. Brain Res. 190: 139–152.
40. Barber, R. P. & Saito, K., 1976. In: GABA in Nervous System Function (Roberts, E., Chase, T. N. & Tower, D. B., eds.), pp. 113–132. Raven Press, New York.

41. Wood, J. G., McLaughlin, B. J. & Vaughn, J. E., 1976. In: GABA in Nervous System Function (Roberts, E., Chase, T. N. & Tower, D. B., eds.), pp. 133–148, Raven Press, New York.

42. Krantis, A., 1979. Proc. Austral. Physiol. Pharmacol. Soc. 10: 290P.

43. Jessen, K. R., Saffrey, M. J., Van Noorden, S., Bloom, S. R., Polak, J. M. & Burnstock, G., 1980. Neurosci. 5: 1717–1735.

44. Coocks, T. & Burnstock, G., 1979. Eur. J. Pharmacol. 54: 251–259.

45. Levy, R. A., 1977. Progr. Neurobiol. 9: 211–267.

46. Vizi, E. S., 1979. Progr. Neurobiol. 12: 181–290.

Received December 22, 1980.

Post-translational carboxylation of preprothrombin

B. Connor Johnson, Ph. D.
Oklahoma Medical Research Foundation and The University of Oklahoma Health Sciences Center, Dept. of Biochemistry and Molecular Biology, Oklahoma City, OK 73104, U.S.A.

Contents

Molecular and Cellular Biochemistry 38, 77–121 (1981).   0300–8177/81/0381–0077/$ 9.00.
© 1981, Martinus Nijhoff/Dr. W. Junk Publishers, The Hague.

80

I. Introduction

The determination of the sites of possible regulation in the formation of an active enzyme protein was only possible after the overall pathway of active enzyme synthesis had been established. Regulation may be via the triplet code at the genetic transcription level, or at the translation level from messenger RNA to protein or at a post-translational level via chemical modification and/or polypeptide aggregation. The fact that the role of vitamin K in the formation of the normally pro-active forms of the coagulation proteins (II, VII, IX, and X) was post-translational was shown by Goswami and Munro (1) in 1962, and further confirmed by Hill, et al. (2), Babior (3), Lowenthal and Simmons (4), Ranhotra, et al. (5), and Shah and Suttie (6). In these studies total enzyme activity (prothrombin) recovery in vivo was obtained following administration of vitamin K to vitamin K deficient (7, 8) rats which had received protein synthesis blocking agents. R. E. Olson, et al. (9–12) stated that vitamin K functioned in prothrombin synthesis at a genetic or translation level on the basis of no response to the vitamin after synthesis of protein was inhibited. This, however, became untenable with the finding of carboxylation as the vitamin K dependent step (13–16) in prothrombin 'completion.'

II. The current status of post-translational carboxylation

1. A brief history of vitamin K

a. Discovery

Henrick Dam (17, 18) while investigating the cardiovascular effects of cholesterol-free diets, discovered vitamin K in 1929 as a dietary requirement for normal blood clotting in chicks. The nutritional hemorrhagic disease in chicks was reported by McFarlane, et al. (19) in 1930, and by Holst and Holbrook (20) in 1933. Both Dam (21, 22) and Almquist (23, 24) reported independently that this disease was due to the lack of a new fat-soluble vitamin and Dam proposed the name vitamin K (25, 26) (K for Koagulation). The coagulation defect was shown by Schoenheyder to be due to a lack of prothrombin activity in the blood (27). The vitamin was isolated in 1939 by Dam, et al. (28) from alfalfa and from putrified fish meal by Doisey's group (29). In the same year Almquist and Klose (30) found that phthiocol had vitamin K activity and Ansbacher and Fernholz (31) found the very high activity of 2-methyl-1,4-naphthoquinone. With this information available vitamin K_1 (from alfalfa) was characterized in Doisey's laboratory as 2-methyl-3-phytyl-1,4-naphthoquinone (32). A review of the isolation of vitamin K appeared in 1971 (33).

b. Synthesis

The vitamin was synthesized independently by Karrer, et al. (34), Almquist and Klose (35) and Fieser (36, 37) in 1939. The structure of vitamin K_2 (from putrified fish meal) was published by Doisey's group the next year (38). A review of vitamin K synthesis has been published (39).

c. Structural specificity in nutrition

With these structures known it was possible to systematically examine the specificity of structural requirements for vitamin K activity when the compound was fed to deficient chicks. This was thoroughly done by Fieser, et al. (40) and later further data on structural requirements was published by Isler, et al. (41, 42), Weber and Wiss (43), Pennock (44), Griminger (45), Dunphy and Brodie (46), and many others.

The structure of vitamin K_1 or phylloquinone is:

This compound, 2-methyl-3-phytyl-1,4-naphthoquinone is the form of vitamin K originally isolated from alfalfa. As it occurs naturally the β,γ double bound is in the trans configuration.

The structure of vitamin K_2 and the menaquinones is:

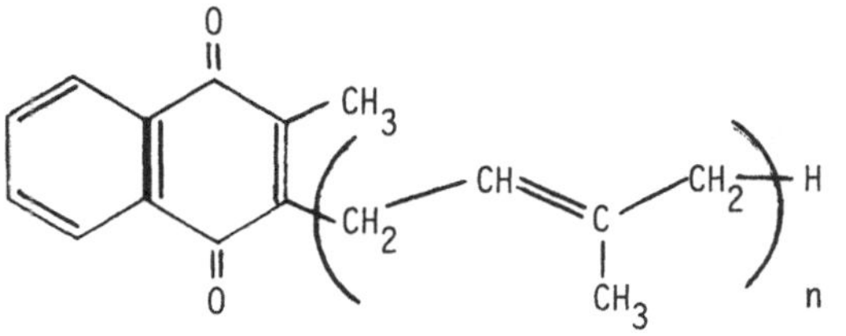

n = 1 to 14

The menaquinones are in general derivatives of 2-methyl-1,4-naphthoquinone which have an unsaturated side-chain of variable length containing 5 to 70 carbon atoms at position three. The compound isolated originally from putrified fish meal was a menaquinone, shown by Isler, et al. (41) to be menaquinone-7 (i.e. n = 7). This series of compounds has been designated (IUPAC) by the term MK plus the number of isoprene units in the side-chain, thus in this case MK-7. In general the menaquinones are made in bacteria, where the most common bacterial form is MK-8, while phylloquinone (vitamin K_1) is made by higher plants. Many modified forms occur in various microorganisms.

Since the intact animal uses equally well menadione (2-methyl-1,4-naphthoquinone) or vitamin K_1 it appears that the isoprenoid side chain at position three can be made by the animal. However, the principle form made under these conditions is not known. Matschiner and co-workers have found in bovine liver primarily MK-9 to MK-12 and the 2,3-epoxides (47–49) and principally MK-4 in rat liver (58). Martius, et al. also report MK-4 (51–53) in the liver. Dialameh, et al. have reported the enzymatic alkylation of menadione to menaquinones by microsomes from chicken liver (54). They found that the menaquinone homologue synthesized dependend on the isoprenyl pyrophosphate available.

One of the most commercially useful water soluble compounds has been the bisulfite addition product whose structure (55, 56) is:

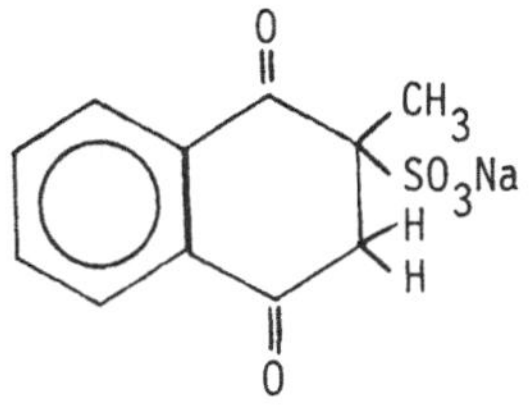

Another water soluble vitamin K compound is the tetrasodium salt of the diphosphate ester of menadione hydroquinone (57).

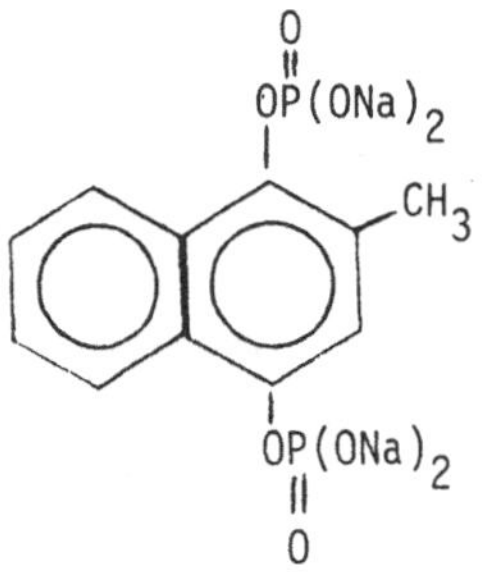

While menadione and vitamin K_1 are equally active on a molar basis when fed to vitamin K-deficient chicks (40), when various vitamin K analogs were given by intracardial injection into vitamin K-deficient rats, MK-9 was the most active compound found, being 25 × as active as vitamin K_1 (58). Menadione was still active but at a much slower rate which could indicate that conversion of menadione to forms with a side chain in position 3 is necessary for function in vivo. The addition of the side chain may be made by bacteria of the intestinal tract and in the body. The conversion of menadione has been demonstrated in vivo in the rat where 18 h after ^{3}H-menadione administration the label was found in MK-4 (58) in all tissues examine. Vitamin K_1 yields similar results (59). Similar results are also reported for the dog (60).

d. Functions proposed prior to 1974

The original overall function of vitamin K was shown to be in the formation of the blood coagulation protein prothrombin (27). Later it was found that there were four vitamin K-dependent blood coagulation proteins – Factor II – prothrombin, Factor VII – proconvertin, Factor IX – Christmas factor and Factor X – Stuart factor (61–68). Other functions proposed for vitamin K included, in particular, mitochondrial respiration and oxidative-phosphorylation (69–73).

Many mechanistic papers on the role of the transfer of phosphate by 3-ring chromanol derivatives of vitamin K appeared between 1958 and 1968 (e.g., 74–82). Vitamin K has also been studied with regard to general protein synthesis following Martius, et al.'s postulation (83) that the reason for the failure of formation of prothrombin, etc., was due to failure to form ATP with the coagulation proteins being the first to show the deficiency in protein synthesis due to the lack of ATP.

Amino acid incorporation experiments and experiments on the effect of severe vitamin K deficiency in various species showed no effect either on total protein synthesis (2, 84, 85) nor on oxidative phosphorylation in the animal (86–88).

Other vitamin K function proposals have included glycosylation of prothrombin and other vitamin K dependent blood coagulation proteins (89–92), although removal of carbohydrate moieties from prothrombin does not affect its ability to be activated to thrombin (93, 94) as does vitamin K deficiency. Sloane (95) has proposed hydroxylation as a role for vitamin K. At the molecular level this may turn out to be the same role as that involved in protein carboxylation, i.e., oxidation to remove a hydrogen. Lev and Milford have reported that in bacteria vitamin K stimulates sphingolipid synthesis (96) while Brodie, et al. (46, 97) using *M. phlei* have indicated that the role of vitamin K is in oxidative phoshorylation.

2. 1974 – year of discovery

a. Post-translational modification

One line of evidence that the role of vitamin K in the formation of the blood clotting proteins was post-translational was the non-inhibitory effect of protein synthesis blocking agents in vivo on the response of the animal to vitamin K (2, 4, 98) and the in vitro formation of prothrombin non-protein synthesizing liver homogenates (1) or cell cultures (3); containing protein-synthesis antagonists (3, 5).

b. Early antibody research

During the time that the work referred to in section ld was being carried out, data using prothrombin fluorescent-antibody indicated a rapid prothrombin formation response to vitamin K by the liver hepatocyte (99, 100). This was taken as implying that vitamin K was inducing synthesis and thus, that there was no inactive precursor present since if there were it should have also reacted with prothrombin antibody. However, a number of papers have appeared since 1968 showing that a prothrombin precursor demonstrable by prothrombin antibody (101–104), is present in liver and blood of vitamin K deficient animals. These results are in complete agreement with those of section 2a above and 2c below and is further discussed under section 16.

c. Discovery of 'abnormal' prothrombin

While a number of inherited altered prothrombins which are nonfunctional due to genetic mutations are known, we will use here the term 'abnormal prothrombin' to refer only to isoprothrombin, warfarin prothrombin, dicoumarol prothrombin, PIVKA II, decarboxyprothrombin precursor, etc.; that is the moral prothrombin polypeptide chain which has not undergone the vitamin K dependent post-translational modification. The existence of such an abnormal prothrombin was first reported by Hemker's laboratory at Leiden in 1963 (105). He reported that under conditions of vitamin K deficiency or following administration of a vitamin K antagonist, plasma contained an anomalous prothrombin-like protein which they postulated to be a prothrombin precursor and termed PIVKA. They later reported similar abnormal proteins (PIVKA, VII, PIVKA IX, and PIVKA X on the basis of immunological techniques (106–109).

Suttie's group (6, 110) showed that bovine dicoumarol-prothrombin has a lower calcium binding affinity than does 'completed' prothrombin and they purified this inactive prothrombin from the plasma of dicoumarol-treated cows (111). In addition to being non-activatable by the usual prothrombin-assay (i.e., factor Xa + factor V + phospholipid) and having a lower calcium-binding activity this abnormal prothrombin is not adsorbed onto barium salts and all three differences are due to lack of the vitamin K dependent completion step (111). Sonicated liver microsomes prepared from vitamin K deficient rats contain a protein which liberates thrombin activity when incubated with *Echis carinatus* venom (112) and is thus presumably the prothrombin precursor protein found by the earlier immunological procedures by Ganrot and

Nilehen (102), Hemker, et al. (113), Josso, et al. (103), Stenflo (104), Schieck, et al. (114), Malhotra (115), Denson (116), and others, and which is synthesized in the liver independently of vitamin K. This prothrombin precursor-abnormal prothrombin has been studied quite extensively, including its purification (117, 118) not only from bovine but also from rat (119) and human liver (120, 121) and from bovine blood (122). It has subsequently been shown that there are at least two forms of the rat liver prothrombin precursor with pI's of 5.8 and 7.2 (123). Abnormal prothrombin also shows differences to prothrombin in phospholipid binding (124). It has been found in bovine, human, chick, rat and mouse plasma and in the liver microsomes of rats, mice, guinea pigs, hamsters, rabbits, dogs and chickens but not the bovine (125).

d. Demonstration of in vivo vitamin K-dependent carboxylation of prothrombin in vitamin K-deficient rats

Eventually in 1974 the different lines of study regarding the function of vitamin K were resolved totally independently in three different laboratories. Based on the finding that the finalization of clotting factors by liver cells (126) was dependent upon the presence of bicarbonate (127) we demonstrated in vivo that the completion step in vitamin K-dependent prothrombin formation was carboxylation (13). This new reaction, protein carboxylation, occurred on glutamyl residues.

For perhaps six months we 'rejoiced' in the thought that we alone knew that the 'strange' role of vitamin K in clotting protein formation was the post-translational carboxylation of a preformed polypeptide. As in many cases our excitement was soon dampened by the finding that 1974 was in fact the year of discovery and two other widely separated laboratories had made the same discovery by totally different means. In fact, at the time of the FEBS meeting in Budapest we found that not only had the discovery been made in two other laboratories but that the work showing which glutamyl residues in bovine prothrombin were carboxylated had already been done. So let us return now to these elegant and essentially simultaneous discoveries. In all cases the work was based logically on the previous work of the various laboratories.

e. Proof of carboxylation by chemical characterization of the product

Stenflo at Lund had shown an abnormal prothrombin by antibody cross-reaction (104) and proceeded to determine the difference between normal and abnormal prothrombin. He found in 1973 (128) that an amino terminal fragment of approximately 27 000 MW prepared from purified normal prothrombin had an identical amino acid and carbohydrate composition to the same fragment prepared from dicoumarol-prothrombin. However, the fragment from normal prothrombin had Ca^{2+}-dependent antigenic determinants missing in the fragment from dicoumarol-prothrombin. In peptide maps the difference between normal and dicoumarol-prothrombins was clearly shown in thermolysin digests of the amino-terminal fragments. The definitive work of this group isolated a calcium binding tetrapeptide consisting of residues 6 to 9 from the amino terminal end of normal prothrombin (14). They showed on the basis of NMR spectroscopy and by mass spectrometry that this tetrapeptide contained two residues of a new modified glutamic acid, γ-carboxyglutamic acid. Abnormal dicoumarol administration lacked the modified amino acid residues in positions 7 and 8.

Similarly, Nelsestuen and Suttie (129) had isolated in 1973 an unusual tryptic peptide from normal prothrombin and had shown it to contain part of the vitamin K-dependent region. In 1974 Nelsestuen, et al. (15) isolated from proteolytic digests of this 'vitamin K-dependent peptide', a modified glutamylserine dipeptide and characterized it as a peptide of serine plus γ-carboxyglutamic acid. They thus showed that the incorporation of the γ-carboxyl group is dependent on vitamin K.

f. Structure of carboxylated glutamic acid

The structure of this derivative was shown by Stenflo, et al. (128) and Nelsestuen, et al. (15) on the basis of mass spectra and NMR analysis to be:

$$H_2N - CH - COOH$$
$$|$$
$$CH_2$$
$$|$$
$$CH$$
$$\diagup \quad \diagdown$$
$$COOH \quad COOH$$

a malonic acid derivative. This is a rather unstable structure and heating in acidic solution will regenerate glutamic acid. The two γ-carboxyls appear equal and 1/2 the ^{14}C-label incorporated in ^{14}C-bicarbonate incorporation experiments reported above is lost on acid hydrolysis.

3. Carboxylation of vitamin K-dependent proteins by various in vitro systems

a. Liver microsomes

Once the step in the vitamin K-dependent completion of prothrombin and presumably other similarly dependent proteins was known to be protein carboxylation, methods were found for carrying on the reaction in vitro. Shah and Suttie (130) had already shown that post-mitochondrial supernates from vitamin K deficient rats produce prothrombin when vitamin K is added in vitro. This prothrombin production, as in vivo, was not affected by addition of cycloheximide. This pushed the research another step beyond that of Chung (127) who had added the vitamin K to the animal prior to killing rather than to a liver homogenate preparation.

This in vitro prothrombin formation and the knowledge that the reaction of vitamin K was protein carboxylation led rapidly to the establishment of vitamin K-dependent microsomal, cell-free, carboxylation systems (131–133). These in vitro systems employed microsomes from the livers of vitamin K-deficient rats plus ^{14}C-NaHCO$_3$, vitamin K$_1$ and NADH and were carried out in air. Detailed conditions for the reaction are described in part III.

b. Solubilization of carboxylation system

We found that this microsomal enzyme complex system could be 'solubilized' (extracted) from the vitamin K-deficient microsomes by various detergents such as Triton X100, Lubrol PX, sodium deoxycholate, etc. (134, 135). A number of different detergents have been successfully used over the past five years. A very similar procedure was later published by Esmon and Suttie (136).

c. Microsomal carboxylation systems from other species

Using fractionated bovine liver Vermeer, et al.

(137) have developed an in vitro cell-free prothrombin carboxylation system. This system is very interesting in that it appears to have a much longer time course than the rat microsomal carboxylation. Bovine liver microsomes were shown to contain inhibitor activity which must first be eliminated. Similar inhibitors apparently also exist in rat microsomes but do not prevent the reaction. In 1977 Lowenthal and Jaeger (138) reported a cell-free system from rat liver which made clotting factors in response to vitamin K and in 1978 Garvey and Olson (139) carried out the in vitro reation in chick liver.

d. Cell culture, vitamin K-dependent systems

A cell culture system for vitamin K-dependent protein carboxylation was developed by Munns, et al. (140) using cultured H-35 hepatoma cells. Prothrombin synthesis was demonstrated by radioimmunoassay and selective barium salt adsorption to separate carboxylated (normal) prothrombin from non-carboxylated precursor. Like the perfused liver synthesis of prothrombin carried out by J. P. Olson, et al. (141) the hepatoma cells would synthesize precursor in the absence of vitamin K and normal (i.e., carboxylated) prothrombin in its presence.

Poggi, et al. (142) showed with Lewis lung carcinoma cell cultures that addition of warfarin to the cell culture lowered factor X activating activity. Oesterud, et al. (143) have shown that macrophages also produce the blood coagulation factors.

e. ATP-biotin requirements

As the protein carboxylation system was being developed, several requirements were proposed. These included NADH, ATP, biotin, oxygen, polypeptide substrate from the microsomes and a CO$_2$ source. NADH and oxygen will be discussed in more detail later, however, ATP plus its generating system and biotin can be dealt with at this time. The ATP response turned out to be primarily a response to the salt of the generating system. The optimum level for the Triton X100 solubilized system appears to be approximately 200 mM with NaCl and Na phosphate possessing equal activity (134). In addition adenine and various adenine nucleotides appear to have a protective effect (about 20%) greater stability) on the enzyme system (144).

There is no requirement for ATP as a chemical

energy source, the energy for the reaction being provided by the oxidation of the reduced form of vitamin K.

Historically carboxylation in animals has been an ATP plus biotin catalyzed reaction, however, all attempts to show an effect of biotin, for example, biotin deficiency, or the in vitro addition of avidin have not shown any biotin involvement in the reaction (132, 145, 146). As early as 1973 Petrelli and Marsili (147) had shown that biotin deficiency with adequate vitamin K in the diet did not affect prothrombin activity levels.

f. Vitamin K and protein carboxylation

All of us involved in the discovery of protein carboxylation as the vitamin K-dependent step in prothrombin completion feel, I am sure, real satisfaction in the agreement among all the research groups. The function discovered in 1974 was the same in all laboratories and now six years later is a part of textbook nutrition and biochemistry.

4. Prothrombin structure and structure of other vitamin K-dependent blood clotting proteins

The work of Magnusson, et al. (148) in 1974 immediately added immensely to this feeling of gratification of an important breakthrough – the function of one more vitamin accounted for! Magnusson, et al. (148), who had already sequenced thrombin, elucidated the primary structure of the vitamin K-dependent part of prothrombin. His laboratory showed that all ten of the first glutamyl residues of prothrombin were actually γ-carboxy-glutamyl (gla) residues.

5. Vitamin K quinone versus hydroquinone

While the oral form of vitamin K is the quinone, pimarily due to the instability of the hydroquinone, the finding that for either particulate microsomes or detergent solubilized microsomes to operate with anything like optimum efficiency NADH (or NADPH) was also needed, immediately pointed to the probability that the functional form used in the carboxylation reaction was the reduced hydroquinone (or a semiquinone) form. This was demonstrated by at least three laboratories independently (136, 149, 150). All three papers were received in March or April 1976.

With requirements for oxygen (see Section 6) and vitamin K hydroquinone established as initiator of the reaction, this indicated a new mixed function type of reaction. One of the first questions considered was whether vitamin K semiquinone would replace vitamin K hydroquinone + oxygen just as the hydroquinone replaced the quinone plus NADPH. However, when semiquinone was made and identified by its ESR spectrum (151), it was found that it like the hydroquinone would not function in the absence of oxygen (152, page 205). This meant that the obligatory presence of oxygen was not to convert hydroquinone to some intermediate state between quinone and hydroquinone, however, it still left open the possibility that the semiquinone could be as functional as the hydroquinone. However, semiquinone would probably lead immediately to formation of a charge transfer complex, thus providing plenty of hydroquinone for the reaction. Since the various intermediate oxidation forms between the hydroquinone and the quinone are so fleeting, so unstable, we use vitamin K hydroquinone as the compound of preference in carrying out the in vitro carboxylation reaction.

6. Requirements and conditions for the solubilized liver microsomal vitamin K-dependent carboxylation

a. Liver microsomes

For rat liver the microsomal preparation is best prepared from vitamin K deficient rats, however, an entirely functional preparation can be made from the livers of warfarin treated animals. These preparations contain both the carboxylase system and the endogenous polypeptide substrates. To date it has not been found feasible to isolate exogenous preprothrombin protein add it to the solubilized rat liver carboxylation system and obtain significant vitamin K-dependent carboxylation of it.

In the bovine liver system Veermer, et al. (153) have been able to add back separately purified decarboxyprothrombin obtained from coumarin-treated cows, and find increased prothrombin formation (154). The course of the reaction is very slow (2 to 3 h) as compared to the rat liver microsomal solubilized carboxylation system (2 to 3 min.) at 37° and the relationship between the two has not been established. Shah and Suttie (155) have compared the vitamin K-dependent carboxylation of endogenous precursor present in liver microsomes from eight species after warfarin treatment, and in the case of the rat and hamster also in vitamin K-deficient animals. The most active preparations were obtained from the livers of vitamin K deficient warfarin-resistant rats. The vitamin K-dependent protein carboxylase reaction has been confirmed by Zurbin in Kiev (169).

b. CO_2

A source of carbon dioxide or bicarbonate is required for the reaction and Jones, et al. (156), have shown that the active species is CO_2 rather than HCO_3^-.

c. pH optimum

The reaction proceeds very well at all pH's between 7 and 8 and falls off rapidly above 8 and below 7. The optimum is approximately pH 7.4 (134, 157, 158).

d. Temperature

While the original in vitro solubilized vitamin K-deficient liver microsomal carboxylation systems were run at 37° the enzymatic reaction can satisfactorily be carried out at temperatures from 0° to 37° and many different temperatures have been used. Maximum carboxylation occurs in the range 20° to 25°. At 37° the reaction system is completely inactivated after about 2 min and results in about 1/2 the carboxylation obtained at 20°. At 0° the reaction continues linearly for about 2 h, eventually reaching values approaching those obtained at 37° (see for example – fig. 4 reference 159).

e. Oxygen

Probably the most interesting current aspect of this vitamin K-dependent carboxylation is the mixed-function nature of the reaction in which both a reducing compound (the naphthohydroquinone) and oxygen are required. Total omission of either one completely blocks the reaction. The oxygen requirement was shown by Esmon and Suttie (136) for the reaction initiated by vitamin K and NADH and also for the reaction initiated by vitamin K hydroquinone. The former reaction appears more sensitive to oxygen lack than is the latter which may indicate an oxygen function in phylloquinone reductase as well as in protein

carboxylase (150) or merely that in the crude system being (160) used NADH plus oxygen carries out many reactions not related to vitamin K hydroquinone. The role of oxygen does not appear to be replaceable by other types of oxidant since neither FAD, ferricyanide nor H_2O_2 will replace molecular oxygen (152, 161).

During the carboxylation incubation the major metabolite of vitamin K formed is vitamin K-2,3-epoxide (162). However, the question of whether the reaction is, in fact, an oxidative carboxylation in which there is a coupled reaction analogous to oxidative phosphorylation has not been solved despite the efforts of many laboratories. (This is discussed more fully in section 23).

f. Hydroquinones

A review of hydroquinone dehydrogenases was published by Crane (163), however, it is essentially devoted to ubiquinone hydroquinone and does not discuss the various oxidation forms of vitamin K hydroquinone. Of more interest is the series of papers by Weissberger, et al. (e.g., 164, 165, 166) on the auto oxidation of hydroquinones. These workers point out that, in general, the oxidation of hydroquinones procedes in univalent steps and that the intermediate semiquinones are in equilibrium with reduced and oxidized forms and their dimers. Their overall reaction produces $O_2^=$ anion which will then produce, O_2^- superoxide radical, or H_2O_2. As will be discussed later under *Mechanisms proposed* (Sect. 12), we have shown that H_2O_2 will not substitute for vitamin K hydroquinones plus oxygen (277), however, it has been postulated that $O_2^=$ anion may be able to remove the γ-hydrogen from stabilized glutamyl residues (279). Whether charge-transfer complexes are involved is still an area of conjecture. Wallin (167) has reported that there is no strict coupling of vitamin K dependent carboxylation and epoxidation of vitamin K.

Further study of the carboxylation system has not added additional requirements unless possibly a role for manganese which could logically be a possible oxygen 'activator-carrier', however, the amount required appears inordinately high (10 mM) (168).

7. Other vitamin K-dependent proteins

a. Blood proteins in addition to the well established vitamin K-dependent clotting factors II, VII, IX and X

While prothrombin and clotting factor proteins VII, IX, and X have long been established as vitamin K-dependent, other gla-containing proteins have now been reported in blood. These include protein C found by Stenflo in bovine plasma in 1976 (171) and confirmed by Kisiel, et al. in the same year (172). It is a glycoprotein composed of a heavy chain (MW 41 000) and a light chain (MW 21 000) held together by disulfide bonding (173). Davie's group have reported isolation of a fifth vitamin K-dependent (i.e., gla-containing) protein (protein S) from human plasma (174). A possible sixth vitamin K dependent protein in bovine plasma is Protein Z reported by Prowse and Esnouf (175). Seegers, et al. (176) have proposed a blood protein M which they postulate may also be vitamin K-dependent. It is possible that this is the same protein as the humoral factors proposed by Trauber, et al. (177) and by Shah, et al. (178). The homology of the new proteins C, S, and Z with the previously known gla-containing plasma proteins will be reviewed in section 8.

b. Osteocalcin, a bone protein

Hauschka, Lian and Gallop (179) have identified a non-blood plasma gla-containing protein in proteins solubilized from chicken bone. The same protein was found independently by Price and co-workers in bovine calcified tissue (180–181) and shown to contain 3 gla residues in a small (6800 M.W.) protein. The properties of this protein called osteocalcin have been presented by Lian, et al. (182) as well as its in vitro carboxylation by bone microsomes (183–185). Hauschka, et al. (186–188) have shown that the protein appears in embryonic chick bone at the same time as the first deposition of bone mineral 8 to 12 days after fertilization and increases markedly in quantity during bone development. The ability of bone gla-protein to inhibit hydroxyapatite crystallization is lost if the osteocalcin is decarboxylated (see below) indicating that it is the gla-region which associates with mineral (189, 190). γ-Carboxyglutamyl residues have been found in calcified turkey tendon but not in uncalcified tendon (191), while present in the collagenous proteins of bovine cementum (192). Price, et al. (193) have shown that fetal rat bone contains less than 0.1% of the adult rats level of extractable gla-containing protein of bone, however, the fetal rat bone does contain 30% of the adult level of gla but the gla-protein is not extracted during demineralization and may differ from the adult bone protein.

In a survey of various species, King (194) has shown that gla is not detectable in the calcified skeletons of six invertebrate species and he raises the possibility that invertebrates lack the carboxylase enzyme. He has found gla-proteins in shark tooth and aragonitic fish otolith.

Price and Baukol (195) have evidence that the vitamin K carboxylated protein of rat osteosarcoma cells in culture responds with a six fold rise to the administration of 1,25-dihydroxyvitamin D_3 added at less than 1 ng/ml. This appears to be a specific effect of the vitamin D compound in that there is no change in total protein synthesis by these cells. This makes a very interesting connection between two vitamins and calcium (all requires nutrients).

c. Atherocalcin

Lian, et al. (196) have found gla-proteins in calcified skin, calcified atheromatous plaques from aorta and in other ectopic calcification proteins. Acid proteins, which may be the same proteins, have been found in atheromatous plaque by Keeley (197). Is this finding related to the report by Sharaev and Bogdanov of a reduction in total glycosaminoglycans in the aortic walls of vitamin K-deficient rats (198)?

The gla-protein from human atherosclerotic plaque has been purified and named atherocalcin (199). The protein is not present in the normal aorta wall nor the pre-atherosclerotic fatty streak but increases dramatically with calcification. The protein has a molecular weight of approximately 80 000, 16 gla residues/molecule and is different from other known gla-proteins. On the other hand, Deyl, et al. (200) report that the gla-protein of rat atheromatous plaque has the same amino acid make-up as osteocalcin and essentially the same as the gla-protein of turkey tibial tendon.

Two applied studies show this calcification by a gla-protein to be of practical significance. Levy, et al. (201) have studied the pathogenesis of valvar calcification and report increased acidic proteins with increases in valvar calcification. Pierce, et al. (202) report calcification inside artificial hearts and its inhibition by warfarin. Sharaev, et al. have found that the mechanical properties of the aorta are related to the vitamin K supply (203).

d. Chorioallantoic membrane

Tuan, et al. (204) have reported the purification of the calcium binding protein of the chorioallantoic membrane of the chick embryo. This protein is composed of four subunits of identical molecular weight (22 000–25 000) and contains γ-carboxyglutamic acid whose formation required vitamin K and was blocked by warfarin (205). While the number of gla-residues in the protein remains uncertain (2 to 10) the membrane does contain vitamin K-dependent carboxylase (206).

In addition to this membrane protein the suggestion has been made that there is an effect of vitamin K on the protein of rat erythrocyte membrane (207).

e. Kidney proteins

Hauschka, et al. (208) in 1976 identified gla as a constituent of renal tissue in chicken, rat, and rabbit. The gla-protein is not a blood protein and appears to be located in the cortex. The authors also demonstrated vitamin K dependent post-translational glutamyl carboxylation in vitro by kidney microsomes. Griep and Friedman (209) have isolated a gla-protein from kidney and shown it to be different from blood proteins or osteocalcin. It contains 26 gla residues/1000 amino acids while bone contains about 50 (3/molecule). At the same time Buchthal and Bell (210) have found vitamin K-dependent protein-carboxylation in both kidney and spleen.

Renal calculi also contain a gla-protein (211). This protein has a molecular weight of about 17 000, contains about 40 gla residues/1000 amino acids and is different from both the kidney gla-protein and osteocalcin.

A gla-protein has been reported in the urine by Fernlund (212) but whether it is related to the gla-protein of the kidney has not been established.

f. Ovocalcin

Krampitz, et al. (213) have recently reported that chicken egg shells also contain a gla-protein which they have named ovocalcin. It has an apparent molecular weight of about 2500. An apparently related protein has been reported in oyster shells (214).

g. Lung

Bell (215) has reported vitamin K-dependent carboxylation by lung microsomes.

h. Placenta

Friedman, et al. (216) have similarly found the vitamin K-dependent carboxylating system in human placenta.

i. Tumor cells

We have found that at least some tumor cell lines contain gla-proteins (217–220) and this lends some credence to the rather numerous suggestions that vitamin K antagonists may be able to influence tumor metastasis perhaps by preventing cell membrane protein carboxylation and, hence, cell lodgement (221–227).

j. Microsomal proteins

Gla-proteins have now been found among the proteins of mammalian ribosomes (228–230). The amounts are small per total microsomal protein (6–10 gla-residues/1000 amino acids).

Similarly, gla-proteins have been found in bacteria (R. Delaney, unpublished data), and Lee and Brodie (231) have shown that E. coli ribosomes will carry out vitamin K-dependent protein carboxylation. Interestingly, as Dallam has shown when studying oxidative phosphorylation in bacteria (82) the vitamin K content can be destroyed by irradiation and in this work the carboxylation reaction could be inhibited both by warfarin treatment and by irradiation.

8. The functional significance of the post-translational vitamin K-dependent protein carboxylation

As was originally suggested by Esmon, et al. (124) the carboxylation converts a gene-product polypeptide into a protein which can also bind calcium and phospholipid. These properties of carboxylated proteins have been studied particularly by Nelsestuen and co-workers (110, 232–235) who have reported that the calcium-dependent

Table 1. Structure of vitamin K-dependent region of carboxylated protein.

AMINO ACID SEQUENCE

Protein	1 A	2 N	3 K	4 G	5 F	6 L	7 X	8 X	9 X	10 V	11 R	12 K	13 G	14 N	15 L	16 X	17 R	18 X	19 C	20 L	21 X	22 X	23 P	24 C	25 S	26 R	27 X	28 X	29 A	30 F	31 X	32 A	33 L	34 X	35 S	36 L	37 S	38 A	39 T	40 D	41 A	42 F	43 W	Reference
Bovine Prothrombin (1 ltr code)	A	N	K	G	F	L	X	X	X	V	R	K	G	N	L	X	R	X	C	L	X	X	P	C	S	R	X	X	A	F	X	A	L	X	S	L	S	A	T	D	A	F	W	148, 240, 242
Bovine Prothrombin	ala	asn	lys	gly	phe	leu	GLA	GLA	GLA	val	arg	lys	gly	asn	leu	GLA	arg	GLA	cys	Leu	GLA	GLA	pro	cys	ser	arg	GLA	GLA	ala	phe	GLA	ala	leu	GLA	ser	leu	ser	ala	thr	asp	ala	phe	trp	244, 247, 250, 257, 260
Human Prothrombin	ala	asn	thr	–	phe	leu	GLA	GLA	–	val	arg	lys	gly	asn	leu	GLA	arg	GLA	cys	ser	GLA	GLA	thr	cys	ser	tyr	GLA	GLA	ala	phe	GLA	ala	leu	GLA	ser	ser	thr	ala	thr	asp	val	phe	trp	174, 260
Rat Prothrombin	ala	asn	asn	gly						ile																																		259, 493
Chicken Prothrombin	ala	asn	lys	gly	phe	leu	GLA	GLA	met	ile	–	lys	gly	asn	leu	GLA	arg	GLA	cys	leu	GLA	GLA	thr	cys	asn	tyr	GLA	GLA	ala	phe	GLA	ala	leu	GLA	ser	thr	val	asp	thr	asp	ala	phe	trp	260
Factor VII Bovine	ala	asn	–	gly								pro	gly	ser	leu	GLA																												250, 253, 257
Factor IX Human	tyr	asn	ser	gly	lys	leu	GLA	GLA	phe	val	gln	–	gly	asn	leu	GLA	arg	GLA	cys	lys	GLA	GLA	lys	cys	ser	phe	GLA	GLA	ala	arg	GLA	val	phe	GLA	asn	thr	GLA	lys	thr	thr	GLA	phe	trp	174, 253
Factor IX Bovine	tyr	asn	ser	gly	lys	leu	GLA	GLA	phe	val	arg	–	gly	asn	leu	GLA	arg	GLA	cys	leu	GLA	GLA	lys	cys	ser	phe	GLA	GLA	ala	arg	GLA	val	phe	GLA	asn	thr	GLA	asp	thr	thr	GLA	phe	trp	244, 250, 253
Protein C Bovine Light Chain	ala	asn	ser	–	phe	leu	GLA	GLA	–	leu	arg	pro	gly	asn	val	GLA	GLA	arg	GLA	ser			val	cys	GLA	phe	GLA	GLA	ala	arg	GLA	ile	phe	gln	asn	thr	GLA	asp	thr	met	ala	phe	trp	172, 249, 257 / 258
Protein S Human	ala	asn	thr	–	leu	leu	GLA	GLA	–	thr	lys	lys	gly	asn	leu	GLA	arg	GLA	cys																									174, 250
Protein S Bovine	ala	asn	thr	–	leu	leu	GLA	GLA	–	thr	lys	lys	gly	asn	leu	GLA	arg	GLA	cys																									250, 251, 257
Protein Z Bovine	ala	gly	ser	tyr	leu	leu	GLA	GLA	–	leu	phe	GLA	gly	X	leu																													252
Factor X, Bovine	ala	asn	ser	–	phe	leu	GLA	GLA	val	lys	gln	gly	asn	leu	GLA	arg	GLA	cys	leu	GLA	GLA	ala	cys			leu	GLA	GLA	ala	arg	GLA	val	phe	GLA	asp	ala	GLA	gln	thr	asp	GLA	phe	trp	254, 255, 257
Factor X, Bovine	ala	asn	ser	–	phe	leu	GLA	GLA	val	lys	gln	gly	asn	leu	GLA	arg	GLA	cys								leu	GLA	GLA	ala	arg	GLA	val	phe	GLA	asp	asp	GLA	gln	thr	asp	GLA	phe	trp	244
Factor X₂ Bovine	ala	asn	ser	–	phe	leu	GLA	GLA	val	lys	gln	gly	asn	leu	GLA	arg	GLA	cys							ser	leu	GLA	GLA	ala	arg	GLA	val	phe	GLA	asp	asp	GLA	gln	thr	asp	GLA	phe	trp	256
Factor X Human	ala	asn	ser	–	phe	leu	GLA	GLA	met	lys			ly		leu																	met	lys											174

There are a few cases where the sequence is not agreed on by different investigators, however, none of these are in homologous region.

Table 2. Structure of vitamin K-dependent region of non-plasma proteins.

Amino Acid Sequence

Protein	1	2	3	4	5	6	7	8	9	10	11	12	13	14	15	16	17	18	19	20	21	22	23	24	25	26	27	28	29	30	31	32	33	34	35	36	37	38	39	40	41	42	43	Reference
Calf Bone Protein	tyr	leu	asp	his	trp	leu	gly	ala	hyp	ala	pro	tyr	pro	asp	pro	leu	GLA	pro	lys	arg	GLA	val	cys	GLA	leu	asn	pro	asp	cys	asp	glu	leu	ala	asp	his	ile	gly	phe	gln	glu	ala	tyr	arg etc.	(148, 241, 242; 494, 495)
Human Bone	tyr	leu	tyr	gln	trp	leu	gly	ala	pro	val	pro	tyr	pro	asp	pro	leu	glu*	pro	arg	arg	GLA	val	cys	GLA	leu	asn	pro	asp	cys	asp	glu	leu	ala	asp	asp	thr	ala	gly	ile	val	ala	tyr	ile etc.	(261, 495)
Swordfish Bone	tyr	leu	tyr		ala	thr	arg	ala	gly	asp	asp	leu	thr	pro	leu	gln	GLA	ser	leu	arg	GLA	val	cys	GLA	leu	asn	val	ala	ala	glu	glu			met	ala	asp			val		ala	tyr	ile etc.	(181, 261; 494, 495)

* The one peculiarity is the glutamyl residue at position 17, closer to the amino terminal than the γ-carboxylated glutamyl residues at positions 21 and 24. The glu residue at position 17 is reported[261] to be 9% carboxylated while 21 and 24 are 100% carboxylated. This protein was isolated from a 79 year old man and decarboxylation at position 17 seems the most probable explanation.

interaction of carboxylated proteins with membranes is a complex process including calcium binding to the carboxyl groups and to the membrane to form a protein-membrane complex. For example, the prothrombinase complex can be considered as a dissociable aggregate of factor Xa, factor V, and phospholipid which activates prothrombin via a calcium dependent binding. Similar conclusions are reached by Lindhout and Hemker (236).

Hauschka, et al. (237) concluded that this calcium binding carboxylation modification is particularly important in mineralized tissues, and may involve regulation of calcium metabolism in such tissues. Similarly, Robertson, et al. (238) have studied the binding of calcium and magnesium to gla-proteins using NMR spectroscopy. This appears to be a useful method for the study of metal binding and the determination of dissociation constants. In the case of gla-peptides this constant appears to be in the millimolar range (approximately 0.6 mM for a synthetic gla-gla containing peptide).

The practical outcome is some explanation of the fact that uncarboxylated abnormal prothrombin is not activated to thrombin by factor Xa, factor V and phospholipid in the prothrombin clotting assay (although it can be hydrolyzed to thrombin by various other proteolytic enzymes such as *Echis carinatis* venom or trypsin).

Recently, Osterberg, et al. (239) have shown by x-ray scattering that calcium binding to the prothrombin molecule gives it a more extended conformation. This change is pictured as two ellipsoids which increase in angle between major axes upon binding calcium.

9. Homology

Almost immediately upon the discovery of glutamyl residue carboxylation as the vitamin K-dependent step came the announcement from Magnusson's laboratory at Aarhus that the first ten glutamyl residues of prothrombin were carboxylated, (i.e., amino acid residues 7, 8, 15, 17, 20, 21, 26, 27, 30, 33 from the amino terminal end) (148, 240). Since then his group has completely sequenced bovine prothrombin and human prothrombin (241–243). Matthes (244) at the same time showed that many serine proteases have a high degree of homology. He compared the amino acid sequences of bovine prothrombin with trypsinogen,

plasminogen, chymotrypsinogen, elastase, as well as factor X and the amino terminal portion of factor IX, while Hewett-Emmet (245) has used Gibbs and McIntyre diagonal plots (246) to compare bovine prothrombin to human prothrombin, bovine factor X, bovine osteocalcin, bovine factors IX and VII and protein C (see also 247).

As can be seen from Tables 1 and 2 while there is a great deal of homology among the plasma vitamin K-dependent proteins, and a great deal between the bone gla-proteins of various species there appears to be none between the blood and the bone gla-proteins. Comparison of Tables 1 and 2 indicates no common ancestor for the two groups of carboxylated proteins.

Walz, et al. (260) have partially sequenced chicken prothrombin and their data indicate (see Table 2) a high degree of structural conservation through 300 million years of evolution (the split of birds and mammals). In addition to these data on sequence homology of the blood vitamin K-dependent proteins, Magnusson's group has published a great deal on configuration and regional structure within the molecule (241–243). Most characteristic has been the finding of the kringle structures. Baskova, et al. (262) have found that prothrombin contains 14% α-helix, 46% β-helix, and 50% random regions.

10. Exogenous substrates for the in vitro vitamin K-dependent protein carboxylation assay

a. Small peptides

After many unsuccessful attempts in many laboratories to prepare a preprothrombin or a decarboxylated prothrombin which would be carboxylated in vitro, a major breakthrough (263) was made when it was found that the crude liver carboxylating system would use as substrate the pentapeptide Phe-Leu-Glu-Glu-Val (the sequence 5–9 of bovine prothrombin). Houser, et al. (264) have found that the (5–9) sequence from rat prothrombin, which contains an Ile in place of Val in position 9, is an ever superior substrate for the rat liver derived systems. The pentapeptide most often used currently in this assay is Phe-Leu-Glu-Glu-Leu (a sequence from factor X).

More recently Finnan and Suttie (265) have shown that the simpler glutamic acid derivative N-t-BOC-Glu-α-benzyl ester will also serve as a carboxylation substrate. While less active it is very much cheaper and, hence, is currently the substrate

Table 3. Relative activity of some peptides for carboxylation.

										Relative activity
			Phe	Leu	Glu	Glu	Leu			100
			Phe	Ala	Glu	Glu	Leu			72
			Phe	Gly	Glu	Glu	Leu			4
			Phe	Leu	Glu	Glu	Ile			123
			Phe	Leu	Glu	Glu	Val			72
Val	His	Leu	Ser	Ala	Glu	Glu	Lys	Glu	Ala	26
Val	His	Leu	Ser	Ala	Glu	Glu	Lys	Glu	Ala	17
		Phe	Glu	Ala	Leu	Glu	Ser	Leu		5
				Leu	Glu	Glu	Leu			8
			BOC	Leu	Glu	Glu	Leu	O	Me	77
CH_3	CH_2	CO	Phe	Leu	Glu	Glu	Leu	O	Me	149
		BOC	Phe	Leu	Glu	Glu	Leu	O	Me	24
	C_6H_5	CO	Phe	Leu	Glu	Glu	Leu	O	Me	27
				BOC	Glu	Glu	Leu	O	Me	107
					BOC	Glu	Leu	O	Me	0
					BOC	Glu	OCH_2	C_6H_5*		5
			Phe	Glu	Leu	Glu	Leu			0
			Phe	Leu	Glu	Leu				0
		Phe	Glu	Ala	Leu	Glu	Ser	Leu		5
				BOC	Asp	Asp	Leu	O	Me	0
				BOC	Glu	Asp	Leu	O	Me	11
				BOC	Asp	Glu	Leu	O	Mè	11
				BOC	Glu	Glu	Leu	O	Me	0

All peptides were compared at the same concentration in the same soluble system.
These data are taken from references 265, 268, 362, 364.
* benzyl ester of α-carboxyl of glutamyl residue

of choice for many carboxylation reactions concerned with enzyme purification and enzyme mechanism.

Considering further the pentapeptide carboxylation, four areas of interest have appeared. (i) Comparison of various pentapeptides, (ii) the stimulation of pentapeptide carboxylation by pyridoxal phosphate, (iii) the sequence of carboxylation events, (iv) requirement for a free γ-carboxyl on the glutamyl residue.

i) Comparison of peptides. In Table 3 are given a series of peptides that have been compared as exogenous substrates in the carboxylation reaction (265, 268). When these different peptides are compared, it appears that hydrophobicity is a major factor in extent of carboxylation. This is presumably why covering both the α-amino and l-carboxy groups of glutamic acid makes it into a substrate. On the other hand as one examines Table 1 it is clear that many of the gla residues formed by glu-carboxylation are not in obviously hydrophobic regions of the endogenous protein sequences and thus other considerations (probably related to conformation) must also be important. D-glutamic acid is not carboxylated in peptide nor is aspartic acid.

ii) The effect of pyridoxal phosphate. It was shown by Suttie, et al. (263) that pyridoxal-5′-phosphate (PLP) stimulated about two-fold the carboxylation of exogenous peptide (Phe-Leu-Glu-Glu-Leu) but had no effect on carboxylation of the endogenous protein precursors. Dubin, et al. (266) have been able to show clearly that this stimulation is not due to Schiff's base formation between peptide and pyridoxal phosphate but is due to binding of the pyridoxal phosphate to the microsomal enzyme(s). In agreement with this finding is the report of Griffith (267) that pyridoxal phosphate binds and modifies human α-thrombin. Rich, et al. (268) have also reported that amino protected peptides which could not form Schiff's bases with pyridoxal phosphate are still stimulated by pyridoxal phosphate. Huang, et al. (269, 294) have reported that while pyridoxal phosphate stimulates carboxylation of pentapeptide it does not effect carboxylation of t-BOC-glu-α-benzyl ester and they also concluded that the action of pyridoxal phosphate in stimulating pentapeptide carboxylation is interaction with manganous ion at the active site of the enzyme. Suttie, et al. (270) have also continued to study the stimulation of pentapeptide carboxylation and agree with the suggestion that PLP is possibly reacting with the enzyme.

iii) Sequence of events after carboxylation. Finnan and Suttie (265, 271) have shown that carboxylation of the pentapeptide, Phe-Leu-Glu-Glu-Leu proceeds via essentially complete carboxylation of the first (from amino end) glu with essentially none of the second glu carboxylated to give Phe-Leu-Gla-Glu-Leu. A post carboxylation non-vitamin K-dependent modification of this monocarboxylated peptide apparently on the gla residue, indicates some further reaction, possibly ester formation at some stage in the reaction. Decottignies-Le Marechal et al. (272) confirms Phe-Leu-Gla-Glu-Val as the chief product of carboxylation of the Val-terminal pentapeptide. They too find a small amount of another monocarboxylated peptide product formed in a non-vitamin K-dependent reaction.

iv) Requirement for a free γ-carboxyl on the glutamyl residue. The other finding of interest is that if the t-BOC-Glu-α-benzyl ester is methylated in the γ-position the diester so formed is essentially inactive as a substrate. This may indicate that the free γ-carboxyl of the glutamyl residue must take part in the reaction, possibly by forming an ester-type linkage affecting the active site of the enzyme (273).

11. Site of action of vitamin K hydroquinone in the carboxylation reaction

The overall carboxylation reaction can be written as:

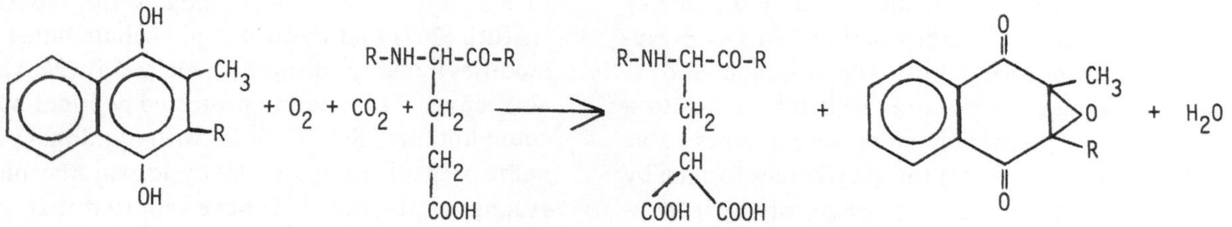

This obviously involves a series of at least three reactions unless a 3 point concerted (S_N2) reaction were postulated. For the usual, 2 molecules at a time reaction, the following sequence is suggested (1) hydroquinone reacts with oxygen, (2) an 'activated' oxygen removes a hydrogen from the γ-carbon of the glutamyl residue, (3) either CO_2 is 'activated' in some way, or the CO_2, without requiring activation, merely adds to a carbanion left when the γ-hydrogen is removed to yield a γ-carboxyglutamyl residue, and (4) by virtue of a vitamin K epoxidase vitamin K-2,3-epoxide is formed. Whether the carboxylation and epoxidation are mutually interdependent, i.e., tightly coupled, has not been established but will be discussed under section 13.

Friedman, et al. (274, 275) using the pentapeptide Phe-Leu-Glu-Glu-Leu tritiated at the γ-position of each Glu residue have shown that vitamin K is required to remove the hydrogen from the γ-position of the glutamyl residue in the liver microsomal carboxylation system and that in the absence of CO_2 hydrogen exchange takes place without carboxylation. This hydrogen 'withdrawing' reaction requires oxygen as well as vitamin K hydroquinone.

Matthes (244) has stated that the hydroxylation of an alanine residue to a serine at position 36 of prothrombin and position 43 of bovine factor X and protein C (276) is an essential vitamin K-dependent step required for the carboxylation of glutamyl residues, however, osteocalcin and the synthetic peptide substrates are carboxylated in the vitamin K-dependent reaction (removal of a γ-hydrogen from a glutamyl residue) even though neither alanine nor serine are involved. On the other hand, vitamin K is a quinone-hydroquinone pair and perhaps involves electron transport which can also play a role in alanine hydroxylation and in benzopyrene hydroxylation (94).

12. Proposed mechanisms of protein carboxylation

Since Friedman, et al. (274) showed that the vitamin K-dependent step was the removal of a γ-hydrogen from the glutamyl residue, questions include: (1) what product of vitamin K hydroquinone plus oxygen is alkaline enough to remove this hydrogen and (2) is the glutamyl species produced a free radical or is the original glu-γ-carboxyl so bound that a relatively stable carbanion could result at the γ-position of the glutamyl residue, stabilized by the adjacent carbonyl?

The mechanisms proposed for the post-translational carboxylation of the glutamyl residue will be considered under the subheadings (a) a free radical mechanism, (b) a carbanion mechanism with regard to the glutamyl residue, (c) possible 'activation' of the CO_2, (d) role of oxygen in the hydrogen removal reaction, (e) metal oxygen carriers, (f) alkyl carbonates, (g) reducing agent inhibition, (h) possible model organic chemistry reactions, and (i) plant CO_2 fixation.

a. Free radical mechanism

One possible scenario is the incomplete oxidation of the naphthohydroquinone, to the neutral semiquinone radical:

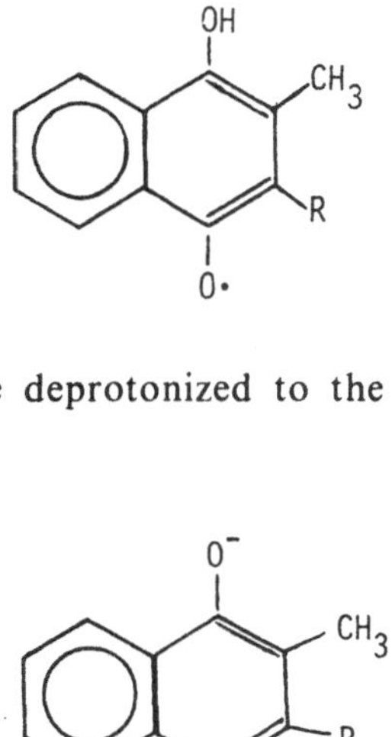

which can be deprotonized to the semiquinone anion radical:

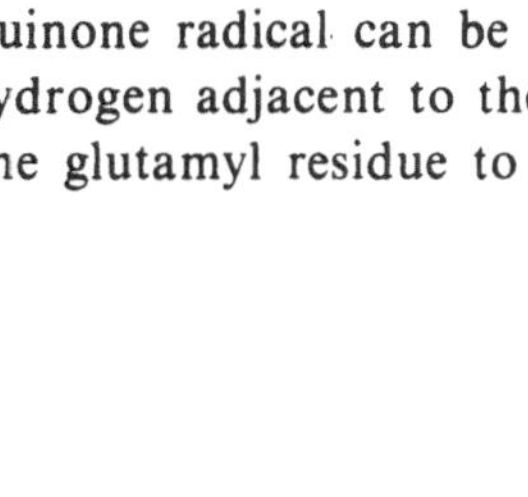

Such a semiquinone radical can be proposed to withdraw a hydrogen adjacent to the γ-terminal carboxyl of the glutamyl residue to leave a free radical:

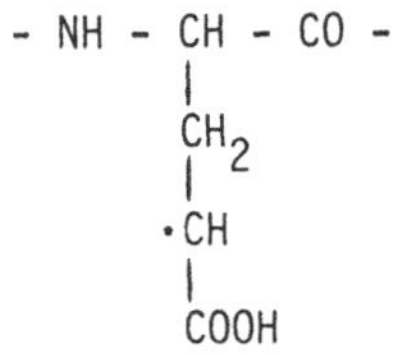

Other reactions which, at least in theory, could account for the formation of such a glutamyl radical are the production of superoxide radical $O_2^{\bar{\cdot}}$ or a hydroxyl radical $[OH \cdot]$ by reaction of vitamin K hydroquinone with molecular oxygen. Such a radical could then serve as the withdrawing group to give this glutamyl radical product.

Evidence against a free-radical reaction is that to date we have not observed any ESR signal during the reaction at temperatures from 0° to 37° (Floyd, R. & Mack, D. O., unpublished data). Other evidence against the semiquinone hypothesis has been mentioned, i.e., even with synthesized semiquinone which shows the proper ESR signal (151), molecular oxygen is required for carboxylation to occur (152). Hence, it appears that a semiquinone radical is not the reactant which removes the γ-hydrogen.

Some support on the other hand is given to a free radical mechanism by the data showing that the spin-trapping agents phenyl-N-tert butyl nitrone, at 100 mM inhibited the carboxylation 94% if the carboxylation reaction were carried out with vitamin K quinone plus NADH but only 20% at levels of 9 to 36 mM if vitamin K hydroquinone were the reactant. Another spin-trapping agent, 5,5-dimethyl-1-pyrroline-N oxide gave 77% inhibition when used at 72 mM in the presence of vitamin K hydroquinone while 2-methyl-2-nitrosopropane gave 41% inhibition at 100 mM of carboxylation initiated by vitamin K quinone plus NADH (145, 150, 152). The levels required of these spin-trapping agents to block the carboxylation seem high if this were a free radical reaction. The stable nitroso free radicals, 4-hydroxy-2,2,6,6-tetramethylpiperid-1-yloxy (tempol) and 4-oxo-2,2,6,6-tetramethylpiperid-1-yloxy (tempone), however, gave efficient blocking of carboxylation at 10 mM suggesting that a free radical mechanism is still a viable hypothesis. Lu Valle and Weissberger (165, 166) and numerous other investigators have shown that almost all hydroquinone oxidations proceed in univalent steps and that the intermediate semiquinones, (i.e., free

Figure I

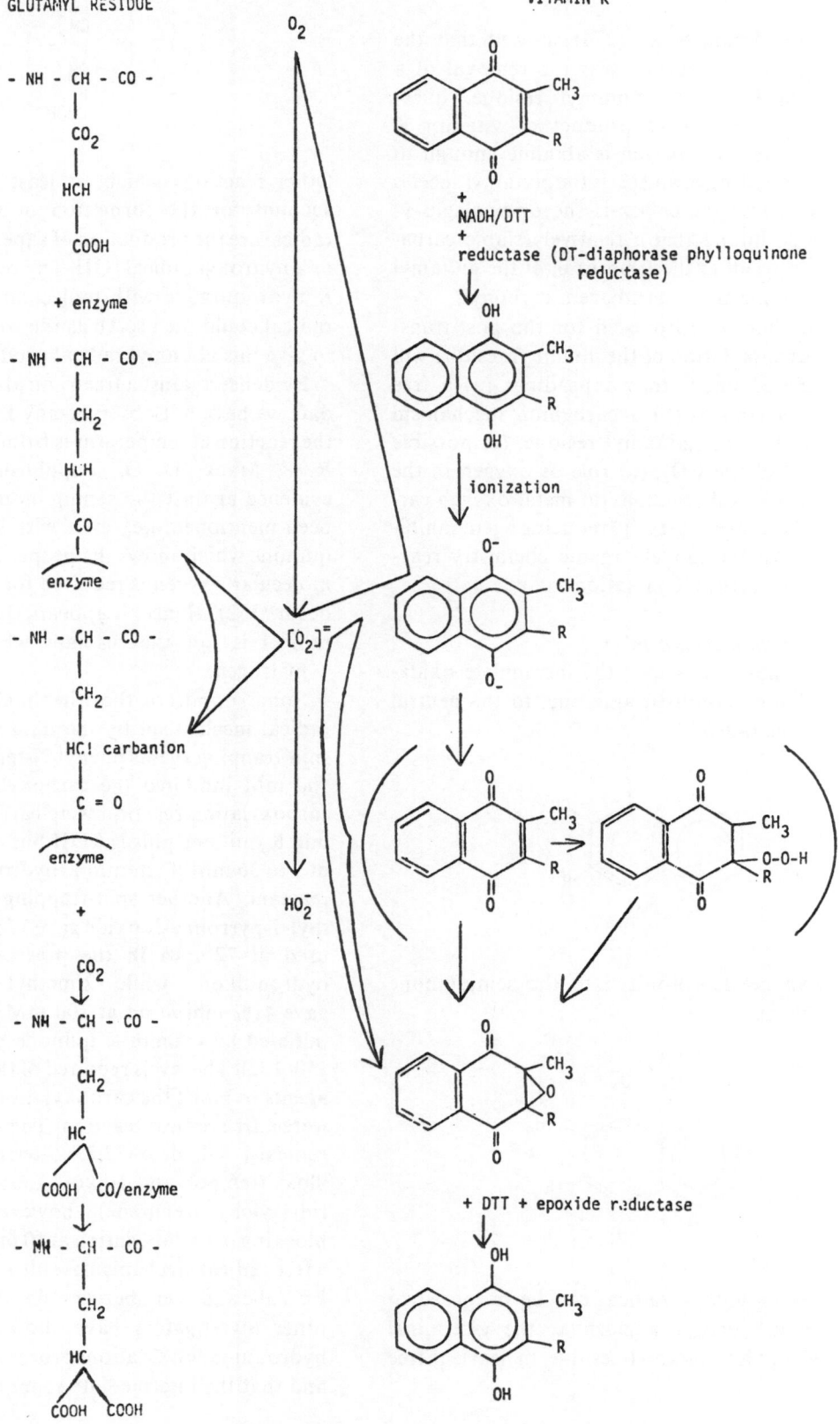

radicals) equilibrate with the reduced and oxidized forms and their dimers and thus the semiquinones are stabilized by resonance. This would lead from the hydroquinone to the semiquinone plus $O_2^{\bar{\;}}$. This $O_2^{\bar{\;}}$ ion could perhaps serve as the withdrawing agent for glutamyl residue and for the oxidizing agent to form vitamin K-2,3-epoxide.

b. Carbanion mechanism

The other related possibility is that the glutamyl residue intermediate after γ-hydrogen removal is the glutamyl carbanion. For this hypothesis to be reasonable it is necessary to tie up the –OH of the γ-carboxyl group so that the resulting carbonyl could serve as stabilizing agent for the adjacent carbanion. Evidence that this γ-carboxyl group takes part in the reaction has already been presented (273, 278). In addition, the lack of ESR signal supports such a mechanism. A tentative proposal is given as follows (279).

Proof that the γ-carboxyl actually participates in the reaction would support such a model. H_2O_2 which is a product of hydroquinone plus oxygen and the source of the $[O_2]^=$ anion neither serves as an inhibitor of the reaction nor as a substitute for the oxygen requirement if the catalase of the microsomal solution is blocked by azide (161). The mechanism as written does not fit the usual quinone oxidation reduction which proceeds by univalent steps (e.g., 281). However, the flavoprotein reductase DT-diaphorase (NAD(P)H:quinone oxidoreductase) which has been extensively studied by Ernster's groups (c.f., 283) has been shown to be a two-electron transfer enzyme (282). This would be expected to limit autooxidation and thus superoxide ($O_2^{\bar{\;}}$ formation). This has been demonstrated by Ernster, et al. (283).

This mechanism does not account for the specificity with regard to the 2-methyl group or the naphthoquinone ring system that has been demonstrated since it would seem that any hydroquinone plus molecular oxygen should yield H_2O_2. However, the specificity is presumably conferred by the enzyme.

An argument which might favor the formulation given in Fig. 1 includes the early report of Sadowski and Suttie (280) that the 2,3-epoxide was only produced from vitamin K hydroquinone plus molecular oxygen and not from the quinone. This formulation provides for a different oxidizing agent derived from molecular oxygen. The main argument against carbanion formulation at present is the requirement for esterification of the γ-carboxyl to provide a carbonyl to stabilize the adjacent carbanion. No energy source for this esterification-desterification reaction is provided for. In addition, when a synthetic γ-carboxyl ester is used it is virtually inactive as a substrate (273). Reaction of the glutamic acid γ carboxyl with the enzyme as part of the reaction is under investigation.

c. Activation of CO₂ mechanism

While numerous attempts have been made to find a CO_2 derivative of vitamin K which would serve as carboxylating agent, no such derivative has been found. If the reaction does proceed via a carbanion of the glutamyl residue this would add CO_2 directly without CO_2 'activation' in a nucleophilic reaction (284). This type of reaction in microsomes has been described by Ullrich and Schnabel (285). However, their reaction involved cytochrome P450 linkage and cytochrome P450 does not appear to be involved in the protein carboxylation (145).

On the other hand, Esnouf, et al. (286, 287) have reported that in the presence of superoxide dismutase (SOD), the carboxylation of both endogenous protein and exogenous peptide substrates is inhibited and they have suggested that superoxide is produced which reacts with CO_2 to form an intermediate in the carboxylation reaction. Using microsomes plus vitamin K hydroquinone + 1 mg/ml superoxide dismutase they report a 30% inhibition of peptide carboxylation (20% inhibition of endogenous protein carboxylation). At 10 mg/ml they reported 60% inhibition. Under similar conditions using the Triton X100 solubilized system we obtain approximately 50% inhibition of carboxylation at 20 mg/ml of SOD while other inhibitors such as Cu^{2+} ion or parahydroxymercurobenzoate (PHMB) give essentially total blocking at 1.0 mM. Esnouf, et al. suggest generation of an active $CO_3^{\bar{\;}}$ radical which gives rise to an ESR signal. If a CO_2 hydroperoxide ($CO_3^{\bar{\;}}$) were involved the 50% inhibition obtainable with SOD should be prevented by xanthine oxidase + xanthine which should reverse the SOD inhibition by continuous superoxide production. However, we found no effect of xanthine oxide plus xanthine on the SOD inhibited carboxylase (Mack, D. O. & Curtis, T. A., unpublished data). The suggestion is also contrary to the results found with the luminescence that accompanies the aerobic xanthine oxidase reaction which is also inhibited by SOD and by scavengers of hydroxyl radicals but is entirely dependent upon carbonate (288).

The reaction of superoxide with vitamin K_1 and related compounds gave the epoxide rather than a hydroperoxide derivative in the work of Saito, et al. (289). Winterbourn, et al. (290) feel that SOD could be involved in controlling the levels of various free radicals (including a superoxide radical) and that the role of vitamin K is involved at this level. Gallop, et al. (490) also currently favor a free-radical carboxylation reaction.

d. Role of oxygen

As shown by Lu Valle and Weissberg in 1947 (165, 166), the organic chemical reaction of hydroquinones with oxygen results in the formation of H_2O_2. Thus if the 'activation' of CO_2 as postulated by Esnouf does not occur (286, 287) the molecular oxygen perhaps must be 'activated' to, for example, superoxide anion or some organic [perhaps vitamin K derivative (291)] superoxide or hydroperoxide. What is the evidence for superoxide versus hydroperoxide or some other oxygen activation? Larson and Suttie (291–293) have reported that glutathione peroxidase is a potent inhibitor of the carboxylation reaction and on this based their postulation of a vitamin K hydroperoxide as the glu-γ-hydrogen withdrawing agent. They have reported that the vitamin K hydroquinone could be replaced in vitro by t-butyl hydroperoxide (291, 293). However, both of these claims have been contended. Highly purified glutathione peroxidase has been found (294) not to inhibit carboxylation, and the $^{14}CO_2$ incorporation seen with t-butyl hydroperoxide (293) has been found not to be glutamyl residue carboxylation (491).

We have been unable to obtain either endogenous or exogenous substrate carboxylation when H_2O_2, t-butyl hydroperoxide or cumene hydroperoxide replaced vitamin K hydroquinone plus oxygen (161) as initiator of the reaction. Thus, it appears that the form of oxidation product formed by the reaction between vitamin K hydroquinone and molecular oxygen is not yet established. While we currently favor the carbanion reaction sequence outlined in Fig. 1, another oxidant intermediate we have considered many times, particularly in view of

the abstract of Sadowski and Suttie (280) showing (^{18}O incorporated into epoxide only from vitamin K hydroquinone but not from its quinone, is a mixed function compound such as the epoxide or peroxide (held by the enzyme):

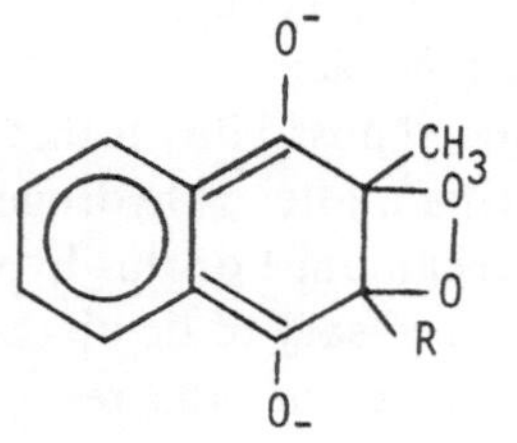

Vire, et al. (295) studying the degradation of menadione at the dropping mercury electrode have suggested that above pH 6.0 oxidation of vitamin K hydroquinone may procede via the 2,3-epoxide of the hydroquinone. If by virtue of the enzyme such a compound could be derived directly from the hydroquinone the vitamin K hydroquinone oxide molecule held in the hydroquinone configuration by the enzyme could be postulated as the hydrogen withdrawing agent. Its conversion to, for example, a 3-OH derivative would immediately precede the quinone epoxide formation with further oxygen. This could explain the epoxide of the quinone as the 'final' metabolic product of vitamin K found in the liver. It would also mean tight coupling of carboxylation and epoxidation.

e. Metal catalysis of the oxidation step

Metal catalysis seems to be a natural mechanism to function with oxygen as a hydrogen withdrawing agent. The idea of a metal chelate led many of us to look for cytochrome P450 involvement but all blocking agents tried for this reaction have proved inactive. More recently with the suggestion of manganese involvement, a Mn^{2+} complex with oxygen has been suggested (e.g. 294). However, the manganese level used to affect the carboxylation is so high (10 mM) (168) that this mechanism is viewed with some skepticism. Nevertheless, it may turn out to be the most important postulation yet.

f. Alkyl carbonate as carboxylation agent

One of the first mechanisms claimed was the formation of a carbonic acid half-ester of a vitamin K hydroquinone hydroxyl, however, the formation of such a co$_2$ donor no longer appears plausible (296). Alkyl monocarbonates as 'activated Co$_2$' in biological systems require ATP for formation (297). The organic chemistry of some carbonic acid half-esters has been reviewed by Williams and Douglas (298).

g. Effect of certain reducing agents on vitamin K-dependent protein carboxylation

In 1979, Suzuki, et al. (299) reported vitamin K deficiency in male rats fed diets containing the antioxidant butylated hydroxy toluene (BHT). In the same year Olson and Jones (300) found that the function of vitamin K was inhibited by giving the animals 'megadose' levels of α-tocopherol. Benson, et al. (301) have now reported a striking increase in DT-diaphorase activity in livers of mice fed BHA (butylated hydroxyanisole, a commercial antioxidant). We compared in vitro a number of highly potent antioxidants and showed that of the antioxidants of Kappus, et al. (302) the very active antioxidants 2-hydroxyestradiol and 7,8-dihydroxy-choropromazine totally blocked the carboxylation reaction in vitro when added at 10 mM. Although another antioxidant 7-hydroxychloropromazine was non-inhibitory at 10 mM (145, 161). The finding that even in vitro (161) the carboxylation can be blocked by lipid soluble antioxidants supports the theory that the initial reaction is between vitamin K hydroquinone and oxygen.

Kahl (303) has recently shown that the antioxidant ethoxyquin leads to an increase in epoxide hydrolase activity in liver microsomes. This may be the basis of the vitamin K deficiency found when BHT is fed (299). Dansette (304) in a study of microsomal epoxide hydrolase points out that this enzyme is inactive in polysubstituted epoxides which might explain the need for substitutions at positions 2 and 3 to have a stable epoxide which functions in carboxylation.

h. Organic model reactions

Backvall and Karlson (305) have carried out a very interesting organic reaction which may be pertinent to the vitamin K-dependent carboxylation. They have shown that copper and nickel both may catalyze the insertion of CO$_2$ into epoxides. An analogous reaction could be hypothesized in which a stabilized vitamin K hydroquinone epoxide, for example, forms an alkene carbonate which both removes the hydrogen and adds the carboxyl to the glutamyl residue.

Bottaccio, et al. (306) studied the carboxylation of organic substrates with CO$_2$ in the presence of different phenoxides. They reported that organic substrates possessing an active hydrogen could be easily carboxylated under very mild conditions in the presence of alkali phenoxides. For example, one mole acetophenone + CO$_2$ + 3.6. mole 2,6-di (tertbutyl)-p-cresol at 20° (i.e., 1 M phenoxide in toluene under carbon dioxide) gave a 73% yield of benzol acetic acid. They write the general reaction as:

$$C_6H_5 + RH \text{ (acceptor)} \rightarrow C_6H_5OH + RM$$
$$RM + CO_2 \text{ (donor complex)} \rightarrow RCOOM$$

A specific example given is:

In this case the alkali salt of a hydroquinone is catalyzing carboxylation of a benzene ring.

i. Plant CO₂ – fixation

Is there any analogy between the ability of the plant to utilize CO_2 and the hydroquinone catalyzed carboxylation of glutamyl residues in peptide linkage?

Nakajima, et al. (307) have been able to carry out carboxylation using artificial photosynthetic models with known iron sulfur complexes as catalyst. Their carboxylation reaction involved the use of a single alkyl mercaptan, an iron-sulfur complex and sodium dithionite.

$$RCH_2 \; \underset{\underset{O}{\|}}{C} - S - C_8H_{17} + CO_2 \quad \xrightarrow[\substack{Na_2S_2O_4 \\ NaHCO_3}]{Fe \; complex} \quad RCH_2 - \underset{\underset{O}{\|}}{C} - COOH$$

The higher plant reaction involves a reaction catalyzed by ribulose-1,5-diphosphate carboxylase, a bifunctional enzyme which catalyzes the carboxylation reaction in the reductive pentose phosphate cycle and the oxidation of ribulose-1,5-diphosphate. The reactive oxygen species involved is superoxide anion (O_2^-) (308). Christeller and Laing (309) and Miziorko and Sealy (310) have reported that manganese ion gives the lowest Km for soyabean ribulose diphosphate carboxylase with CO_2 and O_2. Thus, as is possible in the vitamin K hydroquinone-dependent carboxylase the oxygenation reaction appears dependent on a divalent cation. Miziorko and Sealy (310) suggest that there is an ordered addition of Co_2 and divalent cation to the carboxylase and that upon formation of this ternary complex the enzyme becomes catalytically competent.

Whether or not the apparent similarities are real and helpful must await purification of the vitamin K hydroquinone dependent carboxylase.

13. Protein synthesis and the post-translational site of protein carboxylation

From the sequencing of so many of the gla-containing proteins has come the observation that there is no carboxylation after about amino acid 35 from the amino terminal. This must be due to some change which occurs between the carboxylation of

the last residue carboxylated (before amino acid residue 40) and the next glu residue (amino acid 65 in prothrombin). All subsequent glu residues are non-carboxylated. Matthes has suggested (276) that carboxylation is dependent on prior alanine hydroxylation and that there is no carboxylation beyond the last point of alanine hydroxylation. However, other explanations come readily to mind. Since the carboxylase complex is very hydrophobic it appears quite possible that carboxylation can only occur within the lipophyllic membrane. Suttie in 1967, on the basis of the effect of puromycin or actinomycin on prothrombin peptide synthesis suggested that the site of vitamin K action is somewhere between the formation of nascent peptide and transport of the completed glycoprotein from the liver cell (311). Similarly J. P. Olson, et al. using perfused liver formation of prothrombin suggested that vitamin K acts between ribosomal synthesis and the appearance of active prothrombin (141). These results are in agreement with the work of Hill, et al. that the site of vitamin K action is after peptide bond formation (2). Sheinbuks (230) has presented evidence that vitamin K-dependent carboxylation occurs at the level of nascent polypeptide chain formation.

Two possibilities appear most probable. (1) The growing peptide chain remains within or attached to the hydrophobic carboxylase containing area as long as it remains attached to its signal peptide. As translated, preprothrombin contains a signal peptide of 23 amino acids: [Met]-Ala-X-Val-X-X-Pro-X-Leu-Pro-X-X-Leu-Ala-Leu-Ala-Ala-Leu-Phe-X-Leu-Val-X-(312,313) and appears highly hydrophobic. The postulation can then be made that once the signal peptide is lost, attachment to the membrane is lost and carboxylation no longer will occur. (2) Another possibility is that further carboxylation will be prevented by removal of the growing peptide chain into a hydrophyllic environment far from the carboxylase once the first glycosylation occurs. However, the first amino acid residue glycosylated in prothrombin is Asn residue 77 and five uncarboxylated glu residues occur between the last Gla residue at 33 and the Asn residue at 77.

Thus, it appears more probable that the signal peptide is involved in the positioning of the nascent peptide chain for carboxylation through the first 33 to 36 residues. In prothrombin the first non-carboxylated Glu-residue is residue 49 (the other Glu-residues before 77 are residues 56, 60, 63, 68).

However, it is quite possible that the inability of the in vitro system to carboxylate isolated abnormal (non-carboxylated) prothrombin is due to the hydrophyllic nature of its four glycosyl residues.

14. Structural specificity of vitamin K for the in vitro carboxylation

The nutritional activity of various analogs of vitamin K was discussed earlier under section 1c. In this section the vitamin K structural requirements for function in the solubilized microsomal vitamin K dependent carboxylation system will be reviewed.

The most striking difference was the finding that menadione is inactive in vitro although in vivo it is as active on a molar basis as vitamin K_1 or the various K_2's. Friedman and Shia (149) compared several analogs and found that not only was menadione inactive but so was vitamin K_1 in which the β-γ double bond was in the cis rather than the naturally occurring trans configuration while we found (Girardot, J-M. and Johnson, B. C. (160)) hydrogenation of this double bond also destroyed activity. The methyl group at position 2 and the naphthoquinone ring sysem are essential in vitro as in vivo. Jones, et al. (314) also reported no activity for menadione, nor for 2,3-dimethyl-1,4-naphtho-quinone. Later after the dithiothreitol (DTT) stimulation of the quinone + NADH + CO_2 + O_2 reaction had been established (149, 157) it was shown that menadione plus DTT was active in vitro (170).

Since these earlier reports many different analogs of vitamin K have been synthesized (145, 315). It has been found that 3-thioethers of menadione are active if the side chain so added is uncharged but apparently does not have to be completely hydrophobic and may be aliphatic or aromatic. The most active thio adducts are those of dithiol compounds such as DTT, dithioerythritol (DTE) and dithiobutane. 3-0-ethers are also active, particularly when used as the hydroquinones, rather

than as the quinone plus NADH with or without DTT. As the hydroquinones even such compounds as the 2,3-dimethyl-1,4-naphtohydroquinone are functional (145, 315).

In addition to finding a wide range of structural analogs of vitamin K with carboxylating activity a number of menadione derivatives were found to be inhibitory. Some of the most active of these which gave essentially complete inhibition of carboxylation initiated by vitamin K hydroquinone are listed in Table 4.

In all of the cases listed in Table 3 the inhibition could be totally reversed by the addition of 10 mM DTT. Thus, these compounds were not competing for the vitamin K function but were blocking an SH essential for the carboxylation (see Section 15).

Substitution at position 5 of the naphthalene ring by a hydroxyl or alkoxy group eliminates carboxylation activity as does replacement of the 2-methyl group by hydroxy or methoxy groups.

Table 4. Menadione derivatives which block protein carboxylation initiated by vitamin K hydroquinone.[a]

Compound[b]	Levels	% Inhibition
1,4-naphthoquinone	0.3 mM	98
Menadione	0.3 mM	94
Vitamin K-S (II)[c]	0.2 mM	95
2,3-dichloro-1,4-naphthoquinone	0.3 mM	100
2-methyl-(3-thioethylamine)-1,4-naphthoquinone	0.3 mM	94
3-methyl-5-ethoxy-1,4-naphthoquinone	0.3 mM	97

[a] –0.11 mM
[b] in all these cases inhibition was completely reversed by 10 mM DTT.
[c] -3-(1,4-dihydro-3-methyl-1,4-dioxo-2-naphthylthio) propionic acid.

Table. 5. Carboxylation inhibitors (carboxylation initiated by vitamin K hydroquinone*).

Compound	Levels	% Inhibition
Duroquinone	2.0 mM	99
2-methyl-5-hydroxy-1,4-naphthoquinone (plumbagin)	0.3 mM	100
2-hydroxy-3-(3-methyl-2-butenyl)-1,4-naphthoquinone (lapachol)	15.0 mM	95

* –0.11 mM

In Table 5 are listed these and some other quinones which blocked the carboxylation and the block was not removed by DTT.

Surprisingly while the compounds listed in both Table 3 and Table 4 were still without activity in when used as the hydroquinones the carboxylation reaction, they showed much less inhibitory activity. This gives the impression that neither as the quinones nor as the hydroquinones were they competing for a vitamin K hydroquinone binding site but rather that as quinones they were oxidizing the required hydroquinone or not being reduced by phylloquinone reductase or in some other manner interfering with the reaction of the required hydroquinone with molecular oxygen to produce the hydrogen-withdrawing species.

In a recent reexamination of the in vitro activity of menaquinones and vitamin K_1 (149, 315), in the soluble system, Yen and Mack (316) have found that there is really very little difference in functional activity between MK-1 through MK-10 and vitamin K_1, or even 2,3-dimethyl-1,4-naphthoquinone, when the reaction was carried out with the quinone plus NADH plus adequate DTT. MK-3 and MK-4 appear to show slightly the highest activity.

15. Dicoumarol, warfarin and related anticoagulants compared to chloro-K and tetrachloropyridinol

In 1941 Link and co-workers isolated, characterized and synthesized the compound from 'toxic-sweet clover' which caused the hemorrhaging in cattle (317, 318). This compound, dicoumarol (I) is produced during spoilage from the natural coumarin of the plant. Many modifications of the original dicoumarol structure have been synthesized, of which the most commonly used is the rat-poison warfarin II (319).

Another related class of anticoagulants are the indandiones, of which an example is phenindione (III).

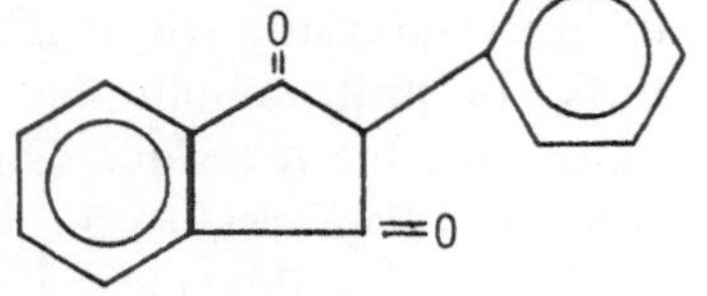

III

These chemical compounds are anticoagulants whose in vivo administration causes lowered blood prothrombin. This effect can be reversed by administration of vitamin K to the animal.

However, when used in vitro in the detergent solubilized microsomal carboxylation system initiated with vitamin K hydroquinone these 'anti-vitamin K' compounds do not inhibit carboxylation unless added at very high levels. On the other hand these compounds do block DT-diaphorase (phylloquinone-reductase) and also vitamin K epoxide reductase (320, 321). This is presumably how they work in vivo, producing reduced prothrombin levels by preventing formation of vitamin K hydroquinone from vitamin K epoxide.

In addition to the effect of warfarin on plasma prothrombin level, when administered at higher levels the compound is very toxic, uncoupling oxidative phosphorylation. At 50 mg warfarin/ 100g/ body weight the rat will die in a about 2 h with no symptoms of hypoprothrombinemia (2).

There are, however, two antagonists of vitamin K which do block the soluble system carboxylation reaction, these are chloro-K in which a chlorine replaces the methyl group in the 2 position and 2,3,5,6-tetrachloro-4-pyridinol (TCP) and many of its analogs (322).

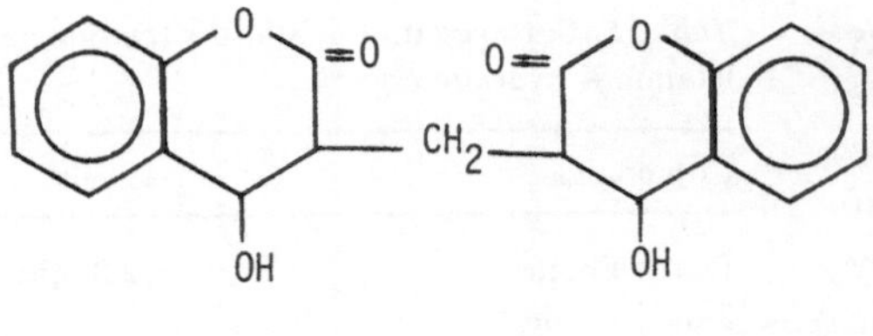

dicoumarol
I

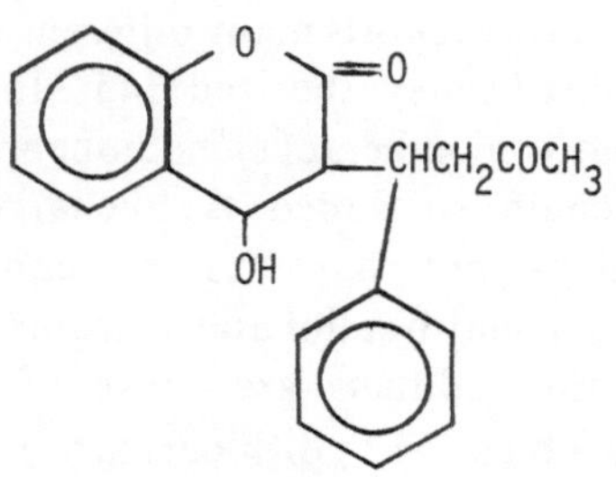

warfarin
II

When TCP is given to a normal rat, prothrombin time reaches a maximum about 48 h after giving the drug. It, like the dicoumarins, is highly toxic and requires about the same length of time for pro-thrombin reduction. This time is related to pro-thrombin turnover time (see Section 21). The chloro analog of vitamin K first made by Lowen-thal and Chowdhury (323) and acts as a non-competitive inhibitor of vitamin K (324).

Friedman and Griep (325) have shown that TCP and the related imidazopyridines, e.g., 1-hydroxy-2-trifluoromethyl - imidazo[4,5 - b] - 3 - chloro-pyridine, (1-H-IP)

1-H-IP

are potent inhibitors in vitro of vitamin K depen-dent post-translational glutamyl-residue carboxyl-ation. These compounds also inhibit vitamin K epoxidase but are less inhibitory of the vitamin K and vitamin K epoxide reductase enzyme(s). How-ever, all four types of inhibitors, coumarins, indan-diones, TCP and 1-H-IP are competitive inhibitors with respect to NAD(P)H, of the NAD(P)H-vitamin K (and epoxide) reductase(s).

The 50% carboxylase inhibition obtained by 10^{-5} M TCP is not competitive with respect to pentapep-tide substrate, nor with respect to pyridoxalphos-phate, imidazole buffer, DTT, salts, oxygen or vitamin K hydroquinone. Inhibition is reversed by dissociation of inhibitor-enzyme complex, e.g., if TCP is added to resuspended acetone powder (381) prior to other reactants and the carboxylase activity is then pelleted by centrifuga-tion and resuspended in fresh buffer lacking TCP, carboxylation is equal to that found in the prior control incubation.

A warfarin-binding protein has been isolated from liver endoplasmic-reticulum (326) which

bound 0.7 mole warfarin per mole of protein. This warfarin binding was inhibited by vitamin K_1. While this warfarin binding is apparently due to a specific protein which has been assumed to be the reductase proteins blocked by warfarin, Otagiri, et al. (327) have shown the interaction of warfarin with serum albumin. Fehske, et al. (328) state that a tryptophane of serum albumin is part of the warfarin binding site. Wilting, et al. (329) have shown warfarin binds to serum albumin and have shown that albumin has a single high affinity site for warfarin with the affinity increased by calcium.

Valente, et al. (330) suggest that the activity of warfarin is due to its open side-chain tautomeric form. Whitlon, et al. (331) have found that the vitamin K-dependent carboxylase system will utilize vitamin K epoxide for the carboxylation reaction in intact microsomes if DTT, but not NADH, is used as reducing agent. Using the epoxide plus DTT, the reaction is inhibited by warfarin, simi-larly the vitamin K reductase while using either DTT or NADH in the particulate microsomes, is inhibited by warfarin only when DTT is the re-ductant. Solubilizing the microsomes by a deter-gent eliminates both the ability of DTT to catalyze vitamin K reductase and also the inhibitory effect of warfarin on the reaction (157).

While Esnouf, et al. (332) have reported the inhibition of carboxylase by some copper com-plexes we have shown (145) that simple copper salts are very active inhibitors of the reaction of 1.0 mM, 90% inhibition.

Meeks and Couri (92) while agreeing that war-farin does not directly block carboxylation, state that it inhibits prothrombin glycosylation 80–90% and that this inhibition is reversed by vitamin K_1.

Park, et al. (333) have studied the effect of dicoumarin anticoagulants as well as chloro-K on vitamin K metabolism (see Section 20) and pro-thrombin activity. In the intact animal all five antagonists inhibited clotting factor synthesis with the same rate of prothrombin decline. Most in-terestingly the coumarol derivatives increased the plasma ratio of vitamin K epoxide to vitamin K while chloro-K had the opposite effect. They inter-pret these data as showing that interruption of the vitamin K epoxide cycle at either the epoxidase or reductase step will result in lowered prothrombin carboxylation. That is, the vitamin goes through a cycle $KH_2 \rightarrow KO \rightarrow (K) \rightarrow KH_2$ as a part of its normal functioning. These data suggest that TCP and 1-H-IP have the same binding site on carboxylase and/or vitamin K epoxidase while the coumarin and indandione anticoagulants have a common binding site on the vitamin K + DTT reductase and the vitamin K epoxide reductase which may also be related enzymes. These latter enzymes are also inhibited by TCP and 1-H-IP.

Phenprocoumon and warfarin (335 and many earlier papers from Matschiner's and Bell's laboratories) cause on increased accumulation of vitamin K epoxide in the liver suggesting again that the epoxide formation cycle is closely linked to prothrombin formation (335, 331) and its inhibition. Fig. 2 gives a possible scheme of the vitamin K function-metabolism cycle based on evidence with intact microsomes.

16. Abnormal (undercarboxylated) prothrombins

In 1963 Hemker, et al. (105) first reported an anomalous prothrombinlike protein in the plasma of vitamin K deficient or phenprocoumon treated animals. They later named this protein PIVKA and have since reported the occurrence of PIVKA-II, PIVKA-IX and PIVKA-X (106) and suggested these proteins were precursors of the blood vitamin K dependent clotting proteins II, IX, and X (they also postulated a PIVKA-VII). The work of Shah and Suttie (6) supported this as well as supporting the results of Hill, et al. (2) that the vitamin K action was post-translational modification of an already formed (or being formed) polypeptide. In the same year, 1972, before carboxylation had been discovered, Nelsestuen and Suttie (111) purified an inactive-prothrombin from the plasma of dicoumarol-treated cows. Similarly Morrison and Esnouf (338) isolated dicoumarol-prothrombin from human plasma and indicated that this inactive-prothrombin is, in fact, a complex mixture. Cesbron, et al. (120) isolated abnormal prothrombin from plasma of patients on coumarin therapy and showed it reacted with prothrombin antisera as had Nilehn and Ganrot (101) and Josso, et al. (103) in 1968. Both Cesbron, et al. (120) and Suttie (112) showed that this abnormal prothrombin yielded thrombin upon hydrolysis with various proteinases including *Echis carinatus* venom. Suttie suggested at that time that the vitamin K-dependent step involved attachment of some unrecognized prosthetic-group

to a precursor protein. Using affinity chromatography warfarin-prothrombin was also isolated from rat liver (117–119). It yields thrombin on protease treatment. Eight other species have been shown to produce abnormal prothrombin following warfarin treatment and except for the bovine all species showed increased levels in their liver microsomes as well as in plasma (125). Wallin and Prydz have developed a simple and rapid method for the purification of the warfarin prothrombin from bovine blood (122) using prothrombin antiserum coupled to Sepharose 4B as immunoadsorbent. Abnormal prothrombin as well as not binding calcium nor binding to barium salts has also lost the ability to bind to phospholipid surfaces (124). As a result of these changes in binding ability, activation by factor Xa, factor V and Ca^{2+} is not accelerated by phospholipid. The rate of activation brought about by factor Xa, Ca^{2+}, and factor V only is affected by the lack of carboxylation (slowed) and the pathway of activation to thrombin remains unchanged (118, 124, 338, see also the prior papers of Cesbron, etc.).

Ever since Magnusson's proof of 10 γ-carboxyglutamic acid residues in prothrombin (148) we have all wondered whether the glutamyl residues are carboxylated sequentially or simultaneously, and do there occur a series of vitamin K-deficient prothrombins with different numbers of the glutamyl residues 1 through 10 carboxylated. By 1976 evidence began to appear on the second of these questions. Grant and Suttie (123) as mentioned earlier found two 'prothrombin precursors' with PI's of 5.0 and 5.8 in vitamin K-deficient rat liver. The new, PI-5.0, protein while it yields thrombin by protease action does not bind phospholipid. Other forms of prothrombin have been reported by Prowse, et al. (339) from cows on long term warfarin treatment and they suggest the existence of partially carboxylated forms of prothrombin. From humans on prolonged warfarin treatment the same group (340) report two undercarboxylated prothrombins one containing an average of 7 out of 10 possible gla-residues the other containing only 4 gla-residues.

Friedman, et al. (341) have also shown not only that partially carboxylated prothrombins exist but that in the plasma of coumarin-treated patients there are a spectrum of such 'preprothrombins'. They found all normal prothrombin bound to phospholipid and separated the coumadin-induced prothrombins into a group averaging 6.5 mole of γ-carboxyglutamic acid/mole protein which still bound phospholipid and a second group averaging 2.8 mole γ-carboxyglutamic acid/mole protein which failed to bind phospholipid. There is considerable electrophoretic heterogeneity in these groups of plasma 'preprothrombins' presumably due to a range of proteins containing different amounts of γ-carboxyglutamic acid/mole. Malhotra (342–344) has isolated a number of undercarboxylated prothrombins from the plasma of dicoumarol treated cows. These include a 'preprothrombin' with 7 gla-residues (342), one with 5 gla-residues (343) and one with 2 gla-residues (344). Malhotra (345, 346) has reported evidence that the gla-residues cause conformational changes in the prothrombin molecule at the Arg-156-Ser and Arg-52-Asn residues which may help explain the resistance of abnormal prothrombins to normal activation by factor Xa, factor V, calcium and phospholipid. Studying the relative rates of activation (conversion to thrombin) of the 10 gla, 7 gla, 5 gla, and 2 gla prothrombins, he reported relative activation times of 1.5, 3–5, and 7–9 h for the last three (the undercarboxylated prothrombins) compared to 6–8 min for normal prothrombin. These data all indicate while with dicoumarol treatment carboxylation can be interrupted at several points during the post-translational carboxylation only the completed prothrombin is assayed in the usual clotting assay. The amount of carboxylation which occurs appears related to the relative levels of antagonist and vitamin K available to the liver microsomal carboxylating system.

As would be expected similar results have been reported for factor X (108) except that in this case the protein isolated appears to be completely non-carboxylated.

Lindhout, et al. in 1976 (109) by the use of specific antibodies to factors II, IX, and X demonstrated the presence of not only a dicoumarol prothrombin but also, a dicoumarol-factor IX (PIVKA-IX) and a dicoumarol-factor X (PIVKA-X) in bovine plasma after phenprocoumon.

Lewis, et al. (347) prepared highly specific antibody to human factor IX, sensitive at 1/1280 dilution and showed that the binding of calcium to factor IX increased (up to twofold) the antibody titre. Furie's group (348–351) and Guillin, et al.

(121) have made conformational antibodies to investigate the tertiary structural differences between abnormal prothrombins and between their activation fragments. They have isolated a population of antibodies specific for the carboxylated fragment 1 region of prothrombin. This implies that this region is exposed to the surface of the protein where the γ-carboxyglutamic acid residues are accessible. They have been able to isolate an antibody subpopulation from anti-abnormal prothrombin antisera which binds to abnormal prothrombin but not to prothrombin. As in the work of Lewis, et al. (347) above they also found a calcium dependent antibody subpopulation in anti-prothrombin antisera, however, the binding of abnormal prothrombin antibody was not influenced by calcium. These data suggest that there are major conformational differences in the tertiary structure of the fragment 1 region between prothrombin and abnormal prothrombin (352).

Lutes and Shapiro (353) have also prepared antisera directed to determinants in the amino terminal half of prothrombin and shown that reactivity to it is unaltered by desialation. They suggest that this approach can be an aid in the determination of structural changes in the abnormal prothrombins. Most recently Furie's group in continuation of earlier work (351, 354) have been able to prepare antibody to calcium-prothrombin, antibody which bound tightly in the presence of calcium but not in the absence of metal ions (352). This antibody bound to prothrombin-fragment 1 (the activation sequence fragment containing all the gla-residues), but did not bind to abnormal (uncarboxylated) prothrombin. This indicates that normal prothrombin changes conformation in the presence of calcium and that this change is recognized by the antibody and is located in the amino terminal region of prothrombin. Carlisle and Suttie on the other hand have been able to prepare antiserum to prothrombin precursor which was not influenced by calcium and contains apparently antibodies to at least two undercarboxylated precursors (355).

17. Chemical decarboxylation of prothrombin

We found that half of the carboxyl groups of labeled prothrombin were removed by heating in acid solution (Girardot, J. M., unpublished data).

This is to be expected of a malonic acid derivative and has been reported several times. Most recently, Tuhy, et al. (336) and Poser and Price (189) have proposed a better decarboxylation system which has proven very useful in laboratory work. Poser and Price (189) have been able to completely decarboxylate osteocalcin by heating the protein freeze-dried from 0.1 M NH_4HCO_3 for 5 h at 110°. This heating of the dry protein does not hydrolyze any peptide bonds nor significantly denature the protein. The protein can also be freeze-dried from 0.05 M HCl and quantitatively decarboxylated in 3 h at 110°. Tuhy, et al. (336) have used a similar procedure heating the lyophilized protein in vacuo at 110° for several hours.

18. Localization of the microsomal carboxylation system and the effect of inducers of microsomal enzymes

a. Localization

In 1977 Helgeland (356) presented evidence that the submicrosomal site of vitamin K dependent precursor-protein carboxylation was located in the rough microsomes and was associated with the luminal side of the membrane while the protein substrate appeared to be localized in both luminal and membrane fractions. This was confirmed by Carlisle and Suttie (357, 358) who found over twice as much pentapeptide carboxylase activity in the rough as in the smooth microsomal fraction. It was not present in the mitochondria or cytosol of hepatocytes. A similar distribution has been reported by Wallin and Prydz (359). The vitamin K epoxidase activity appears to be localized similarly to the carboxylase activity (358). Hassouna and Leach (360) state that immunological methods are more specific than clotting assays for the determination of the vitamin K-dependent proteins. In contrast to the site of carboxylation, Janson and Helgeland (361) have shown by antibody methods three- to fourfold higher levels of prothrombin in sonicates from smooth microsomes than from rough microsome fractions.

b. Inducers

In view of the known effect of phenobarbital, methylphenanthrene and other reagents to increase the level of many microsomal proteins the effect of phenobarbital administration on carboxylase levels has been studied and shown to increase the carboxylase level about twofold (158, 454) (see also section 24d).

Shah and Suttie (363) report that vitamin K deficiency or warfarin administration also causes a two- to threefold increase in protein carboxylase activity as measured by pentapeptide carboxylation. This increase after warfarin was inhibited by cycloheximide suggesting that enzyme protein synthesis had been induced by the deficiency. However, during the same time that carboxylase enzyme activity appeared to increase microsomal prothrombin precursor level also increases. These data and those of Dubin, et al. (365) show that this increase in peptide carboxylase due to lack of vitamin K is not necessarily related to an increase in carboxylase enzyme. That is, a decrease in peptide carboxylation activity occurs following in vivo injection of vitamin K to deficient rats, the decrease, however, can also be produced by adding prothrombin antiserum to remove prothrombin precursor. In both cases adding back in vitro decarboxylated vitamin K-dependent proteins restores the level of pentapeptide carboxylation. Similarly the warfarin 'induction' of pentapeptide carboxylation blocked by cycloheximide is reversed by in vitro addition of decarboxylated protein. These results suggest that the increased endogenous carboxylation after warfarin treatment is primarily due to increase in the precursor proteins rather than of enzyme protein.

19. Obligate SH nature of the protein carboxylation reaction

There are important functions of SH compounds or groups in this post translation modification. We will discuss these under: (a) are sulfhydryl derivatives of menadione functional compounds? (b) does the reduction of KO require of sulfhydryl group? (c) is vitamin K-dependent carboxylase an SH enzyme? (d) are b and c related functions of the SH requirement?

a. SH requirement for carboxylation; SH enzyme(s)

Mack, et al. (134, 157) and Friedman and Shia (149) showed that carboxylation initiated by vitamin K quinone plus NADH is stimulated by DTT and that DTT (or DTE) will replace NADH when the carboxylation is carried out by intact microsomes. These di-SH compounds cannot be replaced in this function by mono-SH compounds (145). The carboxylation initiated by vitamin K hydroquinone in both intact microsomes and solubilized microsomes is completely blocked by PHMB (134, 145, 366) at 1.0 mM (139) and also by such SH inhibitors as 5,5'-dithiobis-(2-nitrobenzoic acid) (DTNB) and quinone analogs of vitamin K with a free three-position such as menadione (145, 315), but less by N-ethy maleimide and little by iodoacetic acid or iodoacetamide. All these inhibitions are reversed by DTT (and DTE), and the same SH anagonists inhibit both endogenous protein and exogenous peptide substrate carboxylation. This leads to the conclusion that the carboxylation includes an SH enzyme.

Considering the possible cycle $K \rightarrow KH_2 \rightarrow KO \rightarrow K$, and the comparative carboxylation reaction data for intact microsomes and detergent solubilized microsomes which we submitted to the Journal of Biol. Chem. in 1975 t which was not accepted and was later mostly incorporated into other publications (134, 145) and the very careful study by Whitlon, et al. (331) in 1978 the following points seem clear. (1) The vitamin K hydroquinone dependent carboxylation is blocked by SH reagents such as PHMB. (2) The vitamin K epoxide reduction in the suggested vitamin K cycle requires DTT and is blocked by warfarin, while the the vitamin K-dependent glutamyl-carboxylation is not. In further support of a cycle in which the epoxide plays a vital part (i.e., the epoxidase and reductase are required for continued carboxylation) we have found that by carrying out the reaction at 0° we can show sequential stimulation of carboxylation by vitamin K hydroquinone additions (155). This cycle can perhaps be formulated somewhat as in Fig. 2. I have written vitamin K quinone (K) in brackets because there is no real evidence that vitamin K epoxide reductase yields the quinone rather than the hydroquinone. The DTT dependent, warfarin and pHMB blocked reductase of the epoxide may yield again vitamin K hydroquinone or may yield the quinone. The functional system in the liver is probably:

$$K \rightarrow KH_2 \underset{DTT}{\overset{O_2}{\rightleftharpoons}} KO$$

and the driving force for the H removal and thus the carboxylation is the potential between KH_2 and KO.

Robert Freedman (367) has reviewed in general terms the SH enzyme concept (a proteinthiol-proteindisulfide interchange) and feels that despite

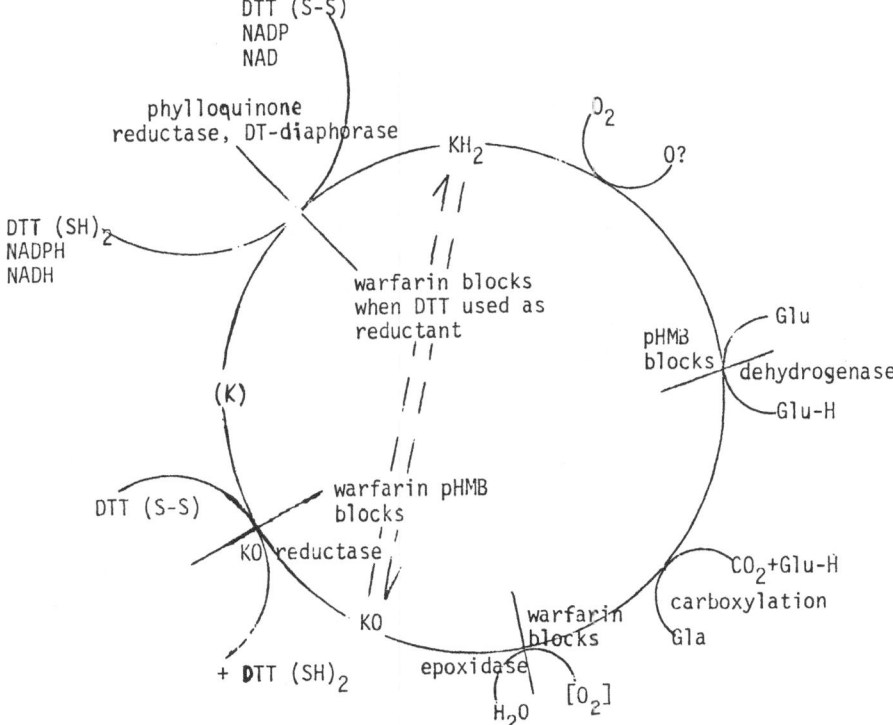

knowledge of an SH requirement and of blocking by SH blocking agents it is still necessary to isolate in pure form each enzyme which may belong to the group of SH-enzymes in order to assign the -SH role in the enzyme.

b. Thioethers of menadione

Another important thiol function in carboxylation is the ease with which the three position of the 2-methyl-1,4-naphthoquinone ring system reacts with SH compounds. The two functions may or may not be related. Fieser and Turner in 1947 (368) showed that mercaptans add to menadione. T. C. Stadtman has found a menadione thioether as a cofactor for a phosphatase from *Cl. sticklandii* (369). Nickerson, et al. (370) showed that glutathione (SH) reacts with menadione by nucleophilic substitution to form a thiol addition compound.

It is most interesting that in this latter reaction to form thiodione the H eliminated is taken up by a second quinone molecule and oxidation results in H_2O, production [c.f., formation H_2O_2 in the reactions of a hydroquinone with oxygen (166, 371)]. Related thioethers have been made, 2-solanesyl-1,4-naphthoquinone and 2-mercaptoethanol (157). We have prepared a large number of thioethers of menadione and shown them to be highly active in the carboxylation reaction, both when used as the quinones plus NADH with the quinone reductase and when used as the hydroquinones. When the thioether side-chain carries a charge or when there are other alterations to the 2-methyl-1,4-naphthoquinone ring this activity is lost.

In terms of mechanism of the reaction the useful information from this series of compounds is that the compounds from menadione and a dithiol have the greatest in vitro carboxylase activity and are considerably more active than the corresponding mono-thio products which are in turn more active than the oxygen ethers which are in their turn more active than hydroquinones such as the 2,3-dimethyl, the 2-methyl-3-monoprene or the 2-methyl-3-pentadecyl-1,4-naphthohydroquinone, indicating perhaps a thiol role at the 3-position in vitamin K function.

20. *Isolation and purification of the carboxylase enzyme(s)*

At this stage of the work on vitamin K and post-translational protein carboxylation, very little can be reported in terms of real success in isolation of the enzymes involved. It is obvious that if the cycle given in Fig. 2 is all required for the carboxylation system to operate, at least two reductases and two oxidative steps plus a carboxylation step must be considered. On the other hand if it is possible to separate and assay on a routine basis the vitamin K hydroquinone plus molecular oxygen step which produces the oxidative compound which withdraws the γ-hydrogen from glutamyl residues to give the glu minus hydrogen compound [i.e., 'the 1/2 reaction' (274)] purification of a single enzyme may be possible. The ability to use simple exogenous substrates greatly facilitates this possibility.

A number of attempts at concentration of the carboxylase system from the microsome have been reported. However, until real solubilization, rather than micellar solutions can be obtained, little can be accomplished. Factors such as ionic strength have proven of great importance in the assay (372). Houser, et al. (373) have reported about a 200 fold increase in carboxylase activity, although in very small yield. Canfield, et al. (374) have reported some concentration of a stable lipoprotein complex containing the vitamin K dependent carboxylase by removal of other proteins from the microsomes.

Wallin, et al. (359, 375–377) and Canfield, et al. (378) have published a series of articles on carboxylase purification. Wallin (377) has suggested that when vitamin K reductase (DT-diaphorase, E. C. 1.6.99.2) was removed from a microsomal carboxylation system it lost its carboxylation activity but in those experiments vitamin K quinone plus NADH was used as a source of vitamin K hydroquinone. Other papers of this group show about a 15 to 20 fold purification of carboxylase activity over the original microsomes. The enzyme is a tightly bound integral membrane protein and the increases in specific activity thus far obtained represent primarily removal of hemoglobin and other proteins or inhibitors. This preparation has lost its vitamin K and KO reductase activity and now requires the hydroquinone form of vitamin K. Their results and ours (379) are in agreement that lipid is required for activity. Price and Johnson have been able to fractionate the crude system into two required components (50).

Most recently Wallin and Suttie (380) have reported that not only do liver microsomes contain the vitamin K-dependent carboxylation system but that a pyridine nucleotide-dependent carboxylase of unknown endogenous compounds also occurs apparently brought about by a totally different enzyme. This latter carboxylation is most active following addition of NADP and can be removed by dialysis. This non-vitamin K-dependent carboxylase does not appear to be a problem in purification of the vitamin K-dependent enzyme.

One of the frequently used procedures for tissue preparation prior to isolation of many enzymes is the preparation of an acetone powder. In the case of the vitamin K-dependent carboxylase we recovered only 20% of soluble activity from acetone powder preparations solubilized by sodium deoxycholate and adjusted to pH 7.4. Friedman and Shia (381) have, however, been able to prepare acetone powder preparations with essentially undamaged activity for pentapeptide carboxylation. The vitamin K-dependent carboxylase activity is dissolved back in non-ionic detergent (Triton X 100).

In contrast to all the work on the rat microsomal vitamin K-dependent carboxylase, Vermeer, et al. (153) have reported the partial purification of the bovine carboxylase. However, the system is still not purified in that non-vitamin K dependent CO_2 fixation also occurs. They report the enzyme to be inhibited by prothrombin.

21. γ-Carboxyglutamic acid detection, determination, synthesis and metabolism

a. Detection in intact polypeptide

One of the most important recent contributions to this field has been the method of Hauschka whereby each gla-residue in gla-containing protein is converted to a tritiated glutamyl residue (382). In this procedure each gla residue is tritiated by drying from TDCl (0.05 M) in D_2O and the dry protein heated at 110° for 3 to 6 h in vacuo. This decarboxylation procedure results in tritium replacing the carboxyl on each gla-residue. All of the tritium incorporated is in glutamic acid and the efficiency of the exchange decarboxylation is practically theoretical.

Earlier detection procedure included Zytkovicz

and Nelsestuen's procedure of reduction of vitamin K-dependent proteins by ^{3}H-diborane to yield 5,5'-^{3}H-dihydroxyleucine which is released by acid hydrolysis of the protein (383). A very similar pocedure is that of Rose, et al. (384) in which the protein or peptide is decarboxylated in D_2O forming γ-D-glutamic acid. The protein is hydrolyzed and the ratio of D-glu to H-glu is determined by mass spectrometry.

b. Determination of gla-residues

Hauschka in 1977 (385) first formalized the alkaline hydrolysis which all laboratories were using to search for γ-carboxyglutamic acid. He reported that hydrolysis of the protein by 2 M KOH at 110° for 22 h gave quantitative recovery of gla. Tabor and Tabor (386) and Yamagata, et al. (387) have also analyzed directly for gla by an amino acid analyzer modification, after alkaline hydrolysis. Direct analysis has been preferred by Madar, et al. (388) who state that preliminary reduction to 5,5'-dihydroxyleucine with tritium labelled diborane allows only partial recovery and low sensitivity. Madar, et al., acknowledge, the 'gla-doublet' problem in cases of potassium contamination but eliminate it with a 'few drops' of 5% $HClO_4$. James (389) has adapted the procedure to the Technicon Autoanalyzer to present a method capable of separating gla from all other amino acids except taurine.

Five different procedures for gla detection-determination were presented at the Steenbock Symposium in June, 1979. These include detection by dansylation (390), automated sequenator methods (391) and two-dimensional high-voltage paper electrophoresis (392). In addition Grundberg, et al. (393) have developed a detection method useful at the nanomole level for gla analysis by selective anion exchange elution and fluorescence detection. This method is based on prior alkaline hydrolysis, column purification and detection by the sensitive O-phthalaldehyde fluorescent derivative rather than by ninhydrin and can be used for the determination of gla in protein alkaline hydrolysates (394) and in urine (393).

A novel procedure presented in this same symposium was the use of β-carboxyglutamic acid as an internal standard for the quantitative determination of free gla in urine (395) at concentration of 10–50 μmol/l.

c. Cleavage of gla-peptide bonds

Katayama and Titani (396) have found that structural research on the gla-proteins can be facilitated by the fact that not only single methionyl peptide bonds but also gla-peptide bonds are cleaved by cyanogen bromide and related reagents.

d. Metabolism of γ-carboxyglutamic acid

It has been found that when proteins containing gla are degraded in the body, gla appears in the urine primarily as the free amino acid (212, 397). Work with the rat shows that gla (whether free or in a protein) is not degraded metabolically but is quantitatively excreted unchanged (398).

Surprisingly, this amino acid (gla) is a powerful competitive inhibitor of oxidative deamination of glutamate by the enzyme glutamate dehydrogenase (399), [E.C. 1.4.1.3], and is an activator of reductive amination of ketoglutarate by the same enzyme, although it is not metabolized by the enzyme.

e. γ-Carboxyglutamic acid synthesis

In order to establish the structure of gla and to have it available as a standard and as a substrate precursor a number of synthetic methods for gla have been developed (400–406). These methods are particularly important to research on the mechanism of the carboxylation reaction.

22. Vitamin K determination, synthesis and metabolism

a. Detection and determination

Many vitamin K assay procedures have been suggested over the years, however, they were insensitive and of no great interest since food vitamin K deficiency is not an important disease. However, with the discovery of the function of vitamin K there has been a resurgence in interest in assay methods for vitamin K, and the many naturally occurring, 1,4-naphthoquinones. Some of the more recent procedures include the titanium reduction and spectrophotometric assay of Vire, et al. (295), a number of HPLC methods including those of Lefevere, et al. (407) Donnahey, et al. (408) and Haroon, et al. (409) which detect as little as 500 picograms and separate cis and trans isomers as well as the epoxides and the various menaquinones. Mack (410) has separated the menaquinones by HPLC using silver ion as modifier.

Gas-liquid chromatography has been applied to the quantitative analysis of vitamin K and its epoxide in blood (411), in leafy vegetables (412), and in photodegradation products (413), while Collins, et al. (414) have separated natural mixtures of bacterial menaquinones by reverse phase thin-layer chromatography.

With the proposal that both vitamin K hydroquinone and vitamin K epoxide ae involved in the carboxylation (see section 16) several HPLC methods have been developed for the determination of the epoxide. This is a requirement for the study of the epoxidase phase of the reaction. Bjornsson, et al. (415) separated vitamin K from vitamin K epoxide by HPLC using radiolabeled compounds as markers. Bechtold and Jahnchen (411) carried out the same separation by gas-liquid chromatography and electron-capture detection.

b. Vitamin K synthesis

While the very basic and important synthetic work of Fieser and co-workers on the synthesis of vitamin K and many, many analogs has already been referred to (Section 1b), new methods continue to appear. Naruta (416) has used allyltin reagents to synthesize quinone derivatives. This procedure has given vitamin K_2 (MK-5) in almost 80% yield.

Snatzke, et al. (417) have prepared the 2,3-epoxide of menadione in enantiomerically pure form.

c. Vitamin K metabolism

Shearer and Barkhan (418) investigated the metabolites of vitamin K_1 and found urinary water soluble glucuronide conjugates as the major excretion product. One of the aglycones prepared from the glucuronides appears to be phylloquinone.γ-lactone previously identified by Wiss and Gloor (419). In vitro the one metabolic product formed from vitamin K_1 appears to be the 2,3-epoxide (280). The epoxide also appears to be the major metabolite formed in vivo (420, 421) and the latter authors suggest that the epoxide or its formation is involved in the carboxylation reaction.

In man warfarin administration results in a two-fold increase in the urinary excretion of vitamin K metabolites (422) apparently because it blocks the recycling of vitamin K epoxide back to vitamin K hydroquinone. Bjornsson, et al. (423, 424) report a rapid turnover of vitamin K_1 in man (about 150 min) and the major liver metabolite as the epoxide which accumulates with warfarin administration.

Of most interest and importance in terms of vitamin K function is the report by Vire, et al. (295) of the formation of epox naphthohydroquinone anion:

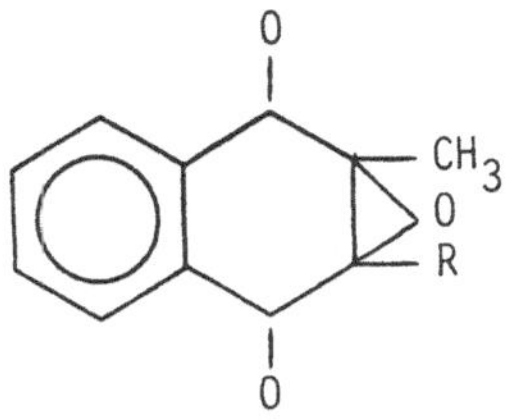

If in fact such an intermediate is formed in the liver this could possibly serve as a logical withdrawing group for the γ-hydrogen of glutamyl residues (see section 12d).

23. Prothrombin turnover

On the basis of the rate of disappearance of blood prothrombin following high-level cycloheximide treatment to normal rats we published (425, 426) an approximate 6–8 h turnover-time for prothrombin. This is not inconsistant with the report of Bell and Matschiner (427) of 5–7 h inactivation time. These are much shorter times that those previously reported by Josso, et al. (428). The recovery of prothrombin formation by vitamin K administration to vitamin K deficient rats, immediately after cycloheximide administration proved that the vitamin is acting at a site later than polypeptide synthesis. Siegfried, et al. (429) indicate a faster rate of formation of prothrombin in the female than the male rat due to a faster rate of precursor synthesis. They obtained optimal rates of vitamin K promoted recovery and fastest prothrombin disappearance rates with high levels of cycloheximide as did we. However, the more cycloheximide used and the more vitamin K deficient the animal the quicker will be both degradation of the remaining prothrombin and the more rapid the response to vitamin K thus I feel more confident of the 7–8 h life time of prothrombin found after giving normal rats levels of cycloheximide just sufficient to stop synthesis yet not kill the animal and to permit recovery. Owen, et al. (430) used 125_I labeled canine prothrombin given to adult dogs and obtained

about 80% catabolism per day which appears slow compared with the cycloheximide-treated-rat results, however, this may be related to animal size.

24. Other enzymes of the vitamin K carboxylation cycle

If such a cycle, with regard to vitamin K reuse exists some attention should be given in this review to (a) vitamin K reductase (DT-diaphorase), (b) vitamin K epoxidase [E.C. 1.14.99.20] and (c) vitamin K epoxide reductase in addition to the vitamin K dependent oxidative glu-γ-hydrogen removal and glu-carboxylation reaction.

a. Vitamin K reductase

This enzyme has been known for a number of years and has been variously termed phylloquinone reductase (431), NADH-quinone reductase, menadione reductase, DT-diaphorase [E.C. 1.6.99.2] (432), etc. According to Wosilait and Nason (433) there are at least two enzymes, menadione reductase and quinone reductase in *E. coli* and in rat liver. Koli, et al. (492) claim there are three quinone dehydrogenases in pig liver, a D-diaphorase [E.C. 1.6.99.5], a T-diaphorase [E.C. 1.6.99.6], and a DT-diaphorase [E.C. 1.6.99.2]. The latter two are blocked by dicoumarol while the first is not. Menadione is a good substrate and sensitivity of the reductase to coumarin and indandione antagonists of vitamin K has been well documented (431, 434, 437). Ernster, et al. (438) propose that warfarin-resistant strains of rats possess a lowered DT-diaphorase activity which is responsible for their genetically determined resistance to warfarin. According to Hosoda, et al. (439) who purified the enzyme to homogeneity, it has a molecular weight of approximately 50 000 and has one mole of FAD/mole of enzyme. Lind and Ernster (440) have explored the relationship between DT-diaphorase and the aryl hydrocarbon hydroxylase system. They showed that treatment of rats with 3-methylcholanthrene causes a several fold increase in liver DT-diaphorase activity. The enzyme occurs both in the microsomes and the cytosol, the majority being in the latter fraction. The enzyme is inhibited by 7,8-benzoflavone (which has no effect on carboxylase) indicating the diaphorase to be a cytochrome P450 enzyme. A simple three-step method for the purification of NAD(P)H dehydrogenase (DT-diaphorase) from rat liver has been presented by Wallin, et al. (376). The final enzyme preparation was electrophoretically homogenous and made up of two monomers of about 27 000 M. W. each but with different amino-terminal amino acids suggesting that the enzyme is made up of two non-identical subunits. Recently, Fasco and Principe (441) have been able to tie the reductase system even more closely to the carboxylation system by showing very high activity in hydroquinone formation from both the quinone and the quinone and the quinone epoxide of vitamin K_1. DTT provided reducing equivalents for the reductase system directly rather than indirectly via a DT-diaphorase. Thus, it again appears that there are two or more reductases, one used DTT and is blocked by warfarin and others use NAD(P)H. None of these data completely solve the problems of the postulated vitamin K and carboxylation cycle as to number of reductases, their cofactors, their substrates, and their blocking agents.

b. Vitamin K-2,3-epoxide reductase

Is this the same enzyme as vitamin K quinone reductase? On the basis of a di-SH required cofactor to yield the hydroquinone from the epoxide while NAD(P)H will serve as cofactor for an enzyme which yields the hydroquinone from the quinone it appears that there must be at least two enzymes. These are both reductions, however, the reduction of vitamin K-2,3-epoxide could proceed from epoxide directly to hydroquinone or to quinone and then to hydroquinone. This latter pathway could require two enzymes.

A major pathway of vitamin K metabolism is conversion of its hydroquinone to the quinone-2,3-epoxide and reduction of the epoxide back to the hydroquinone. Earlier work by Matschiner and co-workers (49, 421, 444) and by Bell, et al. (321, 335, 443) proposed that coumarin and indandione anti-coagulants inhibited vitamin K dependent pro-thrombin completion by preventing the regeneration of vitamin K from its 2,3-epoxide. The epoxide accumulates in rat, man and bovine in the presence of coumarin and indandione antagonists. These results are consistent with the hypothesis that continuous vitamin K hydroquinone regeneration from its major metabolite the 2,3-epoxide is required. Whitlon, et al. (331) in further study of the

significance of vitamin K epoxide to the action of the coumarin drugs and the role of vitamin K hydroquinone in protein carboxylation are in agreement with the work of Mack, et al. (134) that vitamin K-dependent carboxylase activity of intact microsomes is dependent primarily on DTT and the reaction is blocked by warfarin. However, when the microsomes are solubilized by detergent the DTT-epoxide reductase and warfarin blocking activity are lost, while NADH reduction of vitamin K quinone [E.C. 1.6.99.5] is not lost. The vitamin K epoxide reductase will use DTT but not NADH. The DTT requiring epoxide reductase is strongly inhibited by warfarin.

Siegfried has reported the solubilization by potassium cholate of vitamin K epoxide reductase from rat liver microsomes (444, 445) and again shown its DTT dependence. In a similar metabolic cycle present in the membranes of plant chloroplasts ascorbate has been shown to act as the reducing agent of violaxanthin de-epoxidase (446). Silverman (447) has provided experimental evidence supporting a molecular hypothesis that the 3-substituted-4-hydroxycoumarin drugs block vitamin K function by inactivation of vitamin K epoxide reductase. This hypothesis is based upon the fact that this epoxide reductase requires thiol not replaceable by NAD(P)H as reductant. He has used the compound:

as a model for the dicoumarins in the study of their possible reaction with SH-enzymes.

c. Vitamin K epoxidase

The accumulation of vitamin K epoxide in warfarin treated rats and the in vitro inhibition of epoxide reduction (442) by warfarin led Matchiner's group (449, 450) and later Bell's (451–453) to study the epoxidation and assert that vitamin K-dependent protein carboxylation is linked to the metabolism of the vitamin and in particular to its conversion to its epoxide. As already stated this could be because vitamin K hydroquinone is an intermediate in the conversion of the quinone to the quinone epoxide. The direct relationship between warfarin injection level and vitamin K epoxide formation in rabbit plasma over about 5 h has been shown by Park, et al. (448).

Unlike the coumarins, tetrachloro (TCP) and chloro-K inhibit both in vivo and in vitro vitamin K epoxidation and vitamin K-dependent oxidative-carboxylation.

Properties of the epoxidase have been studied by Sadowski, et al. (454) who showed the enzyme to be located primarily in the rough microsomes (455) where it produces vitamin K epoxide from vitamin K hydroquinone plus molecular oxygen. While most of the above discussion seems to favor the suggestion that the protein carboxylation and the vitamin hydroquinone epoxidation are a coupled oxidative-carboxylation, this is still an unresolved hypothesis. Friedman and Smith (456) and Suttie, et al. (292) support this hypothesis. However, Wallin (167) feels that the two reactions are not coupled based on his data that NADH plus vitamin K reductase plus vitamin K quinone can bring about carboxylation after separating out the epoxidase. On the other hand Egeberg and Helgeland (455) and Suttie, et al. (457) have presented circumstantial evidence that the two events are coupled. This evidence includes the finding that removal of a portion of the epoxidase activity by prothrombin antisera also lowers carboxylase activity as well as lowering epoxidase activity. The low epoxidase activity found in rats given vitamin K is consistent with low quantities of endogenous substrates being available for carboxylation. It appears plausible that the treatment with the immunoadsorbent may have removed some of a 'carboxylase/epoxidase' activity to give the decreases found. When the carboxylation level was increased by increasing the substrate concentration (c.f., 365) the epoxidase activity also increased.

d. Microsomal enzyme inducers and carboxylation

It is well established that agents such as phenobarbital and 3-methylcholanthrene increase many microsomal enzymes including the cytochrome P450 system and DT-diaphorase. We found that in a similar way phenobarbital given to the animal increases the carboxylating ability of rat liver microsomes (158). Fasco and Cashin (458) have studied the effect of both phenobarbital and 3-methylcholanthrene and shown that they both

diminish the response to warfarin. This has also been reported for glutethimide (459).

Huggins, et al. (460), Lind and Ernster (440), and Lind, et al. (461) have found that 3-methylcholanthrene in particular is a potent inducer of DT-diaphorase which they state to be the preferred quinone reductase in connection with conjugation reactions.

e. Antagonists to vitamin K and cancer

As referred to earlier there is currently considerable interest between the vitamin K-dependent reaction and tumor metastases. Coumarin compounds have been stated to reduce lung metastasis in Lewis lung carcinoma (466) perhaps by virtue of inhibition of carboxylation (463). On the other hand, Poggi, et al. (142) also using Lewis lung carcinoma showed that cells from warfarin treated mice had uniformly lower factor X-activating activity than controls so that any antimetastatic role might just be related to coagulation at the site of cell lodgement.

III. Methodology of carrying out the in vitro carboxylation reaction in a solubilized microsomal abstract

This procedure has been given in detail in Methods in Enzymology (135) and hence will be given in abbreviated form here. Nevertheless, with the following outline one should be able readily to carry out not only the post-transcriptional carboxylation of endogenous protein but also the carboxylation of exogenous peptide and the epoxidation of vitamin K hydroquinone and determine these activities.

For satisfactory in vitro carboxylation it is necessary to start with vitamin K deficient animals or if these are not available warfarin treated animals, although in the latter case less carboxylation is obtained.

1. Vitamin K-deficient rats

The deficiency is produced in white male rats by feeding them a vitamin K-deficient diet (5) made up of: purified soy protein 20% (Teklad or equivalent) (this level can vary from 15 to 35% satisfactorily) tionlein 6.0%, methyl linoleate 1.0%, AIN meneral mix 3.5% (464), Alphacel 4%, AIN vitamin mix (minus menaquinone) (464) 1%, DL-methionine 0.5% and sucrose 63.8% (this level will, of course, vary with the soy protein level to keep the total 100) plus choline chloride 0.2%. They are housed in coprophagy prevention cages (8) which may be built in square, circular or linear form. The production of the deficiency requires about seven days for 150–250 g rats if water bottles are kept clean and access to feces is avoided. Partridge (465) and Barber and Colvin (466) have both reported that a nutritional vitamin K deficiency is more readily produced as the protein content of the diet is decreased while Matschiner and Doisey (467) obtain their most severe deficiency at their highest (35%) soy protein level.

If warfarin is used it should be administered at the level of 1–5 mg/kg body weight, 18–24 h before killing.

2. Vitamin K-deficient rat liver microsomes

The livers are excised and homogenized in twice their volume of 0.25 M sucrose, containing 2 mM benzamidine-HCl in 0.1 M imidazole or 50 mM phosphate buffer, pH 7.4. The homogenate is centrifuged for 15 min at $10\,000 \times g$, 3–4°. The post mitochondrial supernate is re-centrifuged at $105\,000 \times g$, 3–4° for 1 h. The fluffly top layer is removed from the pellet and the pellet is suspended in 1/2 the original volume of the post mitochondrial supernatant and re-centrifuged. The top layer is removed as before and the pellet resuspended in 1/5 the original volume.

3. Preparation of soluble carboxylation system

One ml of the microsomal suspension is diluted with 1 ml of a solution containing 4.0% Triton X100 (many other detergents may also be used), 800 mM NaCl and 8 mM benzamidine-HCl, in the starting buffer, pH 7.4. The supernatant after centrifugation at $105\,000 \times g$ for 1 h contains the proteins required for carboxylation.

4. Carboxylation assay

The assay is carried out in capped tubes using 0.15 ml of the solubilized microsomal solution (from 0.25 g liver)/tube. The final assay volume of 0.2 ml (the assay can readily be scaled up or down) contains 5 μCi $Na_2\,^{14}CO_3$ (S.A. 40–60 mCi/mmole and 0.1 mM vitamin K_1 hydroquinone. If the vitamin K_1 quinone form is used the final solution should be made 1 mM with respect to NADH and 2 mM with DTT. All additions are made in the starting buffer. The vitamin K compound (normally KH_2) may be added in ethanol. Maximum carboxylation occurs at 20°–25° and is essentially complete in 5 min. The reaction, however, will occur even at 0° where it will continue linearly for at least 2 h.

5. Determination of carboxylation

After incubation, 0.9 ml 10% trichloroacetic acid (TCA) and 0.1 ml of 1.0% w/v BSA solution are added, the TCA pellet is twice dissolved in 2% sodium carbonate and reprecipitated with 10% TCA. After a final 5% TCA wash the pellet is dissolved in 0.5 ml 2% Na_2CO_3 solution and transferred with 5 ml (if using small counting tubes) or 14 ml (if using the larger counting tubes) of Scintisol (Aquasol, Handifluor, etc., etc.) to a liquid scintillation vial and counted in a liquid scintillation counter. Chemiluminescence is inhibited by adding 0.2 ml of N HCl to the vial.

6. Preparation of vitamin K hydroquinone

The hydroquinone to be used is made by treatment of the quinone with sodium dithionite as described by Fieser (468). The hydroquinone can also readily be made by reduction of the quinone with sodium borohydride $NaBH_4$. Since sodium dithionite at the levels used does not influence the assay, the solution of vitamin K hydroquinone containing sodium dithionite can be used to initiate the assay. Sodium dithionite does, however, give a strong ESR signal. $NaBH_4$, on the other hand, does function as a reducing agent in the assay. The preferred procedure is to reduce with $HaBH_4$, store the pure hydroquinone under petroleum ether and make up solutions in ethanol or detergent as needed. It is more stable in detergent.

7. Substrates

The procedure outlined above gives good data on the carboxylation of endogenous protein precursors. However, simultaneous assays can be carried out on exogenous substrates such as Phe-Leu-Glu-Glu-Leu or N-t-BOC-glu-α-benzyl ester by adding these substrates at from 1 to 4 mM to the assay mixture. The carboxylation of these exogenous substrates gives a soluble product which remains in solution after the TCA precipitation. Hence, the supernatant must be thoroughly bubbled with CO_2 to constant count, in order to eliminate $^{14}CO_2$ and measure actual exogenous carboxylation.

IV. Summary

In summary, in this review on the function of vitamin K in post-translational modification of precursor proteins by carboxylation of certain glutamyl residues, I have tried to cover in particular the recent work on the reaction, the enzymes involved and the mechanisms being considered.

In doing this I have also considered vitamin K, its discovery, its functional form and the possible relation of its metabolism to the carboxylation reaction. Equally the various vitamin K-dependent gla-containing proteins currently known have been described. The carboxylation of synthetic small molecule exogenous substrates and the synthesis and metabolism of the products of carboxylation are of great help in studying the reaction.

Structural specificity of vitamin K analogs in vivo and in vitro has been compared and the use of various antagonists in vivo and in vitro considered in attempts to gain an understanding of the overall reaction.

The reactions subsequent to carboxylation, e.g., the activation of prothrombin to thrombin via serine proteases and the related activation of the other vitamin K-dependent proteins have not been considered in this review. The review has not covered prothrombin or other vitamin K-dependent protein isolation, nor the determination of these proteins.

As the vitamin K-dependent protein carboxylation story has developed over the past six years, a number of reviews have been written which help in keeping up with the various aspects of the field as it has expanded. These reviews refer to many of the papers I have had to eliminate due to space limitations. They are referenced as 469–489.

The review is in no sense comprehensive and many papers have been missed or only mentioned. I have tried to concentrate on the more recent work and, thus, much of the very fine work of the 1940's on vitamin K chemistry is hardly mentioned.

Some redundancy has been built into the organization of the review so that a reader can obtain a reasonable view of any one section without having to search the whole review for all possible relevant information on any particular part of the field.

Acknowledgement

The work described from our laboratories was carried out by Dr. Donald Mack, Dr. Jean-Marie Girardot, Dr. Max Wolfensberger, Dr. Adam Dubin, Dr. Joy Price, Dr. Eric Suen, Dr. Shunsuke Yuyama, post-doctoral fellows and/or graduate students with the help of the technicians Julie Miller, Doug Bayless, Betty Wiseman, Tom Curtis, Mary Ann Vaughan, Vicki Bartels, and Julie Watson at various times during the 7 years 1973 to the present.

References

1. Goswami, P. & Munro, H. N., 1962. Biochim. Biophys. Acta 55: 410–412.
2. Hill, R. B., Gaetani, S., Paolucci, A. M., Rama Rao, P. B., Alden, R., Ranhotra, G. S., Shah, D. V., Shah, V. K., & Johnson, B. C., 1968. J. Biol. Chem. 243: 3930–3939.
3. Babior, B. M., 1966. Biochim. Biophys. Acta 123: 606–610.
4. Lowenthal, J. & Simmons, E. L., 1967. Experientia 23: 421–422.
5. Ranhotra, G. S. & Johnson, B. C., 1969. Proc. Soc. Exp. Biol. Med. 132: 509–513.
6. Shah, D. V. & Suttie, J. W., 1972. Arch. Biochem. Biophys. 150: 91–95.
7. Mameesh, M. S. & Johnson, B. C., 1959. Proc. Soc. Exp. Biol. Med. 101: 467–469.
8. Metta, V. C., Nash, L., & Johnson, B. C., 1961. J. Nutr. 74: 473–476.
9. Olson, R. E., 1964. Science 145: 926–928.
10. Johnston, M. F. N., Kipfer, R. K., & Olson, R. E., 1972. J. Biol. Chem. 3987–3993, 3994, 4000, 4001–4007.
11. Olson, R. E., Kipfer, R. K., & Li, L. F., 1969. Adv. Enzyme Regulation 7: 83–94.
12. Olson, R. E., 1974. Vitamins and Hormones 32: 483–511.
13. Girardot, J.-M., Delaney, R., & Johnson, B. C., 1974. Biochem. Biophys. Res. Commun. 59: 1197–1203.
14. Stenflo. J., Fernlund, P., Egan, W., & Roepstorff, P., 1974. Proc. Nat. Acad. Sci., USA 71: 2730–2733.

114

15. Nelsestuen, G. L., Zytokovicz, T. H. & Howard, J. B., 1974. J. Biol. Chem. 249: 6347–6350.
16. Anonymous, 1975. Nutr. Rev. 33: 25–28.
17. Dam, H., 1929. Biochem. Z. 215: 475–492.
18. Dam, H., 1930. Biochem. Z. 220: 158–163.
19. McFarlane, W. D., Graham, W. R. & Richardson, F., 1931. Biochem. J. 25: 358–366.
20. Holst, W. F. & Halbrook, E. R., 1933. Science 77: 354.
21. Dam, H., 1934. Nature 133: 909–910.
22. Dam, H. & Schoenheyder, F., 1934. Biochem. J. 28: 1355–1359.
23. Almquist, H. J., 1935. Nature 136: 31.
24. Almquist, H. J., 1975. Am. J. Clin. Nutr. 28: 656–659.
25. Dam, H., 1935. Nature 135: 652–653.
26. Dam, H., 1935. Biochem. J. 29: 1273–1285.
27. Schoenheyder, F., 1936. Biochem. J. 30: 890–896.
28. Dam, H., Geiger, A., Glavind, J., Karrer, P., Karrer, W., Rothschild, E. & Salomon, H., 1939. Helv. Chim. Acta 22: 310–313.
29. MacCorquodale, D. W., Binkley, S. B., McKee, R. W., Thayer, S. A. & Doisey, E. A., 1939. Proc. Soc. Exp. Biol. Med. 40: 482–483.
30. Almquist, H. J. & Klose, A. A., 1939. J. Am. Chem. Soc. 61: 1610–1611.
31. Ansbacher, S. & Fernholz, E., 1939. J. Am. Chem. Soc. 61: 1924–1925.
32. MacCorquodale, D. W., McKee, R. W., Binkley, S. B., Cheney, L. C., Holcomb, W. F., Thayer, S. A. & Doisey, E. A., 1939. J. Biol. Chem. 130: 433.
33. Mayer, H. & Isler, O., 1971. Methods in Enzymology XVIII(C), 469–491.
34. Karrer, P., Geiger, A., Ruegg, R. & Salomon, H., 1939. Helv. Chim. Acta 22: 1513–1516.
35. Almquist, H. J. & Klose, A. A., 1939. J. Am. Chem. Soc. 61: 2557–2558.
36. Fieser, L. F., 1939. J. Am. Chem. Soc. 61: 2559–2561.
37. Fieser, L. F., 1939. J. Am. Chem. Soc. 61: 2561.
38. Binkley, S. B., McKee, R. W., Thayer, S. A. & Doisey, E. A., 1940. J. Biol. Chem. 133: 721–729.
39. Mayer, H. & Isler, O., 1971. Methods in Enzymology XVIII (C), 491–547.
40. Fieser, L. F., Tishler, M. & Sampson, W. L., 1941. J. Biol. Chem. 137: 659–692.
41. Isler, O., Ruegg, R., Chopard-dit-Jean, L. H., Winterstein, A. & Wiss, O., 1958. Helv. Chim. Acta 41: 786–807.
42. Isler, O. & Wiss, O., 1959. Vitamins and Hormones 17: 53–90.
43. Weber, F. & Wiss, O., 1971. The Vitamins (W. H. Sebrell, Jr. & R. S. Harris, eds.) Vol. III, 2nd Edition, Academic Press, New York, pp. 457–466.
44. Pennock, J. F., 1966. Vitamins and Hormones 24: 307–329.
45. Griminger, P., 1966. Vitamins and Hormones 24: 605–618.
46. Dunphy, P. S. & Brodie, A. F., 1971. Methods in Enzymology XVIII (C), pp. 407–461.
47. Matschiner, J. T., Taggart, W. V. & Amelotti, T. M., 1967. Biochemistry 6: 1243–1248.
48. Matschiner, J. T. & Amelotti, J. M., 1968. J. Lipid Res. 9: 176–179.
49. Matschiner, J. T., Bell, R. G., Amelotti, J. M. & Knauer, T. E., 1970. Biochim. Biophys. Acta 201: 309–315.

50. Price, J. A., Bartels, V. L., Chiu, A., Delaney, R. & Johnson, B. C., 1980. J. Biol. Chem. 255: 1808–1811.
51. Martius, C. & Esser H., 1958. Biochem. Z. 331: 1–9.
52. Billeter, M., Bolliger, W. & Martius, C., 1964. Biochem. Z. 340: 290–303.
53. Martius, C., Semadeni, E. C. & Alvino, C., 1965. Biochem. Z. 342: 492–494.
54. Dialameh, G. H., Yekundi, K. G. & Olson, R. E., 1970. Biochim. Biophys. Acta 223: 332–338.
55. Moore, M. B., 1941. J. Am. Chem. Soc. 63: 2049–2051.
56. Carmack, M., Moore, M. B. & Balis, M. E., 1950. J. Am. Chem. Soc. 72: 844–847.
57. Fieser, L. F. & Fry, E. M., 1940. J. Am. Chem. Soc. 62: 228–229.
58. Taggart, W. V. & Matschiner, J. T., 1969. Biochemistry 8: 1141–1146.
59. Matschiner, J. T., 1969. Fat Soluble Vitamins (H. F. DeLuca & J. W. Suttie, editors) University of Wisconsin Press, Madison, Wisconsin, pp. 377–397.
60. Duello, T. J. & Matschiner, J. T., 1971. Int. J. Vit. Nutr. Res. 41: 180–188.
61. Owen, C. A., Jr., Magath, T. B. & Bollman, J. L., 1951. Am. J. Physiol. 166: 1–11.
62. Koller, F., Loeliger, A. & Duckert, F., 1951. Acta Haematol. 6: 1–18.
63. Aggeler, P. M., White, S. G., Glendening, M. B., Page, E. W., Leake, T. B. & Bates, G., 1952. Proc. Soc. Exp. Biol. Med. 79: 692–694.
64. Biggs, R., Douglass, A. S., MacFarlane, R. G., Dacie, J. V., Pitney, W. R., Merskey, C. & O'Brien, J. R., 1952. Brit. Med. J. 2: 1378–1382.
65. Hougie, C., Barrow, E. M. & Graham, J. B., 1957. J. Clin. Invest. 36: 485–496.
66. Owren, P. A. & Aas, K., 1951. Scand. J. Clin. Lab. Invest. 3: 201–208.
67. Naeye, R. L., 1956. Proc. Soc. Exp. Med. 91: 101–104.
68. McElfresh, A. E. & Ozge, A., 1957. J. Lab. Clin. Med. 49: 753–755.
69. Ball, E. G., Anfinsen, C. B. & Cooper, O., 1947. J. Biol. Chem. 168: 257–270.
70. Fieser, L. F. & Heymann, N., 1948. J. Biol. Chem. 176: 1363–1370.
71. Martius, C. & Nitz-Litzow, D., 1953. Biochim. Biophys. Acta 12: 134–140.
72. Martius, C. & Nitz-Litzow, D., 1954. Biochim. Biophys. Acta 13: 289–290.
73. Martius, C., 1966. Vitamins and Hormones 24: 441–445.
74. Chmielewska, A. & Cieslak, T., 1958. Tetrahedron Lett. 4: 135–146.
75. Clark, V. M., Hutchinson, D. W., Kirby, G. W., Clark, M. & Todd, A., 1961. J. Chem. Soc. 715–721: 722—725.
76. Andrews, K. J. M., 1961. J. Chem. Soc. 1808–1816.
77. Vilkas, M. & Lederer, E., 1962. Experientia 18: 546–549.
78. Asano, A., Brodie, A. F., Wagner, A. F., Wittreich, P. E. & Folkers, K., 1962. J. Biol. Chem. 237: 2411–2412.
79. Erickson, E. R., Wagner, A. F. & Folkers, K., 1963. J. Am. Chem. Soc. 85: 1534–1535; 1535–1537.
80. Watanabe, T. & Brodie, A. F., 1966. Proc. Nat. Acad. Sci. USA 56: 940–945.

81. Dallam, R. D. & Anderson, W. W., 1957. Biochim. Biophys. Acta 25: 439.

82. Dallam, R. D. & Hamilton, J. W., 1964. Radiation Res. 22: 548–555.

83. Martius, C. & Nitz-Litzow, D., 1954. Biochim. Biophys. Acta 13: 152–153.

84. Shah, D. V. & Suttie, J. W., 1971. Proc. Nat. Acad. Sci. USA 68: 1653–1657.

85. Suttie, J. W., Nelsestuen, G. L. & Shah, D. V., 1973. Thromb. Diath. Haemorrhag. Supp. 54: 37–49.

86. Bayer, R. E. & Kennison, R. E., 1951. Arch. Biochem. Biophys. 84: 63–70.

87. Colpa-Boonstra, J. P. & Slater, E. C., 1958. Biochim. Biophys. Acta 27: 122–133.

88. Paolucci, A. M., Rama Rao, P. B. & Johnson, B. C., 1963. J. Nutr. 81: 17–22.

89. Johnson, H. V., Martinovic, J. & Johnson, B. C., 1971. Biochem. Biophys. Res. Commun. 43: 1040–1048.

90. Martius, C., Burkart, W. & Stalder, R., 1971. FEBS Lett. 18: 257–260.

91. Johnson, B. C. & Valkovich, G., 1972. Biochem. Biophys. Res. Commun. 48: 1437–1443.

92. Meeks, R. G. & Couri, D., 1978. Biochim. Biophys. Acta 544: 634–637.

93. Nelsestuen, G. L. & Suttie, J. W., 1971. Biochem. Biophys. Res. Commun. 45: 198–203.

94. Henriksen, A., Christensen, T. B. & Helgeland, L., 1976. Biochim. Biophys. Acta 421: 348–352.

95. Sloane, N. H., 1978. Arch. Biochem. Biophys. 186: 401–405; 1979, Fed. Proc. 38: 723.

96. Lev, M. & Milford, A. F., 1971. Biochem. Biophys. Res. Commun. 45: 358–362.

97. Brodie, A. F. & Watanabe, T., 1966. Vitamins and Hormones 24: 447–463.

98. Suttie, J. W., 1970. Arch. Biochem. Biophys. 141: 571–578.

99. Barnhart, M. I. & Anderson, G. F., 1962. Biochem. Pharmacol. 9: 23–27.

100. Anderson, G. F. & Barnhart, M. I., 1964. Am. J. Physiol. 206: 929–938.

101. Nilehn, J. E. & Ganrot, P. O., 1968. Scand. J. Clin. Lab. Invest. 22: 17–22.

102. Ganrot, P. O. & Nilehn, J. E., 1968. Scand. J. Clin. Lab. Invest. 22: 23–28.

103. Josso, F., Lavergne, J. M., Gouault, M., Prou-Wartelle, O. & Soulier, J. P., 1968. Thromb. Diath. Haemorrhag. 20: 88–98.

104. Stenflo, J., 1970. Acta Chem. Scand. 24: 3762–3763.

105. Hemker, H. C., Veltkamp, J. J., Hensen, A., & Loeliger, E. A., 1963. Nature 200: 589–590.

106. Reekers, P. P. M., Lindhout, M. J., Kop-Klaassen, B. H. M. & Hemker, H. C., 1973. Biochim. Biophys. Acta 317: 559–562.

107. Hemker, H. C. & Reekers, P. P. M., 1974. Thromb. Diath. Haemorrhag. Supp. 57: 83–86.

108. Lindhout, M. J., Kop-Klaassen, B. H. M., Kop, J. M. M. & Hemker, H. C., 1978. Biochim. Biophys. Acta 533: 302–317.

109. Lindhout, M. J., Kop-Klaassen, B. H. M., Reekers, P. P. M. & Hemker, H. C., 1976. J. Mol. Med. 1: 223–235.

110. Nelsestuen, G. L. & Suttie, J. W., 1972. Biochemistry 11: 4961–4964.

111. Nelsestuen, G. L. & Suttie, J. W., 1972. J. Biol. Chem. 247: 8176–8182.

112. Suttie, J. W., 1973. Science 179: 192–193.

113. Hemker, H. C., Muller, A. D. & Loeliger, E. A., 1970. Thromb. Diath. Haemorrhag. 23: 633–637.

114. Schieck, A., Kornalik, F. & Habermann, E., 1972. Naunyn-Schmiedebergs Arch. Pharmacol. 272: 402–416.

115. Malhotra, O. P., 1972. Nature New Biol. 239: 59–60.

116. Denson, K. W. E., 1971. Brit. J. Haematol. 20: 643–648.

117. Shah, D. V., Suttie, J. W. & Grant, G. A., 1973. Arch. Biochem. Biophys. 159: 483–491.

118. Esmon, C. T., Grant, G. A. & Suttie, J. W., 1975. Biochemistry 14: 1595–1600.

119. Morrissey, J. J., Jones, J. P. & Olson, R. E., 1973. Biochem. Biophys. Res. Commun. 54: 1075–1082.

120. Cesbron, N., Boyer, C., Guillin, M-C. & Menache, D., 1973. Thromb. Diath. Haemorrhag. 30: 437–450.

121. Guillon, M-C., Aronson, D. L., Bezéaud, A., Menache, D., Schlegel, N. & Amar, M., 1977. Thromb. Res. 1: 223–233.

122. Wallin, R. & Prydz, H., 1975. Biochem. Biophys. Res. Commun. 62: 398–406.

123. Grant, G. A. & Suttie, J. W., 1976. Biochemistry 15: 5387–5393.

124. Esmon, C. T., Suttie, J. W. & Jackson, C. M., 1975. J. Biol. Chem. 250: 4095–4099.

125. Carlisle, T. L., Shah, D. V., Schlegel, R. & Suttie, J. W., 1975. Proc. Soc. Exp. Biol. Med. 148: 140–144.

126. Babior, B. M. & Kipnes, R. S., 1970. Biochemistry 9: 2564–2569.

127. Chung, G. C. H., Delaney, R., Mack, D. & Johnson, B. C., 1975. Biochim. Biophys. Acta 386: 556–566.

128. Stenflo, J., 1973. J. Biol. Chem. 248: 6325–6332.

129. Nelsestuen, G. L. & Suttie, J. W., 1973. Proc. Nat. Acad. Sci. USA 70: 3366–3370.

130. Shah, D. V. & Suttie, J. W., 1974. Biochem. Biophys. Res. Commun. 60: 1397–1402.

131. Mack, D. O., Girardot, J-M., Chung, G., Delaney, R. & Johnson, B. C., 1975. Fed. Proc. 34: 258.

132. Esmon, C. T., Sadowski, J. A. & Suttie, J. W., 1975. Fed. Proc. 34: 221.

133. Esmon, C. T., Sadowski, J. A. & Suttie, J. W., 1975. J. Biol. Chem. 250: 4744–4748.

134. Mack, D. O., Suen, E. T., Girardot, J-M., Miller, J. A., Delaney, R. & Johnson, B. C., 1976. J. Biol. Chem. 251: 3269–3276.

135. Johnson, B. C., 1980. Methods in Enzymology 67F: 165–180.

136. Esmon, C. T. & Suttie, J. W., 1976. J. Biol. Chem. 251: 6238–6243.

137. Vermeer, C., Soute, B. A. M., Govers-Riemslag, J. & Hemker, H. C., 1976. Biochim. Biophys. Acta 444: 926–930.

138. Lowenthal, J. & Jaeger, V., 1977. Biochem. Biophys. Res. Commun. 74: 25–33.

139. Garvey, W. T. & Olson, R. E., 1978. J. Nutr. 108: 1078–1086.

140. Munns, T. W., Johnston, M. F. M., Liszewski, M. K. & Olson, R. E., 1976. Proc. Nat. Acad. Sci. USA 73: 2803–2807.

141. Olson, J. Pl., Miller, L. L. & Troup, S. B., 1966. J. Clin. Invest. 45: 690–701.

142. Poggi, A., Colucci, M., Delaini, F., Semeraro, N. & Donati, M. B., 1980. Europ. J. Cancer 16: 1641–1642.

143. Oesterud, B., Lindahl, U. & Seljelid, R., 1980. FEBS Lett. 120: 41–43.

144. Mack, D. O., Miller, J. A., Delaney, R. & Johnson, B. C., 1977. Fed. Proc. 36: 306.

145. Johnson, B. C., Mack, D. O., Delaney, R., Wolfensberger, M. R., Esmon, C., Price, J. A., Suen, E. & Girardot, J-M., 1980. (see reference 482) pp. 455–466.

146. Friedman, P. A. & Shia, M. A., 1977. Biochem. J. 163: 39–43.

147. Petrelli, F. & Marsili, G., 1973. Boll. Soc. Ital. Biol. Sper. 49: 1114–1119.

148. Magnusson, S., Sottrup-Jensen, L., Petersen, T. E., Morris, H. R. & Dell, A., 1974. FEBS Lett. 44: 189–193.

149. Friedman, P. A. & Shia, M., 1976. Biochem. Biophys. Res. Commun. 70: 647–654.

150. Girardot, J-M., Mack, D. O., Floyd, R. A. & Johnson, B. C., 1976. Biochem. Biophys. Res. Commun. 70: 655–661.

151. Blois, M. S., Jr. & Maling, J. E., 1960. Biochem. Biophys. Res. Commun. 3: 132–135.

152. Johnson, B. C., Girardot, J-M., Suen, E. T., Mack, D. O., Floyd, R. A. & Delaney, R., 1978. World Rev. Nutr. Diet 31: 202–209.

153. Vermeer, C., Soute, B. A. M., Hemker, H. C., 1978. Biochim. Biophys. Acta 523: 494–505.

154. Vermeer, C., Hemker, H. C. & Soute, B. A. M., 1978. Bibliotheca Haematol. 44: 54–60.

155. Shah, D. V. & Suttie, J. W., 1979. Proc. Soc. Exp. Biol. Med. 161: 498–501.

156. Jones, J. P., Gardner, E. J., Cooper, T. G. & Olson, R. E., 1977. J. Biol. Chem. 252: 7738–7742.

157. Mack, D. O., Suen, E. T., Girardot, J-M., Miller, J. A., Delaney, R. & Johnson, B. C., 1976. Fed. Proc. 35: 1763.

158. Suen, E. T., 1979. Studies on Vitamin K Dependent Carboxylase, Ph. D. Dissertation, University of Oklahoma.

159. Mack, D. O., Curtis, T. A. & Johnson, B. C., 1980. (see reference 482) pp. 467–470.

160. Girardot, J-M., Mack, D. O., Price, J., Suen, E. & Johnson, B, C., 1977. Fed. Proc. 36: 307.

161. Johnson, B. C., Bartels, V. L., Watson, J. J. & Mack, D. O., 1980. Fed. proc. 39: 1669.

162. Sadowski, J. A., 1975. Fed. Proc. 34: 898.

163. Crane, F. L., 1977. Ann. Rev. Biochem. 46: 439–469.

164. James, T. H. & Weissberger, A., 1938. J. Am. Chem. Soc. 60: 98–104.

165. LuValle, J. E. & Weissberger, A., 1947. J. Am. Chem. Soc. 69: 1567–1575.

166. LuValle, J. E. & Weissberger, A., 1947. J. Am. Chem. Soc. 69: 1576–1582.

167. Wallin, R., 1979. Biochem. J., 178: 513–519.

168. Larson, A. E. & Suttie, J. W., 1980. FEBS Lett. 118: 95–98.

169. Zurbin, G. I., 1979. Ukr. Biokhim. Zh. 51: 552–559.

170. Olson, R. E., Houser, R. M., Searcy, M. T., Gardner, E. J., Scheinbuks, J., Subba Rao, G. N., Jones, J. P. & Hall, A. L., 1978. Fed. Proc. 37: 2610–2614.

171. Stenflo, J., 1976. J. Biol. Chem. 251: 355–363.

172. Kisiel, W., Ericsson, L. H. & Davie, E. W., 1976. Biochemistry 15: 4893–4900.

173. Kisiel, W., Canfield, W. M., Ericsson, L. H. & Davie, E. W., 1977. Biochemistry 16: 5824–5831.

174. Di Scipio, R. G., Hermodson, M. A., Yates, S. G. & Davie, E. W., 1977. Biochemistry 16: 698–706.

175. Prowse, C. V. & Esnouf, M. P., 1977. Biochem. Soc. Trans. 5: 255–256.

176. Seegers, W. H., Ghosh, A. & Wu, V-Y., 1980. (see reference 482) pp. 96–101.

177. Trauber, D., Hawkins, K., Karpatkin, M. & Karpatkin, S., 1979. J. Clin. Invest. 64: 1713–1716.

178. Shah, D. V., Nyari, L. J., Swanson, J. C. & Suttie, J. W., 1980. Thromb. Res. 19: 111–118.

179. Hauschka, P. V., Lian, J. B., & Gallop, P. M., 1975. Proc. Nat. Acad. Sci., USA 72: 3925–3929.

180. Price, P. A., Otsuka, A. S., Poser, J. W., Kristaponis, J. & Raman, N., 1976. Proc. Nat. Acad. Sci., USA 73: 1447–1451.

181. Price, P. A., Poser, J. W. & Raman, N., 1976. Proc. Nat. Acad. Sci., USA 73: 3374–3375.

182. Lian, J. B., Hauschka, P. V. & Gallop, P. M., 1978. Fed. Proc. 37: 2615–2620.

183. Lian, J. B. & Friedman, P. A., 1978. J. Biol. Chem. 253: 6623–6626.

184. Nishimoto, S. K. & Price, P. A., 1980. J. Biol. Chem. 255: 6579–6583.

185. Lian, J. B. & Heroux, K. M., 1980. (see reference 4 82) pp. 245–254.

186. Hauschka, P. V. & Reid, M. L., 1978. Develop. Biol. 65: 426–434.

187. Hauschka, P. V. & Reddi, A. H., 1980. Biochem. Biophys. Res. Commun. 92: 1037–1041.

188. Hauschka, P. V., 1980. (see reference 482) pp. 227–236.

189. Poser, W. J. & Price, P. A., 1979. J. Biol. Chem. 254: 431–436.

190. Poser, J. W., 1979. Dissertation Abst. Int. B 40: 1696.

191. Glimcher, M. J., Brickley-Parsons, D. & Kossiva, D., 1979. Calcif. Tissue Int. 27: 281–284.

192. Glimcher, M. J., Lefteriou, B. & Kossiva, D., 1979. Calcif. Tissue Int. 28: 83–86.

193. Price, P. A., Lothringer, J. W. & Nishimoto, S. K., 1980. J. Biol. Chem. 255: 2938–2942.

194. King, K., Jr., 1978. Biochim. Biophys. Acta 542: 542–546.

195. Price, P. A. & Baukol, S. A., 1980. J. Biol. Chem. 255: 11660–11663.

196. Lian, J. B., Skinner, M., Glimcher, M. J. & Gallop, P., 1976. Biochem. Biophys. Res. Commun. 73: 349–355.

197. Keeley, F. W., 1977. Biochim. Biophys. Acta 494: 384–394.

198. Sharaev, P. N & Bogdanov, N. G., 1979. Byull. Eksp. Biol. Med. 88: 53–55.

199. Levy, R. J., Lian, J. B. & Gallop, P., 1979. Biochem. Biophys. Res. Commun. 91: 41–49.

200. Deyl, Z., Macek, K., Vancikova, O. & Adam, M., 1979. Biochim. Biophys. Acta 581: 307–315.

201. Levy, R. J., Zenker, J. A. & Lian, J. B., 1980. J. Clin. Invest. 65: 563–566.

202. Pierce, W. S., Donachy, J. H., Rosenburg, G. & Baier, R. E., 1980. Science 208: 601–603.

203. Sharaev, P. N., Bogdanov, N. G. & Yamoldinov, R. N., 1980. Vopr. Pitaniya 1980 (3): 75–76.

204. Tuan, R. S., Scott, W. A. & Cohn, Z. A., 1978. J. Biol. Chem. 253: 1011–1016.

205. Tuan, R. S., Scott, W. A. & Cohn, Z. A., 1978. J. Cell Biol. 77: 752–761.

206. Tuan, R. S., 1979. J. Biol. Chem. 254: 1356–1364.

207. Bronshtein, L. M., Anisimov, A. A., Oblizina, G. V., Dubovskaya, S. S. & Rabinovich, I. S., 1978. Vopr. Med. Khim. 24: 80–84.

208. Hauschka, P. V., Friedman, P. A., Traverso, H. P. & Gallop, P. M., 1976. Biochem. Biophys. Res. Commun. 71: 1207–1213.

209. Griep, A. E. & Friedman, P. A., 1980. (see reference 482) pp. 307–310.

210. Buchthal, S. D. & Bell, R. G., 1980. (see reference 482) pp. 299–302.

211. Lian, J. B., Prien, E. L., Jr., Glimcher, M. J. & Gallop, P. M., 1977. J. Clin. Invest. 59: 1151–1157.

212. Fernlund, P., 1976. Clin. Chim. Acta 72: 147–155.

213. Krampitz, G., Meisel, H., Witt-Krause, W., 1980. Naturwissenschaften 67: 38–39.

214. Samata, T., 1979. Ph. D. Dissertation, University of Bonn.

215. Bell, R. G., 1980. (see reference 482) pp. 286–293.

216. Friedman, P. A., Hauschka, P. V., Shia, M. A. & Wallace, J. K., 1979. Biochim. Biophys. Acta 583: 261–265.

217. Delaney, R., Gray, P. N. & Johnson, B. C., 1978. Proc. Southwest Oncology Group Meeting, San Antonio, Texas, November 7–9, 1978.

218. Delaney, R. & Gray, P. N., 1979. Fed. Proc. 38: 710.

219. Gray, P. N. & Delaney, R., 1979. Proc. 11th Int. Congress. Biochem., Toronto, Canada, July, 1979, p. 482.

220. Gray, P. N., Delaney, R. & Johnson, B. C., 1979. Proc. 11th Int. Congress Biochem., Toronto, Canada, July, 1979, p. 666.

221. Lacour, F., Oberling, Ch. & Guerin, M., 1957. Bull. Assoc. Franc. Etude Cancer 44: 88–91.

222. Michaels, L., 1964. Lancet 1964 (2): 832–836.

223. Hilgard, P. & Thornes, R. D., 1976. Europ. J. Cancer 12: 755–762.

224. Hilgard, P., 1977. Brit. J. Cancer 35: 891–892.

225. Hilgard, P., Schulte, H., Wetzig, G. & Schmidt, C. G., 1977. Brit. J. Cancer 35: 78–85.

226. Hilgard, P., 1979. Thromb. & Haemost. 42: 353.

227. Zacharski, L. R. Henderson, W. G., Rickles, F. R., Forman, W. B., Cornell, C. J., Jr., Forcier, R. J., Harrower, H. W. & Johnson, R. O., 1979. Cancer 44: 732–741.

228. Van Buskirk, J. J. & Kirsch, W. M., 1978. Biochem. Biophys. Res. Commun. 80: 1033–1038.

229. Van Buskirk, J. J., Low, M. & Kirsch, W. M., 1980. (see reference 482) pp. 274–278.

230. Scheinbuks, J., 1980. (see reference 482) p. 279–285.

231. Lee, S-H. & Brodie, A. F., 1980. Biochem. Biophys. Res. Commun. 95: 499–506.

232. Nelsestuen, G. L., Broderius, M. & Martin, G., 1976. J. Biol. Chem. 251: 6886–6893.

233. Nelsestuen, G. L., Kisiel, W. & Di Scipio, R. G., 1978. Biochemistry 17: 2134–2138.

234. Nelsestuen, G. L., 1978. Fed. Proc. 37: 2621–2625.

235. Nelsestuen, G. L., 1977. Calcium-Binding Proteins and Calcium Function. Elsevier North Holland, Inc., New York and Amsterdam, pp. 323–332.

236. Lindhout, M. J. & Hemker, H. C., 1978. Biochim. Biophys. Acta 533: 318–326.

237. Hauschka, P. V., Lian, J. B. & Gallop, P. M., 1978. TIBS 3: 75–78.

238. Robertson, P., Jr., Hiskey, R. G. & Koehler, K. A., 1978. J. Biol. Chem. 253: 5880–5883.

239. Osterberg, R., Sjoberg, B., Osterberg, P., and Stenflo, J., 1980. Biochemistry 19: 2283–2286.

240. Morris, H. R., Dell, A., Petersen, T. E., Sottrup-Jensen, L. & Magnusson, S., 1976. Biochem. J. 153: 663–679.

241. Magnusson, S., Petersen, T. E., Sottrup-Jensen, L. & Claeys, H., 1975. Cold Spring Harbor Conf. on Cell Proliferation (E. Reich, D. B. Rifkin, an E. Shaw, eds.) 2: 123–149.

242. Magnusson, S., Sottrup-Jensen, L., Petersen, T. E. & Claeys, H., 1975. Prothrombin and Related Coagulation Factors (H. C. Hemker & J. J. Veltkamp, eds.) University of Leiden Press, p. 25–46.

243. Magnusson, S., 1976. Plasma Proteins (B. Blomback and L. A. Hansen, eds.) John Wiley & Sons, New York, pp. 254–276.

244. Matthes, K. L., 1975. Die Medizinische Welt (N.F.) 26: 1777–1782.

245. Hewett-Emmett, D., 1978. Bibliotheca Haemostas. 44: 94–104.

246. Gibbs, A. J. & McIntyre, G. A., 1970. Eur. J. Biochem. 76: 1–11.

247. Young, C. L., Barker, W. C., Tomaselli, G. M. & Dayhoff, M. O., 1978. Atlas of Protein Sequence and Structure 5 (Suppl. 3), (M. W. Dayhoff, ed.) National Biomedical Research Foundation, Georgetown University, Washington, D.C. pp. 73–85.

248. Stenflo, J., Fernlund, P. & Roepstorff, P., 1975. Cold Spring Harbor Conferences on Cell Proliferation (E. Reich, D. B. Rifkin, & E. Shaw, editors) 2, 111–112.

249. Fernlund, P., Stenflo, J. & Tufvesson, A., 1978. Proc. Natl. Acad. Sci. USA 75: 5889–5892.

250. Stenflo, J. & Jonsson, M., 1979. FEBS Lett. 101: 377–381.

251. Di Scipio, R. G. & Davie, E. W., 1979. Biochemistry 18: 899–904.

252. Petersen, T. E., Thogersen, H. C., Sottrup-Jensen, L., Magnusson, S. & Jornvall, H., 1980. FEBS Lett. 114: 278–282.

253. Katayama, K., Ericsson, L. H., Enfield, D. L., Walsh, K. A., Neurath, H., Davie, E. W. & Titani, K., 1979. Proc. Nat. Acad. Sci. USA 76: 4990–4994.

254. Enfield, D. L., Ericsson, L. H., Walsh, K. A., Neurath, H. & Titani, K., 1975. Proc. Natl. Acad. Sci., USA 72: 16–19.

255. Titani, K., Fujikawa, K. Enfield, D. L., Ericsson, L. H., Walsh, K. A. & Neurath, H., 1975. Proc. Natl. Acad. Sci., USA 72: 3082–3086.

256. Thøgersen, H. C., Petersen, T. E., Sottrup-Jensen, L., Magnusson, S. & Morris, H. R., 1978. Biochem. J. 175: 613–627.

257. Davie, E. W., 1980. (see reference 482) pp. 3–7.

258. Fernlund, P. & Stenflo, J., 1980. (see reference 482) pp. 84–88.

259. Grant, G. A. & Suttie, J. W., 1976. Arch. Biochem. Biophys. 176: 650–662.

260. Walz, D. A., 1978. Bibliotheca Haemostas. 44: 8–14.

118

261. Poser, J. W., Esch, F. S., Ling, N. C. & Price, P., 1980. J. Biol. Chem. 255: 8685–8691.
262. Baskova, I. P., Memon, M. S., Ramanov, V. V. & Rusak, A. F., 1977. Biokhimiya 42: 95–99.
263. Suttie, J. W., Hageman, J. M., Lehrman, S. R., & Rich, D. H., 1976. J. Biol. Chem. 251: 5827–5830.
264. Houser, R. M., Carey, D. J., Dus, K. M., Marshall, G. R. & Olson, R. E., 1977. FEBS Lett. 75: 226–230.
265. Finnan, J. L. & Suttie, J. W., 1980. (see reference 482) pp. 509–517.
266. Dubin, A., Suen, E. T., Delaney, R., Chiu, A. & Johnson, B. C., 1979. Biochem. Biophys. Res. Commun. 88: 1024–1029.
267. Griffith, M. J., 1979. J. Biol. Chem. 254: 3401–3406.
268. Rich, D. H., Lehrman, S. R., Kawai, M., Goodman, H. L. & Suttie, J. W., 1980. (see reference 482) pp. 471–479.
269. Huang, J. S., Huang, S. S. & Olson, R. E., 1980. Fed. Proc. 39: 788, 1855.
270. Suttie, J. W., Gewecke, L. O., Finnan, J. L., Lehrman, S. R. & Rich, D. H., 1980. (see reference 482) pp. 450–454.
271. Finnan, J. L. & Suttie, J. W., 1979. Fed. Proc. 38: 876.
272. Decottignies-Le Maréchal, P., Rikong-Adie, H., Azerad, R. & Gaudry, M., 1980. Biochem. Biophys. Res. Commun. 90: 700–707.
273. Johnson, B. C., Sridhar, R., Delaney, R. & Watson, J., 1980. Fed. Proc. 39: 788.
274. Friedman, P. A., Shia, M. A., Gallop, P. M. & Griep, A. E., 1979. Proc. Nat. Acad. Sci., USA 76, 3126–3129.
275. Friedman, P. A., 1980. (see reference 482) pp. 401–407.
276. Matthes, K. J., 1980. (see reference 482) pp. 13–15.
277. Gorman, K., Floyd, R. A., Watson, J. J., Mack, D. O., Delaney, R. & Johnson, B. C., 1980. Fed. Proc. 37: 1893.
278. Johnson, B. C., Mack, D. O. & Delaney, R., 1980. Proc. 6th Int. Cong. Thromb., Monte-Carlo, October, 1980, p. 39.
279. Wolfensberger, M., Delaney, R., Mack, D. O., Esmon, C. & Johnson, B. C., 1978. Fed. Proc. 37: 1443.
280. Sadowski, J. A. & Suttie, J. W., 1976. Fed. Proc. 35: 662.
281. Bachur, N. R., Gordon, S. L., Gee, M. V. & Kon, H., 1979. Proc. Nat. Acad. Sci. USA 76: 954–957.
282. Iyanagi, T. & Yamazaki, I., 1970. Biochim. Biophys. Acta 216: 282–294.
283. Ernster, L., Nordenbrand, K. & Orrenius, S., 1980. First. Int. Symp. Lipid Peroxidation in Biol. & Med., Nagoya, Japan (K. Yagi, editor) Academic Press, New York, in press.
284. Schlenk, H. & Bergmann, G., 1928. Liebigs Ann. Chem. 463: 98–227 (p. 193).
285. Ullrich, V. & Schnabel, K. H., 1973. Arch. Biochem. Biophys. 159: 240–245.
286. Esnouf, M. P., Green, M. R., Hill H. A. O., Irvine, G. B. & Walter, S. J., 1978. Biochem. J. 174: 345–348.
287. Esnouf, M. P., Burgess, A. I., Walter, S. J., Green, M. R., Hill, H. A. O. & Okolow-Zubkowska, M. J., 1980. (see reference 482) pp. 422–432.
288. Hodgson, E. K. & Fridovich, I., 1976. Arch. Biochem. Biophys. 172: 202–205.
289. Saito, I., Otsuki, T. & Matsuura, T., 1979. Tetrahedron Lett. 19: 1693–1696.
290. Winterbourn, C. C., French, J. K. & Claridge, R. F. C., 1978. FEBS Lett. 94: 269–272.
291. Larson, A. E. & Suttie, J. W., 1978. Proc. Nat. Acad. Sci. USA 75: 5413–5416.

292. Suttie, J. W., Larson, A. E., Canfield, L. M. & Carlisle, T. T., 1978. Fed. Proc. 37: 2605–2609.
293. Larson, A. E., McTigue, J. J. & Suttie, J. W., 1980. (see reference 482) pp. 413–421.
294. Olson, R. E., Huang, J. S., Zee-Cheng, R. K. Y., Huang, S. S., Hall, A. L., O'Brian, J. K., Kloepper, R. & Chiu, Y. J. P., 1980. Fed. Proc. 39: 1669.
295. Viré, J. C., Patriarche, G. J. & Christian, G. D., 1979. Anal. Chem. 51: 752–757.
296. Dunkle, B. F., Turner, P. M., Hall, A. L., Wing, D. A., Houser, R. M. & Olson, R. E., 1979. Fed. Proc. 38: 723.
297. Sauers, C. K., Jencks, W. P. & Grok, S., 1975. J. Am. Chem. Soc. 97: 5546–5553.
298. Williams, A. & Douglas, K. T., 1975. Chem. Rev. 75: 640.
299. Suzuki, H., Nakao, T. & Hiraga, K., 1979. Toxicol. Appl. Pharmacol. 50: 261–262.
300. Olson, R. E. & Jones, J. P., 1979. Fed. Proc. 38: 710.
301. Benson, A. M., Hunkeler, M. J. & Talalay, P., 1980. Proc. Nat. Acad. Sci. USA 77: 5216–5220.
302. Kappus, H., Kieczka, H., Scheulen, M. & Remmer, H., 1977. Naunyn-Schmiedebergs Arch. Exp. Pathol. Pharmacol. 300: 179–187.
303. Kahl, R., 1980. Biochem. Biophys. Res. Commun. 95: 163–169.
304. Dansette, P. M., 1980. Ann. Biol. Clin. 38: 25–34.
305. Bäckvall, J. E. & Karlsson, O., 1980. Tetrahedron Lett. 21: 4985–4988.
306. Bottaccio, G., Marchi, M. & Chiusoli, G. P., 1977. Gazz. Chim. Ital. 107: 499–500.
307. Nakajima, T., Yabushita, Y. & Tabashi, I., 1975. Nature 256: 60–61.
308. Bhagwat, A. S. & Sane, P. V., 1978. Biochem. Biophys. Res. Commun. 84: 865–873.
309. Christeller, J. T. & Laing, W. A., 1979. Biochem. J., 183: 747–750.
310. Miziorko, H. M. & Sealy, R. C., 1980. Biochemistry 80: 1167–1171.
311. Suttie, J. W., 1967. Arch. Biochem. Biophys. 118: 166–171.
312. MacGillivray, R. T. A., Chung, D. W. & Davie, E. W., 1980. (see reference 482) pp. 546–552.
313. Chung, D. W., MacGillivray, R. T. A. & Davie, E. W., 1980. Ann. N. Y. Acad. Sci. 343: 210–215.
314. Jones, J. P., Fausto, A., Houser, R. M., Gardner, E. J. & Olson, R. E., 1976. Biochem. Biophys. Res. Commun. 72: 589–597.
315. Mack, D. O., Wolfensberger, M., Girardot, J-M., Miller, J. A. & Johnson, B. C., 1979. J. Biol. Chem. 254: 2656–2664.
316. Yen, C. S. & Mack, D. O., 1980. Proc. Soc. Exp. Biol. Med. 165: 306–308.
317. Link, K. P., 1944. Harvey Lectures 39: 162–216.
318. Overman, R. S., Stahmann, M. A., Sullivan, W. R., Huebner, C. F., Campbell, H. A. & Link, K. P., 1942. J. Biol. Chem. 142: 941–955; Campbell, H. A. & Link, K. P., 1941. J. Biol. Chem. 138: 21–34; Stahmann, M. A., Huebner, C. F. & Link, K. P., 1941. 138: 513–527; Huebner, C. F. & Link, K. P., 1941. J. Biol. Chem. 138: 529–534.
319. Stahmann, M., Ikawa, M. & Link, K. P., 1947. U.S. Patent 2: 427, 578.
320. Ernster, L., Danielson, L. & Ljunggren, M., 1962. Biochim. Biophys. Acta 58: 171–188.

321. Bell, R. G. & Caldwell, P. T., 1973. Biochemistry 12: 1759-1762.

322. Marshall, F. N., 1972. Proc. Soc. Exp. Biol. Med. 139: 223-227.

323. Lowenthal, J. & Chowdhury, M. N. R., 1970. Can. J. Chem. 48: 3957-3958.

324. Shah, D. V. & Suttie, J. W., 1973. Proc. Soc. Exp. Biol. Med. 143: 775-779.

325. Friedman, P. A. & Griep, A. E., 1980. Biochemistry 19: 3381-3386.

326. Searcey, M. T., Graves, C. & Olson, R. E., 1977. J. Biol. Chem. 252: 6260-6267.

327. Otagiri, M., Matsumoto, U. & Perrin, J. H., 1980. J. Pharm. Dynamics 3 (9) S2.

328. Fehske, K. J., Mueller, W. E., Wollert, U. & Velden, L. M., 1979. Mol. Pharmacol. 16: 778-789.

329. Wilting, J., van der Giesen, W. F., Janssen, L. H. M., Weideman, M. M., Otagiri, M. & Perrin, J. H., 1980. J. Biol. Chem. 255: 3032-3037.

330. Valente, E. J., Porter, W. R. & Trager, W. F., 1978. J. Med. Chem. 21: 231-234.

331. Whitlon, D. S., Sadowski, J. A. & Suttie, J. W., 1978. Biochemistry 17: 1371-1377.

332. Esnouf, M. P., Green, M. R., Hill, H. A. O. & Walter, S. J., 1979. FEBS Lett. 107: 146-150.

333. Park, B. K., Leck, J. B., Wilson, A. C., Serlin, M. J. & Breckenridge, A. M., 1979. Biochem. Pharmacol. 28: 1323-1329.

334. Schmidt, W., Beermann, D., Oesch, F. & Jähnchen. E., 1979. J. Pharm. Pharmacol. 31: 490-491.

335. Ren, P., Stark, P. Y., Johnson, R. L. & Bell, R. G., 1977. J. Pharmacol. Exp. Ther. 201: 541-546.

336. Tuhy, P. M., Bloom, J. W. & Mann, K. G., 1979. Biochemistry 18: 5842-5848.

337. Morrison, S. A. & Esnouf, M. P., 1973. Nature New Biol. 242: 92-94.

338. Malhotra, O. P., 1975. Thromb. Diath. Haemorrhag. 34: 592.

339. Prowse, C. V., Mattock, P., Esnouf, M. P. & Russell, A. M., 1976. Biochim. Biophys. Acta 434: 265-279.

340. Esnouf, M. P. & Prowse, C. V., 1977. Biochim. Biophys. Acta 490: 471-476.

341. Friedman, P. A., Rosenberg, R. D., Hauschka, P. V. & Fitz-James, A., 1977. Biochim. Biophys. Acta 494: 271-276.

342. Malhotra, O. P., 1979. Thromb. Res. 15: 427-437.

343. Malhotra, O. P., 1979. Thromb. Res. 15: 439-448.

344. Malhotra, O. P., 1979. Thromb. Res. 15: 449-463.

345. Malhotra, O. P., 1980. (see reference 482) pp. 62-65.

346. Cassen, J. & Malhotra, O. P., 1980. (see reference 482) pp. 388-391.

347. Lewis, R. M., Reisner, H. M., Chung, K-S., & Roberts, H. R., 1980. Blood 56, 608-614.

348. Furie, B., Provost, K. L., Blanchard, R. A. & Furie, B. C., 1978. J. Biol. Chem. 253: 8980-8987.

349. Furie, B. & Furie, B. C., 1979. J. Biol. Chem. 254: 9766-9771.

350. Blanchard, R. A., Furie, B. & Furie, B. C., 1980. (see reference 482) pp. 66-71.

351. Sperling, R., Furie, B. C., Blumenstein, M., Keyt, B. & Furie, B., 1978. J. Biol. Chem. 253: 3898-3906.

352. Tai, M. M., Furie, B. C. & Furie, B., 1980. J. Biol. Chem. 255: 2790-2795.

353. Lutes, R. T. & Shapiro, S. S., 1979. Thromb. Res. 16: 129-145.

354. Furie, B. C., Blumenstein, M. & Furie, B., 1979. J. Biol. Chem. 254: 12521-12530.

355. Carlisle, T. L. & Suttie, J. W., 1980. Thromb. Res. 18: 405-416.

356. Helgeland, L., 1977. Biochim. Biophys. Acta 499: 181-193.

357. Carlisle, T. L. & Suttie, J. W., 1980. Biochemistry 19: 1161-1167.

358. Carlisle, T. L., Shah, D. V. & Suttie, J. W., 1980. (see reference 482) pp. 443-449.

359. Wallin, R. & Prydz, H., 1979. Thromb. Haemostas. 41: 529-536.

360. Hassouna, H. I. & Leach, R. E., 1978. Bibliotheca Haemostas. 44: 28-38.

361. Janson, T. L. & Helgeland, L., 1975. Biochim. Biophys. Acta 379: 598-605.

362. Finnan, J. L., Goodman, H. L. & Suttie, J. W., 1980. (see reference 482) pp. 480-483.

363. Shah, D. V. & Suttie, J. W., 1978. Arch. Biochem. Biophys. 191: 571-577.

364. Suttie, J. W., Lehrman, S. R., Geweke, L. O., Hageman, J. M. & Rich, D. H., 1979. Biochem. Biophys. Res. Commun. 86: 500-507.

365. Dubin, A., Suen, E. T., Delaney, R., Chiu, A. & Johnson, B. C., 1980. J. Biol. Chem. 255: 349-352.

366. Mack, D. O., Wolfensberger, M., Price, J. A. & Suen, E. T., 1978. Fed. Proc. 37: 1443.

367. Freedman, R., 1979. FEBS lett. 97: 201-210.

368. Fieser, L. F. & Turner, R. B., 1947. J. Am. Chem. Soc. 69: 2335-2338.

369. Stadtman, T. C., 1959. J. Biol. Chem. 234: 636-640.

370. Nickerson, W. J., Falcone, G. & Strauss, G., 1963. Biochemistry 2: 537-543.

371. Baxendale, O. H. & Hardy, H. R., 1953. Trans. Faraday Soc. 49: 1433-1437.

372. Dolin, M. I. & Baum, R. H., 1965. Biochem. Biophys. Res. Commun. 18: 202-205.

373. Houser, R. M., Hall, A. H. & Olson, R. E., 1978. Fed. Proc. 37: 1588.

374. Canfield, L. M., Sinsky, T. A. & Suttie, J. W., 1979. Fed. Proc. 38: 710.

375. Wallin, R. & Suttie, J. W., 1980. Fed. Proc. 39: 789.

376. Wallin, R., Gebhardt, O. & Prydz, H., 1978. Biochem. J. 169: 95-101.

377. Wallin, R., Canfield, L. M., Sinsky, T. A. & Suttie, J. W., 1980. (see reference 482) pp. 490-499.

378. Canfield, L. M., Sinsky, T. A. & Suttie, J. W., 1980. Arch. Biochem. Biophys. 302: 515-524.

379. Price, J. A. & Johnson, B. C., 1980. (see reference 482) pp. 500-504.

380. Wallin, R. & Suttie, J. W., 1980. Biochem. Biophys. Res. Commun. 94: 1374-1380.

381. Friedman, P. A. & Shia, M. A., 1980. Biochim. Biophys. Acta. 616: 362-370.

382. Hauschka, P. V., 1979. Biochemistry 18: 4992–4998.

383. Zytkovicz, T. H. & Nelsestuen, G. L., 1975. J. Biol. Chem. 250: 2968–2972.

384. Rose, K., Priddle, J. D., Offord, R. E. & Esnouf, M. P., 1980. Biochem. J. 187: 239–243.

385. Hauschka, P. V., 1977. Anal. Biochem. 80: 212–223.

386. Tabor, H. & Tabor, C. W., 1977. Anal. Biochem. 78: 554–556.

387. Yamagata, F., Kasai, H. & Okuyama, T., 1977. Bunseki Kagaku 26: 819–824.

388. Madar, D. A., Willis, R. A., Koehler, K. A. & Hiskey, R. G., 1979. Anal. Biochem. 92: 466–472.

389. James, L. B., 1979. J. Chromatogr. 175: 211–215.

390. Low, M., Van Buskirk, J. J. & Kirsch, W. M., 1980. (see reference 482) pp. 150–152.

391. Fernlund, P. & Stenflo, J., 1980. (see reference 482) pp. 161–165.

392. Petersen, T. E., Thøgersen, H. C., Magnusson, S. & Sottrup-Jensen, L., 1980. (see reference 482) pp. 171–174.

393. Grundberg, C. M., Lian, J. B. & Gallop, P. M., 1980. (see reference 482) pp. 153–156.

394. Grundberg, C. M., Lian, J. B. & Gallop. P. M., 1979. Anal. Biochem. 98: 219–225.

395. Fernlund, P., 1980. (see reference 482) pp. 166–170.

396. Katayama, K. & Titani, K., 1978. FEBS Lett. 95: 157–160.

397. Lian, J. B., Glimcher, M. J. & Gallop, P. M., 1977. Calcium-Binding Proteins and Calcium Functions (R. H. Wasserman, et al., editors) Elsevier North-Holland, New York, pp. 379–381.

398. Shah, D. V., Tews, J. K., Harper, A. E. & Suttie, J. W., 1978. Biochim. Biophys. Acta 539: 209–217.

399. Federici, G., Ricci, G., Matarese, R. M., Spoto, G., Dupré, S. & Cavallini, D., 1979. Arch. Biochem. Biophys. 196: 304–306.

400. Boggs, N. T., III, Gawley, R. E., Koehler, K. A. & Hiskey, R. G., 1975. J. Org. Chem. 40: 2850–2851.

401. Oppliger, M. & Schwyzer, R., 1977. Helv. Chim. Acta 60: 43–47.

402. Boggs, N. T., III, Goldsmith, B., Gawley, R. E., Koehler, K. A. & Hiskey, R. G., 1979. J. Org. Chem. 44: 2262–2269.

403. Danishefsky, S., Berman, E., Clizbe, L. A., Hirama, M., 1979. J. Am. Chem. Soc. 101: 4385–4386.

404. Bory, S., Gaudry, M., Marquet, A. & Azerad, A., 1979. Biochem. Biophys. Res. Commun. 87: 85–91.

405. Juhasz, A. & Bajusz, S., 1980. Inter. J. Pept. 15: 154–158.

406. Zee-Cheng, R. K-Y. & Olson, R. E., 1980. Biochem. Biophys. Res. Commun. 94: 1128–1132.

407. Lefevere, M. F., De Leenheer, A. P. & Claeys, A. E., 1979. J. Chromatogr. 186: 749–762.

408. Donnahey, P. L., Burt, V. T., Rees, H. H. & Pennock, J. F., 1979. J. Chromatogr. 170: 272–277.

409. Haroon, Y., Shearer, M. J., Barkhan, P., 1980. J. Chromatogr. 200: 293–299.

410. Mack, D. O., 1980. J. Liq. Chromatogr. 3: 1005–1021.

411. Bechtold, H. & Jaehnchen, E., 1979. J. Chromatogr. 164: 85–90.

412. Seifert, R. M., 1979. J. Agr. Food Chem. 27: 1301–1304.

413. Nakata, Y. & Tsuchida, E., 1980. Methods in Enzymology 67F: 148–160.

414. Collins, M. D., Shah, H. N. & Minnikin, D. E., 1980. J. Appl. Bact. 48: 277–282.

415. Bjornsson, T. D., Swezey, S. E., Meffin, P. J. & Blaschke, T. F., 1978. Thromb. Haemostas. 39: 466–473.

416. Naruta, Y., 1980. J. Am. Chem. Soc. 102: 3774–3783.

417. Snatzke, G., Wynberg, H., Feringa, B., Marsman, B. G., Greydanus, B. & Pluim, H., 1980. J. Org. Chem. 45: 4094–4096.

418. Shearer, M. J. & Barkhan, P., 1973. Biochim. Biophys. Acta 297: 300–312.

419. Wiss, O. & Gloor, U., 1966. Vitamins & Hormones 24: 575–586.

420. Bell, R. G. & Matschiner, J. T., 1970. Arch. Biochem. Biophys. 141: 473–476.

421. Burt, V. T., Bee, V. & Pennock, J. F., 1977. Biochem. J. 162: 297–302.

422. McBurney, A., Shearer, M. J. & Barkhan, P., 1978. Biochem. Pharmacol. 27: 273–278.

423. Bjornsson, T. D., Meffin, P. J., Swezey, S. E. & Blaschke, T. F., 1979. J. Pharmacol. Expo. Ther. 210: 322–326.

424. Bjornsson T. D., Meffin, P. J., Swezey, S. E. & Blaschke, T. F., 1980. (see reference 482) pp. 328–332.

425. Johnson, B. C., Hill, R. B., Alden, R. & Ranhotra, G. S., 1966. Life Sci. 5: 385–392.

426. Johnson, B. C., 1970. Nutrition (J. Masek, K. Osancova, & D. P. Cuthbertson, editors) Excerpta Medica, pp. 125–135.

427. Bell, R. G. & Matschiner, J. T., 1969. Arch. Biochem. Biophys. 135: 152–159.

428. Josso, F., Prou-Wartelle, O. & Soulier, J. P., 1962. Nouvelle Rev. Franc. Hematol. 2: 647–672.

429. Siegfried, C. M., Knauer, G. R. & Matschiner, J. T., 1979. Arch. Biochem. Biophys. 194: 486–495.

430. Owen, C. A., Mann, K. G. & McDuffie, F. C., 1979. Thromb. Haemostas. 42: 548–555.

431. Martius, C. & Strufe, R., 1954. Biochem. Z. 326: 24–27.

432. Ernster, L., 1966. Methods in Enzymology X, 309–317.

433. Wosilait, W. D. & Nason, A., 1954. J. Biol. Chem. 208: 785–798.

434. Marki, F. & Martius, C., 1960. Biochem. Z. 333: 111–135.

435. Marki, F. & Martius, C., 1961. Biochem. Z. 334: 293–303.

436. Ernster, L. & Navazio, F., 1958. Acta Chem. Scand. 12: 595.

437. Ernster, L., Ljunggren, M. & Danielson, L., 1960. Biochem. Biophys. Res. Commun. 2: 88–92.

438. Ernster, L., Lind, C. & Rase, B., 1972. Europ. J. Biochem. 25: 198–206.

439. Hosoda, S., Nakamura, W. & Hayashi, K., 1974. J. Biol. Chem. 249: 6416–6423.

440. Lind, C. & Ernster, L., 1974. Biochem. Biophys. Res. Commun. 56: 392–400.

441. Fasco, M. J. & Principe, L. M., 1980. Biochem. Biophys. Res. Commun. 97: 1487–1492.

442. Matschiner, J. T., Zimmerman, A. & Bell, R. G., 1974. Thromb. Diath. Haemorrhag. Supp. 52: 45–52.

443. Ren, P., Laliberte, R. E. & Bell, R. G., 1974. Mol. Pharmacol. 10: 373–380.

444. Siegfried, C. M., 1978. Biochem. Biophys. Res. Commun. 83: 1488–1495.

445. Siegfried, C. M., 1980. (see reference 482) pp. 354–360.

446. Siefermann, D. & Yamamoto, H. Y., 1975. Arch. Biochem. Biophys. 171: 70–77.

447. Silverman, R. B., 1980. J. Am. Chem. Soc. 102: 5421–5423.

448. Park, B. K., Leck, J. B. & Breckenridge, A. M., 1980. Biochem. Pharmacol. 29: 1601–1602.

449. Willingham, A. K. & Matschiner, J. T., 1974. Biochem. J. 140: 435–441.

450. Willingham, A. K., Laliberte, R. E., Bell, R. B. & Matschiner, J. T., 1976. Biochem. Pharmacol. 25: 1063–1066.

451. Bell, R. G., Caldwell, P. T. & Holm, E. E. T., 1976. Biochem. Pharmacol. 25: 1067–1070.

452. Bell, R. G. & Stark, P., 1976. Biochem. Biophys. Res. Commun. 72: 619–625.

453. Bell, R. G., 1978. Fed. Proc. 37: 2599–2604.

454. Sadowski, J. A., Schnoes, H. K. & Suttie, J. W., 1977. Biochemistry 16: 3856–3863.

455. Egeberg, K. & Helgeland, L., 1980. Biochim. Biophys. Acta 627: 225–229.

456. Friedman, P. A. & Smith, M. W., 1977. Biochem. Pharmacol. 26: 804–805.

457. Suttie, J. W., Gewecke, L. O., Martin, S. L., & Willingham, A. K., 1980. FEBS Lett. 109: 267–270.

458. Fasco, M. J. & Cashin, M. J., 1980. Toxicol. Appl. Pharmacol. 56: 101–109.

459. Corn, M., 1966. Thromb. Diath. Haemotol. 16: 606–612

460. Huggins, C., Ford, E., Fukunishi, R. & Jensen, E. V., 1964. J. Exp. Med. 119: 943–954.

461. Lind, C., Vadi, H. & Ernster, L., 1978. Arch. Biochem. Biophys. 190: 97–108.

462. Hilgard, P., Schulte, H., Wetzig, C., Schmitt, G. & Schmidt, C. G., 1977. Brit. J. Cancer 35: 78–85; 891–892.

463. Hilgard, P. & Maat, B., 1979. Eur. J. Cancer 15: 183–187.

464. Am. Inst. Nutr. Ad Hoc Comm. on Standards for Nutritional Studies, 1977. J. Nutr. 107: 1340–1348.

465. Partridge, G. G., 1980. Lab. Anim. 14: 193–195.

466. Barber, D. L. & Calvin, H. W., Jr., 1980. Toxicol. Appl. Pharmacol. 56: 8–15.

467. Matschiner, J. T. & Doisey, E. A., Jr., 1965. J. Nutr. 8: 93–99.

468. Fieser, L., 1940. J. Biol. Chem. 133: 391–396.

469. Johnson, B. C., 1970. The Fat-Soluble Vitamins (H. F. De Luca & J. W. Suttie, eds.) University of Wisconsin Press, Madison, Wisconsin, pp. 491–519.

470. Suttie, J. W. & Jackson, C. W., 1977. Physiol. Rev. 57: 1–70.

471. Stenflo, J., 1977. New Engl. J. Med. 296: 624–625.

472. Suttie, J. W., 1977. Seminars in Hematology 14: 365–374.

473. Prydz, H., 1977. Seminars in Thrombosis & Hemostasis 4: 1–14.

474. Stenflo, J. & Suttie, J. W., 1977. Ann. Rev. Biochem. 46: 157–172.

475. Suttie, J. W., 1978. World Rev. Nutr. Diet. 31: 196–201.

476. Olson, R. E., 1978. World Rev. Nutr. Diet. 31: 216–225.

477. Stenflo, J., 1978. Adv. in Enzymol. 46: 1–32.

478. Olson, R. E. & Suttie, J. W., 1978. Vitamins and Hormones 35: 59–108.

479. Olson, R. E., 1979. TIBS 4: 118–120.

480. Esnouf, M., 1979. Biochem. Soc. Trans. 7: 624–627.

481. Suttie, J. W., 1978. The Fat Soluble Vitamins (H. F. De Luca, ed.) Plenum Press, New York, pp. 211–277.

482. Suttie, J. W., editor, 1980. Vitamin K Metabolism and Vitamin K Dependent Proteins, University Park Press, Baltimore, Maryland.

483. Suttie, J. W., Canfield, L. M. & Shah, D. V., 1980. Methods in Enzymology 67F: 180–185.

484. Helgeland, L., 1980. Biochem. Educ. 8: 66–69.

485. Pugh, D. M., 1980. Vet. Sci. Comm. 4: 15–28.

486. Gallop, P. M., Lian, J. B. & Hauschka, P. V., 1980. New Engl. J. Med. 302: 1460–1466.

487. Suttie, J. W., 1980. CRC Crit. Rev. Biochem. 8: 191–223.

488. Suttie, J. W., 1980. TIBS 5: 302–304.

489. Suttie, J. W., 1978. Handbook of Lipid Research 2, The Fat Soluble Vitamins (H. F. De Luca, ed.) Plenum Press, New York, pp. 211–277.

490. Gallop, P. M., Friedman, P. A. & Henson, E., 1980. (see reference 482) pp. 408–412.

491. Hall, A. L., Turner, P. M., Dunkle, B. F., Wing, D. A. & Olson, R. E. (see reference 482) pp. 433–442.

492. Koli, A. K., Yearly, C., Scott, W. & Donaldson, K. O., 1969. J. Biol. Chem. 244: 621–629.

493. Houser, R. M., Carey, D. J., Dus, K. M., Marshall, G. R. & Olson, R. E., 1977. FEBS Lett. 75: 226–230.

494. Price, P. A., Otsuka, A. S. & Poser, J. W., 1977. Calcium Binding Proteins and Calcium Function (R. H. Wasserman, editor) pp. 333–337.

495. Price, P. A., Epstein, D. J., Lothringer, J. W., Nishimoto, S. K., Poser, J. W. & Williamson, M. K., 1980. (see reference 482) pp. 219–226.

Received March 12, 1981.

Glutamate and aspartate agonists structurally related to ibotenic acid

Tage Honoré[+], Povl Krogsgaard-Larsen, Jan J. Hansen and Jørn Lauridsen

The Royal Danish School of Pharmacy, Department of Chemistry BC, Universitetsparken 2, DK-2100 Copenhagen ø, Denmark

Summary

This mini-review describes a noval class of excitatory heterocyclic amino acid. The selective interactions of these synthetic amino acids with the central glutamic acid (GLU) and aspartic acid (ASP) receptors have been established on the basis of microelectrophoretic techniques using glutamic acid diethyl ester (GDEE) and α-aminoadipic acid (α-AA) as selective antagonists for GLU and ASP, respectively. The parent compound, ibotenic acid (IBO) preferentially activates ASP receptors, but elongation of the side chain of IBO afforded homoibotenic acid (homo-IBO), a GLU agonist. The introduction of bulky substituents into the heterocyclic ring of homo-IBO resulted in a dramatic increase in potency. Alteration of the position of the side chain in IBO to give α-amino-5-methyl-3-hydroxy-4-isoxazoleacetic acid (AMAA), preserved the ASP agonism. However, elongation of the side chain of AMAA gave α-amino-5-methyl-3-hydroxy-4-isoxazolepropionic acid (AMPA), which is a very powerful neuronal excitant with selective interaction with the GLU receptors.

None of the new compounds are inhibitors of the binding of ^{3}H-kainic acid (^{3}H-KAIN) to rat brain membranes, indicating that the mechanism of action of these compounds is different from that of the neurotoxic compound KAIN. The described compounds may be important tools in future investigations of the physiological role and the mechanism of action of ASP and GLU in the central nervous system (CNS).

Introduction

Besides being important compounds as protein precursors and metabolic intermediates, ASP and GLU have received much attention as putative excitatory neurotransmitters in the mammalian CNS (for reviews, see 1–4).

A considerable amount of evidence supports the existence of receptors for ASP and GLU in the CNS (for reviews, see 5, 6). The existence of different receptors for GLU and ASP has been demonstrated using GDEE and α-AA as selective antagonists for GLU and ASP, respectively (7, 8). Fig. 1 shows the formulas of GLU and ASP as well

as those of their antagonists. Various structural analogues of GLU and ASP have been tested for excitatory effects after microelectrophoretic application near central neurones (9–13). Some of these

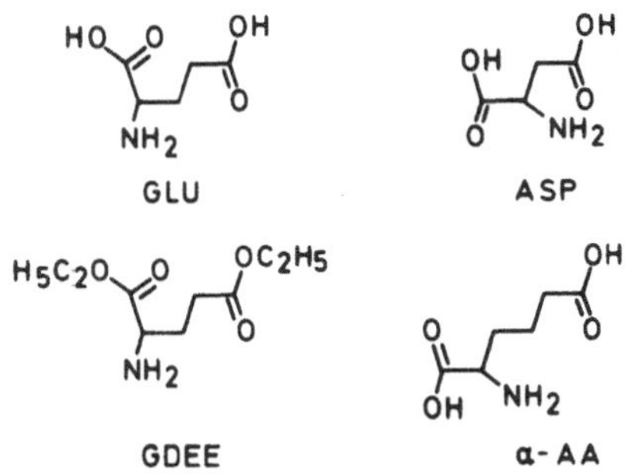

Fig. 1. The structures of GLU and ASP, and of their antagonists GDEE and α-AA.

[+] Present address: Ferrosan A/S Sydmarken 5, DR-2860, Søborg, Denmark.

Molecular and Cellular Biochemistry 38, 123–128 (1981). 0300–8177/81/0381–0123/$ 1.20.
© 1981, Martinus Nijhoff/ Dr. W. Junk Publishers, The Hague.

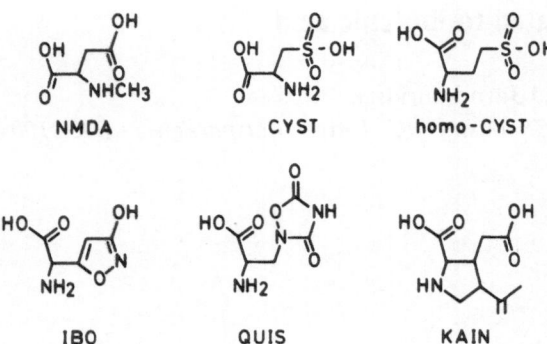

Fig. 2. The structures of excitatory compounds structurally related to GLU and ASP.

Table 1. A summary of different GLU binding sites as obtained by *in vitro* receptor-binding techniques.

Preparation	Numbers of binding sites	K_D (μM)	b_{max} nmol/mg
Synaptic membranes from rat brain (15)	2	0.2	0.002
	4		0.009
Solubilized glycoprotein from rat brain 16	1	0.8	66
Synaptic membranes from rat brains (17)	1	8	0.03
Proteolipid fraction from rat cerebral cortex (18)	3	0.3	0.5
		5	32
		55	166
Synaptic membranes from rat cerebral cortex (19)	1	0.744	0.073
Synaptic membranes from rat striatum (20)	1	0.2	0.006

are illustrated in Fig. 2. From a structural point of view the compounds in Fig. 2 can be divided into two main groups: Flexible compounds, and compounds with reduced conformational mobility. Acidic amino acid with a high degree of molecular flexibility might be expected to interact with both types of receptors for excitatory amino acids as a consequence of their ability to adopt several conformations, whereas the more rigid compounds are likely to exhibit more selective actions.

Based on microelectrophoretic experiments using GDEE and α-AA selective antagonists, the compounds illustrated in Fig. 2 could be divided into three sub-groups (8), 1) compounds relatively sensitive to α-AA, but not to GDEE (N-methyl-D-aspartic acid (NMDA) and IBO), 2) compounds relatively sensitive to GDEE, but not to α-AA (GLU and quisqualic acid (QUIS)), and 3) compounds moderately sensitive to both antagonists (cysteic acid (CYST), homocysteic acid (homo-CYST), and ASP). The potent neuronal excitant, KAIN, which is a structural analogue of GLU, was only moderately sensitive to α-AA and insensitive to GDEE antagonism, and it seems unlikely that KAIN and GLU activate the same receptor (14).

If the previously mentioned excitatory effects of the compounds in microelectrophoretic experiments are a consequence of activation of receptors for GLU and ASP in the mammalian CNS, it might be possible to identify and characterize the receptor sites concerned using ligand-binding techniques.

Several attempts to detect sodium-independent binding of GLU to fractions from rat brain have revealed a variety of binding sites (15-20). Binding constants of these sites are shown in Table 1. These studies might be evidence for the possible existence of a GLU-receptor, although none of the binding sites show as low a K_D for the ligand as has been demonstrated in other related neurotransmitter receptor systems (21, 22). In all these studies, however, GLU is a more potent inhibitor than ASP of ^{3}H-GLU binding.

A single study (23), which has dealt with the binding of ASP to a protolipid fraction from rat cerebral cortex, has revealed three binding sites for ASP: $K_D = 0.2\ \mu$M, $b_{max} = 3$ nmol/mg, $K_D = 10\ \mu$M, $b_{max} = 132$ nmol/mg, and $K_D = 50\ \mu$M, $b_{max} = 617$ nmol/mg. In this study ASP is a more potent inhibitor than GLU of ^{3}H-ASP binding. The fact that GLU selectively interferes with ^{3}H-GLU binding, and that ASP selectively interferes with ^{3}H-ASP binding might indicate different binding sites for GLU and ASP.

KAIN did not significantly inhibit the binding of ^{3}H-GLU and ^{3}H-ASP in any of the above mentioned experiments, supporting the conclusion from electrophoretic experiments, that KAIN does not act at a receptor for either GLU or ASP, in spite of its structural relationship with GLU.

Binding experiments using ^{3}H-KAIN as the ligand have revealed binding sites with receptor properties (24-28). In these experiments QUIS was a potent inhibitor, whereas GLU and IBO were only moderately potent inhibitors, and ASP was almost inactive as an inhibitor of ^{3}H-KAIN binding. Although GLU was an inhibitor of ^{3}H-KAIN,

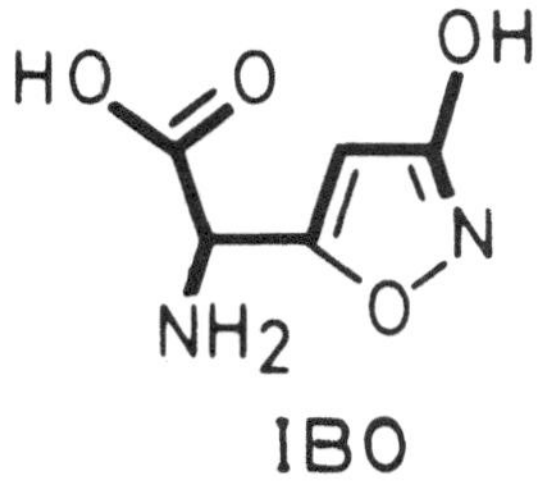

Fig. 3. The structure of IBO with the GLU structure indicated.

it was concluded that KAIN binding may not represent binding to a GLU receptor. Recently, the existence of negative cooperation between the KAIN and GLU binding sites has been demonstrated (29), which might indicate an allosteric interaction of GLU at the KAIN receptor. Thus, it is possible that KAIN activates a receptor for an unidentified endogenous ligand.

The above mentioned studies may represent evidence for distinct GLU and ASP receptors and their possible multiplicity. However, further evidence can only be obtained by using more potent and specific agonists and antagonists for acid amino acids. This minireview describes the development of a new class of compound with selective GLU or ASP agonist activities, using IBO (Fig. 3) as a lead structure.

IBO is a constituent of *Amanita muscaria* (30), with a structural similarity to GLU, since the 3-isoxazolol nucleus can be regarded as a masked carboxyl group. As previously mentioned, however, IBO seems to be an ASP agonist rather than a GLU agonist. The structural manipulations of IBO involve elongation and/or change of the position of the side chain of the 3-isoxazolol nucleus. Furthermore, the introduction of substituents into the 3-isoxazolol nucleus will favour some conformations, due to steric hindrance in the molecule.

Materials and methods

The following IBO analogues were prepared by published procedures: homo-IBO and 4-bromo-homoibotenic acid (4-Br-homo-IBO) (31, 32), 4-methylibotenic acid (4-CH$_3$-IBO) (32), 4-methyl-homoibotenica acid (4-CH$_3$-homo-IBO) (33), AMPA (32, 33), and AMAA (34).

The preparation of the following IBO analogues

will be described elsewhere α-amino-3-hydroxy-5-isoxazolebutanoic acid (A) and α-amino-3-hydroxy-5-isoxazolepentanoic acid (B) (T. Honoré and J. Lauridsen). IBO was a gift from Drs N. Nakamura and C. H. Eugster, NMDA from Dr J. C. Watkins and Mr B. Twitchin and α-AA from Mr B. Twitchin.

[G-^{3}H]-KAIN (spec. act. 2.6 Ci/mmol) was purchased from The Radiochemical Centre, Amersham, England.

All other chemicals were of the purest grade available from regular commercial sources.

Microelectrophoretic experiments

Experiments were carried out on lumbar dorsal horn interneurones and Renshaw cells of cats anaesthetized with pentobarbitone sodium. Extracellular potentials were recorded by means of the centre barrel of seven barrel micropipettes, and the compounds tested were adminstered electrophoretically as anions from aqueous solutions in the outer barrels of the micropipettes (35, 36). The approximate potency of each excitant was assessed relative to that of GLU on the basis of the electrophoretic current required to produce equal and submaximal excitatory effect. Antagonism of amino acid induced excitation by GDEE and α-AA was tested as previously described (8, 37), using GLU and NMDA as reference excitants.

Inhibition of ^{3}H-KAIN binding to rat brain membranes

The method is essentially that of Simon *et al.* (24). Aliquots of synaptic membranes (0.8–1.2 mg of protein) prepared as earlier described (38) were incubated in triplicates at 4 °C for 20 min in 2 ml of 50 mM tris-citrate buffer (pH 7.1), which was 40 nM with respect to ^{3}H-KAIN, and which contained varying concentrations of the indicated inhibitors. Bound radioactivity was separated from free by centrifugation at 48 000 *g* for 10 min followed by rinsing of the pellet with 2 × 5 ml of icecold distilled water, and was measured by conventional methods. Specifically bound ^{3}H-KAIN was obtained by subtracting from the total bound radioactivity in the absence of inhibitor the amount not displaced by 100 μM KAIN. IC$_{50}$-values were estimated by examining the effects of at least four different

Table 2. Structures of the IBO analogues and their effects as neuronal excitants after microelectrophoretic application and as inhibitors of ³H-KAIN binding.

COMPOUND	PREFERENTIALLY ANTAGONIZED BY	INHIBITION OF KAIN BINDING IC$_{50}$-values (µM)
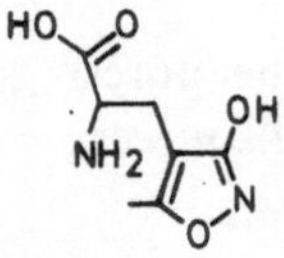 AMPA	GDEE	>100
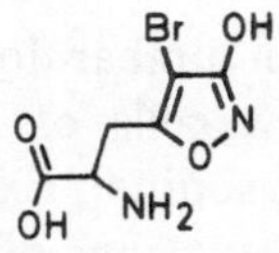 4-Br-homo-IBO	GDEE	>100
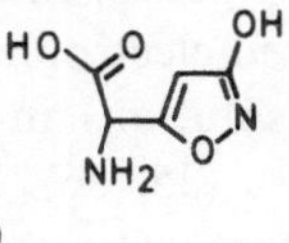 IBO	α-AA	12.2
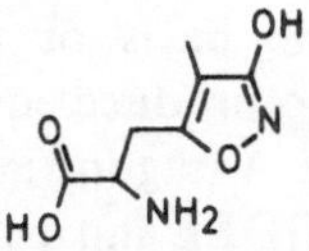 4-CH$_3$-homo-IBO	GDEE	>100
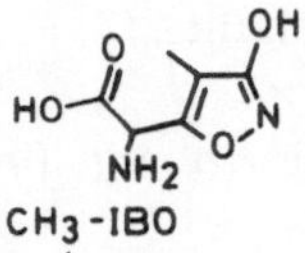 4-CH$_3$-IBO	α-AA	10.0
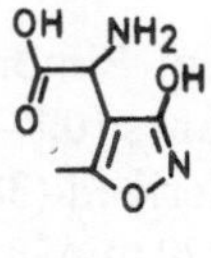 AMAA	α-AA	>100
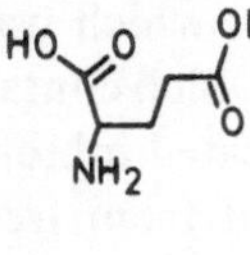 GLU	GDEE	0.41
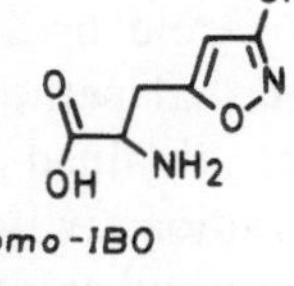 homo-IBO	GDEE	>100

The compounds are presented in decreasing order of excitatory potency after microelectrophoretic application.

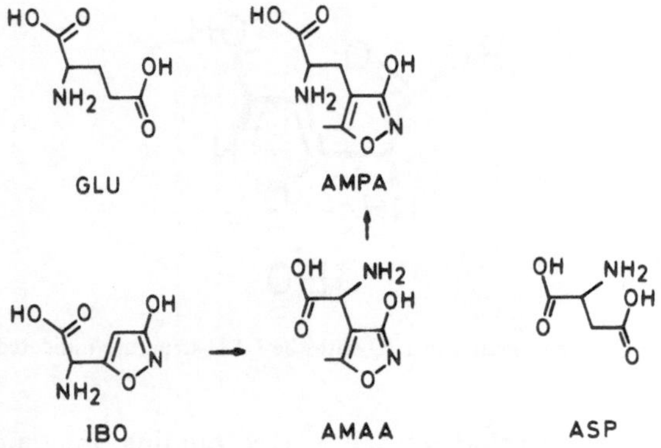

Fig. 4. An illustration of the change of IBO into the ASP analogue AMAA and the GLU analogue AMPA.

concentrations of the inhibitor and performing log-probit analyses of the results. Protein measurements were carried out using the method of Lowry (39) using bovine serum albumin as a standard.

Results and discussion

Table 2 presents the new compounds in decreasing order of relative potency, furthermore the antagonist of the excitation produced and the inhibition of ³H-KAIN binding (36).

IBO seems to activate the ASP receptors in spite of its similitude to GLU. When the amino acid side chain of the 3-isoxazolol nucleus is moved from the 5- to the 4-position, and a methyl group is introduced into the 5-position, IBO is changed into AMAA, which is a structural analogue of ASP (Fig. 4). AMAA is moderately potent as an excitatory substance, being equipotent with GLU. Based on the selective antagonism of the excitatory action of AMAA by α-AA, AMAA seems preferentially to activate the ASP receptors. Elongation of the side chain of AMAA with one carbon atom gave the GLU analogue AMPA (Fig. 4). AMPA is a very potent excitatory compound, which seems to activate the GLU receptors (antagonism by GDEE).

Elongation of the side chain of IBO gave homo-IBO (Fig. 5), which is a weak GLU agonist (antagonism by GDEE). The potency of homo-IBO could be enhanced by replacement of the hydrogen atom in the 4-position of the isoxazole nucleus by bulky groups to give 4-CH$_3$-homo-IBO and 4-Br-

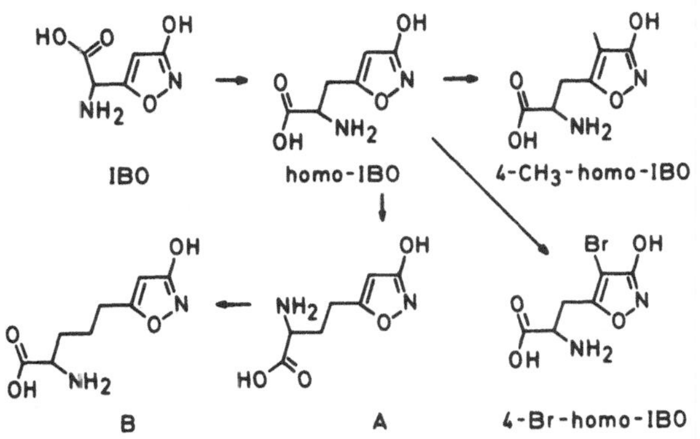

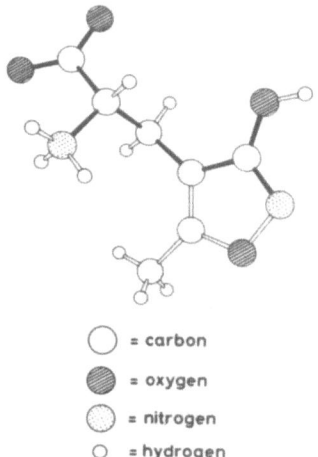

Fig. 5. An illustration of the systematic elongation of the amino acid side chain of IBO.

○ = carbon
◉ = oxygen
◌ = nitrogen
○ = hydrogen

Fig. 6. The conformation of AMPA as obtained by X-ray crystallographic structure determination.

homo-IBO (Fig. 5). The powerful excitatory effects of these compounds apparently result from activation of the central GLU receptors, as both compounds are specifically antagonized by GDEE. The enhancement of the potency seen in 4-CH₃-homo-IBO and 4-Br-homo-IBO may be explained by the steric influence of the substituents in the ring. These groups force the amino acid side chains into conformations which are easily recognized by the GLU receptors (36).

The 4-substituted compounds homo-IBO and AMPA have qualitatively the same mode of action. This might reflect conformational simmilarities of the active conformations of these compounds, the active conformations of which might be identical with the low-energy conformation of AMPA de-

monstrated by X-ray crystallographic methods (Fig. 6) (33), although this investigation only showed one of probably many low-energy conformations of AMPA.

Further elongation of the side chain of homo-IBO produced the compounds A and B (Fig. 5) which, based on preliminary microelectrophoretic experiments (Curtis, D. R., personal communication), are very weak as excitatory substances. These compounds are, however, weak antagonists of NMDA-induced excitations. In this respect the compounds are weaker than α-AA.

In conclusion to the microelectrophoretic experiments it can be concluded that stepwise elongation of the side chain of ASP-agonists (ASP, IBO and AMAA) produces compounds, which are GLU-agonists (GLU, homo-IBO, and AMPA) followed by compounds, which are ASP-antagonists (α-AA, A, α-aminopimelic acid, and B).

Recently it has been demonstrated, that AMPA is a potent neurotoxic compound when injected locally into the caudate (Di Chiara, personal communication) with a potency of ca. one tenth of that of the neurotoxic compound KAIN. Neuronal degeneration induced by other excitatory compounds such as GLU, QUIS, and IBO has previously been reported (40–42). These compounds are moderate to potent inhibitors of ³H-KAIN binding to membranes from rat brains, and it has been suggested, although there are some disgreements (26–29), that neuronal degeneration induced by acid amino acids might be related to the KAIN binding site. When tested in the KAIN binding test AMPA showed no affinity for the KAIN binding site, as shown in Table 2. Consequently AMPA might represent a useful tool in the search for an understanding of the mechanism of the neuronal degeneration induced by KAIN and other 'excitotoxic' amino acids.

The fact that none of the new GLU-agonists presented in Table 2 are active as inhibitors of ³H-KAIN binding add further evidence to the hypothesis that KAIN and GLU binding site are different.

The potent excitatory effects of the new compounds taken together with their apparent specificity make them valuable model compounds in the study of acid amino acid neurotransmitters.

Acknowledgements

This work was supported by the Danish Medical Research Council. The close collaboration of Professor D. R. Curtis, Canberra, Australia is gratefully acknowledged. The authors wish to thank Mrs B. Hare and Mr S. Stilling for skillful secretarial and technical assistance.

References

1. Curtis, D. R. & Johnston, G. A. R., 1974. Ergeb. Physiol. Biol. Chem. Exp. Pharmakol. 69: 97–188.
2. Krnjević, K., 1974. Physiol. Rev. 418–540.
3. Curtis, D. R., 1979. Glutamic Acid: Advances in Biochemistry and Physiology Eds., L. J. Filer, Jr., S. Garattini, M. R. Kare, W. A. Reynolds & R. J. Wurtman, Raven Press, New York, pp. 163–175.
4. Nistri, A. & Constanti, A., 1979. Prog. Neurobiol. (Oxford), 13: 117–235.
5. Watkins, J. C., 1978. Kainic Acid as a Tool in Neurobiology Eds., E. G. McGeer, J. W. Olney & P. L. McGeer, Raven Press, New York, pp. 37–69.
6. Johnston, G. A. R., 1979. Glutamic Acid: Advances in Biochemistry and Physiology Eds., L. J. Filer, Jr., S. Garattine, M. R. Kare, W. A. Reynolds & R. J. Wurtman, Raven Press, New York, pp. 177–185.
7. Hicks, T. P., Hall, J. G. & McLennan, H., 1978. Can. J. Physiol. Pharmacol. 56: 901–907.
8. McLennan, H. & Lodge, D., 1979. Brain Res. 169: 83–90.
9. Curtis, D. R. & Watkins, J. C., 1963. J. Physiol. (London), 166: 1–14.
10. Cox, D. W. G., Headley, P. M. & Watkins, J. C., 1977. J. Neurochem. 29: 579–588.
11. Johnston, G. A. R., Curtis, D. R., De Groat, W. C. & Duggan, A. W., 1968. Biochem. Pharmacol. 17: 2488–2489.
12. Johnston, G. A. R., Curtis, D. R., Davies, J. & McCulloch, R. M., 1974. Nature (London), 248: 804–805.
13. Biscoe, T. J., Evans, R. H., Headley, P. M., Martin, M. R. & Watkins, J. C., 1976. Br. J. Pharmacol. 58: 373–382.
14. Hall, J. G., Hicks, T. P. & McLennan, H., 1978. Neurosci. Lett. 8: 171–175.
15. Michaelis, E. K., Michaelis, M. L. & Boyarsky, L. L., 1974. Biochim. Biophys. Acta 367: 338–348.
16. Michaelis, E. K., 1975. Biochem. Biophys. Res. Commun. 65: 1004–1012.
17. Roberts, P. J., 1974. Nature (London) 252: 399–401.
18. De Robertis, E. & Fiszer de Plazas, S., 1976. Neurochem. 26: 1237–1243.
19. Foster, A. C. & Roberts, P. J., 1978. J. Neurochem. 31: 1467–1477.
20. Baudry, M. & Lynch, G., 1979. Eur. J. Pharmacol. 57: 283–285.
21. Enna, S. J. & Snyder, S. H., 1977. Mol. Pharmacol. 13: 442–453.
22. Bennett, J. P., Jr. & Snyder, S. H., 1976. Mol. Pharmacol. 12: 373–389.
23. Fiszer de Plazas, S. & De Robertis, E., 1976. J. Neurochem. 27: 889–894.
24. Simon, J. R., Contrera, J. F. & Kuhar, M. J., 1976. J. Neurochem. 26: 141–147.
25. London, E. D. & Coyle, J. T., 1979. Mol. Pharmacol. 15: 492–505.
26. Vincent, S. R. & McGeer, E. G., 1979. Life Sci. 24: 265–270.
27. Schwarcz, R. & Fuxe, K., 1979. Life Sci. 24: 1471–1480.
28. Henke, H., 1979. Neurosci. Lett. 14: 247–251.
29. London, E. D. & Coyle, J. T., 1979. Eur. J. Pharmacol. 56: 287–290.
30. Eugster, C. H., 1969. Fortschr. Chem. Org. Naturst. 27: 261–321.
31. Hansen, J. J. & Krogsgaard-Larsen, P., 1979. J. Chem. Soc. Chem. Commun. 87–88.
32. Hansen, J. J. & Krogsgaard-Larsen, P., 1980. J. Chem. Soc. Perkin Trans. I, 1826–1833.
33. Honoré, T. & Lauridsen, J., 1980. Acta Chem. Scand. (in B 34, 235–240.
34. Christensen, S. B. & Krogsgaard-Larsen, P., 1978. Acta Chem. Scand. B32: 27–30.
35. Curtis, D. R., Duggan, A. W., Felix, D. & Johnston, G. A. R., 1971. Brain Res. 32: 69–96.
36. Krogsgaard-Larsen, P., Honoré, T., Hansen, J. J., Curtis, D. R. & Lodge, D., 1980. Nature (London) 284: 64–66.
37. Lodge, D., Headley, P. M. & Curtis, D. R., 1978. Brain Res. 153: 603–608.
38. Honoré, T., Hjeds, H., Krogsgaard-Larsen, P. & Christiansen, T. R., 1978. Eur. J. Med. Chem. 13: 429–434.
39. Lowry, O. H., Rosebrough, N. J., Farr, A. L. & Randall, R. J., 1951. J. Biol. Chem. 193: 265–275.
40. Olney, J. W., 1978. Kainic Acid as a Tool in Neurobiology Eds., E. G. McGeer, J. W. Olney & P. L. McGeer, Raven Press, New York, pp. 95–121.
41. Kizer, J. S., Nemeroff, C. B. & Young Blood, W. W., 1978. Pharmacol. Rev. 29: 301–318.
42. Schwarcz, R., Hökfelt, T., Fuxe, K., Jonsson, G., Goldstein, M. & Terenius, L., 1979. Exp. Brain Res. 37: 199–216.

Received April 30, 1980.

GABA agonists
Development and interactions with the GABA receptor complex

Povl Krogsgaard-Larsen and Erik Falch
The Royal Danish School of Pharmacy, Department of Chemistry BC, Universitetsparken 2, DK-2100 Copenhagen Ø, Denmark

Summary

This review describes the development of GABA receptor agonists with no detectable affinity for other recognition sites in GABA-mediated synapses. The key compounds are THIP, isoguvacine, and piperidine-4-sulphonic acid (P4S), developed via extensive structural modifications of the potent but not strictly specific GABA agonist muscimol. The structural parameters, which have to be considered in the design of GABA agonists are discussed on the basis of the structures and biological activities of these GABA agonists and a number of related compounds.

A model, which summarizes our present knowledge of the structure of the postsynaptic GABA receptor complex, is presented, and the interaction of GABA agonists with various sites in this complex is discussed. Of particular interest are the effects of GABA agonists on the binding of diazepam to the benzodiazepine binding site, assumed to be a structural unit of the GABA receptor complex. While rigid molecules like THIP are capable of activating the GABA receptors, a certain degree of conformational mobility of GABA agonists apparently is a prerequisite for stimulation of diazepam binding in vitro at $0\,^{\circ}C$. These findings suggest that GABA receptor functions involve conformational changes of certain elements of the receptor complex.

Some aspects of the pharmacology of GABA agonists are discussed, including the attempts to develop GABA agonists with desirable pharmacokinetic and toxicological characteristics. While muscimol is a toxic compound, THIP is well tolerated by animals, and in contrast to isoguvacine, THIP penetrates into the brain after systemic administration to animals, a difference which can be explained on the basis of their protolytic properties. The attempts to develop pro-drugs of isoguvacine capable of penetrating the blood-brain barrier with subsequent decomposition in the brain tissue to isoguvacine are described.

Introduction

Studies of the central receptors operated by γ-aminobutyric acid (GABA) play an important role in the elucidation of the neurotransmitter function of this amino acid. Our knowledge about the structures, functions, and locations of the GABA receptors is still very incomplete, but extensive physiological and biochemical studies during the past few years (1–5) have shed some light on these key problems. In addition, these studies have provided substantial evidence of the existence of multiple GABA receptors in the mammalian central nervous system (CNS).

Using electrophysiological techniques, which offer the most direct approach to studies of receptors, two populations of GABA receptors have been identified and characterized, the 'presynaptic' (axo-axonic) and the postsynaptic (axo-somatic and axo-dendritic) receptors (6–9). Activation of these receptors result in depolarization and hyperpolarization of the respective postsynaptic membranes. In both cases the physiological mechanisms result in increases in membrane permeability to chloride ions (6, 7), indicating that both types of

Molecular and Cellular Biochemistry 38, 129–146 (1981). 0300-8177/81/0381-0129/$ 3.60.
© 1981, Martinus Nijhoff/Dr. W. Junk Publishers, The Hague.

130

GABA receptor are coupled to chloride ionophores. However, the relative contributions of pre- and postsynaptic mechanism to GABA-mediated inhibition in different parts of the mammalian CNS are not known (8).

The development of radioreceptor binding techniques (10–12) has resulted in a dramatic acceleration of the in vitro studies of GABA receptor mechanisms. The original GABA receptor binding technique (10) has been subjected to various modifications (13–15), and in addition to GABA, the GABA agonists muscimol (16–18) and isoguvacine (19, 20) have been used as radioactive ligands. Both electrophysiological methods and radioreceptor binding techniques have inherent limitations. While the former technique allows studies of alterations of synaptic membranes resulting from activation or blockade of the receptors, physiological experiments are normally not sufficiently quantitative to clarify the receptor mechanisms involved (9, 21). Electrophysiological studies on cultured neurones can provide more precise information about GABA receptor functions (22, 23), although cell cultures must necessarily be different from cells in intact nervous tissue. The receptors studied in radioreceptor binding experiments probably represent more or less disintegrated forms of the physiological GABA receptors. Consequently, interpretations of kinetic data derived from such studies in terms of molecular mechanisms of the receptors in the intact synaptic environments must be performed with great care. The receptor binding technique has been used for studies of the interaction of GABA with the isolated and partially purified GABA receptor macromolecule(s) (24–27). Detailed studies along these lines and combined uses of different techniques will provide more precise information about GABA receptor mechanisms.

The postsynaptic GABA receptor complex

The fundamental elements of the GABA receptor complex is a receptor site, which binds GABA, and a chloride channel regulated by an as yet unknown mechanism. However, studies along different lines indicate that the postsynaptic GABA receptor is actually a multiunit complex containing a number of membrane units, some of which may be involved in the control and modulation of the GABA receptor functions.

While only one class of binding site with a relatively low affinity for GABA can be detected on crude synaptic membranes (10), treatment of these membranes with low concentrations of detergents (13, 14, 28–32) or extensive purification of the membranes by repeated washings (30) reveal the presence of two populations of GABA binding sites (Fig. 1). On crude membranes the high-affinity GABA binding sites are occupied by substance(s) assumed to be endogenous inhibitors or modulators of the GABA receptors. The inhibitor appears to be an acidic protein (31, 32), although the activity concerned may in part be associated with phospholipids (29, 33) or GABA itself (30). The high- and low-affinity binding sites for GABA may represent two distinct macromolecules, or they may be part of the same molecular entity (14).

The mechanism of interaction of the 'classical' GABA antagonists bicuculline and picrotoxinin (6) (Fig. 2) with the GABA receptors is different. Bicuculline and bicuculline methochloride (BMC) seem to interact directly with the GABA receptors, possibly to an 'antagonist conformational state' of the receptor (34–36). While picrotoxinin also antagonizes the physiological action of GABA (6, 37), it does not compete directly with GABA for binding to the receptor recognition site (15, 38–40). Picrotoxinin apparently interacts directly with the chloride channel or a membrane structure closely associated with this ionophore (41–43) (Fig. 1). A variety of convulsant and anticonvulsant drugs interfere with this picrotoxinin binding site (43), the physiological role of which is unknown.

Radioactive diazepam binds to a high affinity recognition site in the brain (44–48). It has been established that at least some of the therapeutical effects of the benzodiazepines are the results of 'facilitation' of GABA-mediated neurotransmission (49–51), and although the benzodiazepines are not acting as GABA agonists (52), the GABA receptor complex appears to be the essential site of action of these compounds. This functional interaction between the GABA receptors and the benzodiazepine binding sites is supported by the observations that GABA stimulates the binding of [3H]-diazepam in vitro (53–55). Furthermore chloride ions modulate the binding of both GABA and benzodiazepines (54, 56–58) in agreement with the proposed close association between the benzodiazepine binding site and the GABA receptor-

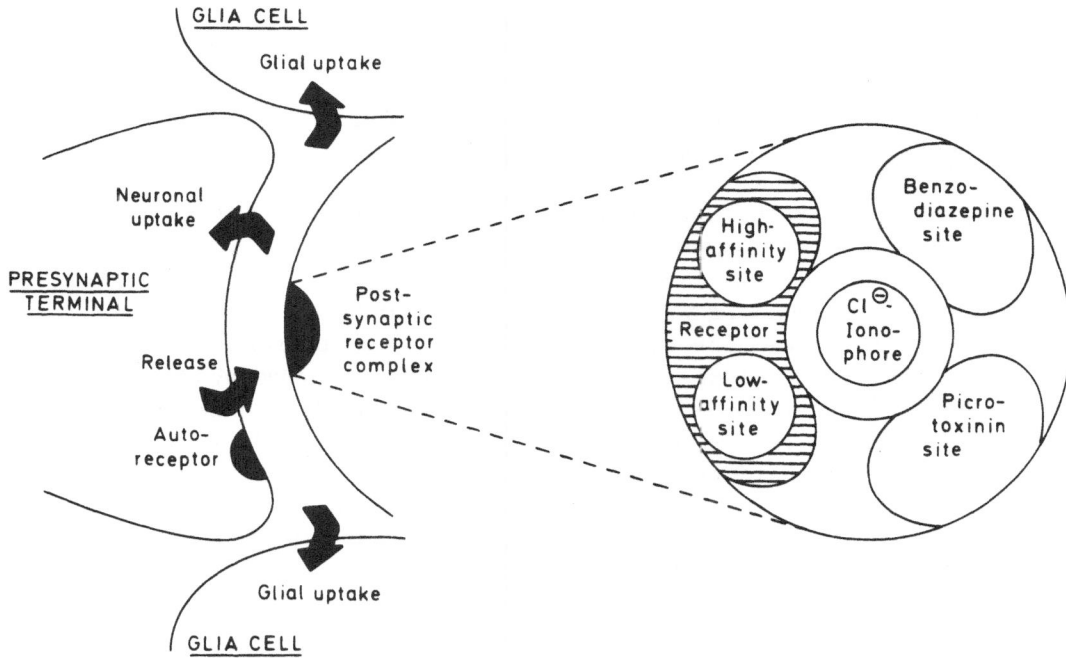

Fig. 1. A schematic illustration of a central axo-somatic GABA-mediated synapse. The GABA transport processes in the nerve terminal and in the glial cells and also the GABA release system, assumed to be regulated by presynaptic autoreceptors, are indicated by arrows. The multiunit postsynaptic GABA receptor complex consists of a chloride channel regulated by a receptor site, which apparently includes a high- and a low-affinity binding site for GABA. The GABA receptor functions seem to be regulated by at least two subunits, which selectively bind the benzodiazepines and picrotoxinin, respectively, *in vitro*.

ionophore complex (Fig. 1). The physiological role of this benzodiazepine site is, however, unknown. There is some evidence that the benzodiazepines and the proposed GABA receptor modulator(s) bind to the same site in the receptor complex (31, 32, 59), and a variety of other compounds have been proposed as natural ligands for the benzodiazepine binding site, including nicotinamide (60) and various purine derivatives (61–63).

In spite of extensive studies our knowledge of the structural and functional interactions between the different units of the GABA receptor complex is still limited. More detailed information about the physiological role of the benzodiazepine binding site may be obtained after isolation and partial characterization of the bio-macromolecule(s) involved (25, 64–67). The functional interaction between the GABA receptors and the benzodiazepine binding sites has been further supported (68, 69), but the complexity of this research field is emphasized by the fact that not all benzodiazepine recognition sites are coupled to the GABA receptors (70).

Presynaptic GABA receptors and autoreceptors

The GABA analogue baclofen (Fig. 2), which is used in the treatment of human spasticity (71),

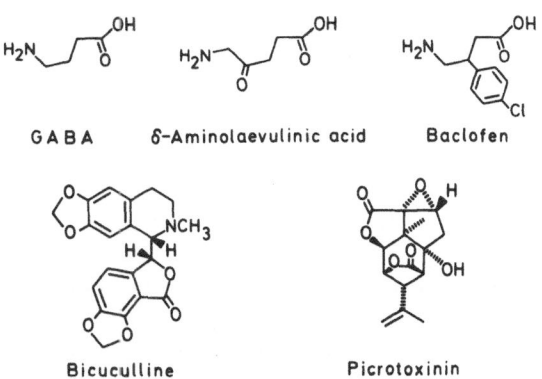

Fig. 2. The structures of GABA, δ-aminolaevulinic acid, and baclofen. The last-named compounds are putative selective agonists for presynaptic GABA autoreceptors (77) and for presynaptic GABA receptors on sympathetic nerve terminals (75), respectively. The structures of the GABA antagonists bicuculline and picrotoxinin are illustrated.

132

depresses the firing of cat spinal neurones (72), and it is a very weak and non-stereoselective inhibitor of GABA receptor binding in vitro (73). Since the depressant effect of baclofen is insensitive to the GABA antagonist bicuculline (72), baclofen is assumed to interact with a unique class of GABA receptors (74). Baclofen and GABA have recently been shown to inhibit the release of biogenic amines from tissue preparations in vitro in a bicuculline-insensitive manner, (–)-baclofen being much more potent than the optical antipode (75). Based on these observations baclofen is assumed to be a selective agonist for a population of GABA receptors on sympathetic nerve terminals, which are involved in the regulation of transmitter release (75).

Studies in vitro have revealed the existence of presynaptic GABA autoreceptors (39, 76–78) (Fig. 1). GABA and GABA agonists inhibit the release of radioactive GABA accumulated in the tissue preparations, and δ-aminolaevulinic acid (Fig. 2) appears to be a selective agonist for this population of GABA receptors (77), which in contrast to the GABA receptors on sympathetic terminals are sensitive to bicuculline and picrotoxinin. Based on comparative studies, using a variety of specific GABA agonists, the ligand specificities of these proposed autoreceptors and the postsynaptic GABA receptors are identical (M. J. W. Brennan and P. Krogsgaard-Larsen, unpublished). These findings together suggest that the physiological release of GABA is subject to negative feedback control through presynaptic autoreceptors with properties similar to those of the postsynaptic receptors (39, 76–78).

Design of GABA agonists

A prerequisite for satisfactory identification and pharmacological characterization of the different populations of GABA receptors is the availability of potent and specific agonists and antagonists for each type of receptor. As already mentioned certain GABA analogues interact selectively with the different classes of GABA receptor so far known, but the above condition is still far from being satisfactorily fulfilled. Furthermore, GABA agonists and antagonists should preferably have pharmacokinetic characteristics which make animal behavioural experiments possible and ideally also

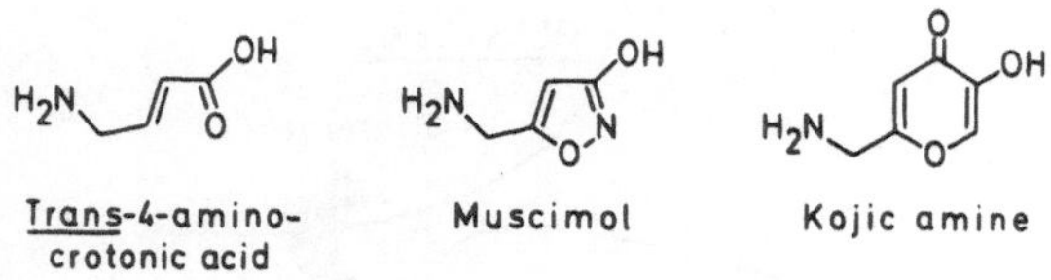

Fig. 3. The structures of the GABA analogues trans-4-aminocrotonic acid, muscimol, and kojic amine.

toxicological properties acceptable for administration of the compounds to man.

A variety of simple GABA analogues have been prepared and tested as inhibitors of GABA receptor binding, GABA uptake, and of the activity of the GABA-metabolizing enzyme (GABA-T) (42, 74, 79). These compounds including trans-4-aminocrotonic acid (80) (Fig. 3), which interfere more or less effectively with all recognition sites in GABA mediated synapses, are not useful as tools for GABA receptor studies.

Certain heterocyclic compounds like muscimol and kojic amine, which have some structural resemblance to GABA (Fig. 3), are selective GABA agonists capable of penetrating the blood-brain barrier (81–83). Both compounds have been subjected to structural modifications, and in particular muscimol has been extensively used as a model compound for the development of GABA uptake inhibitors (84) and of GABA agonists and antagonists (81, 85).

This review describes the conversion of muscimol, which is a powerful GABA agonist and a substrate for GABA transport carriers and apparently also for GABA-T, into very potent and specific GABA agonists.

Materials

GABA analogues

The following GABA analogues were prepared by published procedures: Muscimol (86); dihydromuscimol ((RS)-5-aminomethyl-2-isoxazolin-3-ol), 4-methylmuscimol, 4-methylhomomuscimol, (S)- and (R)-5'-methylmuscimol ((S)- and (R)-5-(1-aminoethyl)-3-isoxazolol) (87); thiomuscimol (88); isomuscimol, azamuscimol, 2-methylazamuscimol (89); (RS)-5'-methylmuscimol ((RS)-5-(1-aminoethyl)-3-isoxazolol), (RS)-5'-ethylmuscimol ((RS)-

5-(1-aminopropyl)-3-isoxazolol (90); 4-ethylmuscimol (91); 4-aminomethyl-5-methyl-3-isoxazolol (1), 4-(2-aminoethyl)-5-methyl-3-isoxazolol (2) (92); (S)- and (R)-4-methyl-trans-ACA ((S)- and (R)-trans-4-amino-2-pentenoic acid) (93); THIP (4, 5, 6, 7-tetrahydroisoxazolo[5, 4-c]pyridin-3-ol), THAO (5, 6, 7, 8-tetrahydro-4H-isoxazolo[4, 5-c]azepin-3-ol, 5, 6, 7, 8-tetrahydro-4H-isoxazolo[5, 4-c]azepin-3-ol (3) (94); THPO (4, 5, 6, 7-tetrahydroisoxazolo[4, 5-c]pyridin-3-ol), THAZ (5, 6, 7, 8-tetrahydro-4H-isoxazolo[4, 5-d]azepin-3-ol) (95); iso-THAZ (5, 6, 7, 8-tetrahydro-4H-isoxazolo[3, 4-d]azepin-3-ol) (96); iso-THIP (4, 5, 6, 7-tetrahydroisoxazolo[3, 4-c]pyridin-3-ol), aza-THIP (4, 5, 6, 7-tetrahydropyrazolo[3, 4-c]pyridin-3-ol), 2-methylaza-THIP (2-methyl-4, 5, 6, 7-tetrahydropyrazolo[3, 4-c]pyridin-3-ol, isoguvacine, cis-3-OH-isonipecotic acid ((3RS, 4RS)-3-hydroxypiperidine-4-carboxylic acid), 4-OH-isonipecotic acid (4-hydroxypiperidine-4-carboxylic acid), (RS)-perhydroazepine-3-carboxylic acid (6), 2, 3, 6, 7-tetrahydro-1H-azepine-4-carboxylic acid (4), 2, 5, 6, 7-tetrahydro-1H-azepine-4-carboxylic acid (5) (97); guvacine (98); P4S (piperidine-4-sulphonic acid) (99).

The preparation of the following compounds will be published elsewhere: 3-Pyrroline-3-carboxylic acid (7) (P. Thorbek, H. Hjeds and K. Schaumburg); (S)- and (R)-4-methyl-GABA ((S)- and (R)-4-aminovaleric acid) (P. Krogsgaard-Larsen); O-methyl-THIP (3-methoxy-4, 5, 6, 7-tetrahydroisoxazolo[5, 4-c]pyridine (P. Krogsgaard-Larsen and J. S. Johansen); isoguvacine methyl ester (13), isoguvacine acetyloxymethyl ester (8), isoguvacine propionyloxymethyl ester (9), isoguvacine valeroyloxymethyl ester (10), isoguvacine 2-ethylbutyryloxymethyl ester (11), isoguvacine pivaloyloxymethyl ester (12) (E. Falch, P. Krogsgaard-Larsen and A. V. Christensen).

Radioisotopes and chemicals

[2, 3-³H]GABA (specific activity 58 Ci/mmol) and [aminomethyl-³H]muscimol (specific activity 9.5 Ci/mmol) were purchased from The Radiochemical Centre, Amersham, England, where [2, 6-³H]isoguvacine (specific activity 18.7 Ci/mmol) was also prepared using a published procedure for labelling of isoguvacine (100). All other amino acids and chemicals were of the purest grade available from regular commercial sources.

Methods

Microelectrophoretic experiments

The determination of the depressant effects of the described GABA analogues on mammalian central neurones were performed as described elsewhere (99, 101–103) using microelectrophoretic techniques (104). Experiments were performed on lumbar dorsal horn interneurones and Renshaw cells of cats anaesthetized with pentobarbitone sodium (35 mg/kg intraperitoneally initially, supplemented intravenously when required). Extracellular action potentials were recorded by means of the centre barrel of seven barrel micropipettes. The compounds tested were administered electrophoretically from the outer barrels of the micropipettes, which contained solutions of the compounds (100–200 mM, adjusted to pH 3–4) or the GABA antagonist BMC (10 mM in 165 mM-NaCl). In some experiments the most potent GABA agonists were used as dilute solutions (50 mM) in 165 mM-NaCl. Firing of the cells was induced by electrophoretically administered (RS)-homocysteic acid (200 mM, adjusted to pH 7.5).

The depressant effects are expressed relative to that of GABA (---). The number of symbols indicates greater, equal, or less activity on an approximately linear scale (cf. Table 1 and Figs. 5, 6). Zero indicates no activity, and effects of doubtful significance are cited in brackets. The specificity of the depressant effects as the results of activation of GABA receptors was examined by simultaneous ejection of the GABA analogues and BMC or strychnine, a glycine antagonist (104, 105). Thus, a GABA agonist is defined as a BMC-sensitive, strychnine-insensitive neuronal depressant (6). Antagonism by BMC is indicated by +, whereas 0 indicates no significant reduction of the depressant effect by BMC. None of the compounds described in this review, which have been tested microelectrophoretically, showed strychnine-sensitive depressant effects.

Inhibition of GABA receptor binding

In an attempt to estimate the affinity of the

GABA analogues for the *low-affinity* binding sites of the GABA receptors in vitro the compounds listed in Table 1 were tested as inhibitors of the binding of radioactive GABA to 'crude' rat brain synaptic membranes (103, 106), prepared by a published procedure (10). Since the high-affinity GABA binding sites on these membranes apparently are occupied by 'endogenous inhibitor(s)' (13, 14, 28–32) and/or artificial products formed during disintegration of the rat brain tissue, the test compounds are assumed to compete with GABA primarily for binding to the low-affinity binding sites on these membranes.

The 'crude' synaptic membranes were prepared as described in detail elsewhere (10). The membranes were frozen at $-20\,^\circ$C for at least 18 h. Frozen pellets were after thawing resuspended in water, maintained at $25\,^\circ$C for 20 min and centrifuged at 48 000 g for 10 min, and the pellets were then suspended in Tris-citrate buffer for GABA binding assay. For the standard [³H]GABA binding assay procedure, aliquots of the synaptic membranes (0.8–1.2 mg of protein) were incubated in triplicate at $4\,^\circ$C for 5 min in 2 ml of 50 mM Tris-citrate buffer (pH 7.1) containing 6 nM-[³H]GABA (10). Total specific GABA binding was obtained by subtracting from the total bound radioactivity the amount not displaced by 1 mM-GABA. In routine experiments approximately 4000 cpm/mg of protein were bound in the absence of displacer, whereas only 1800 cpm/mg of protein were bound in the presence of 1 mM-GABA. Thus, 2200 cpm/mg of protein, corresponding to 55% of the totally bound radioactivity represent specifically bound [³H]GABA. Protein was measured by a described procedure (107). The GABA analogues were tested initially at a concentration of 100 000 nM, and if GABA binding was inhibited by more than 50% at this concentration, an estimate was made of the IC_{50} value (the concentration of inhibitor producing 50% inhibition of specifically bound [³H]GABA) by examining the effects of at least four different concentrations of inhibitor and performing log-probit analyses of the results.

In order to test the effect of the GABA analogues on the *high-affinity* GABA receptor sites, membranes prepared by a modified procedure (103) were utilized. The isolation procedure for this type of membranes is similar to that (10) outlined above. However, the membranes were frozen rapidly at $-70\,^\circ$C, and before freezing and after thawing the pellets were submitted to at least two additional resuspensions in water and subsequent centrifugations at 48 000 g for 20 min. These more rapidly frozen and extensively washed membranes have binding characteristics similar to those of membranes treated with low concentrations of detergents (13, 14, 28–32). Under incubation conditions identical with those used for the 'crude' synaptic membranes, the present membranes bind approximately 5700 cpm/mg of protein in the absence of displacer, whereas only 1200 cpm/mg of protein were bound in the presence of 1 mM-GABA (103). Thus, the modifications of the isolation procedure have resulted in an increase in the total [³H]GABA binding capacity of the membranes of approximately 40%, and 79% of the bound radioactivity represent specifically bound GABA. Also in accordance with the findings for membranes treated with detergents (13, 14, 28–32), the present type of membranes display biphasic binding of [³H]GABA with K_D values (20 and 150 nM), comparable with those measured for detergent-treated membranes. The standard [³H]GABA binding procedure based on these membranes was identical with that described for the 'crude' synaptic membranes, the incubation medium containing 6 nM-[³H-GABA] (103). Under these conditions the inhibitors are assumed to compete with radioactive GABA primarily for binding to the high-affinity receptor sites (cf. Table 1).

While the compounds listed in Table 1 were tested as inhibitors of the binding of [³H]GABA to 'crude' as well as to rapidly frozen and more extensively washed rat brain membranes, the binding data shown in Figs. 5, 6 and Table 2 were obtained using the latter type of membrane. Consequently, the IC_{50} values concerned are comparable with those listed in the column 'Inhibition of High-Affinity GABA Receptor Binding' in Table 1.

Similarly, studies on the inhibition of the binding of [³H]muscimol and of [³H]isoguvacine to the GABA receptors in vitro were performed using the more extensively washed membranes. These experiments were performed under conditions identical with those used in the [³H]GABA binding experiments, the concentrations of [³H]muscimol and of [³H]isoguvacine in the incubation media being 3 nM and 5 nM, respectively (20).

Activation of [³H]diazepam binding

The procedure for the measurement of stimulation of [³H]diazepam binding to rat brain membranes is described in detail elsewhere (108). The isolated synaptic membranes were suspended in 100 mM-Tris-citrate buffer (pH 7.1) to 160 vol (vol/weight rat brain tissue). Aliquots of 2.5 ml were incubated with 0.4 nM-[³H]diazepam (14.4 Ci/mmol) for 20 min at 0 °C in a total of 2.75 ml. GABA agonists were added in duplicate immediately before the radioactive diazepam. Samples were diluted to 10 ml in cold buffer after the incubation and immediately filtered through GF/C glass-fibre filters and washed with 10 ml of buffer. The radioactivity on the filters was measured by scintillation counting. All binding values were calculated as specific binding, which is total binding minus binding in the presence of 3000 nM-diazepam. Control specific binding averaged approximately 700 cpm/15 mg of tissue; specific binding in the presence of 3000 nM-muscimol was approximately 1000 cpm/15 mg of tissue; non-specific binding was approximately 150 cpm/15 mg of tissue. The EC_{50} values (the concentrations of GABA analogues required for 50% activation of [³H]diazepam binding) were calculated as earlier described (108).

Inhibition of GABA uptake in mouse brain 'mini-slices'

Mouse brain 'mini-slices' ('prisms', $0.5 \times 0.1 \times 0.1$ mm) were prepared as described elsewhere (109). This tissue preparation primarily represents the neuronal GABA uptake system (110), and to study the effects of GABA analogues on this high-affinity transport system mouse brain 'mini-slices' corresponding to approximately 200 µg of protein were incubated as earlier described (109). The IC_{50} values for inhibition of high-affinity neuronal GABA uptake at 1000 nM-GABA and without preincubation of the tissue in the presence of inhibitor were determined as earlier described in detail (109).

Relationship between structure and biological activity of GABA agonists

Monocyclic muscimol analogues

Muscimol and a number of muscimol analogues were tested as inhibitors of the binding of radioactive GABA to GABA receptor sites on two different preparations of rat brain synaptic membranes. On one type of membranes (10) the high-affinity binding sites appear to be masked by substances assumed to be endogenous inhibitors or modulators of the physiological GABA receptors (31–32). Only a low-affinity receptor site seems to be available for binding GABA and GABA analogues to these membranes (10), and Table 1 illustrates the relative affinity of the muscimol analogues concerned for this receptor site. The compounds were also tested as inhibitors of GABA binding using membranes isolated under conditions (103), which apparently unmask the high-affinity receptor sites without use of detergents. Under the test conditions used these sites presumably are mainly responsible for the binding of GABA and of inhibitors.

It is evident from Table 1 that the relative potencies of the compounds in these two series of experiments are similar but not identical. The affinity of the muscimol analogues concerned for the high-affinity GABA receptor site is typically 5–10 times higher than the affinity for the low-affinity site in reasonable agreement with the ratios between the K_D values of the respective receptor sites (13, 14, 28–32).

With a few exceptions there is a good correlation between the affinity of the compounds listed in Table 1 for the GABA receptor sites in vitro and their intrinsic activity on the receptors in vivo, measured as BMC-sensitive depressant effects on cat spinal neurones. Azamuscimol and (RS)-5'-ethylmuscimol represent the most notable exceptions to this apparent correlation. The former compound interferes with the receptors in vitro and in vivo, but the moderately potent depressant action of azamuscimol is insensitive to BMC (103). The latter muscimol analogue exhibits BMC-insensitive depressant effects (101), but this compound has no detectable affinity for the GABA receptors in vitro (106). These effects, and in particular those of (RS)-5'-ethylmuscimol, are similar to those of

Table 1. Structures and effects on the GABA receptors in vivo and in vitro of some muscimol analogues.

COMPOUND	STRUCTURE	DEPRESSION OF THE FIRING OF SPINAL NEURONES		INHIBITION (IC_{50}, nM) OF		ANTAGONISM OF GABA
		RELATIVE POTENCY	ANTAGONISM BY BMC	HIGH-AFFINITY GABA RECEPTOR BINDING	LOW-AFFINITY GABA RECEPTOR BINDING	
GABA		– – –	+	33	340	
Muscimol		– – – –	+	6	24	
Dihydro-muscimol		– – – –	+	9	56	
Thio-muscimol		– – – –	+	19	120	
Iso-muscimol		–	0	29000	>100000	
Aza-muscimol		– –	0	16000	>100000	
2-Methyl-azamuscimol		n.t.		>100000	>100000	
(RS)-5'-Methyl-muscimol		– – –	+	2000	7000	
(RS)-5'-Ethyl-muscimol		– –	0	>100000	>100000	
4-Methyl-muscimol		–	0	26000	>100000	
4-Ethyl-muscimol		0		>100000	>100000	0
4-Methyl-homomuscimol		0		>100000	>100000	0
1		0		>100000	>100000	0
2		0		>100000	>100000	0

The GABA agonist and antagonist activities of the compounds were tested on cat spinal neurones using microelectrophoretic techniques (101, 103, 104). The relative potencies of the compounds as neuronal depressants were assessed relative to that of GABA (–––) (for details see 'Methods'). The potencies of the compounds as preferential inhibitors of low- and high-affinity GABA receptor binding were measured using rat brain synaptic membranes exhibiting low-affinity (10) and both high- and low-affinity (103) binding sites, respectively (for details see 'Methods'). n.t., not tested.

baclofen (72, 73) suggesting that these compounds interfere with the BMC-insensitive GABA receptors assumed to be present on sympathetic nerve terminals (75).

From the lowest half of Table 1 it appears that alterations of the structure and position of the side chain of muscimol typically result in dramatic loss of effects on the GABA receptors (81, 85, 101, 111). Direct steric hindrance of the additional groups may prevent the alkylated muscimol analogues from interacting with the GABA receptors. Alternatively, these groups may introduce high rotational energy barriers, which prevent these compounds from adopting conformations recognizable by the GABA receptors. Structure-activity studies on cyclic GABA analogues and bicyclic muscimol analogues, in which the 'GABA structure elements' are locked in different conformations (cf. Figs. 5, 6) indicate that the latter effect is of major importance. In other words, a necessary condition for interaction of a GABA analogue with the GABA receptor is an ability to adopt a 'receptor-active conformation' different from the low-energy conformations of GABA and muscimol (81, 111).

In the compounds listed in the upper half of Table 1 the isoxazole ring of muscimol has been replaced by related 5-membered heterocyclic rings. In these compounds the fundamental structural elements of muscimol are preserved including the presence of an acidic hydroxy group in the 3-position of the rings, responsible for the zwitterionic structures of all of these compounds (cf. Fig. 4). In spite of an immediate structural similarity of these muscimol analogues, their activities are strictly dependent on the structures of the heterocyclic rings (103). While the pronounced differences between the biological activities of these compounds can not be correlated with the differences in

their protolytic properties, there is a correlation between the GABA agonist activities and the degrees of delocalization of the negative charges of these compounds (81, 103) (Fig. 4). The charged structures of the potent GABA agonists muscimol, dihydromuscimol, and probably also thiomuscimol (81, 112) are similar to that determined for GABA (113). On the other hand, the negative charges of isomuscimol and apparently also those of azamuscimol and 2-methylazamuscimol are highly delocalized (81, 114) (Fig. 4), and the affinity of these compounds for the postsynaptic GABA receptors are more than three orders of magnitude lower than that of muscimol (103). These studies emphasize the importance of ionic forces for GABA agonist-receptor interactions. Since the dispersion of the negative charges of some heterocyclic GABA analogues over the greater part of the molecules reduces their receptor affinity, it may be concluded that the complementary areas of the GABA receptors have hydrophobic properties.

THIP and related bicyclic muscimol analogues

THIP, a conformationally immobilized analogue of muscimol (Fig. 5), is a potent and specific GABA agonist (102, 103, 106), which strongly suggests that THIP reflects the 'receptor-active conformation' of muscimol (81, 111). Accordingly, even minor alterations of the structure of THIP result in considerable reduction or complete loss of GABA agonist activity (Fig. 5). THPO is a weak inhibitor of high-affinity GABA receptor binding and a weak depressant of neuronal firing (101). This latter effect may, however, be indirect. THPO is an inhibitor of GABA uptake (84, 115), and the observed depressant effect may be a consequence of inhibition of the re-uptake of synaptically released GABA after microelectrophoretic administration of THPO. A similar depressant effect is observed after microelectrophoretic application on central neurones of nipecotic acid (101), a potent GABA uptake inhibitor with little or no affinity for the GABA receptors (84, 109).

THIP is even more sensitive than muscimol to variations of the hydroxylated 5-membered ring. While aza-THIP and 2-methylaza-THIP have no detectable affinity for GABA receptors in vitro (97) (Fig. 5), iso-THIP and iso-THAZ are weak inhibitors of high-affinity GABA binding, but

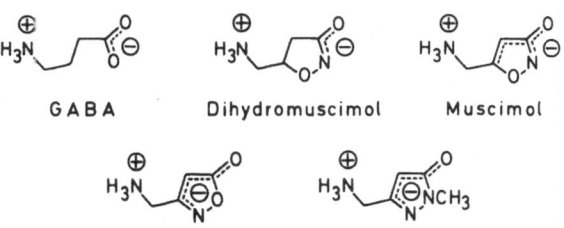

Fig. 4. The approximate charge delocalizations in the zwitterionic structures of GABA, dihydromuscimol, muscimol, isomuscimol, and 2-methyl-azamuscimol (103).

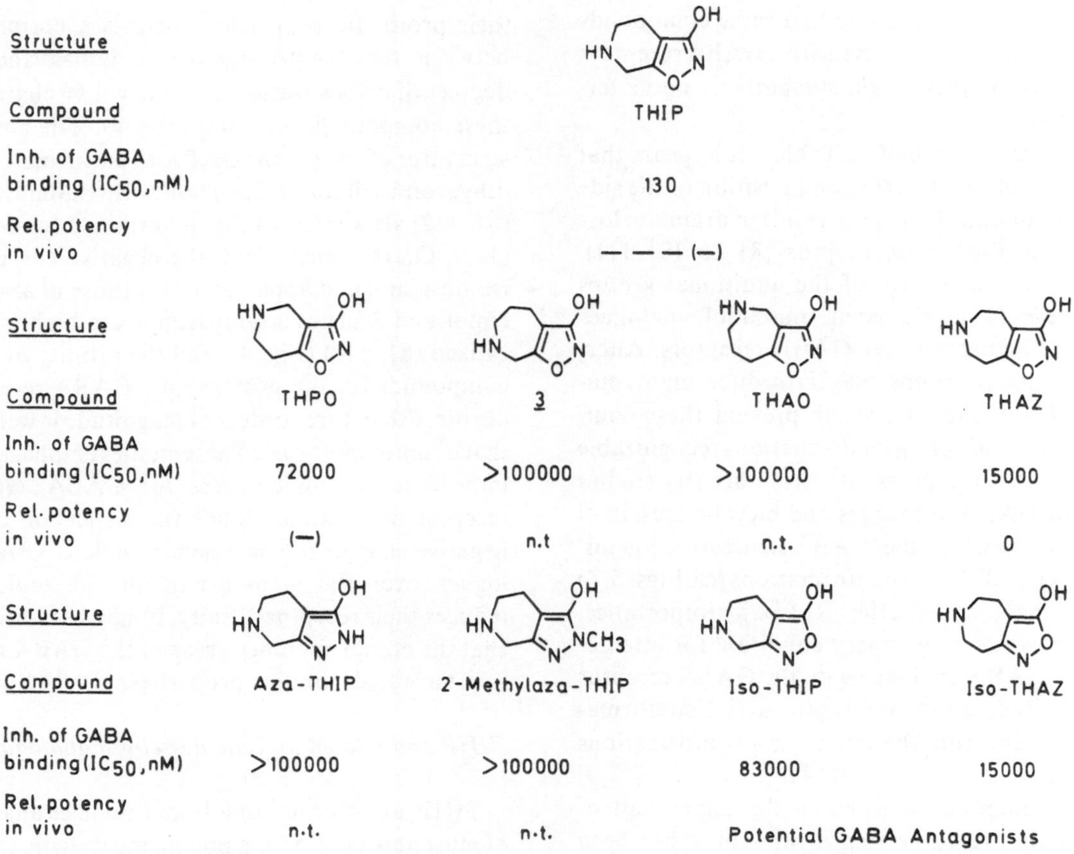

138

Structure	THIP			
Compound	THIP			
Inh. of GABA binding (IC$_{50}$,nM)	130			
Rel. potency in vivo	— — — (—)			

Structure	THPO	3	THAO	THAZ
Compound	THPO	3	THAO	THAZ
Inh. of GABA binding (IC$_{50}$,nM)	72000	>100000	>100000	15000
Rel. potency in vivo	(—)	n.t	n.t.	0

Structure	Aza-THIP	2-Methylaza-THIP	Iso-THIP	Iso-THAZ
Compound	Aza-THIP	2-Methylaza-THIP	Iso-THIP	Iso-THAZ
Inh. of GABA binding (IC$_{50}$,nM)	>100000	>100000	83000	15000
Rel. potency in vivo	n.t.	n.t.	Potential GABA Antagonists	

Fig. 5. The relationship between structures and GABA agonist activities of THIP and a number of structurally related bicyclic muscimol analogues. The inhibition of GABA binding to rat brain synaptic membranes, prepared by a published procedure (103), are expressed as IC$_{50}$ values (nM). The relative potencies of the compounds as depressants of the firing of cat spinal neurones were determined microelectrophoretically (101, 102, 104) and assessed relative to that of GABA (---) (for details, see 'Methods'). n.t., not tested.

these two compounds have GABA antagonistic properties (116).

Isoguvacine and related cyclic amino acids

The 3-isoxazolol unit of muscimol and THIP can be regarded as a masked carboxyl group, and accordingly isoguvacine, which is the amino carboxylic acid analogue of THIP, is a specific and very potent GABA agonist (102, 103, 106). The structure-activity studies illustrated in Fig. 6 further emphasize the remarkable ligand specificity of the GABA receptors. A necessary but obviously not sufficient condition of interaction of these cyclic amino acids with the GABA receptors is the presence of a 'GABA structure element' in the molecules (81). In contrast to isoguvacine, guvacine is not a GABA analogue in the strict sense of the word, and while guvacine is a potent inhibitor of the GABA transport systems (84, 109, 117), it has little or no affinity for the receptors. In general, the compounds having a double bond in the α,β-position of the ring and consequently a planar structure of the vicinity of the carboxyl group have a higher affinity for the GABA receptors than the corresponding saturated cyclic amino acids, and introduction of polar groups into these compounds further reduce the receptor affinity (97) (Fig. 6).

P4S is a notable exception to the above-mentioned rule that amino acids with a planar structure around the acid groups are 'preferred' by the GABA receptors. The piperidine ring of P4S is not planar, and furthermore the structure of the sulphonate group, in contrast to that of the carboxylate group, is not planar. Nevertheless, P4S is equipotent with isoguvacine and an order of magnitude more potent than isonipecotic acid as a GABA agonist (99).

Structure		Isoguvacine	P4S
Compound		Isoguvacine	P4S
Inh. of GABA binding (IC$_{50}$, nM)		37	34
Rel. potency in vivo		— — — —	— — — —

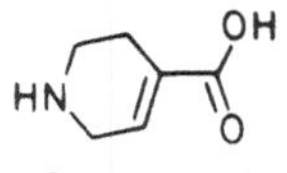

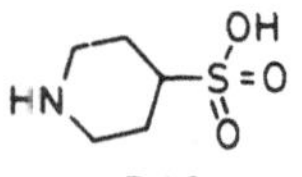

Structure	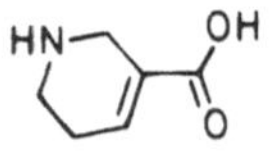 Guvacine	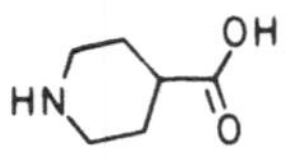 Isonipecotic acid	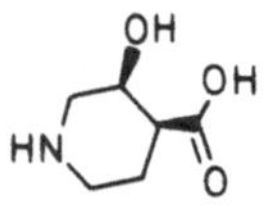 Cis-3-OH-isonipecotic acid	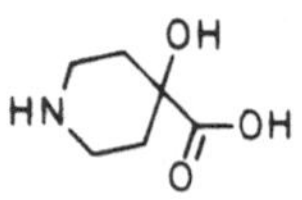 4-OH-isonipecotic acid
Compound	Guvacine	Isonipecotic acid	Cis-3-OH-isonipecotic acid	4-OH-isonipecotic acid
Inh. of GABA binding (IC$_{50}$, nM)	>100000	330	12000	>100000
Rel. potency in vivo	n.t.	— — —	—	n.t.

Structure	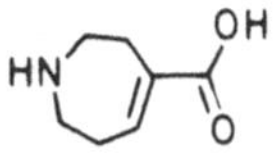 4	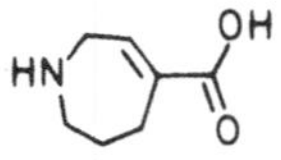 5	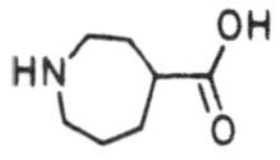 6	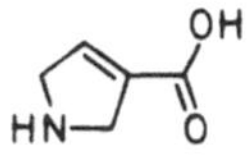 7
Compound	4	5	6	7
Inh. of GABA binding (IC$_{50}$, nM)	15000	23000	>100000	1900
Rel. potency in vivo	n.t.	n.t.	n.t.	n.t.

Fig. 6. The relationship between structure and GABA agonist activities of isoguvacine, P4S (piperidine-4-sulphonic acid), and a number of structurally related cyclic amino acids. The inhibition of GABA binding to rat brain synaptic membranes, prepared by a published procedure (103), are expressed as IC$_{50}$ values (nM). The relative potencies of the compounds as depressants of the firing of cat spinal neurones were determined microelectrophoretically (97, 99, 102, 104) and assessed relative to that of GABA (———) (for details, see 'Methods'). n.t., not tested.

GABA agonist-benzodiazepine interactions

The conformationally restrained GABA agonists THIP (102), isoguvacine (102), and P4S (99) (Fig. 7) are capable of activating the GABA

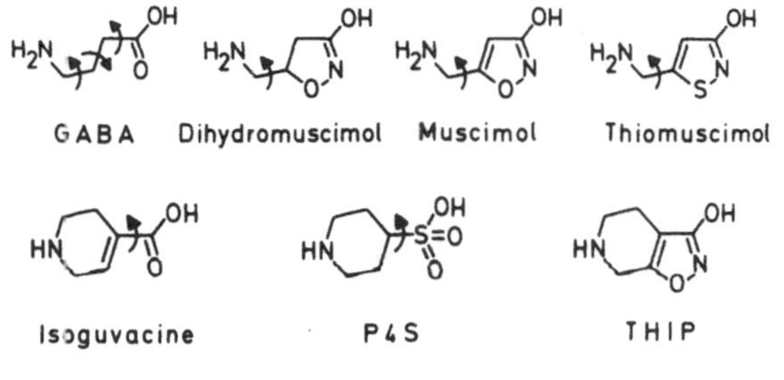

Fig. 7. An illustration of the conformational mobility of GABA and a number of GABA agonists more potent than GABA. The arrows indicate relatively free rotation round carbon-carbon bonds.

receptors in vivo in a manner similar to that of GABA and the flexible GABA agonists muscimol and dihydromuscimol (101, 103) (cf. Table 1 and Figs. 5, 6), suggesting that agonist-induced activation of the receptor is not accompanied by a conformational change of the complex between the GABA agonist and the receptor recognition site.

In contrast to these findings, only GABA agonists with a certain degree of conformational mobility (Fig. 7) are capable of activating the binding of radioactive diazepam to the benzodiazepine binding site in vitro at 0 °C. Thus, muscimol, dihydromuscimol, and thiomuscimol are at least as potent as GABA in this test system (20, 53, 55, 108), whereas THIP and isoguvacine have little or no effect (20, 55, 108, 118). Surprisingly, P4S is a de-activator of the binding of [³H]diazepam under the conditions used (108).

In general the concentrations of GABA and the flexible GABA agonists required for 50% increase of diazepam binding are considerably higher than those producing the same degree of inhibition of [³H]GABA receptor binding (cf. Table 2). This difference may be explained by the fact that the vigorous procedure for isolation of the membranes may cause partial disintegration of the attached GABA receptor complexes. While the binding of GABA and GABA agonists to the receptor macromolecules may not imply the presence of intact membrane receptors, a certain degree of integrity of the receptor complex may be a prerequisite for detection of the interaction between the GABA receptors and the benzodiazepine binding sites in vitro (20).

Based on the observation that THIP, isoguvacine, and P4S in addition are capable of reversing the stimulation of diazepam binding induced by GABA and muscimol in a manner similar to that of bicuculline, it has been proposed that these GABA agonists actually have partial agonist properties (108). While THIP can reverse the anticonvulsant effects of benzodiazepines in some animal experiments (119), it has, however, not yet been possible to detect partial GABA agonist/antagonist or antagonist properties of THIP (20) (J. Arnt, unpublished).

The relative potencies of the GABA agonists depicted in Fig. 7 as BMC-sensitive neuronal depressants and as inhibitors of [³H]GABA and [³H]isoguvacine binding are very similar (20), and these findings, supported by the results listed in Table 2, indicate that the stimulation of [³H]diazepam binding is mediated by the physiologically relevant GABA receptor (20). It appears that the

Table 2. Structures and effects on various recognition sites in GABA-mediated synapses in vitro of some GABA analogues of known absolute configuration.

COMPOUND	FORMULA	INHIBITION (IC_{50}, nM) OF				ACTIVATION (EC_{50}, nM) OF THE BINDING OF
		NEURONAL GABA UPTAKE (Mouse brain slices)	THE GABA RECEPTOR BINDING OF ^{3}H-GABA	^{3}H-MUSCIMOL	^{3}H-ISOGUVACINE	^{3}H-DIAZEPAM
(S)-(−)-5'-Methyl-muscimol		>1 000 000	640	510	1600	230 000
(R)-(+)- —"—		>1 000 000	19 000	8900	8200	2 300 000
(S)-(−)-4-Methyl-trans-ACA		>5 000 000	4100	3500	2500	390 000
(R)-(+)- —"—		160 000	148 000	145 000	84 000	>2 000 000
(S)-(−)-4-Methyl-GABA		750 000	4700	2500	5200	550 000
(R)-(+)- —"—		200 000	5000	4300	6100	410 000

The inhibition of neuronal GABA uptake in mouse brain slices was determined and the IC_{50} values (nM) calculated as earlier described (109). The inhibition of the binding of [³H]GABA, [³H]muscimol, and [³H]isoguvacine to GABA receptor sites was determined (20) using rat brain membranes prepared by a published procedure (103) (for details, see 'Methods'). Stimulation of the binding of [³H]diazepam to rat brain membranes was measured as earlier described (108).

relative potencies of the listed GABA analogues of known absolute configuration as inhibitors of radioactive GABA, muscimol, and isoguvacine and as activators of diazepam binding are very similar. If GABA, muscimol, and isoguvacine bind to different receptors, the inhibitors would have to compete with these radioactive ligands for binding to different biomolecules, which would be expected to possess different degrees of asymmetry. In that case, different relative potencies of the asymmetric inhibitors would have been observed. Accordingly, the characteristics of [³H]muscimol (16, 17) and of [³H]isoguvacine (19, 20) binding have been shown to be compatible with these ligands binding to the GABA receptor. The relative potencies of the compounds depicted in Table 2 as inhibitors of neuronal GABA uptake are evidently different from those observed in the four series of binding experiments supporting the generally accepted view that the presynaptic GABA uptake mechanisms are not involved in mediating the effects of the benzodiazepines.

The observation that a certain degree of conformational mobility of GABA agonists is a necessary condition for the activation of [³H]diazepam binding, but not for the physiological activation of the GABA receptors, have shed some light on the molecular mechanisms of the postsynaptic GABA receptor complex (20). It is possible that the binding site for the benzodiazepines (Fig. 1) is identical with the membrane structures, which bind the proposed GABA receptor modulator(s) (31, 32). The initial step in the re-establishment of the resting state of the GABA receptor, activated by a GABA agonist, may involve a conformational change of the GABA agonist-receptor complex. This conformational change possibly increases allosterically the affinity of the modulator for its binding site and consequently that of the benzodiazepines if present (20). If the re-binding of the modulator(s) to the GABA receptor really locks, physically or biochemically, the receptor in a resting state with the chloride ionophore closed, and if the described conformational changes play a role during this process, it is understandable that the benzodiazepines are capable of prolonging GABA neurotransmission and that stimulation of the binding of [³H]diazepam in vitro can be accomplished by flexible but not by rigid GABA agonists, at least not at low temperatures. It has recently been demonstrated that THIP and P4S do display potent chloride-dependent stimulation of [³H]flunitrazepam binding at elevated temperatures (30 or 37 °C) (P. Supavilai and M. Karobath, unpublished), supporting the above proposal that conformational changes of agonist-receptor macromolecule complexes do play a role during the function of the GABA receptors.

Conversion of GABA agonists into antagonists

Even minor structural modifications of muscimol frequently result in compounds with no detectable intrinsic activity on the GABA receptor, and such compounds might be expected to exhibit GABA antagonist properties. However, in no case have simple muscimol analogues without GABA agonist properties been shown to be GABA antagonists (101) (Table 1). Muscimol analogues with a high degree of delocalization of the negative charge, like isomuscimol (Fig. 4), have very low affinity for the GABA receptors, but these compounds are GABA agonists (103, 116).

The spectroscopic properties of THIP (94) are compatible with this bicyclic compound having an electronic structure (Fig. 8) similar to that of muscimol (Fig. 4), and the GABA agonist actions of these compounds are qualitatively very similar (102, 116). Interchange of the heterocyclic oxygen and nitrogen atoms of THIP gives iso-THIP (97), and the charge delocalizations in this compound and in the corresponding 7-membered ring homologue iso-THAZ (Fig. 8) are analogous with that in isomuscimol. Iso-THIP and iso-THAZ still have some affinity for the GABA receptors in vitro (85, 97, 116), but iso-THAZ has been shown not to possess significant intrinsic activity on GABA receptors in vivo after microelectrophoretic application on cat spinal neurones (D. R. Curtis and P. Krogsgaard-Larsen, unpublished). However, these

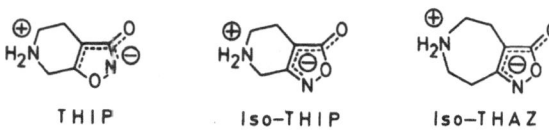

Fig. 8. The approximate charge delocalizations in the zwitterionic structures of the GABA agonist THIP (103) and the potential GABA antagonists iso-THIP and iso-THAZ (116).

two compounds have GABA antagonistic properties, iso-THAZ being the more potent antagonist, although they are considerably weaker than BMC (116).

Pharmacological and pharmacokinetic aspects of GABA agonists

Decreased functions of the central GABA system and disturbed balance between GABA and other neurotransmitters seem to play a role in the development of certain neurological and psychiatric diseases (for references see (1–5)). There is direct or indirect evidence that impaired GABA neurotransmitter functions contribute to the pathogenesis of Huntington's chorea, Parkinson's disease, spasticity, and schizophrenic and epileptic diseases. Decreased GABA activities seem to be involved in the development of these diseases, and consequently there is a considerable interest in the development of drugs capable of stimulating GABA neurotransmission. Direct stimulation of pre- and postsynaptic receptors may be therapeutically relevant, and controlled and selective pharmacological manipulations of the GABA system using GABA agonists is a realistic possibility (120). However, a prerequisite for progress in this potential new field of psychotherapy is the development of GABA agonists with pharmacokinetic and toxicological properties acceptable for use in the human clinic.

Muscimol has been extensively used as a pharmacological tool (2–5, 120). Muscimol, which is capable of penetrating the blood-brain barrier, is, however, very rapidly metabolized after systemic administration to animals (121, 122), the aminomethyl side chain being susceptible to metabolic decomposition. Since the muscimol metabolite(s) have not yet been identified, the possibility of formation of pharmacologically active muscimol metabolites must be kept in mind. Muscimol is also a weak substrate for the neuronal GABA transport carrier (123) and an inhibitor of glial GABA uptake (109), and consequently the toxicological (124, 125) and pharmacological profiles of muscimol may not exclusively be the consequences of activation of the central GABA receptors. Dihydromuscimol and thiomuscimol also have aminomethyl side chains (Table 1), which may be just as susceptible to metabolic transformation as that of muscimol. Consequently, these compounds have not been subjected to extensive animal behavioural studies.

In THIP (Fig. 5) and isoguvacine (Fig. 6) the amino groups are incorporated into additional ring structures, and accordingly these compounds do not interfere with GABA-T in vitro (103). However, in spite of the structural resemblance of these compounds, THIP, but not isoguvacine, penetrates the blood-brain barrier after systemic administration (126). Since both muscimol and THIP are 3-isoxazolol zwitterions (Figs. 4, 8), the ability to cross the lipophilic blood-brain barrier appears to be a specific property of this unique class of compound. However, the different penetrating abilities of THIP and the amino acid zwitterion isoguvacine can be explained exclusively on the basis of their different protolytic properties (126).

As illustrated in Fig. 9 the pK_A values of THIP and isoguvacine are quite different, the difference between the pK_A-I and pK_A-II values of THIP (94)

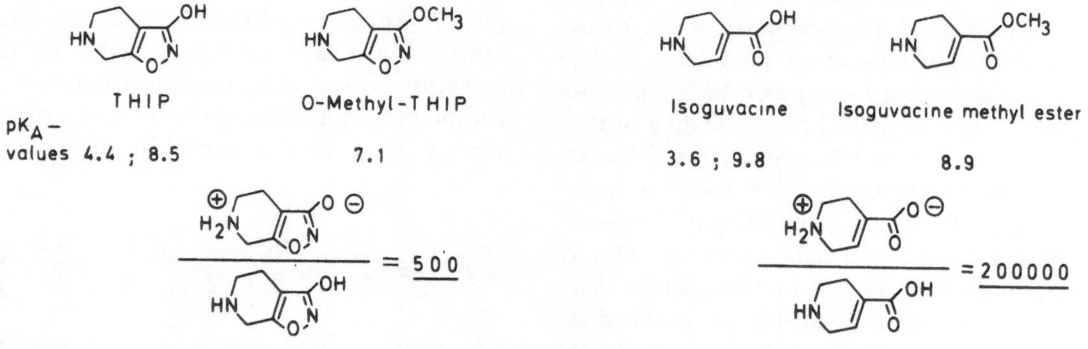

Fig. 9. The structures and pK_A values of THIP, O-methyl-THIP, isoguvacine, and isoguvacine methyl ester and an illustration of the approximate ratios between the ionized and unionized forms of THIP and isoguvacine in aqueous solutions (126), calculated using Wegscheider's method (127).

being considerably smaller than that measured for isoguvacine (97). Using these pK_A-I values and the pK_A values for O-methyl-THIP and isoguvacine methyl ester, in which the acidic groups of THIP and isoguvacine, respectively, have been masked, Wegscheider's method (127) allows calculations of the ratios between the ionized and unionized forms of THIP and isoguvacine (126). As illustrated in Fig. 9 this ratio for THIP (500) is much lower than that for isoguvacine (200 000), indicating that an aqueous solution of THIP contains approximately 0.2% of unionized THIP, whereas isoguvacine in aqueous solution is almost exclusively in the ionized form (126). Since both compounds probably pass the blood-brain barrier as the unionized forms, it is understandable that THIP enters the brain much more easily than isoguvacine after systemic administration to animals.

The pK_A values of muscimol (4.8; 8.4) (103) are similar to those of THIP, and consequently the ratio between ionized and unionized muscimol in aqueous solutions must be of the same order of magnitude as that determined for THIP. However, since muscimol is very rapidly decomposed in the blood stream (121, 122), a calculation of this value for muscimol would be rather meaningless. In the case of THIP it has been shown that one hour after oral administration of a single dose of radioactive THIP to rats (5 mg/kg) approximately 0.1% of the dose is found in the brain, and about 70% of the radioactivity in the brain represent unchanged THIP (126).

In agreement with the described pharmacokinetic properties of THIP, this GABA agonist is pharmacologically active in a variety of animal models (119, 128, 129). THIP is well tolerated by rats, dogs, and baboons and clinical studies on THIP are now in progress (120). In the light of the specificity of THIP as a GABA agonist these studies are of considerable theoretical interest and are expected to provide useful information about the therapeutical usefulness of this class of compound.

While both isoguvacine and THIP affect spinal cord activities in cats after systemic administration (130), isoguvacine has no significant effect on audiogenic seizures after intraperitoneal injection (124). These findings and the described pharmacokinetic properties of isoguvacine (126) compared with the specificity and potency of its GABA agonist activity (102, 103, 106) have prompted the development of a series of potential 'pro-drugs' of isoguvacine (E. Falch, P. Krogsgaard-Larsen and A. V. Christensen, unpublished). A selected number of the acyloxymethyl esters of isoguvacine concerned are depicted in Fig. 10. These derivatives of isoguvacine were designed with the intention of developing 'pro-drugs' capable of penetrating the blood-brain barrier. Furthermore the compounds should be proof against extensive hydrolysis in the blood stream but sufficiently susceptible to hydrolysis in the brain tissue to give isoguvacine. The rates of hydrolysis of the compounds were examined in vitro, and the half-lives ($T_{1/2}$) of the compounds determined under approx-

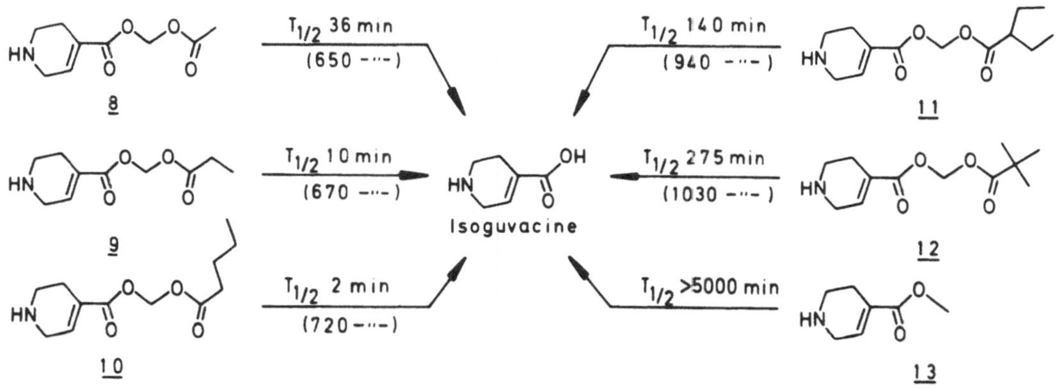

Fig. 10. The structures of a number of acyloxymethyl esters of isoguvacine, designed as potential 'pro-drugs' of isoguvacine capable of penetrating the blood-brain barrier with subsequent hydrolysis in brain tissue to isoguvacine. The rates of hydrolysis of the compounds in vitro under approximate physiological conditions in the absence (values in brackets) and presence of 10% human serum are expressed as half-lives ($T_{1/2}$, min).

imate physiological conditions in the absence (values in brackets) and presence of 10% human serum. As illustrated in Fig. 10, the susceptibility of the compounds to hydrolysis with formation of isoguvacine is strictly dependent on the structure of the acyl group in the side chain. The compounds were tested for anticonvulsant activity in a number of animal models (E. Falch, P. Krogsgaard-Larsen and A. V. Christensen, unpublished). While the compounds were relatively weak in antagonizing convulsions induced by bicuculline and isoniazide, a good correlation between in vitro rates of enzymatic hydrolysis and the times of onset of antagonism of electroshock convulsions was found. Further animal studies on these compounds are required, before their pharmacological importance can be estimated.

This review has emphasized some of the structural and pharmacokinetic parameters, which have to be considered in the design and development of specific GABA agonists of pharmacological interest. In agreement with other processes and functions in GABA mediated synapses (84, 131) the GABA receptors exhibit a remarkable substrate specificity. Further developments in the field of GABA agonists obviously depend on close collaboration between pharmacologists, chemists, and biochemists.

Acknowledgements

This work is supported by The Danish Medical Research Council. The collaboration of Professor, D. R. Curtis, Canberra and Professor, G. A. R. Johnston, Sydney, Australia, and Drs. A. Schousboe, C. Braestrup, H. Hjeds, and T. Honoré, Copenhagen, is gratefully acknowledged. We wish to thank Mrs B. Hare and Mr. S. Stilling for skillful secretarial and technical assistance.

References

1. Roberts, E., Chase, T. N. & Tower, D. B., Eds., 1976. GABA in Nervous System Function, Raven Press, New York.
2. Fonnum, F. Ed., 1978. Amino Acids as Chemical Transmitters, Plenum Press, New York, London.
3. Krogsgaard-Larsen, P., Scheel-Krüger, J. & Kofod, H. Eds., 1979. GABA-Neurotransmitters. Pharmacochemical, Biochemical and Pharmacological Aspects, Munksgaard, Copenhagen.
4. Pepeu, G., Kuhar, M. J. & Enna, S. J. Eds., 1980. Receptors for Neurotransmitters and Peptide Hormones, Raven Press, New York.
5. Costa, E., DI Chiara, G. & Gessa, G. L., Eds., 1981. GABA and Benzodiazepine Receptors, Raven Press, New York (in press).
6. Curtis, D. R. and Johnston, G. A. R., 1974. Ergeb. Physiol. Biol. Chem. Exp. Pharmakol. 69: 97–188.
7. Krnjević, K., 1974. Physiol. Rev. 54: 418–540.
8. Curtis, D. R., 1978. Amino Acids as Chemical Transmitters Ed., F. Fonnum. Plenum Press, New York, London, pp. 55–86.
9. Nistri, A. & Constanti, A., 1979. Prog. Neurobiol. (Oxford) 13: 117–235.
10. Enna, S. J. & Snyder, S. H., 1975. Brain Res. 100: 81–97.
11. Snyder, S. H. & Bennett, J. P., 1976. Annu. Rev. Physiol. 38: 153–175.
12. Yamamura, H. I., Enna, S. J. & Kuhar, M. J. Eds., 1978. Neurotransmitter Receptor Binding, Raven Press, New York.
13. Enna, S. J. & Snyder, S. H., 1977. Mol. Pharmacol. 13: 442–453.
14. Horng, S. J. & Wong, D. T., 1979. J. Neurochem. 32: 1379–1386.
15. Greenlee, D. V., Van Ness, P. C. & Olsen, R. W., 1978. J. Neurochem. 31: 933–938.
16. Beaumont, K., Chilton, W. S., Yamamura, H. I. & Enna, S. J., 1978. Brain Res. 148: 153–162.
17. Wang, Y.-J., Salvaterra, P. & Roberts, E., 1979. Biochem. Pharmacol. 28: 1123–1128.
18. DeFeudis, F. V., 1980. Neuroscience 5: 675–688.
19. Morin, A. M. & Wasterlain, C. G., 1980. Life Sci. 26: 1239–1245.
20. Krogsgaard-Larsen, P. & Arnt, J., 1980. Brain Res. Bull. 5, Suppl. 2: 867–872.
21. Kelly, J. S., 1975. Handbook of Psychopharmacology, Vol. 2, Eds., L. L. Iversen, S. D. Iversen & S. H. Snyder, Plenum Press, New York, London, pp. 29–67.
22. Barker, J. L. & Ransom, B. R., 1978. J. Physiol. (London) 280: 331–354.
23. Barker, J. L., MacDonald, J. F. & Mathers, D. A., 1980. Brain Res. Bull 5, Suppl. 2: 43–49.
24. Fiszer De Plazas, S. & De Robertis, E., 1975. J. Neurochem. 25: 547–552.
25. Gavish, M., Chang, R. S. L. & Snyder, S. H., 1979. Life Sci. 25: 783–790.
26. Chude, O., 1979. J. Neurochem. 33: 621–629.
27. Greenlee, D. V. & Olsen, R. W., 1979. Biochem. Biophys. Res. Commun. 88: 380–387.
28. Wong, D. T. & Horng, J. S., 1977. Life Sci. 20: 445–452.
29. Johnston, G. A. R. & Kennedy, S. M. E., 1978. Amino Acids as Chemical Transmitters Ed., F. Fonnum. Plenum Press, New York, London, pp. 507–516.
30. Greenlee, D. V., Van Ness, P. C. & Olsen, R. W., 1978. Life Sci. 22: 1653–1662.

31. Guidotti, A., Toffano, G. & Costa, E., 1978. Nature (London) 275: 553–555.
32. Toffano, G., Guidotti, A. & Costa, E., 1978. Proc. Natl. Acad. Sci. USA 75: 4024–4028.
33. Lloyd, K. G., Dreksler, S., Shemen, L. & Davidson, L., 1979. GABA-Biochemistry and CNS Functions (Adv. Exp. Med. Biol., Vol. 123) Eds., P. Mandel & F. V. DeFeudis. Plenum Press, New York, London, pp. 399–418.
34. Möhler, H. & Okada, T., 1977. Nature (London) 267: 65–67.
35. Möhler, H. & Okada, T., 1978. Mol. Pharmacol. 14: 256–265.
36. Möhler, H., 1979. GABA-Biochemistry and CNS Functions (Adv. Exp. Med. Biol., Vol. 123) Eds., P. Mandel & F. V. DeFeudis. Plenum Press, New York, London, pp. 355–362.
37. Takeuchi, A. & Takeuchi, N., 1969. J. Physiol. (London) 205: 377–391.
38. Enna, S. J., Collins, J. F. & Snyder, S. H., 1977. Brain Res. 124: 185–190.
39. Snodgrass, S. R., 1978. Nature (London) 273: 392–394.
40. Olsen, R. W., Ticku, M. K., Van Ness, P. C. & Greenlee, D. V., 1978. Brain Res. 139: 277–294.
41. Kelly, J. S., Krnjević, K., Morris, M. E. & Yim, G. K. W., 1969. Exp. Brain Res. 7: 11–31.
42. Olsen, R. W., Greenlee, D. V., Van Ness, P. C. & Ticku, M. K., 1978. Amino Acids as Chemical Transmitters Ed., F. Fonnum. Plenum Press, New York, London, pp. 467–486.
43. Olsen, R. W., Ticku, M. K., Greenlee, D. V. & Van Ness, P. C., 1979. GABA-Neurotransmitters. Pharmacochemical, Biochemical and Pharmacological Aspects Eds., P. Krogsgaard-Larsen, J. Scheel-Krüger & H. Kofod. Munksgaard, Copenhagen, pp. 165–178.
44. Squires, R. F. & Braestrup, C., 1977. Nature (London) 266: 732–734.
45. Möhler, H. & Okada, T., 1977. Science 198: 849–851.
46. Braestrup, C. & Squires, R. F., 1977. Proc. Natl. Acad. Sci. USA 74: 3805–3809.
47. Williamson, M. J., Paul, S. M. & Skolnick, P., 1978. Life Sci. 23: 1935–1940.
48. Möhler, H., Okada, T., Heitz, P. H. & Ulrich, J., 1978. Life Sci. 22: 985–996.
49. Costa, E., Guidotti, A., Mao, C. C. & Suria, A., 1975. Life Sci. 17: 167–185.
50. Mao, C. C., Guidotti, A. & Costa, E., 1975. Naunyn-Schmiedebergs Arch. Pharmacol. 289: 369–378.
51. Haefely, W., Polc, P., Schaffner, R., Keller, H. H., Pieri, L. & Möhler, H., 1979. GABA-Neurotransmitters. Pharmacochemical, Biochemical and Pharmacological Aspects Eds., P. Krogsgaard-Larsen, J. Scheel-Krüger & H. Kofod. Munksgaard, Copenhagen, pp. 357–375.
52. Curtis, D. R., Lodge, D., Johnston, G. A. R. & Brand, S. J., 1976. Brain Res. 118: 344–347.
53. Tallman, J. F., Thomas, J. W. & Gallager, D. W., 1978. Nature (London) 274: 383–385.
54. Martin, I. L. & Candy, J. M., 1978. Neuropharmacology 17: 993–998.
55. Karobath, M., Placheta, P., Lippitsch, M. & Krogsgaard-Larsen, P., 1979. Nature (London) 278: 748–749.
56. Martin, I. L. & Candy, J. M., 1980. Neuropharmacology 19: 175–179.
57. Supavilai, P. & Karobath, M., 1979. Eur. J. Pharmacol. 60: 111–113.
58. Placheta, P. & Karobath, M., 1980. Eur. J. Pharmacol. 62: 225–228.
59. Guidotti, A., Toffano, G., Baraldi, M., Schwartz, J. P. & Costa, E., 1979. GABA-Neurotransmitters. Pharmacochemical, Biochemical & Pharmacological Aspects Eds., P. Krogsgaard-Larsen, J. Scheel-Krüger & E. Kofod. Munksgaard, Copenhagen, pp. 406–415.
60. Möhler, H., Polc, P., Cumin, R., Pieri, L. & Kettler, R., 1979. Nature (London) 278: 563–565.
61. Marangos, P. J., Paul, S. M., Greenlaw, P., Goodwin, F. K. & Skolnick, P., 1978. Life Sci. 22: 1893–1900.
62. Asano, T. & Spector, S., 1979. Proc. Natl. Acad. Sci. USA 76: 977–981.
63. Marangos, P. J., Paul, S. M. & Goodwin, F. K., 1979. Life Sci. 25: 1093–1102.
64. Asano, T. & Ogasawara, N., 1980. Life Sci. 26: 607–613.
65. Gavish, M. & Snyder, S. H., 1980. Life Sci. 26: 579–582.
66. Möhler, H., Battersby, M. K. & Richards, J. G., 1980. Proc. Natl. Acad. Sci. USA 77: 1666–1670.
67. Sieghart, W., Placheta, P., Supavilai, P. & Karobath, M., 1981. GABA and Benzodiazepine Receptors Eds., E. Costa, G. Di Chiara & G. L. Gessa. Raven Press, New York (in press).
68. Nestoros, J. N. & Nistri, A., 1979. Can. J. Physiol. Pharmacol. 57: 1324–1329.
69. Scott Young, W. & Kuhar, M. J., 1980. J. Pharmacol. Exp. Ther. 212: 337–346.
70. Chang, R. S. L., Tran, V. T. & Snyder, S. H., 1980. Brain Res. 190: 95–110.
71. Burke, D., Andrews, C. J. & Knowles, L., 1971. J. Neurol. Sci. 14: 199–208.
72. Curtis, D. R., Game, C. J. A., Johnston, G. A. R. & McCulloch, R. M., 1974. Brain Res. 70: 493–499.
73. Waddington, J. L. & Cross, A. L., 1979. Neurosci. Lett. 14: 123–127.
74. Johnston, G. A. R., 1976. GABA in Nervous System Function Eds., E. Roberts, T. N. Chase & D. B. Tower. Raven Press, New York, London, pp. 395–411.
75. Bowery, N. G., Hill, D. R., Hudson, A. L., Doble, A., Middlemiss, D. N., Shaw, J. & Turnbull, M., 1980. Nature (London) 283: 92–94.
76. Mitchell, P. R. & Martin, I. L., 1978. Nature (London) 274: 904–905.
77. Brennan, M. J. W. & Cantrill, R. C., 1979. Nature (London) 280: 514–515.
78. Arbilla, S., Kamal, L. & Langer, S. Z., 1979. Eur. J. Pharmacol. 57: 211–217.
79. Beart, P. M. & Johnston, G. A. R., 1973. Brain Res. 49: 459–462.
80. Johnston, G. A. R., Allan, R. D., Kennedy, S. M. E. & Twitchin, B., 1979. GABA-Neurotransmitters. Pharmacochemical, Biochemical & Pharmacological Aspects Eds., P. Krogsgaard-Larsen, J. Scheel-Krüger & H. Kofod. Munksgaard, Copenhagen, pp. 149–164.
81. Krogsgaard-Larsen, P., Honoré, T. & Thyssen, K., 1979. GABA-Neurotransmitters. Pharmacochemical, Biochem-

146

ical & Pharmacological Aspects Eds., P. Krogsgaard-Larsen, J. Scheel-Krüger & H. Kofod. Munksgaard, Copenhagen, pp. 201–216.

82. Yarbrough, G. G., Williams, M. & Haubrich, D. R., 1979. Arch. Int. Pharmacodyn. 241: 266–279.

83. Atkinson, J. G., Girard, Y., Rokach, J., Rooney, C. S., McFarlane, C. S., Rackham, A. & Share, N. N., 1979. J. Med. Chem. 22: 99–106.

84. Krogsgaard-Larsen, P., 1980. Mol. Cell. Biochem. 31: 105–121.

85. Krogsgaard-Larsen, P. & Arnt, J., 1979. GABA-Biochemistry & CNS Functions (Adv. Exp. Med. Biol., Vol. 123) Eds., P. Mandel & F. V. DeFeudis. Plenum Press, New York, London, pp. 303–321.

86. Krogsgaard-Larsen, P. & Christensen, S. B., 1976. Acta Chem. Scand. B30: 281–282.

87. Krogsgaard-Larsen, P., Larsen, A. L. N. & Thyssen, K., 1978. Acta Chem. Scand. B32: 469–477.

88. Lykkeberg, J. & Krogsgaard-Larsen, P., 1976. Acta Chem. Scand. B30: 781–785.

89. Hjeds, H. & Krogsgaard-Larsen, P., 1979. Acta Chem. Scand. B33: 294–298.

90. Krogsgaard-Larsen, P. & Christensen, S. B., 1974. Acta Chem. Scand. B28: 636–640.

91. Bowden, K., Crank, G. & Ross, W. J., 1968. J. Chem. Soc. (C) 172–185.

92. Hjeds, H. & Krogsgaard-Larsen, P., 1976. Acta Chem. Scand. B30: 567–573.

93. Honoré, T., Hjeds, H., Krogsgaard-Larsen, P. & Christiansen, T. R., 1978. Eur. J. Med. Chem. Chim. Ther. 13: 429–434.

94. Krogsgaard-Larsen, P., 1977. Acta Chem. Scand. B31: 584–588.

95. Krogsgaard-Larsen, P. & Hjeds, H., 1974. Acta Chem. Scand. B28: 533–538.

96. Krogsgaard-Larsen, P., Hjeds, H., Christensen, S. B. & Brehm, L., 1973. Acta Chem. Scand. 27: 3251–3258.

97. Krogsgaard-Larsen, P. & Christiansen, T. R., 1979. Eur. J. Med. Chem. Chim. Ther. 14: 157–164.

98. Krogsgaard-Larsen, P., Thyssen, K. & Schaumburg, K., 1978. Acta Chem. Scand. B32: 327–334.

99. Krogsgaard-Larsen, P., Falch, E., Schousboe, A., Curtis, D. R. & Lodge, D., 1980. J. Neurochem. 34: 756–759.

100. Christensen, S. B. & Krogsgaard-Larsen, P., 1980. J. Label. Cpds. 17: 191–202.

101. Krogsgaard-Larsen, P., Johnston, G. A. R., Curtis, D. R., Game, C. J. A. & McCulloch, R. M., 1975. J. Neurochem. 25: 803–809.

102. Krogsgaard-Larsen, P., Johnston, G. A. R., Lodge, D. & Curtis, D. R., 1977. Nature (London) 268: 53–55.

103. Krogsgaard-Larsen, P., Hjeds, H., Curtis, D. R., Lodge, D. & Johnston, G. A. R., 1979. J. Neurochem. 32: 1717–1724.

104. Curtis, D. R., Duggan, A. W., Felix, D. & Johnston, G. A. R., 1971. Brain Res. 32: 69–96.

105. Curtis, D. R., Duggan, A. W. & Johnston, G. A. R., 1971, Exp. Brain Res. 12: 547–565.

106. Krogsgaard-Larsen, P. & Johnston, G. A. R., 1978. J. Neurochem. 30: 1377–1382.

107. Lowry, O. H., Rosebrough, N. J., Farr, A. L. & Randall, R. J., 1951. J. Biol. Chem. 193: 265–275.

108. Braestrup, C., Nielsen, M., Krogsgaard-Larsen, P. & Falch, E., 1979. Nature (London) 280: 331–333.

109. Schousboe, A., Thorbek, P., Hertz, L. & Krogsgaard-Larsen, P., 1979. J. Neurochem. 33: 181–189.

110. Riddall, D. R., Leach, M. J. & Davison, A. N., 1976. J. Neurochem. 27: 835–839.

111. Krogsgaard-Larsen, P., 1978. Amino Acids as Chemical Transmitters Ed., F. Fonnum. Plenum Press, New York, London, pp. 305–321.

112. Brehm, L., Hjeds, H. & Krogsgaard-Larsen, P., 1972. Acta Chem. Scand. 26: 1298–1299.

113. Steward, E. G., Player, R. B. & Warner, D., 1973. Acta Cryst. B29: 2038–2040.

114. Honoré, T. & Brehm, L., 1978. Acta Cryst. B34: 3417–3419.

115. Krogsgaard-Larsen, P. & Johnston, G. A. R., 1975. J. Neurochem. 25: 797–802.

116. Arnt, J. & Krogsgaard-Larsen, P., 1979. Brain Res. 177: 395–400.

117. Johnston, G. A. R., Krogsgaard-Larsen, P. & Stephanson, A., 1975. Nature (London) 258: 627–628.

118. Maurer, R., 1979. Neurosci. Lett. 12: 65–68.

119. Fuxe, K., Köhler, C., Agnati, L. F., Andersson, K., Ögren, S.-O., Eneroth, P., Perez de la Mora, M., Karobath, M. & Krogsgaard-Larsen, P., 1981. GABA and Benzodiazepine Receptors Eds., E. Costa, G. Di Chiara & G. L. Gessa. Raven Press, New York (in press).

120. Krogsgaard-Larsen, P. & Christensen, A. V., 1980. Annu Rep. Med. Chem. 15: 41–50.

121. Maggi, A. & Enna, S. J., 1979. Neuropharmacology 18: 361–366.

122. Baraldi, M., Grandison, L. & Guidotti, A., 1979. Neuropharmacology 18: 57–62.

123. Johnston, G. A. R., Kennedy, S. M. E. & Lodge, D., 1978. J. Neurochem. 31: 1519–1523.

124. Anlezark, G., Collins, J. & Meldrum, B., 1977. Neurosci. Lett. 7: 337–340.

125. Worms, P., Depoortere, H. & Lloyd, K. G., 1979. Life Sci. 25: 607–614.

126. Krogsgaard-Larsen, P., Schultz, B., Mikkelsen, H., Aaes-Jørgensen, T. & Bøgesø, K. P., 1981. Amino Acid Transmitters Eds., DeFeudis, F. V. & Mandel, P. Raven Press, New York, pp. 69–76.

127. Edsall, J. T. & Wyman, J., 1958. Biophysical Chemistry, Vol. I, Academic Press, New York, pp. 485–486.

128. Christensen, A. V., Arnt, J. & Scheel-Krüger, J., 1979. Life Sci. 24: 1395–1402.

129. Meldrum, B. & Horton, R., 1980. Eur. J. Pharmacol. 61: 231–237.

130. Polc, P., 1979. Prog. Neuro-Psychopharmacol. 3: 345–352.

131. Metcalf, B. W., 1979. Biochem. Pharmacol. 28: 1705–1712.

Received July 9, 1980.

Pharmacology of GABA-mediated inhibition of spinal cord neurons in vivo and in primary dissociated cell culture

Robert L. Macdonald and Anne B. Young
Dept. of Neurology, University of Michigan, Ann Arbor, Michigan 48109, U.S.A.

Summary

Organization of the postsynaptic GABA-receptor chloride channel complex on spinal cord neurons

In this paper it is shown that the postsynaptic GABA-receptor chloride ion channel complex is composed of several functional subunits. There are probably at least two stereospecific locations on the receptor for GABA-binding and both must be occupied to obtain an increase in chloride conductance. The interaction between these sites is uncertain but there could be either positive cooperativity between the sites or only a requirement that both sites are occupied without occupation of either site affecting the affinity for GABA of the other site. There is a chloride conductance channel coupled to the GABA receptor which opens for an average of 20 msec and has an average conductance of 18 pS. The GABA-coupled chloride channel may or may not have the same composition as the glycine coupled chloride channel.

In addition to the GABA-recognition site and the chloride ion channel, GABA-receptors must have additional binding sites or modulator sites where drugs can bind to modify GABA activation of the GABA-receptor. The convulsant PICRO binds to a site which is independent of the GABA-recognition site and PICRO reduces GABA responses. Barbiturates and benzodiazepines augment GABA-responses without reducing GABA-binding and thus they must bind to a modulator site independent of the GABA recognition site. Whether or not this is the same site as the PICRO binding site is uncertain. Thus, the GABA-receptor-chloride ion channel complex is composed of at least: 1) two GABA-binding sites; 2) a chloride ion channel; 3) a convulsant binding site (PICRO-binding site) and 4) an anticonvulsant binding site. This organization serves several obvious purposes. First, since two GABA-molecules are required to activate GABA-coupled chloride ion channels, the dose-response relationship for GABA is sigmoidal and steep. Thus minor shifts in GABA affinity will produce large alterations in GABA-responses and the GABA receptor can be easily modulated. Second, since the receptor has binding sites for convulsant and anticonvulsant compounds which decrease and increase GABA-responses, GABAergic inhibition can easily be modulated.

Introduction

The neutral amino acid γ-aminobutyric acid (GABA) was initially identified in brain in 1950 (1, 2, 3). Four years later Hayashi (4) suggested that GABA might play a role in the regulation of neuronal excitability and Florey (5) discovered that an extract of mammalian brain had an inhibitory action on crayfish stretch receptor neurons. When the active component of the brain extract was identified as GABA, Florey and his colleagues (6) suggested that GABA might be an inhibitory neurotransmitter in the mammalian central nervous system (CNS). The inhibitory action of GABA on mammalian CNS neurons was demonstrated by Curtis and coworkers (7) in 1959 using iontophoresis

Molecular and Cellular Biochemistry 38, 147–162 (1981).   0300-8177/81/0381-0147/$ 3.20.

148

of GABA and other amino acids from multibarrel micropipettes. While GABA strongly inhibited firing of spinal cord neurons, they concluded that GABA was not the major inhibitory neurotransmitter in spinal cord. In a later study, Curtis and coworkers (8) demonstrated that GABA produced hyperpolarization and increased conductance and that the GABA-responses had a reversal potential similar to that of inhibitory postsynaptic potentials recorded in spinal cord. It is now well accepted that GABA is a major inhibitory neurotransmitter throughout the CNS (9–12) and modification of GABAergic inhibition has been determined to be involved in the actions of a number of drugs used clinically such as barbiturates (13–18) and benzodiazepines (13, 18–24) and in certain disease states such as epilepsy (25) and Huntington's Disease (26–28).

The purpose of the present article is to review the pharmacology of GABA-mediated inhibition in the spinal cord both *in vivo* and in primary dissociated cell culture. In addition, we will review the pharmacology of several drugs which have actions on GABAergic synaptic transmission with particular emphasis on convulsants, anticonvulsants and anesthetics. While it has been possible to gain much information from studies of spinal cord neurons *in vivo,* considerable technical advantage for investigation of GABA-mediated inhibition can be obtained by growing spinal cord neurons in primary dissociated cell culture. Therefore, we will review: 1) the technique of dissociated cell culture and the properties of spinal cord and dorsal root ganglion neurons in cell culture; 2) the metabolism, uptake, binding, and release of GABA and the action of drugs acting on these systems; 3) the physiology of GABA in both *in vivo* and *in vitro* preparations; and 4) the actions of convulsant, anticonvulsant and anesthetic drugs which antagonize or enhance GABA-responses and the releationship between their actions on GABA-responses and their physiological and pharmacological effects.

Mammalian spinal cord neurons in primary dissociated cell culture

Mammalian spinal cord (SC) and dorsal root ganglion (DRG) neurons can be grown and maintained in primary dissociated cell culture. Cultures

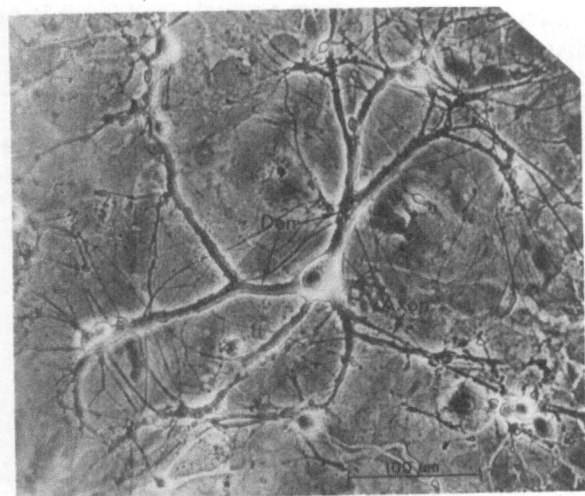

Fig. 1. Spinal cord neuron in primary dissociated cell culture. The large spinal cord neuron is multipolar with four large dendrites (Den) emerging from the soma and a single axon having its origin from a proximal segment of one of the dendrites. Magnification is ×225. (From Ref. (202)).

are prepared from spinal cord and attached dorsal root ganglia obtained from fetal animals using the methods developed by Fischbach (29) and Nelson (30). SC-DRG neuronal cocultures derived from fetal mice contain both SC and DRG neurons which can be unambiguously identified using morphological and electrophysiological criteria (30).

Large SC neurons (>20 μM diameter somata) are multipolar with several dendrites emerging from their somata (Fig. 1). Dendrites are covered with synaptic terminals over most of their membrane surface. A single axon usually emerges from the soma or from a proximal dendritic site and makes numerous synaptic contacts with other SC neurons (31). DRG neurons are round, contain sharply defined nuclei and nucleoli and are usually unipolar or bipolar. DRG neurons receive no synaptic input but DRG axons make synaptic contacts on SC neurons.

Electrophysiological properties of SC and DRG neurons in cell culture are similar to those of neurons *in vivo* (30). SC neurons display considerable spontaneous synaptic activity and depolarization evokes overshooting sodium-dependent action potentials. DRG neurons do not have spontaneous activity and intracellular stimulation evokes over-

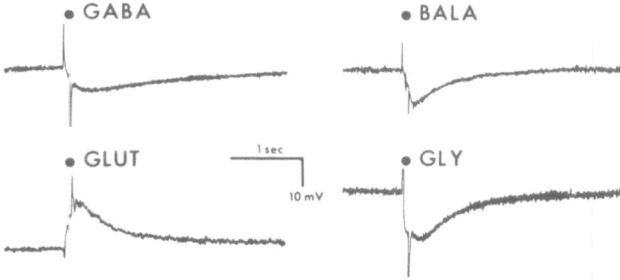

Fig. 2. Spinal cord neurons in cell culture respond to GABA (30 nA), β-alanine (BALA) (60 nA) and glycine (GLY) (30 nA) with a membrane hyperpolarization and to glutamate (GLU) (40 nA) with a depolarization. Amino acids were applied by iontophoresis for 100 msec. All responses were obtained from a single neuron and membrane potential varied from -40 to -44 mV. (From Ref. (36)).

shooting action potentials dependent upon both sodium and calcium.

Since neurons grow in a monolayer in primary dissociated cell culture, it is possible to obtain intracellular recordings under visual control from individual neurons, to apply neurotransmitters or drugs to selected somatic or dendritic locations using iontophoretic or pressure ejection techniques or to superfuse the culture with neurotransmitters or drugs. Individual neurons can also be penetrated by two independent micropipettes to apply the voltage clamp technique.

Synaptic transmission between DRG and SC or between SC and SC neurons can be studied by simultaneously recording from neuron pairs (31–33). Excitatory and inhibitory postsynaptic potentials can be evoked from SC neurons while only excitatory postsynaptic potentials have been evoked by DRG stimulation.

The postsynaptic amino acid pharmacology of SC neurons has been well characterized (34–36). The majority of SC neurons (>90%) respond to iontophoretically applied inhibitory neutral amino acids (GABA, β-alanine, glycine) and to the excitatory acidic amino acid glutamic acid (Fig. 2).

Thus SC and DRG neurons in primary dissociated cell culture have been demonstrated to have typical differentiated neuronal morphology, rich synaptic connectivity and extensive amino acid sensitivity and provide an excellent preparation for study of the physiology and pharmacology of SC and DRG neurons in vivo.

GABA metabolism

GABA has a unique regional distribution in the nervous system as does the enzyme responsible for its synthesis, L-glutamic acid decarboxylase (GAD) (37). Levels are highest in substantia nigra and lowest in brainstem and spinal cord. Within spinal cord, GABA levels are highest in the dorsal and dorsolateral part of dorsal horn (38). The synthesis and degradation of GABA is similar throughout the nervous system.

The immediate precursor for GABA is L-glutamic acid. The formation of GABA from glutamate was described in the first papers reporting the discovery of GABA in CNS tissues (1, 2, 3). L-Glutamate is derived principally from glutamine and α-ketoglutarate, the latter originating from the tricarboxylic acid cycle and glucose. However, alternative pathways have been described and various metabolic compartments of both glutamate and GABA exist (39). GAD (E.C.4.1.1.15) is the enzyme which catalyzes the formation of GABA from glutamate. GAD has a molecular weight of 85 000 daltons and requires pyridoxal phosphate (40). The enzyme is cytoplasmic and is the rate-limiting enzyme in GABA synthesis. It is concentrated in the terminals of GABAergic neurons. The enzyme has been purified, antibodies raised against it and the immunocytochemical localization studied in CNS (41–43). In spinal cord, GAD-positive terminals are concentrated in Rexeds laminae I, II and III and axo-axonic, axodendritic and axosomatic terminals have been demonstrated. All three types of connections are also seen in ventral horn and deep layers of dorsal horn (41–43).

There are a variety of agents that interfere with GAD activity either directly or as antagonists of pyridoxal phosphate. Antagonists of pyridoxal phosphate are primarily carbonyl trapping agents such as isoniazid and thiosemicarbazide. These agents not only inhibit GAD but also GABA-transaminase (GABA-T) (this enzyme is responsible for GABA degradation and also requires pyridoxal phosphate). Depending on which enzyme is inhibited preferentially, GABA levels can be raised or lowered by these agents. Direct inhibitors of GAD, such as 3-mercaptoproprionic acid and allylglycine, are convulsants whose actions appear directly correlated with their abilities to reduce GABA levels (44–46).

GABA is degraded by the enzyme 4-aminobutyrate: 2-oxoglutarate aminotransferase (E.C.2.6.1.19) (GABA-T). The reaction is the transamination of α-ketoglutarate with GABA to form glutamate and succinic semialdehyde. The enzyme (47) is localized to mitochondria and, like GAD, requires pyridoxal phosphate (48). The molecular weight of GABA-T is 109 000 daltons, the K_m for GABA is 1.1 mM and 0.25 mM for α-ketoglutarate (40). The enzyme makes one molecule of glutamate for every molecule of GABA destroyed, thus continually replenishing the precursor supply for GABA. The enzyme has been purified and antibodies raised against it (41–43, 49). Distribution studies have shown the enzyme associated with the mitochondria of synaptic terminals, glia and postsynaptic neuronal regions. Carbonyl trapping agents inhibit GABA-T by interferring with pyridoxal phosphate. One of these is aminooxyacetic acid (AOAA) which has been shown to act preferentially on GABA-T, raising GABA levels at low doses but causing convulsions at higher doses (secondary to inhibitory of GAD). Recently, several irreversible inhibitors of GABA-T have been described and promoted as possible anticonvulsants (50–53). The two agents studied most extensively have been γ-acetylenic GABA (4-amino-hex-5-ynoic acid) and γ-vinyl GABA (4-amino-hex-5-enoic acid). These agents cross the blood brain barrier and thus could be used clinically. Unfortunately, at high doses these drugs also effect GAD and perhaps several other enzymes as well (50, 51, 53). A very potent GABA-T inhibitor, gabaculline ((–)-5-amino-1, 4-cyclohexadienyl carboxylic acid); has a K_i of approximately 1 μM for GABA-T and is only weakly inhibitory on GAD (54).

The last enzyme in GABA degradation is succinic semialdehyde dehydrogenase (E.C. 1.2.1.24) (SSADH). This enzyme is associated with mitochondria and is distributed similarly to GABA-T (48, 55). The reaction converts succinic semialdehyde to succinic acid which enters the tricarboxylic acid cycle (56). Valproic acid (sodium n-dipropylacetic acid), which has been found useful as an anticonvulsant in humans, produced a dose dependent increase in GABA levels in animals. The agent was originally thought to be an anticonvulsant secondary to inhibition of GABA-T (57) but more recently it has been shown to be a more potent inhibitor of SSADH (58) and more importantly to directly augment GABA responses recorded electrophysiologically (59). We have found that valproic acid is a weak inhibitor of GAD, GABA-T and SSADH (IC_{50}'s greater than 15 mM for all three enzymes) in mouse brain and spinal cord neurons in dissociated cell culture. The doses needed to cause 50% inhibition were much above that necessary for anticonvulsant effects (60).

GABA uptake

GABA is actively accumulated into nervous tissues by both high and low affinity transport systems (61, 62). The high affinity uptake is saturable, temperature-sensitive and sodium- and energy-dependent. High affinity uptake has been selectively evaluated by incubating small tissue slices or brain homogenates with low concentrations (10^{-5} to 10^{-8} M) of radioactively labeled GABA for short time periods (less than 10 min) (63, 64). Under these conditions little GABA is metabolized. The high affinity uptake system has a K_m of 5–40 μM depending on the preparation (64). In nervous tissue, it is felt that uptake occurs primarily into GABAergic nerve terminals. It has even been possible to show GABA uptake into specific populations of synaptosomes by sucrose gradient centrifugation (65). Nevertheless, there are several studies which indicate that high affinity uptake systems are also present on glial cells in certain tissues such as rat sensory ganglia and cultured rat glial tumor cells (66–69). There is also controversy over whether GABA uptake actually functions as a mechanism for GABA inactivation. There is evidence that the apparent uptake is really a net exchange. A variety of conflicting studies exist on GABA uptake and the functions of the various transport systems have yet to be resolved (68, 70–73).

Autoradiographic techniques have been the most reliable way of determining which tissue elements accumulate GABA. In brain, the percentage of nerve terminals labeled by ³H-GABA has a regional distribution consistent with the predicted distribution of GABAergic terminals (74, 75). In spinal cord homogenates, it has been demonstrated that approximately 25% of synaptic terminals were labeled when incubated with either ³H-GABA or

[3]H-glycine alone (74). When incubated with both labeled amino acids together, approximately 50% of the terminals were labeled, suggesting that the two amino acids were accumulated into separate populations of terminals. More recently, lesions of specific brain regions or pathways have been shown to selectively decrease GABA uptake in the projection areas of these pathways (63, 70, 76). Thus, measurement of GABA uptake is a valuable technique in the mapping of GABAergic pathways.

GABA uptake has been studied in organ culture and dissociated cell culture of nervous tissue (77–79). In spinal cord cultures, a great number of neurons and almost all glial cells were labeled after incubation with ^{3}H-GABA. In cerebellar cultures, glia, interneurons and Purkinje cells accumulated GABA. In dorsal root ganglia cultures, neurons were labeled only if they had been stripped of glial elements, otherwise only satelite glial cells were labeled (77).

In dissociated cell cultures of embryonic chick spinal cord, GABA uptake has been studied chemically and by autoradiography (79). Both high and low affinity systems were observed with K_ms of 4 and 100 μM respectively. The high affinity system was temperature-sensitive, saturable and sodium-dependent and inhibited more potently by 2,4-diaminobutyric acid than β-alanine. Autoradiography demonstrated uptake into about one half the multipolar neurons and an absence of uptake into glia and nonneuronal cell types.

Blockers of the GABA transport system have been studied rather extensively (80–82). 2,4-Diaminobutyric acid (DABA) and nipecotic acid have been found to be more potent in inhibiting uptake into nerve terminals and neurons than β-alanine (83). Recently, $\pm$-cis-3-aminocyclohexanecarboxylic acid has been found to be a more selective inhibitor of neuronal uptake than DABA or nipecotic acid (84). Of all the uptake blockers that have been studied, the most potent are R-nipecotic acid ($IC_{50} = 8$ μM), and cis-4-hydroxynipecotic acid ($IC_{50} = 12$ μM) (85). The active molecular conformations for inhibition of neuronal GABA uptake differ somewhat from the conformations for optimal inhibition of glial uptake (86, 87). Furthermore, structure activity studies indicate that the conformation of GABA that interacts with the transport system is quite different from that which interacts with GABA synaptic receptors.

Inhibitors of GABA uptake may enhance the neurophysiologic depressant effects of GABA (88, 89). However, they do not cross the blood brain barrier. Ethyl esters of nipecotic acid cross into brain and protect against pentylenetetrazole seizure but their pharmacologic effectiveness in humans is unknown (85).

GABA release

The release of GABA from superfused tissues, glial cells, brain and spinal cord slices and synaptosomes has been studied extensively in recent years (90–96). There have been, however, conflicting data as to whether the release is calcium-dependent and whether certain forms of stimulation (i.e. electrical, potassium or veratradine) are better than others. Potassium evoked release of exogenously labelled GABA has been demonstrated to be calcium dependent in brain slices and synaptosomes (92, 93, 95, 97, 99, 101). Electrical or veratradine induced release of GABA was less consistently calcium-dependent (97, 99, 102). In culture systems, potassium-evoked release of exogenously labeled ^{3}H-GABA has been demonstrated and release was inhibited by reducing the extracellular Ca^{++}/Mg^{++} ratio (78). The pharmacology of the GABA release was not investigated in culture. In mouse neurons in dissociated cell culture, we found that exogenously labelled GABA was released by high-potassium and also was dependent on the Ca^{++}/Mg^{++} ratio. The release was inhibited by GABA but not by DABA, β-alanine, muscimol, barbiturates or bicuculline. Glial preparations have been found to accumulate GABA (see previous section) and to release GABA after potassium stimulation (96, 103, 104, 105). However, glial release did not appear to be calcium dependent (96, 105).

Release of GABA and other neurotransmitters may be regulated by presynaptic GABA receptors (106–109). The calcium-dependent potassium-evoked release of GABA from substantia nigra was inhibited by both GABA and muscimol; however, bicuculline also inhibited the release and additional pharmacology was not reported (108). Recently, GABA has been shown to facilitate the release of ^{3}H-dopamine from caudate nucleus (106, 107) but the effect was not antagonized by bicuculline nor

152

picrotoxin, and others have found an inhibition of ³H-dopamine release from striatal slices by GABA (109). The discrepancies in the results as to whether GABA facilitates or inhibits release may be secondary to technical differences in experimental methodology. It does appear clear, however, that the pharmacology of these presynaptic receptors may be quite different from that of postsynaptic receptors (106–109).

GABA binding

The electrophysiological effects of GABA on neuronal membrane properties have been studied extensively, and it has also been possible to study GABA receptors biochemically by binding studies (110–114). The correlation of biochemical and neurophysiological data hopefully will allow a better understanding of the GABA receptor complex. Most binding studies to date have been performed in different preparations than the physiological studies making comparisons difficult. Mammalian neurons in primary dissociated cell culture provide a single system in which biochemical data and physiological data can be directly compared (115–118).

A variety of ligands have been used to probe the properties of the GABA receptor complex. The two commonly used agonists are ³H-GABA and ³H-muscimol. ³H-GABA binds saturably to synaptic membranes and binding has a pharmacology and a subcellular and regional distribution consistent with that of the synaptic GABA receptor. Two binding sites can be discerned in nervous tissue, a low and a high affinity site with K_Ds of about 20 nM to about 200 nM, respectively (119).

In initial studies of GABA binding, two conditions for binding were demonstrated (110, 120). If nervous tissue membranes were freshly prepared and incubated with ³H-GABA in the presence of sodium, then binding was not bicuculline sensitive and had a pharmacology similar to the uptake site (so-called sodium-dependent binding). If membranes were frozen and assayed for binding in the absence of sodium, binding was bicuculline sensitive and had a pharmacology consistent with the synaptic receptor (so-called sodium-independent binding). Initial studies of these sodium-independent sites suggested one population of

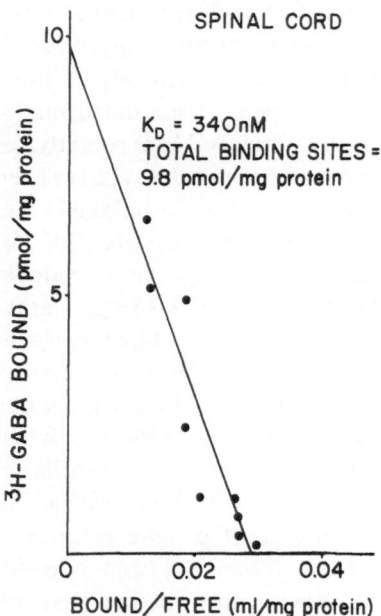

Fig. 3. Scatchard analysis of specific ³H-GABA binding to adult rat spinal cord membranes. Membranes from whole spinal cord homogenized in 50 mM Tris-citrate buffer, pH 7.1 at 4 °C were incubated at 37 °C for 30 min with 0.05% Triton X-100 (v/v) and then centrifuged at 48 000 × g for 10 min. The membranes were washed 3 times with fresh ice cold buffer and finally resuspended in buffer. Aliquots of the suspension (0.2–0.8 mg protein) were incubated in triplicate with increasing concentrations of ³H-GABA (1–500 nM) at 4 °C for 20 min. The assay was terminated by filtration over Whatman GF/B glass fiber filters. Specific binding (●) was obtained by subtracting from the total ³H-GABA bound, that bound in the presence of 0.1 mM GABA (run in triplicate). The experiment has been repeated four times.

binding sites. Subsequent studies, however, demonstrated that two sites became apparent if the tissue was pretreated with the detergent Triton X-100 or if the membranes were repeatedly frozen and thawed and then washed extensively (119). Furthermore, this procedure increased the affinity of GABA for its receptor by at least one order of magnitude. It occurred to several investigators that this phenomenon might represent the removal of an endogenous GABA receptor modulator from the neuronal membranes (GABA-modulin) (121–123). Some of the 'modulator' may be GABA itself but a relatively small protein or peptide has also been implicated. The distribution of the high affinity sites varied quite dramatically throughout the CNS. The number of high affinity sites was highest in the cerebellum and lowest in the spinal cord (124, 125). In our laboratory we have studied ³H-GABA

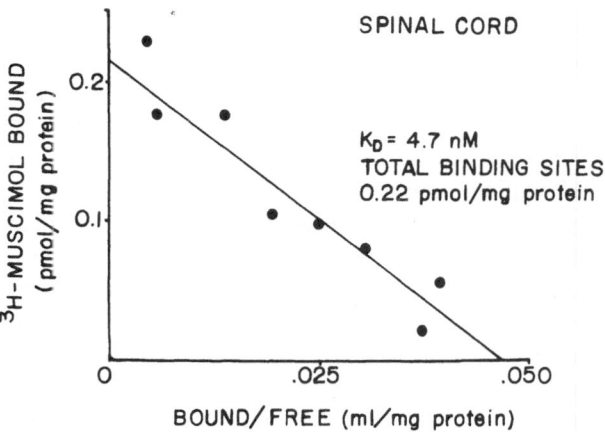

Fig. 4. Scatchard analysis of specific ^{3}H-muscimol binding to adult rat spinal cord membranes. The assay was identical to that described for ^{3}H-GABA in Fig. 3, however, ^{3}H-muscimol was the labeled ligand. The experiment has been replicated four times.

binding in spinal cord and only low affinity sites ($K_D = 340$ nM; $B_{max} = 9.8$ pmol/mg prot) could be demonstrated (Fig. 3) whereas in brain the identical technique indicated two sites (low affinity $K_D = 210$ nM, $B_{max} = 10.1$ pmol/mg prot, and high affinity $K_D = 20$ nM, $B_{max} = 1.5$ pmol/mg prot).

^{3}H-Muscimol also binds to central nervous GABA receptors but only to the high affinity site in tritonized tissue (126–128). We have found that, in

brain, the K_D for ^{3}H-muscimol binding was 6 nM and the B_{max} was 1.7 pmol/mg prot which was similar to the B_{max} of the high affinity GABA receptor binding site. When we studied ^{3}H-muscimol in tritonized spinal cord membranes, only one binding site was found with a $K_D = 6$ nM and $B_{max} = 0.24$ pmol/mg protein (Fig. 4). The ratio therefore of high to low affinity sites in spinal cord was 1:40. Such a ratio precluded accurate quantitation of the high affinity site in spinal cord using ^{3}H-GABA. Even in routine assays at very low concentrations of ^{3}H-GABA, the relative contribution of the low affinity site was substantial.

The high affinity GABA and muscimol binding sites are considered to be associated with the postsynaptic complex (129). Lesions of various nuclei receiving GABAergic input lead to a loss of high affinity receptor sites (129). Also, the high affinity receptor sites are the ones that increased during the development of supersensitivity. In spinal cord in cell culture, we found two binding sites for GABA (Fig. 5) and only a high affinity site for muscimol. The K_Ds for the two GABA binding sites were similar to those found in rat brain and spinal cord although the ratio of high to low affinity sites was higher than that of rat spinal cord. The location of the low affinity sites have not been studied and their significance is unknown.

The pharmacology of the high affinity site revealed that various receptor agonists (as judged by neurophysiological criteria) competed for ^{3}H-

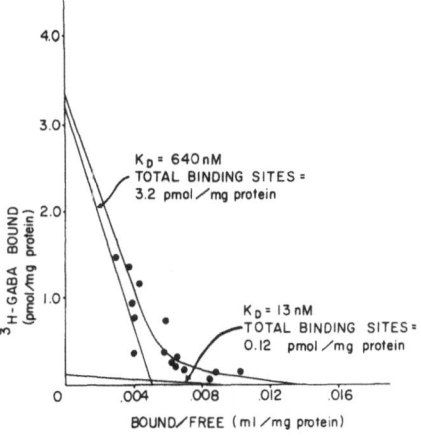

Fig. 5. Scatchard analysis of specific ^{3}H-GABA binding to membranes from mouse spinal cord neurons in dissociated cell culture prepared as described in Fig. 3 except that 0.025% Triton X-100 was used and two washes were carried out and the membranes centrifuged for 20 min at 48 000 × g. The results are the combined data from two experiments and the experiment has been replicated four times.

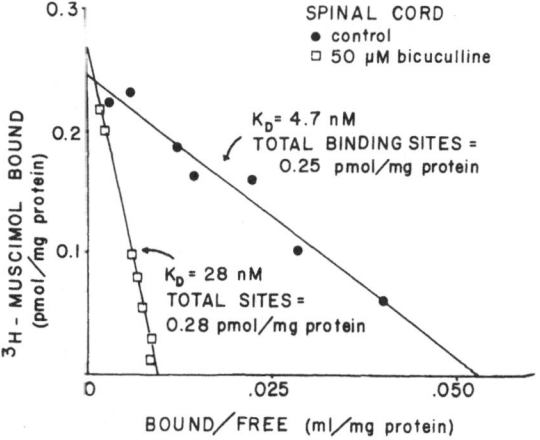

Fig. 6. Scatchard analyses of ^{3}H-muscimol binding in adult rat spinal cord membranes alone (●) and in the presence of 50 μM bicuculline (□). The assay is identical to that in Fig. 3. The experiment has been replicated four times.

GABA binding (130–133). Muscimol, 3-amino-propanesulphonic acid and dihydromuscimol are three potent receptor agonists. Structure activity studies have shown a specific optimal conformation of GABA for interaction with its receptor, different from the conformations which interact with the uptake sites, GAD and GABA-T (134, 135).

Very few GABA antagonists inhibit GABA binding. (+)-Bicuculline is the most potent antagonist with an $IC_{50} = 5\,\mu M$ (134). Other convulsant agents have been investigated and the only ones approaching (+)-bicuculline in potency were (+)-adlumidine, n-propylbicyclophosphate and n-butylbicyclophosphate (136). Bicuculline appeared to be a competitive inhibitor or GABA both by physiological criteria and by biochemical studies (Fig. 6) (136, 137). As indicated earlier, the affinity of GABA receptors could be enhanced dramatically by pretreating membrane fractions with Triton X-100 or by repeated freezing and thawing of the membranes with subsequent extensive washing (119). Such treatment of membranes, however, did not influence the K_I for bicuculline which is difficult to explain if it was indeed interacting strictly competitively with GABA at the receptor site. Furthermore, various anions enhanced the effectiveness of bicuculline in inhibiting GABA binding without changing the affinity of GABA itself (116). Although analysis of the effect of bicuculline on GABA dose response curves indicated competitive inhibition, such studies must be considered carefully. It is possible for a substance to exhibit linear competitive inhibition and nevertheless bind to a site separate from (but closely linked to) the site for the natural substrate (138).

A variety of other agents that antagonized or enhanced GABA responses in physiological experiments had no effect on GABA binding (110, 112, 113). These included picrotoxinin, pentylenetetrazole, penicillin, barbiturates and the benzodiazepines. It is therefore unlikely that these drugs interact directly with the GABA recognition site but rather with a closely related site such as the chloride channel. Several of these agents have been labeled and binding to synaptic membranes studied (139–141). Several studies using ³H-bicuculline methiodide have been published but this agent was not very stable, was difficult to prepare and few detailed studies have been possible. ³H-Dihydropicrotoxinin binding has been reported. Binding

was not displaced by GABA and was weakly displaced by bicuculline (142). However, binding was displaced by picrotoxin analogues, barbiturates and the so-called cage convulsants in potencies similar to their clinical potencies. Finally, benzodiazepine binding studies have demonstrated a class of benzodiazepine receptors intimately related to GABA receptors (143–146). GABA enhanced binding to benzodiazepine receptors as did a variety of GABA analogs. Anions also enhanced benzodiazepine binding suggesting that there may be an association of the receptor with the chloride channel together in the same fractions (145, 147). Diazepam has also been found to interact with GABA modulin and thereby increase the affinity of GABA binding. The GABA receptor and the benzodiazepine receptor can be solubilized together (148, 149).

The GABA receptor complex is certainly far from being completely understood. However, multiple probes are now available to do quite detailed studies on various receptor components and their interactions.

GABA-mediated inhibition in the mammalian spinal cord

In the mammalian spinal cord GABAergic interneurons are presumed to have at least two different sites of action. Release of GABA onto primary afferent terminals would produce presynaptic inhibition while release onto somatic and dendritic locations would produce postsynaptic inhibition.

Stimulation of primary afferents to the spinal cord produced a prolonged depolarization of primary afferent fibers (primary afferent depolarization (PAD)) (150, 151). PAD was associated with reduction of monosynaptic EPSPs recorded in anterior horn cells following orthodromic volleys in muscle and cutaneous afferents and was thought to be due to decreased release of transmitter from the primary afferent terminals. Eccles and coworkers (152) suggested that the reduction in transmitter release was due to release of transmitter from axoaxonic synapses located on the synaptic terminals of primary afferent fibers and also that the neurotransmitter involved might be GABA (153). Application of GABA to isolated spinal cord produced depolarization of dorsal root fibers (154–157) and GABA depolarized dorsal root ganglion cells (158–161). These actions of GABA were blocked by the GABA antagonists picrotoxin and bicuculline (157–161). Thus while GABA did alter membrane potential of primary afferent terminals it produced depolarization rather than the usual hyperpolarization associated with inhibition. Nonetheless, using immunohistochemical techniques Roberts and his colleagues (41–43) demonstrated that GAD-positive (and thus presumably GABAergic) axoaxonic contacts were made on primary afferent terminals. Based on ion substitution experiments, blockade of chloride channels and intracellular recording from dorsal root ganglion neurons it has been demonstrated that GABA increased chloride conductance and that depolarization was produced because the equilibrium potential for chloride ions was depolarized relative to resting membrane potential (159, 161, 162). Thus, there is physiological, pharmacological and anatomical evidence to support the notion that presynaptic inhibition in the dorsal horn is GABA-mediated. PAD, however, may have two different underlying mechanisms. The early picrotoxin-sensitive depolarization is probably due to release of GABA onto presynaptic terminals while the late phase is most likely a consequence of elevated interstitial potassium produced by the large afferent volley (163, 164).

GABA-mediated postsynaptic inhibition is also probably present in the spinal cord. As discussed above, GABA levels are highest in the dorsal and dorsolateral portions of the dorsal horn (38). However, Roberts and his colleagues (41–43) have demonstrated GAD-positive terminals on both dorsal and ventral horn neurons. In the dorsal horn, GAD-positive terminals were identified on the somata of substantia gelatinosa neurons as well as the dendrites of Rexeds layer IV neurons. The lateral portion of the intermediate spinal gray matter and motor nuclei had a light concentration of GAD-positive material. Furthermore, most of the spinal cord neurons studied had at least some GAD-positive terminals on their somata and often on their dendrites. Thus there is immunocytochemical evidence for widespread distribution of GABAergic synaptic terminals. Consistent with this, spinal cord neurons were hyperpolarized by GABA (7–10, 165) and this hyperpolarization was due to an increase in membrane chloride conductance (166). Despite these findings, much post-

synaptic inhibition in the spinal cord was strychnine-sensitive and bicuculline-insensitive implying that it was glycinergic (167). This includes short latency, strychnine-sensitive inhibition of motoneurons produced by single volleys in afferents from cutaneous and muscle nerves, inhibition of spinal interneurons and inhibition of firing of Renshaw cells produced by volleys in hindlimb cutaneous fibers (167–171). Nevertheless, while glycine may be the major neurotransmitter mediating postsynaptic inhibition in the spinal cord, there is substantial evidence that GABA-mediated postsynaptic inhibition is also present in the spinal cord.

GABA-mediated postsynaptic inhibition in spinal cord neurons in cell culture

Application of GABA onto SC neurons in cell culture using iontophoretic or pressure techniques produced both membrane potential and conductance changes (34–36). During intracellular recordings with micropipettes containing 4M potassium acetate, GABA application produced membrane hyperpolarization and an increase in membrane conductance. GABA-response amplitude was a function of membrane potential, and the responses could be reversed by membrane hyperpolarization. The average reversal potential for GABA-responses was –61.1 mV with an average resting membrane potential of –54.6 mV (35). The hyperpolarized reversal potential of GABA-responses associated with increased conductance suggested that either chloride and/or potassium conductance was involved in the response. The role of chloride conductance was examined by altering intra- and extracellular chloride concentrations and determining reversal potentials (35). Injection of chloride ions into SC neurons from intracellular recording micropipettes containing 3M KCl reduced the reversal potential of GABA-responses to –20.3 mV without altering resting membrane potential. Reduction of chloride ions from the bathing medium attenuated GABA-responses but addition of extracellular chloride from a large bore pipette restored the response. Thus, GABA-responses are chloride dependent. Similar experiments which increased extracellular potassium concentration did not alter the GABA-response

156

reversal potential initially, but after sustained potassium induced depolarization, the reversal potential was decreased. This result suggested that potassium was not involved in GABA-responses and that the late changes in GABA-response reversal potential were due to redistribution of chloride ions induced by sustained depolarization. Thus, GABA-mediated inhibitory responses of SC neurons in cell culture are due to an increase in chloride conductance.

Sensitivity to GABA was not uniform over the surface of SC neurons (34, 35) with focal areas of increased sensitivity being distributed over the cell surface. Whether or not these 'hot spots' correspond to localized regions of subsynaptic GABA-receptors is uncertain.

We have used the voltage clamp technique to study membrane currents induced by GABA (168). SC neurons were penetrated by two independent intracellular micropipettes. One micropipette recorded transmembrane potential and the other applied current. The voltage clamp apparatus held membrane potential by applying current through the current micropipette, and it was the applied current that was recorded. Under clamp conditions, the reversal potential for GABA-responses was 8–10 mV more negative than resting membrane potential. We were able to obtain dose-response data during voltage clamp and demonstrate that when the log of the membrane current was plotted as a function of the log of the GABA iontophoretic current, a limiting slope averaged 1.5. This suggested that GABA interacts with the GABA-receptor in a cooperative manner with at least two GABA molecules being required to activate the chloride conductance mechanism.

Since the voltage clamp technique can be applied to SC neurons, conductance fluctuation (or 'noise') analysis can also be applied to investigation of GABA-mediated inhibition (173). Individual SC neurons were impaled with two independent micropipettes and GABA was applied by iontophoresis. Experiments had to be performed at 26 °C to reduce desensitization. The GABA induced increase in noise was analyzed using fluctuation analysis assuming that the noise derived was from statistical variation in the number of open ion channels activated by GABA with a mean level of open channels. Using this analysis, the average conductance of a single channel activated by GABA

was 18 ± 8.2 pS. Using spectral analysis of fluctuations during the plateau phase of the current responses, the average duration of the GABA channel open time was 20 ± 6.6 msec.

Thus, GABA inhibits SC neurons in primary dissociated cell culture by increasing chloride conductance and hyperpolarizing membrane potential. At least two molecules of GABA appear necessary to activate chloride channels. Activation of GABA-receptors briefly opens individual chloride channels with small unitary channel conductance.

Antagonists of GABA-mediated inhibition

The compounds bicuculline (BICUC), picrotoxin (PICRO), pentylenetetrazol (PTZ) and penicillin (PCN) produce convulsions when applied to the mammalian CNS. The action of these agents on SC neurons in cell culture was investigated by applying GABA, other amino acids and convulsants by iontophoresis to focal areas of somata of SC neurons (174, 175). None of the convulsants altered membrane potential or input resistance but all four convulsants rapidly and reversibly antagonized GABA-responses (Fig. 7). The antagonism of GABA-mediated inhibition was selective for GABA since responses to the amino acids β-alanine, glycine and glutamate were unaffected by convulsant concentrations that antagonized GABA-responses. Using spinal cord neurons in cell culture, we have compared the antagonism of GABA-responses by BICUC with the displacement of ^{3}H-GABA by BICUC. BICUC displaced high affinity ^{3}H-GABA binding with an ED_{50} of 15 μM and an ED_{20} of 4 μM (Young, Frere and Macdonald, unpublished work). Antagonism of GABA-responses was produced with an ED_{50} of 1 μM and an ED_{100} of 10 μM. (Macdonald, Nowak and Young, unpublished work). Thus the physiologically relevant displacement of binding occurred over 1 to 10 μM BICUC concentrations and high affinity binding was correlated with antagonism of postsynaptic GABA-responses.

While all of these convulsants (PICRO, BICUC, PCN, PTZ) antagonized GABA-responses, their sites of action are uncertain. Since none of the convulsants antagonized glycine responses, which are also chloride-mediated, it is unlikely that they combine nonspecifically with all chloride channels.

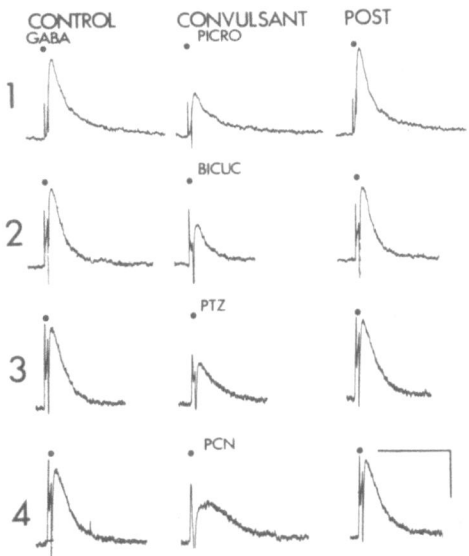

Fig. 7. GABA-responses were antagonized reversibly by the convulsants picrotoxin (PICRO), bicuculline (BICUC), pentylenetetrazol (PTZ) and penicillin (PCN). GABA was applied by iontophoresis (50 msec. pulses) and intracellular recordings were made by glass micropipettes containing 3M KCl. Membrane potential was hyperpolarized to -80 to -90 mV and chloride ions were injected intracellularly. Thus GABA reversal potentials were depolarized to about -20 mV and the GABA-responses were depolarizing rather than hyperpolarizing. Calibration bars are 10 mV × 1 s. (From Ref. (175)).

With intracellular recording techniques applied to invertebrate muscle fibers (176–178) and cat dorsal root ganglion neurons (161), BICUC antagonized GABA-induced increases in conductance noncompetitively. Using extracellular recording from spinal cord interneurons in lamprey (179) and cuneate neurons (180, 181) BICUC antagonism was competitive. Using similar techniques, PICRO antagonized GABA-responses on invertebrate muscle fibers in a competitive (173), noncompetitive (182, 183) and mixed (178) fashion. PICRO antagonized GABA-responses competitively on invertebrate crayfish stretch receptor neurons (184) but noncompetitively on vertebrate dorsal root ganglion neurons (161), spinal cord interneurons (179) and cuneate neurons (180, 181). PCN antagonized GABA-responses primarily noncompetitively in both invertebrate muscle fibers (185) and vertebrate cuneate neurons (186). Dose-response data for PTZ action on GABA-responses has not been published. In summary, BICUC, PICRO and PCN antagonize GABA-mediated inhibition in invertebrate muscle fibers and vertebrate dorsal root ganglion neurons noncompetitively. In studies of vertebrate central neurons PICRO and PCN are also noncompetitive antagonists but BICUC appears to be a competitive antagonist. From a technical point of view, the data from muscle fibers and dorsal root ganglion neurons was obtained using intracellular recording while that from central neurons was either extracellular unit recordings or extracellular d.c. potentials. The intracellular data certainly more accurately reflects the actions of agonists and antagonists than does extracellular recording and therefore the data demonstrating noncompetitive antagonism is more likely to accurately reflect the interaction between convulsants and GABA-responses. Thus, it is likely that in invertebrate muscle the convulsants act on a site other than the GABA-recognition site, either the GABA-coupled chloride channel or the coupling mechanism between the receptor and the channel.

It is likely that these compounds produce convulsions by antagonizing GABA-mediated postsynaptic inhibition. Using the hippocampal slice preparation, Yamamoto (187) demonstrated that paroxysmal depolarizing shifts (PDS) can be recorded from CA$_3$ pyramidal neurons following addition of the convulsant strychnine. PDS are the intracellular correlate of interictal 'spikes' recorded

However, to antagonize GABA-responses each convulsant could combine: 1) with the active site of the GABA-receptor to competitively antagonize GABA-responses, 2) with the GABA-coupled chloride channel to non-competitively antagonize GABA-responses or 3) with a modulator site which either alters the affinity of the receptor for GABA, modifies the coupling between the receptor and chloride channel or changes chloride channel function (decrease unitary channel open time or conductance). While adequate studies of the effect of GABA-antagonists on GABA dose-response curves on spinal cord neurons have not been published, some information is available from other preparations. Much of the quantitative electrophysiological data has been obtained using lobster, crayfish and crab muscle since in these preparations intracellular penetrations can be maintained for the extended time period required for acquisition of dose-response data.

158

in the scalp electroencephalogram of patients with epilepsy (188–190). The PDS are calcium-dependent depolarizations of dendritic origin (191) which are activated by orthodromic stimulation but do not invade the neuronal soma due to orthodromic disynaptic (presumably GABAergic) somatic inhibition (192). Antagonism of the inhibitory postsynaptic potentials by PCN, however, permits somatic invasion by the calcium-dependent depolarization and this results in PDS (193). PCN also produces spinal myoclonus in animals and man, presumably also by blockade of GABA-mediated postsynaptic inhibition. Thus, it is likely that reduction of GABA-mediated inhibition may be involved in the pathogenesis of some forms of human epilepsy and spinal myoclonus.

Augmentors of GABA-mediated inhibition

Barbiturates, benzodiazepines and valproic acid are all used clinically as anticonvulsants. In addition, barbiturates and benzodiazepines are employed therapeutically to reduce anxiety and facilitate sleep. Short acting barbiturates are also useful as anesthetics. The mechanisms of action of these compounds are uncertain but numerous pre- and postsynaptic actions have been described and many of these actions involve GABAergic transmission. Presynaptic actions of barbiturates include: 1) augmentation of GABA-mediated presynaptic inhibition (13, 16); 2) depression of evoked transmitter release from dorsal root afferents (194); 3) augmentation of evoked transmitter release at the neuromuscular junction (195, 196); and 4) direct depolarization of dorsal root afferents which is blocked by the GABA antagonist picrotoxin (16). Postsynaptic effects of barbiturates include: 1) augmentation of GABA-mediated inhibition (15, 17, 18); 2) antagonism of glutamate-mediated excitation (15, 18); 3) reduction of excitatory synaptic transmission; and 4) direct hyperpolarization of spinal cord motoneurons which is blocked by picrotoxin (15).

Benzodiazepines have multiple actions including: 1) augmentation of GABA-mediated presynaptic inhibition (19–21); 2) enhancement (197, 198) and antagonism (199, 200) of GABA-mediated postsynaptic inhibition; and 3) direct depolarization of sympathetic preganglionic nerve terminals (22).

Valproic acid (VPA) has been shown to have a primarily presynaptic action to increase central nervous system GABA levels (57), by antagonizing the major GABA degradative enzymes including GABA-T (57) and, more importantly, SSADH (58). It was suggested that this enhancement of presynaptic GABA would increase GABA-mediated inhibition.

We have used mouse spinal cord neurons in primary dissociated cell culture to investigate the action of these compounds on postsynaptic GABA-responses, other amino acid responses and on resting membrane properties

The anticonvulsant (phenobarbital (PhB) and mephobarbital (MB)) (Fig. 8) and sedative-anesthetic (pentobarbital (PB) and secobarbital (SB)) barbiturates (18, 201), the benzodiazepines (diazepam (DZ) and chlordiazepoxide (CDZ)) (18, 202) and valproic acid (57) all augmented GABA-responses without altering glycine responses. The mechanistic basis for this modulation of GABA-responses is uncertain but it is clear that, since these compounds augmented rather than antagonized GABA-responses, they did not compete with GABA for the GABA-binding site on the GABA receptor. We have proposed that they bind to a modulator site on the GABA-receptor chloride-channel complex to alter GABA-responses (201–203). Since barbiturates, benzodiazepines and valproic acid do not alter the affinity of saturable ^{3}H-GABA binding to spinal cord or brain membranes, it is likely that these compounds do not bind to the GABA recognition site of GABA-receptors but instead bind to a separate site located on the GABA-receptor chloride-channel complex which alters either: 1) the

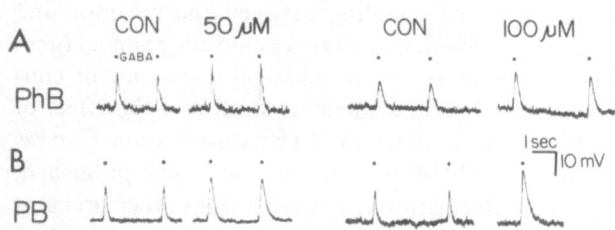

Fig. 8. GABA-responses were augmented by phenobarbital and pentobarbital. GABA was applied by iontophoresis (PhB: 4,5 nA; PB: 3,2.5 nA) for 100 msec, recordings were made with micropipettes containing 3M KCl and membrane potential was hyperpolarized to –60 to –90 mV to achieve large depolarizing GABA-responses. (Macdonald & Schulz, unpublished work.)

coupling between GABA-binding and chloride channels or 2) the GABA-coupled chloride channel properties to increase unitary channel conductance or open time.

Barbiturates, but not benzodiazepines or valproic acid, also antagonized excitatory glutamate-responses (18, 203). For PB and PhB, the two actions occurred at the same drug concentration with PB being somewhat more potent than PhB. In addition, both PB and PhB directly increased neuronal chloride conductance independent of GABA (201, 203). This direct action of the barbiturates was antagonized by the GABA-antagonists PCN and PICRO, suggesting that the barbiturates were 'GABA-mimetic.' However, as discussed above, barbiturates have not been demonstrated to displace ^{3}H-GABA from GABA-binding sites and thus the available evidence suggests that the barbiturates do not bind directly to the GABA-binding site to increase chloride conductance but rather bind to an adjacent site similar to that which PICRO binds. Thus barbiturates could bind: 1) to the GABA-receptor chloride channel complex and activate the GABA-coupled chloride channel independent of the GABA-binding site, 2) to an independent 'barbiturate receptor' which is also coupled to chloride channels or 3) to the GABA-coupled chloride channel with direct activation of the chloride channels.

Despite having multiple actions, it is likely that specific actions of these compounds are responsible for their clinical actions. Augmentation of GABA-mediated postsynaptic inhibition is probably responsible for the anticonvulsant actions of the barbituates and benzodiazepines and possibly for valproic acid. The anesthetic actions of barbiturates are probably due to: 1) direct activation of chloride conductance, 2) augmentation of GABA-mediated inhibition and possibly antagonism of glutamate-mediated excitation and 3) reduction of presynaptic calcium-entry leading to a generalized diminution of synaptic transmission. Thus, the GABA-receptor chloride channel complex is a major site of action for the clinical actions of these compounds.

References

1. Awapara, J., Landua, A. J., Fuerst, R. & Seale, B., 1950. J. Biol. Chem. 187: 35–39.
2. Roberts, E. & Frankel, S., 1950. J. Biol. Chem. 187: 55–66.
3. Udenfriend, S., 1950. J. Biol. Chem. 187: 65–69.
4. Hayashi, T., 1954. J. Med. 3: 183–192.
5. Florey, E., 1954. Arch. Intern. Physiol. 62: 33–53.
6. Bazemore, A. W., Elliott, K. A. C. & Florey, E., 1957. J. Neurochem. 1: 334–339.
7. Curtis, D. R., Phillis, J. W. & Watkins, J. C., 1959. J. Physiol. (Lond.) 146: 185–203.
8. Curtis, D. R., Hosli, L., Johnston, G. A. R. & Johnston, I. H., 1968. Exper. Brain Res. 5: 235–258.
9. Curtis, D. R. & Johnston, G. A. R., 1974. Ergeb. Physiol. 9: 98–188.
10. Krnjevic, K., 1974. Physiol. Rev. 54: 418–450.
11. Roberts, E., 1974. Biochem. Pharmacol. 23: 2637–2649.
12. Krnjevic, K., 1976. In: GABA in nervous system function (Roberts, E., Chase, T. N. & Tower, D. B., eds.), pp. 269–281, Raven Press, New York.
13. Schmidt, R. F., 1971. Ergeb. Physiol. Biol. Chem. Exp. Pharmacol. 63: 20–101.
14. Nicoll, R. A., 1972. J. Physiol. (Lond.) 223: 803–814.
15. Nicoll, R. A., 1975. Brain Res. 96: 119–123.
16. Nicoll, R. A., 1975. Proc. Nat. Acad. Sci. (USA) 72: 1460–1463.
17. Ransom, B. R. & Barker, J. L., 1976. Brain Res. 114: 530–535.
18. Macdonald, R. L. & Barker, J. L., 1979. Brain Res. 167: 323–336.
19. Schlosser, W., 1971. Arch. Int. Pharmacodyn. 194: 93–102.
20. Polc, P., Mohler, H. & Haefely, W., 1974. Arch. Pharmacol. 284: 319–337.
21. Haefely, W., Kulesar, A., Mohler, H., Pieri, L., Polc, P. & Shaffner, R., 1975. Advanc. Biochem. Psychopharmacol. 10: 131–152.
22. Suria, A. & Costa, E., 1975. Brain Res. 87: 102–106.
23. Mohler, H. & Okada, T., 1977. Science 198: 849–851.
24. Squires, R. F. & Braestrup, C., 1977. Nature (Lond.) 266: 732–734.
25. Meldrum, B. S., 1975. Int. Rev. Neurobiol. 17: 1–36.
26. Hornykiewicz, O., 1972. In: Handbook of neurochemistry, Vol. 7 (Lajtha, A., ed.), pp. 465–501, Plenum Press, New York.
27. Hornykiewicz, O., Lloyd, K. G. & Davidson, L., 1976. In: The GABA system, function of the basal ganglia, and Parkinson's disease (Roberts, E., Chase, T. N. & Tower, D. B., eds.), pp. 479–485, Raven Press, New York.
28. Chase, T. N., 1976. The basal ganglia association for research in nervous and mental disease, pp. 337–349, Raven Press, New York.
29. Fischbach, G. D., 1972. Develop. Biol. 28: 407–429.
30. Ransom, B. R., Neale, E., Henkart, M., Bullock, P. N. & Nelson, P. G., 1977. J. Neurophysiol. 40: 1132–1150.
31. Neale, E. A., Macdonald, R. L. & Nelson, P. G., 1978. Brain Res. 152: 265–282.
32. Ransom, B. R., Christian, C. N., Bullock, P. N. & Nelson, P. G., 1977. J. Neurophys. 40: 1151–1162.
33. Nelson, P. G., Neale, E. A. & Macdonald, R. L., 1980. Excitable cells in Tissue culture (Nelson, P. G. & Lieberman, M., eds.), Plenum Press, New York.
34. Ransom, B. R., Bullock, P. N. & Nelson, P. G., 1977. J. Neurophysiol. 40: 1163–1177.

35. Barker, J. L. & Ransom, B. R., 1978. J. Physiol. (Lond.) 280: 331–354.

36. Macdonald, R. L. & Barker, J. L., 1980. Excitable cells in tissue culture (Nelson, P. G. & Lieberman, M., eds.), Plenum Press.

37. Fahn, S., 1976. GABA in nervous system function (Roberts, E., Chase, T. N. & Tower, D. B., eds.), pp. 169–186, Raven Press, New York.

38. Otsuka, M. & Konishi, S., 1976. GABA in nervous system function (Roberts, E., Chase, T. N. & Tower, D. B., eds.), pp. 197–202, Raven Press, New York.

39. Baxter, C. F., 1976. GABA in nervous system function (Roberts, E., Chase, T. N. & Tower, D. B., eds.), pp. 61–87, Raven Press, New York.

40. Wu, J-Y., 1976. GABA in nervous system function (Roberts, E., Chase, T. N. & Tower, D. B., eds.), pp. 7–55, Raven Press, New York.

41. McLaughlin, B. J., Barber, R., Saito, K., Roberts, E. & Wu, J-Y., 1975. J. Comp. Neurol. 164: 305–322.

42. Wood, J. G., McLaughlin, B. J. & Vaughn, J. E., 1976. GABA in nervous system function (Roberts, E., Chase, T. N. & Tower, D. B., eds.), pp. 149–168, Raven Press, New York.

43. Barber, R. P., Vaughn, J. E., Saito, K., McLaughlin, B. J. & Roberts, E., 1978. Brain Res. 141: 35–55.

44. Horton, R. W. & Meldrum, B. S., 1973. Brit. J. Pharmacol. 49: 52–63.

45. Karlsson, A., Fonnum, F., Malthe-Sorenssen, D. & Storm-Mathisen, J., 1974. Biochem. Pharmacol. 23: 3053–3061.

46. Orlowski, M., Reingold, D. F. & Stanley, M. E., 1977. J. Neurochem. 28: 349–353.

47. Salvador, R. A. & Albers, R. W., 1959. J. Biol. Chem. 234: 922–925.

48. Sheridan, J. J., Sims, K. L. & Pitts, F. N., Jr., 1967. J. Neurochem. 14: 571–578.

49. Barber, R. & Saito, K., 1976. GABA in nervous system function (Roberts, E., Chase, T. N. & Tower, D. B., eds.), pp. 113–132, Raven Press, New York.

50. Jung, M. J., Lippert, B., Metcalf, B. W., Schechter, P. J., Bohlen, P. & Sjoerdsma, A., 1977. J. Neurochem. 28: 717–723.

51. Jung, M. J., Lippert, B., Metcalf, B. W., Bohlen, P. & Schechter, P. J., 1977. J. Neurochem. 29: 797–802.

52. Jung, M. J., Lippert, B., Casara, P., Bohlen, P. & Schechter, P. J., 1978. GABA neurotransmitters: pharmacochemical, biochemical and pharmacochemical, aspects (Krogsgaard-Larsen, P., Scheel-Kruger, J. & Kofod, H., eds.), pp. 228–235, Academic Press, New York.

53. Perry, T. L., Kish, S. J. & Hansen, S., 1979. J. Neurochem. 32: 1641–1645.

54. Rando, R. R., 1978. GABA-neurotransmitters: pharmacochemical, biochemical and pharmacological aspects (Krogsgaard-Larsen, P. & Scheel-Kruger, J., eds.), pp. 228–235, Academic Press, New York.

55. Miller, A. L. & Pitts, F. N., Jr., 1967. J. Neurochem. 14: 579–584.

56. Pitts, F. N., Jr & Quick, C., 1965. J. Neurochem. 12: 893–900.

57. Godin, Y., Heiner, L., Mark, J. & Mandel, P., 1969. J. Neurochem. 16: 869–873.

58. Van Der Laan, J. W., DeBoer, T. H. & Bruinvels, J., 1979. J. Neurochem. 32: 1769–1780.

59. Macdonald, R. L. & Bergey, G. K., 1979. Brain Res. 170: 558–562.

60. Frere, R. C., Young, A. B. & Macdonald, R. L., 1980. Neurosci. Abstr. 6: 56.

61. Weinstein, H., Varon, S., Muhleman, D. R. & Roberts, E., 1965. Biochem. Pharmacol. 14: 273–388.

62. Iversen, L. L. & Neal, M. J., 1968. J. Neurochem. 15: 1141–1149.

63. Kuhar, M. J., 1973. Life Sci. 13: 1623–1634.

64. Martin, D. L., 1976. GABA in nervous system function (Roberts, E., Chase, T. N. & Tower, D. B., eds.), pp. 347–386, Raven Press, New York.

65. Iversen, L. L. & Snyder, S. H., 1968. Nature (Lond.) 220: 796–798.

66. Henn, F. A. & Hamberger, A., 1971. Proc. Nat. Acad. Sci. (USA) 68: 2686–2690.

67. Schon, F. & Kelly, J. S., 1974. Brain Res. 66: 289–300.

68. Schrier, B. K. & Thompson, E. J., 1974. J. Biol. Chem. 249: 1769–1780.

69. Hosli, L. & Hosli, E., 1979. GABA - Biochemistry and CNS functions (Mandel, P. & DeFuedis, F. V., eds.), pp. 205–218, Plenum Publishing Corp., New York.

70. Storm-Mathisen, J., Fonnum, F. & Malthe-Sorenssen, D., 1976. GABA in nervous system function (Roberts, E., Chase, T. N. & Tower, D. B., eds.), pp. 387–394, Raven Press, New York.

71. Ryan, L. D. & Roskoski, R., Jr., 1977. J. Pharmacol. Exp. Ther. 200: 285–291.

72. Levi, G., Banay-Schwartz, M. & Raiteri, M., 1978. Amino acids as chemical transmitters (Fonnum, F., ed.), pp. 327–350, Plenum Publishing Corporation, New York.

73. Cutler, R. W. P. & Young, J., 1979. Brain Res. 165: 261–270.

74. Iversen, L. L. & Bloom, F. E., 1972. Brain Res. 41: 131–143.

75. Ljungdahl, A. & Hokfelt, T., 1973. Brain Res. 62: 587–595.

76. Penney, J. B. & Young, A. B., 1980. Brain Res.

77. Hosli, E. & Hosli, L., 1978. Maturation of neurotransmission (Vernadakis, A., Giacobini, E., Filogamo, G. & Karger, S., eds.), pp. 108–115, Basel.

78. Farb, D. H., Berg, D. K. & Fischbach, G. D., 1979. J. Cell. Biol. 80: 651–661.

79. Hosli, E. & Hosli, L., 1980. Exp Brain Res. 38: 241–243.

80. Krogsgaard-Larsen, P. & Johnston, G. A. R., 1975. J. Neurochem. 25: 797–802.

81. Johnston, G. A. R., 1976. GABA in nervous system function (Roberts, E., Chase, T. N. & Tower, D. B., eds.), pp. 395–411, Raven Press, New York.

82. Wood, J. D., Tsui, D. & Phillis, J. W., 1979. Can. J. Physiol. Pharmacol. 57: 581–585.

83. Kelly, J. S. & Dick, F., 1975. Cold Spring Harbor Symp. Quant. Biol. 9: 93–106.

84. Bowery, N. G., Jones, G. P. & Neal, M. J., 1976. Nature (Lond.) 264: 281–284.

85. Brehm, L., Krogsgaard-Larsen, P. & Jacobsen, P., 1978. GABA neurotransmitters: pharmacochemical, biochemical and pharmacological aspects (Krogsgaard-Larsen, P., Scheel-Kruger, J. & Kofod, H., eds.), pp. 247–262, Academic Press, New York.

86. Iversen, L. L. & Kelly, J. S., 1975. Biochem. Pharmacol. 24: 933–938.

87. Schousboe, A., 1978. GABA neurotransmitters: pharmacochemical, biochemical and pharmacological aspects (Krogsgaard-Larsen, P., Scheel-Kruger, J. & Kofod, H., eds.), pp. 263–280, Academic Press, New York.

88. Krogsgaard-Larsen, P., Johnston, G. A. R., Curtis, D. R., Game, C. J. A. & McCulloch, R. M., 1975. J. Neurochem. 25: 803–809.

89. Lodge, D., Johnston, G. A. R., Curtis, D. R. & Brand, J., 1977. Brain Res. 136: 513–522.

90. Hammerstad, J. P., Murray, J. E. & Cutler, R. W. P., 1971. Brain Res. 35: 357–367.

91. Mitchell, J. F. & Roberts, P. J., 1972. Br. J. Pharmacol. 45: 175–176P.

92. Levy, W. B., Redburn, D. A. & Cotman, C. W., 1973. Science 181: 676–678.

93. Mulder, A. H. & Snyder, S. H., 1974. Brain Res. 76: 297–308.

94. Gauchy, C. M., Iversen, L. L. & Jessell, T. M., 1977. Brain Res. 138: 374–379.

95. Vargas, O., DeLorenzo, M., Saldate, M. & Orrego, F., 1977. J. Neurochem. 28: 165–170.

96. Sellstrom, A. & Hamberger, A., 1977. Brain Res. 119: 189–198.

97. Hammerstad, J. P., Cawthon, M. L. & Lytle, C. R., 1979. J. Neurochem. 32: 195–202.

98. Leach, M. J., 1979. J. Pharm. Pharmacol. 31: 533–535.

99. Szerb, J. C., 1979. J. Neurochem. 32: 1565–1573.

100. Collins, G. G. S., 1973. Br. J. Pharmacol. 47: 641P.

101. Cotman, C. W., Haycock, J. W. & White, W. F., 1976. J. Physiol. (Lond.) 254: 475–505.

102. Srinivasan, V., Neal, M. J. & Mitchell, J. F., 1969. J. Neurochem. 16: 1235–1244.

103. Bowery, N. G. & Brown, D. A., 1972. Nature, New Biol. 238: 89–91.

104. Bowery, N. G. & Neal, M. J., 1978. J. Physiol. (Lond.) 275: 58P.

105. Minchin, M. C. W., 1975. J. Neurochem. 24: 571–577.

106. Starr, M. S., 1979. Eur. J. Pharmacol. 53: 215–226.

107. Stoof, J. C., DenBreejen, E. J. S. & Mulder, A. H., 1979. Eur. J. Pharmacol. 57: 35–42.

108. Kamal, L., Arbilla, S. & Langer, S. Z., 1980. Presynaptic receptors (Langer, S. Z. et al., eds.), pp. 193–197, Pergamon Press, New York.

109. Bowery, N. G., Hill, D. R., Hudson, A. L., Doble, A., Middlemiss, D. N., Shaw, J. & Turnbull, M., 1980. Nature (Lond.) 283: 92–94.

110. Zukin, S. R., Young, A. B. & Snyder, S. H., 1974. Proc. Natl. Acad. Sci. (USA) 71: 4802–4807.

111. Enna, S. J. & Snyder, S. H., 1975. Brain Res. 100: 81–97.

112. Olsen, R. W., Greenlee, D., VanNess, P. & Ticku, M. K., 1978. Amino acids as chemical transmitters (Fonnum, F., ed.), Plenum Press, New York.

113. Olsen, R. W., Ticku, M. K., Greenlee, D. & VanNess, P., 1978. GABA neurotransmitters: pharmacochemical, biochemical and pharmacological aspects (Krogsgaard-Larsen, P., Scheel-Kruger, J. & Kofod, H., eds.), pp. 165–178, Academic Press, New York.

114. Olsen, R. W., Ticku, M. K., VanNess, P. C. & Greenlee, D., 1978. Brain Res. 139: 277–294.

115. Young, A. B. & Macdonald, R. L., 1979. Neurosci. Abstr. 5: 602.

116. Macdonald, R. L., Young, A. B. & Nowak, L. M., 1979. Neurosci. Abstr. 5: 593.

117. DeFeudis, F. V., Ossola, L., Schmitt, G., Wolff, P. & Mandel, P., 1980. J. Neurochem. 34: 216–218.

118. Ticku, M. K., Huang, A. & Barker, J. L., 1980. Brain Res. 182: 201–206.

119. Enna, S. J. & Snyder, S. H., 1977. Mol. Pharmacol. 13: 442–453.

120. Young, A. B., Enna, S. J., Zukin, S. R. & Snyder, S. H., 1976. GABA in nervous system function (Roberts, E., Chase, T. N. & Tower, D. B., eds.), pp. 305–317, Raven Press, New York.

121. Greenlee, D. V., VanNess, P. C. & Olsen, R. W., 1978. Life Sci. 22: 1653–1662.

122. Guidotti, A., Toffano, G. & Costa, E., 1978. Nature (Lond.) 275: 553–555.

123. Toffano, G., Guidotti, A. & Costa, E., 1978. Proc. Nat. Acad. Sci. (USA) 75: 4024–4028.

124. Enna, S. J., Ferkany, J. W. & Krogsgaard-Larsen, P., 1978. GABA neurotransmitters: pharmacochemical, biochemical and pharmacological aspects (Krogsgaard-Larsen, P., Scheel-Kruger, J. & Kofod, H., eds.), pp. 191–200, Academic Press, New York.

125. Placheta, P. & Karobath, M., 1979. Brain Res. 178: 580–583.

126. Beaumont, K., Chilton, W. S., Yamamura, H. I. & Enna, S. J., 1978. Brain Res. 148: 153–162.

127. Snodgrass, S. R., 1978. Nature (Lond.) 273: 392–394.

128. Williams, M. & Risley, E. A., 1979. J. Neurochem. 32: 713–718.

129. Guidotti, A., Gale, K., Suria, A. & Toffano, G., 1979. Brain Res. 172: 566–571.

130. Enna, S. J. & Maggi, A., 1979. Life Sci. 24: 1727–1738.

131. Galli, A., Zilletti, L., Scotton, M., Adembri, G. & Giotti, A., 1979. J. Neurochem. 32: 1123–1125.

132. Krogsgaard-Larsen, P., Honore, J. & Thyssen, K., 1978. GABA neurotransmitters: pharmacochemical, biochemical and pharmacological aspects (Krogsgaard-Larsen, P., Scheel-Kruger, J. & Kofod, H., eds.), pp. 201–216, Academic Press, New York.

133. Krogsgaard-Larsen, P., Hjeds, H., Curtis, D. R., Lodge, D. & Johnston, G. A. R., 1979. J. Neurochem. 32: 1717–1724.

134. Krogsgaard-Larsen, P., Johnston, G. A. R., Lodge, D. & Curtis, D. R., 1977. Nature (Lond.) 268: 53–55.

135. Krogsgaard-Larsen, P. & Johnston, G. A. R., 1978. J. Neurochem. 30: 1377–1382.

136. Enna, S. J., Collins, J. F. & Snyder, S. H., 1977. Brain Res. 124: 185–190.

137. Olsen, R. W., Ban, M. & Miller, T., 1976. Brain Res. 102: 283–299.

138. Cleland, W. W., 1963. Biochem. Biophys. Acta 67: 188–196.

162

139. Collins, J. F. & Cryer, G., 1978. Amino acids as chemical transmitters (Fonnum, F., ed.), pp. 499–506, Plenum Press, New York.

140. Mohler, H. & Okada, T., 1977. Nature (Lond.) 267: 65–67.

141. Mohler, H. & Okada, T., 1978. Amino acids as chemical transmitters (Fonnum, F., ed.), pp. 493–498, Plenum Press, New York.

142. Ticku, M. K., Ban, M. & Olsen, R. W., 1978. Mol. Pharmacol. 14: 391–402.

143. Braestrup, C. & Squires, R. F., 1978. Eur. J. Pharmacol. 48: 263–270.

144. Tallman, J. F., Thomas, J. W. & Gallager, D. W., 1978. Nature (Lond.) 274: 383–385.

145. Martin, I. L. & Candy, J. M., 1978. Neuropharmacology 17: 993–998.

146. Tallman, J. F. & Gallager, D. W., 1979. Pharmacol. Biochem. Behav. 10: 809–813.

147. Costa, T., Robard, D. & Pert, C. B., 1979. Nature (Lond.) 277: 315–317.

148. Gavish, M., Chang, R. S. L. & Snyder, S. H., 1979. Life Sci. 25: 783–790.

149. Gavish, M. & Snyder, S. H., 1980. Life Sci. 26: 579–582.

150. Eccles, J. C., 1964. The Physiology of Synapses, Springer-Verlag, Berlin.

151. Levy, R. A., 1977. Prog. Neurobiol. 9: 211–267.

152. Eccles, J. C., Kostyuk, P. G. & Schmidt, R. F., 1962. J. Physiol. (Lond.) 161: 237–257.

153. Eccles, J. C., Schmidt, R. F. & Willis, W. D., 1963. J. Physiol. (Lond.) 168: 500–530.

154. Schmidt, R. F., 1963. Pflugers Arch. Ges. Physiol. 277: 325–346.

155. Tebecis, A. K. & Phillis, J. W., 1967. Comp. Biochem. Physiol. 23: 553–563.

156. Davidoff, R. A., 1972. Science 175: 331–333.

157. Barker, J. L. & Nicoll, R. A., 1972. Science 176: 1043–1045.

158. Feltz, P. & Rasminsky, M., 1974. Neuropharmacol. 13: 553–563.

159. Nishi, S., Minota, S. & Karczmar, A. G., 1974. Neuropharmacol. 13: 215–219.

160. Deschenes, M., Feltz, P. & Lamour, Y., 1976. Brain Res. 118: 486–492.

161. Gallagher, J. P., Higashi, H. & Nishi, S., 1978. J. Physiol. (Lond.) 275: 263–282.

162. Nicoll, R. A., 1978. J. Physiol. (Lond.) 283: 121–132.

163. Sykova, E. & Vyklicky, L., 1978. Neurosciences 3: 1061–1067.

164. Davidoff, R. A., Hackman, J. C. & Osorio, I., 1980. Neurosciences 5: 117–126.

165. Krnjevic, K., Puil, E. & Werman, R., 1977. Can. J. Physiol. Pharmacol. 55: 658–669.

166. Krnjevic, K.; 1976. GABA in nervous system function (Roberts, E., Chase, T. N. & Tower, D. B., eds.), pp. 269–281, Raven Press, New York.

167. Curtis, D. R., Duggan, A. W., Felix, D. & Johnston, G. A. R., 1971. Brain Res. 32: 69–96.

168. Bruggencate, G. ten & Engberg, I., 1968. Brain Res. 11: 446–450.

169. Curtis, D. R., Hosli, L. & Johnston, G. A. R., 1968. Exp. Brain Res. 6: 1–18.

170. Curtis, D. R., Hosli, L., Johnston, G. A. R. & Johnston, I. H., 1968. Exp. Brain Res. 5: 235–258.

171. Werman, R., Davidoff, R. A. & Aprison, M. H., 1968. J. Neurophysiol. 31: 81–95.

172. Barker, J. L., Macdonald, R. L. & Smith, T. G., 1977. J. Gen. Physiol. 70: 1a.

173. McBurney, R. N. & Barker, J. L., 1978. Nature (Lond.) 274: 596–597.

174. Macdonald, R. L. & Barker, J. L., 1977. Nature (Lond.) 267, 720–721.

175. Macdonald, R. L. & Barker, J. L., 1978. Neurology 28: 325–330.

176. Takeuchi, A. & Onodera, K., 1972. Nature New Biol. 236: 55–56.

177. Shank, R. P., Pong, S. F., Freeman, A. R. & Graham, L. T., 1974. Brain Res. 72: 71–78.

178. Constanti, A., 1978. Neuropharmacol. 17: 159–167.

179. Homma, S. & Rovainen, C. M., 1978. J. Physiol. (Lond.) 279: 231–252.

180. Simmonds, M. A., 1978. Br. J. Pharmacol. 63: 495–502.

181. Simmonds, M. A., 1980. Neuropharmacol. 19: 39–45.

182. Takeuchi, A. & Takeuchi, N., 1969. J. Physiol. (Lond.) 205: 377–391.

183. Earl, J. & Large, W. A., 1974. J. Physiol. (Lond.) 236: 113–127.

184. Hori, N., Ikeda, K. & Roberts, E., 1978. Brain Res. 141: 364–370.

185. Hochner, B., Spira, M. E. & Werman, R., 1976. Brain Res. 107: 85–103.

186. Pickles, H. G. & Simmonds, M. A., 1980. Neuropharmacology 19: 35–38.

187. Yamamoto, C., 1972. Exp. Neurol. 35: 154–164.

188. Matsumoto, H., 1964. Electroencephalogr. Clin. Neurophysiol. 17: 294–307.

189. Prince, D. A., 1968. Exper. Neurol. 21: 467–485.

190. Dichter, M. & Spencer, W. A., 1969. J. Neurophysiol. 32: 663–687.

191. Wong, R. K. S. & Prince, D. A., 1978. Brain Res. 159: 385–390.

192. Wong, R. K. S., Prince, D. A. & Basbaum, A. I., 1979. Proc. Natl. Acad. Sci. (USA) 76: 986–990.

193. Wong, R. K. S. & Prince, D. A., 1970. Science 204: 1228–1231.

194. Weakly, J. N., 1969. J. Physiol. (Lond.) 204: 63–77.

195. Thomson, T. D. & Turkanis, S. A., 1973. Br. J. Pharmacol. 48: 48–58.

196. Proctor, W. R. & Weakly, J. N., 1976. J. Physiol. (Lond.) 258: 257–268.

197. Choi, D. W., Farb, D. H. & Fischbach, G. D., 1977. Nature (Lond.) 269: 342–344.

198. Raabe, W. & Gumnit, R. J., 1977. Epilepsia 18: 117–120.

199. Gahwiler, B. H., 1976. Brain Res. 107: 176–179.

200. Steiner, F. A. & Felix, D., 1976. Nature (Lond.) 260: 346–347.

201. Macdonald, R. L. & Barker, J. L., 1978. Science 200: 775–777.

202. Macdonald, R. L. & Barker, J. L., 1978. Nature (Lond.) 271: 563–564.

203. Macdonald, R. L. & Barker, J. L., 1979. Neurology 29: 432–447.

Received October 1, 1980.

Molecular characteristics of glutamate receptors in the mammalian brain

E. K. Michaelis, M. L. Michaelis, H. H. Chang, R. D. Grubbs, and D. R. Kuonen
Neurobiology Section, Dept. of Human Development and Drug Design Program, University of Kansas Lawrence KS 66045, U.S.A.

Summary

The strong excitatory activity of L-glutamic acid on central nervous system neurons is thought to be produced by interaction of this amino acid with specific neuronal plasma membrane receptors. The binding of L-glutamate to these surface receptors brings about an increase in membrane permeability to Na^+ and Ca^{2+} ions presumably through direct activation of ion channels linked to the membrane receptors. The studies described in this paper represent attempts to define the subcellular distribution and pharmacological properties of the recognition site for L-glutamic acid in brain neuronal preparations, to isolate and explore the molecular characteristics of the receptor recognition site, and, finally, to demonstrate the activation of Na^+ channels in synaptic membranes following the interaction of glutamate with its receptors.

Radioligand binding assays with L-[³H] glutamic acid have been used to demonstrate a relative enrichment of these glutamate recognition sites in isolated synaptic plasma membranes. The specific binding of L-[³H] glutamate to these membrane sites exhibits rapid association and dissociation kinetics and rather complex equilibrium binding kinetics. The glutamate binding macromolecule from synaptic membranes has been solubilized and purified and was shown to be a small molecular weight glycoprotein ($M_r \approx 13\,000$). This protein tends to form aggregates which have higher specific activity at low (nM) concentrations of glutamate than the M_r 13 000 protein has. The overall affinity of the purified protein is lower than that of the high affinity sites in the membrane. Nevertheless, the purified protein exhibits pharmacological characteristics very similar to those of the membrane binding sites. On the basis of its pharmacological properties this protein belongs in the category of the physiologic 'glutamate preferring' receptors.

By means of differential solubilization of membrane proteins with Na-cholate, it was shown that this recognition site is an intrinsic synaptic membrane protein whose binding activity is enhanced rather than diminished by cholate extraction of the synaptic membranes. The role of membrane constituents in regulating the binding activity of this protein has been explored and a possible modulation of glutamate binding by membrane gangliosides has been demonstrated. Finally, this glutamate binding glycoprotein is a metalloprotein whose activity is dependent on the integrity of its metallic (Fe) center. This is a clear distinguishing characteristic of this protein vis-à-vis the glutamate transport carriers.

The presence of functional glutamate receptors in synaptosomes and resealed synaptic plasma membranes has also been documented by the demonstration of glutamate-activated Na^+ flux across the membrane of these preparations. The bidirectionality, temperature independence, and apparent desensitization of this stimulated flux following exposure to high concentrations of glutamate are properties indicative of a receptor-initiated ion channel activation. It would appear, then, that the synaptic membrane preparations provide a very useful system for the study of both recognition and effector function of the glutamate receptor complex.

Molecular and Cellular Biochemistry 38, 163–179 (1981). 0300-8177/81/0381-0163/$ 3.40.

Introduction

The dicarboxylic amino acids L-glutamic acid and L-aspartic acid appear to have multiple roles in the central nervous system of both vertebrates and invertebrates. In addition to their known involvement in a number of metabolic processes and in the synthesis of nerve cell proteins, these dicarboxylic amino acids also induce a rather strong electrical depolarization of nerve cell membranes (1, 2, 3). The excitatory effects of L-glutamate and L-aspartate on central nervous system cells were first described by Curtis and Watkins (1). These researchers also outlined the basic structural features of the active site of membrane receptors with which the dicarboxylic amino acids and their structural analogs were thought to interact (1, 4). These early studies of the structure-activity relationships for neuronal excitation outlined the receptor and agonist features that were necessary for optimal receptor activation. Based on the findings from these studies it was proposed that the active site of the receptor must contain two regions which bear positively charged groups which can interact with the α and β or the α and γ carboxyl groups of aspartate and glutamate respectively. A third region with a negatively charged group which can interact with the positively charged α amino group of these two amino acids must also be a component of the receptor active site (1). The presence of such neuronal receptors for the dicarboxylic amino acids which face towards the extracellular environment of the plasma membrane was suggested by the fact that L-glutamate injected intra-neuronally did not produce any electrical excitation while the extracellular application of this amino acid excited almost all neurons within the central nervous system (5).

The biochemical or molecular explorations of the putative receptor sites for the dicarboxylic amino acids in mammalian neurons and in invertebrate muscle preparations was not attempted until recently (6, 7, 8, 9, 10). The definition of receptor activity in these studies relied heavily on the characterization of what is considered to be the first step in receptor activation, that is, the amino acid binding to the recognition site of the receptor macromolecular complex. The binding of radioactively labeled L-glutamic acid (6, 7), of L-aspartic acid (11), or of the potent neuroexcitatory glutamate analog kainic acid (10), to various brain subcellular preparations was determined in these studies and was correlated with the known neurophysiologic and neuropharmacologic specificity of the receptor sites for the dicarboxylic amino acids and their analogs. It is obvious that any attempt to define the molecular characteristics of physiological receptor sites based on the study of the binding of dicarboxylic amino acids to various brain or muscle subcellular fractions would be fraught with ambiguity concerning the specificity of the labeling of such putative physiologic receptors. For example, there are a number of enzymes associated with neuronal and glial membranes and cytoplasm which utilize L-glutamic acid as their substrate, such as glutamate dehydrogenase, glutamine synthetase, γ-glutamyl transpeptidase, or L-glutamic acid decarboxylase (12, 13, 14). In addition, both neuronal and glial membranes are known to contain very active, high affinity ($K_T = 2$-10 μM) transport carriers for the dicarboxylic amino acids (15, 16). Thus, the use of binding sites for the definition of the physiologic receptors for L-glutamic acid (or for L-aspartic acid) would necessitate that some distinction be drawn between the binding of this putative transmitter agent to its receptors and binding to the active sites of various enzymes or uptake carriers.

Furthermore, it would be necessary not only to correlate the pharmacological specificity of such binding interactions with the known pharmacology of glutamate or aspartate-induced neuronal excitation, but also to define the specific subcellular sites for such binding interactions and, ultimately, to purify the binding or recognition macromolecule and to study it in isolation. It is only through the latter type of exploration that one may be able to draw a clear distinction between the molecular characteristics of these putative receptors and those of well-studied enzyme proteins. Finally, the endeavor of receptor identification would be optimized if a functional parameter of the activation of these receptors could be measured in the same preparations which are used for the definition of receptor recognition sites. In invertebrate neuromuscular junctions the interaction of L-glutamic acid with its membrane receptors is known to increase the flux of Na^+ and Ca^{2+} through the plasma membrane into the intracellular space (17, 18). These receptor-mediated increases in ion fluxes are responsible for the electrical depolarization of the cells (17, 18). Therefore, the characterization of the glutamate-stimulated Na^+ or Ca^{2+} flux into the intracellular (or subcellular) space of central nervous system neurons could be used as a measure of receptor function and could be correlated with the specific L-glutamic acid binding activity of the same neuronal preparations. The investigations which have been conducted in our laboratory have involved all of these approaches in an effort to delineate the molecular and supramolecular characteristics of the glutamate receptor sites in neuronal membranes.

Subcellular distribution and kinetics of L-[³H] glutamate binding to brain tissue

In the initial studies which were conducted to determine the presence of specific L-glutamic acid receptor sites in brain preparations (6), an equilibrium dialysis binding assay was used to measure the binding of L-glutamic acid to brain homogenates and other brain subcellular fractions. These studies revealed the presence of Na^+-independent, high affinity ($K_D = 0.2 \mu M$) glutamate binding sites in brain homogenate and in subcellular fractions enriched in plasma membranes. The highest binding activity for radioactively labeled L-glutamate was associated with the synaptic plasma membrane subfraction. The binding of L-glutamic acid as measured in the dilute buffer media used in those studies (10 mM K-phosphate buffer, pH 7.4) exhibited a high degree of stereoselectivity as demonstrated by the fact that an excess of the D-enantiomer brought about only a small inhibition of L-glutamic acid binding. However, the equilibrium dialysis method used in the determination of specific glutamate binding sites in the synaptic membrane preparations provided a high estimate of the total density of such sites. This overestimate of glutamate binding may have been due to a considerable contribution by non-specific glutamate binding interactions with these particulate fractions.

The availability of radioactive L-[³H] glutamic acid of high specific activity (40–50 Ci/mmol), together with the development of a rapid microfuge centrifugation binding assay (19, 20), has led to a more precise estimate of the specific glutamate

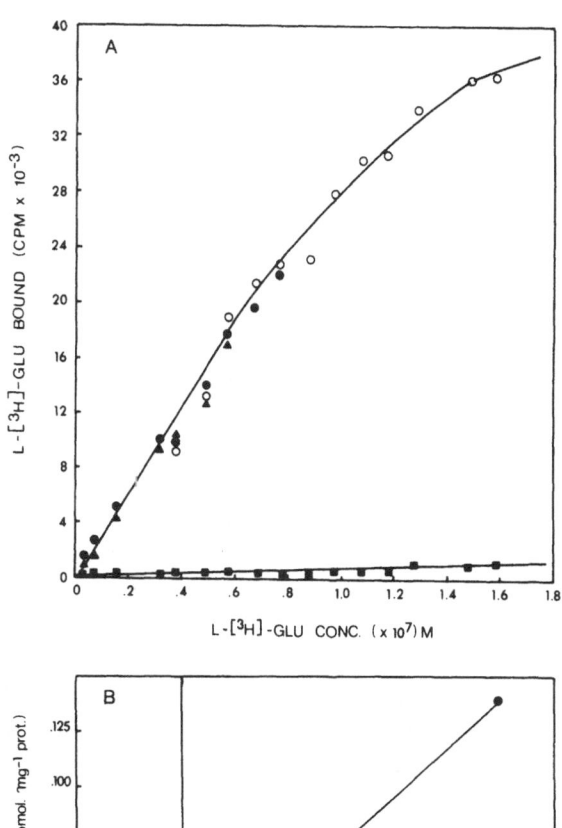

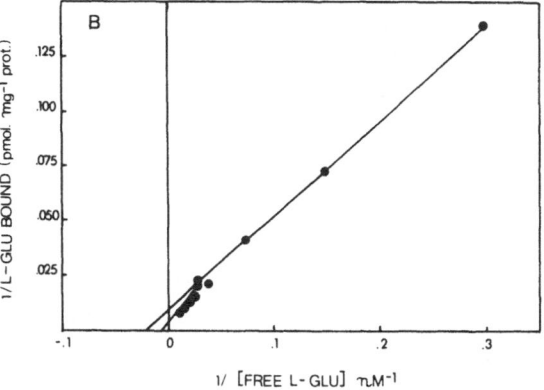

Fig. 1. L-[³H] Glutamic acid binding to brain synaptic membranes. (A) Specific and non-specific binding of L-[³H] glutamic acid at various ligand concentrations was measured by incubating 5 μl aliquots of synaptic membrane preparations (1.68 mg protein/ml) with 95 μl of potassium phosphate buffer for 25 min at 25 °C in the presence of 10^{-4} M p-chloromercuribenzene sulfonate (19). Non-specific (■) binding is the amount of L-[³H] glutamate bound in the presence of 0.1 mM L-glutamate. L-[³H] Glutamate binding was measured by the microfuge centrifugation method (19). Each symbol used for the data points of the specific binding (●, ○, ▲) represents the mean of triplicate determinations from a single experiment. Aliquots from the same batch of synaptic membranes were employed for all binding assays. (B) Inverse plot of L[³H] glutamate binding data obtained from a single experiment conducted as described in (A). Each point is the mean of triplicate determinations, and line fitting for each of the linear segments was done by the method of Least Squares. The estimated K_D's were 60 nM and 208 nM for the high and low affinity sites respectively, and the estimated maximum number of binding sites were 135 and 381 pmol · mg⁻¹ protein respectively.

Table 1. Specific binding of L-glutamate to brain subfractions and liver particulate preparations. The binding of L-[³H] glutamic acid (65.1 nM) was measured under identical conditions for all subfractions. The liver particulate fraction represents the pellet obtained following centrifugation of the homogenate at $39\,000 \times g$ for 25 min. All assays were conducted at 25 °C for 25 min according to the method in (19). Each value is the mean ± S. E. M. of the number of determinations in parentheses.

| Tissue subcellular fraction | L-[³H] glutamate bound (pmol · mg⁻¹ protein) | | | |
	Krebs medium		Phosphate buffer	
Brain Homogenate	0.69 ± 0.20	(3)	0.70 ± 0.06	(3)
Crude mitochondrial	1.59 ± 0.24	(5)	N.D.*	
Synaptosomes	2.32 ± 0.41	(4)	N.D.*	
Synaptic membranes	5.90 ± 0.67	(20)	5.027 ± 0.95	(9)
Liver particulate	0	(4)	0.13 ± 0.08	(4)

* N.D. = not determined.

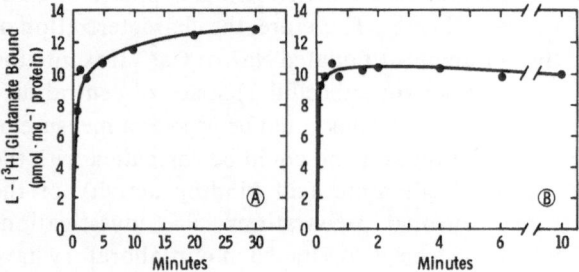

Fig. 2. Time kinetics of specific L-[³H] glutamate binding determined in phosphate buffer systems at 25 °C (A) and 37 °C (B). Each set of binding data was obtained from a single batch of membrane preparations and represents the mean of 3–8 determinations for each data point. L-[³H] Glutamic acid (65.1 nM) and 0.1 mM p-chloromercuribenzene sulfonate were present in all samples. Non-specific binding was determined in triplicate for each time period according to the procedures described for Fig. 1.

binding sites associated with various subcellular preparations and has been valuable in the study of the kinetic characteristics of L-[³H] glutamate binding to specific sites in neuronal membranes. The subcellular distribution of L-[³H] glutamic acid binding as measured by this technique was found to be very similar to that which was previously described (6, 21). The synaptic plasma membrane subfraction consistently has a 7–8 fold enrichment in L-glutamic acid binding activity when compared to that of the brain homogenate preparation (Table 1). In comparison, a particulate fraction from rat liver used as an example of non-neuronal tissue had very low specific glutamate binding activity (Table 1). The two-fold enrichment of specific L-[³H] glutamate binding sites in synaptic membranes as compared to the synaptosomal fraction was paralleled by the nearly two-fold greater activity of (Na⁺–K⁺)-ATPase, a plasma marker enzyme: 6.0 μmol P_i · mg⁻¹ · h⁻¹ in the synaptic membranes compared to 3.4 μmol P_i · mg⁻¹ · h⁻¹ in the synaptosomes (22). This indicates that the glutamate binding sites are co-purified together with the neuronal plasma membrane fractions.

When the glutamate interaction with the synaptic plasma membranes was measured in a K-phosphate buffer medium at 25 °C, there was a clearly distinguishable and quite substantial specific L-[³H] glutamic acid binding component (Fig. 1A). Over the same range of concentrations, the non-specifically bound ligand remained quite low,

usually representing less than 10% of the bound L-[³H] glutamic acid. Inverse plot analysis of the equilibrium binding data from different membrane preparations has revealed the presence of two distinct binding sites, a high affinity group of sites with an apparent $K_D = 60$–70 nM and a lower affinity set of sites with a $K_D = 208$–295 nM. The maximum numbers of binding sites associated with these two binding systems were found to be 70–135 and 208–381 pmol per mg respectively. An example of this is shown in Fig. 1B.

The time kinetics of L-[³H] glutamate binding to the synaptic membranes were found to be dependent on the temperature of the incubation medium (Fig. 2). Binding of glutamate to the synaptic membranes was a rapid process reaching equilibrium within 45–60 sec at 37 °C (Fig. 2B). At 25 °C, there was an early, rapid rate of ligand association with the binding site (80% of equilibrium binding achieved within 60 sec) which was followed by a slower rate of association of glutamate with its binding sites (Fig. 2A). Very similar binding kinetics have been observed when the assays were conducted in the presence of a more physiological medium (Krebs-Henseleit buffer), although the initial rapid phase of binding which occurs in this medium represents only 50–60% of equilibrium binding. Dissociation of L-[³H] glutamic acid from its binding sites measured in a Krebs buffer medium was rapid and complete if excess nonlabeled glutamate was added at an early point in the incubation period (45 sec), and it was somewhat slower and less

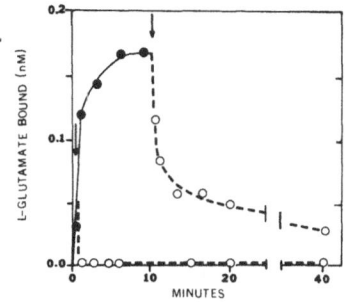

Fig. 3. Association and dissociation kinetics of L-[³H] glutamate binding to synaptic membranes. The membranes (300 μl, 2.0 mg protein/ml) were incubated at 25 °C in Krebs buffer medium which contained 65.1 nM L-[³H] glutamate. At the time periods indicated by the arrows unlabeled L-glutamate was added to an aliquot of the incubation mixture to bring the final concentration to 0.1 mM. Each point is the mean of triplicate determinations of specific L-[³H] glutamate binding determined by the microfuge centrifugation assay method described in (19). Samples which received 0.1 mM L-glutamate are indicated by the symbols (O—O).

complete if nonlabeled ligand was added at a later time (10 min) as shown in Fig. 3. Since the concentration of L-[³H] glutamic acid in the assay (65 nM) was greatly in excess of the concentration of binding sites associated with this membrane preparation (5.6 nM) as estimated from inverse plot analysis, the association of glutamate with its receptor could be considered as a pseudo first-order reaction. The observed rate constant for association, k_{obs}, was 0.379 min⁻¹, and from the equation:

$$k_{assoc} = (k_{obs} - k_{dissoc})/[\text{Glutamate}],$$

the rate constant k_{assoc} was calculated to be $k_{assoc} = 2.61 \times 10^6$ M⁻¹ min⁻¹. The k_{dissoc} was estimated from the rate of dissociation of bound L-[³H] glutamic acid (after 10 min of incubation, Fig. 3) and was found to be $k_{dissoc} = 0.209$ min⁻¹. From these rate constants, an apparent K_D for these sites was obtained, $K_D = 80.06$ nM, a value quite close to that K_D estimated from equilibrium kinetics for L-[³H] glutamate binding to the high affinity sites (Fig. 1).

The presence of a small residual fraction of bound L-[³H] glutamate even 30 min after the addition of excess unlabeled L-glutamic acid (Fig. 3) may be indicative of the formation of a slowly reversible ligand-receptor complex. Results similar to those shown in Fig. 3 were obtained if a 20-fold dilution of the incubation medium which contained

the synaptic membranes and 1 μM L-[³H] glutamate with phosphate or Krebs buffer was introduced. Incubation for 2 min after the dilution with buffer followed by centrifugation at 53 000 × g for 15 min (4 °C) led to the dissociation of 89% of bound L-[³H] glutamate from synaptic membrane sites. It is considered unlikely that the remaining slowly reversible fraction of bound L-[³H] glutamate represents a metabolite of the L-[³H] glutamic acid in the incubation medium since greater than 98% of the L-[³H] glutamic acid added was recovered as unaltered L-[³H] glutamic acid at the end of the incubation period. This was determined by thin layer chromatography of the supernatant from trichloroacetic acid-precipitated tissue suspensions. A somewhat similar slow dissociation of agonists from their binding sites has also been described previously for the dissociation kinetics of β-andrenergic receptor agonists (23) and was thought to represent binding to high affinity sites. This slowly dissociable species may also represent L-[³H] glutamate binding to a subpopulation of high affinity sites.

Pharmacologic characteristics of high affinity glutamate binding

The displacement of bound L-[³H] glutamic acid (65.1 nM) by unlabeled L-glutamate, as well as by unlabeled L-aspartate and L-cysteine sulfinic acid (Fig. 4A), further confirmed the presence of mul-

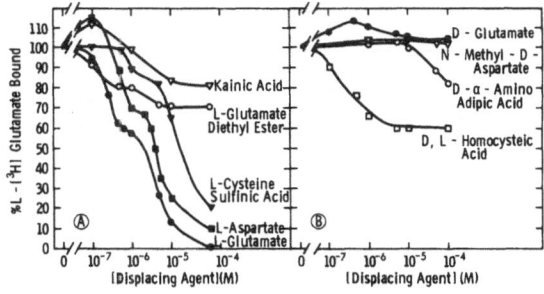

Fig. 4. Displacement of specific L-[³H] glutamate binding to synaptic membranes by glutamate (A) and N-methyl-D-aspartate (B) receptor agonists and antagonists. The displacement of bound L-[³H] glutamic acid (65.1 nM) was determined in phosphate buffer at 25 ° C. Non-specific binding was measured in triplicate samples for the controls and for each concentration of the displacing ligand used. Each data point is the mean of 6–12 determinations from 2–4 separate experiments. The computed standard errors were less than 10% of the mean.

tiple equilibria observed in the direct study of L-[^{3}H] glutamic acid binding (Fig. 1). At least two processes were detected when unlabeled L-glutamic acid was used as the displacing agent in the concentration range of 0.1–100 μM (Fig. 4A). The first displacement process appeared to be complete at a concentration of 1 μM L-glutamate and had an estimated $K_I = 0.16$ μM, whereas the second process, which occurred at glutamate concentrations of 2–100 μM had a $K_I = 2.64$ μM. Since the concentrations of unlabeled glutamate employed in these studies were in a range higher than those used for the direct determination of equilibrium binding kinetics (Fig. 1), and since the concentration of L-[^{3}H] glutamate was very close to the K_D for the high affinity sites, there was apparently no displacement observed from the sites which would correspond to the highest affinity group ($K_D = 60$–70 nM). However, the first K_I which was obtained from the displacement assays (0.16 μM) was quite close to the higher K_D (0.2–0.3 μM) for the group of sites shown in Fig. 1 and almost identical to the lower K_D determined previously by equilibrium dialysis (6). The displacement assays also revealed the presence of a group of sites with an even lower affinity ($K_I = 2.64$ μM), which once again, corresponded very well with the higher K_D for glutamate binding estimated previously by the equilibrium dialysis method ($K_D = 2.08$ μM) (6).

Low concentrations of L-aspartate tended to increase L-[^{3}H] glutamate binding by a process which was suggestive of homotropic cooperative interactions between these two ligands and the specific glutamate binding sites on the membranes (Fig. 4A). The increase in glutamate binding activity observed in the presence of L-aspartate may represent a correlate of the demonstrated enhancement by L-aspartic acid of the physiologic response to L-glutamic acid in invertebrate neuro-muscular preparations (24, 25). The estimated K_I values for all agents tested are summarized in Table 2. It is interesting to note that some agents apparently caused displacement from only one group of L-glutamate binding sites. For example, D,L-homocysteic acid and glutamate diethyl ester appeared to displace glutamate from the higher affinity group of sites (Fig. 4A and 4B).

The excitatory amino acids D-glutamate, L-homocysteic acid, and, to a lesser extent, D-homocysteic acid are thought to interact primarily with receptor sites which are sensitive to the application of N-methyl-D-aspartate (26). These receptor sites are pharmacologically quite distinct from the L-glutamate physiologic receptors (26). The low level of L-[^{3}H] glutamate displacement by N-methyl-D-aspartate, D-glutamate, and even D,L-homocysteic acid (Fig. 4B) would appear to fit the probable labeling by L-[^{3}H] glutamic acid of sites known as 'L-glutamate-preferring' sites (26). This is further supported by the fact that D-α-aminoadipic acid, which is considered to be a specific antagonist of excitation produced by N-methyl-D-aspartate but only a weak antagonist of excitation which is produced by L-glutamate (26), was a relatively weak displacing agent of L-[^{3}H] glutamic acid (Fig. 4B). On the other hand, glutamate diethyl ester, a somewhat stronger glutamate antagonist, was a better inhibitor of glutamate binding, especially at micromolar concentrations (Fig. 4A). Thus it appears, that on the basis of the patterns of ligand displacement, the sites which have previously been designated as the 'L-glutamate-preferring' receptors may be selectively labeled by L-[^{3}H] glutamic acid in these membrane preparations. This selectivity may be due to the fact

Table 2. Apparent K_I values and maximum displacement of L-[^{3}H] glutamate from synaptic membranes by various amino acids and amino acid analogs.

Agonists–antagonists	K_I for glutamate sites		Max. displacement at 0.1 mM
	High affinity	Low affinity	
Glutamate receptors			
L-glutamate	0.16	2.64	100%
L-aspartate	0.36	3.26	89%
L-cysteine sulfinic acid	0.52	14.56	78%
Glutamate diethyl ester	0.16	–	30%
Kainic acid	–	–	18%
N-methyl-D-aspartate receptors			
N-methyl-D-aspartate	–	–	0
D,L-homocysteic acid	0.15	–	40%
D-glutamate	–	–	0%
D-α-amino adipate	–	–	18%
Inhibitory amino acid receptors			
γ-aminobutyric acid	–	–	0%
Glycine	–	–	0%

that the membranes used in the present studies were prepared and stored in a Mg^{2+}-EDTA medium according to procedures published previously (22). This type of preparation may cause decreases in the activity of N-methyl-D-aspartate receptor sites since these receptor sites are known to be easily deactivated by low concentrations of Mg^{2+} ions (27). An alternative possibility is that N-methyl-D-aspartate sites represent only a small proportion of the total sites with which L-[³H] glutamate can interact, and consequently, agents which act on those sites cause the displacement of small amounts of L-[³H] glutamic acid.

The observation that kainic acid, a strong neuro-excitatory amino acid analog (26), did not produce significant displacement of L-[³H] glutamate from its binding sites was also of particular interest. The ineffectiveness of kainic acid in displacing bound glutamate has been observed when displacement assays were conducted in a dilute phosphate buffer (Fig. 4A) or in the more physiologic Krebs buffer medium (data not shown). Thus it is unlikely that the lack of displacing activity by kainate represents an artifact of the conditions of the assay. A probable explanation for this paradoxically low displacing activity will be presented in a later section.

Na^+ channel activation in synaptic membranes by L-glutamic acid

In addition to demonstrating the presence of high affinity binding sites for L-[³H] glutamic acid, we have also been able to show that in both intact synaptosomes, as well as in isolated and resealed synaptic plasma membranes, there is an enhancement of basal Na^+ influx in response to micromolar concentrations of L-glutamic acid (22). Incubation of synaptosomal preparations with 0.01–100 μM L-glutamic acid led to concentration-dependent increases in ^{22}Na uptake (Fig. 5A). The effect of L-glutamate on ^{22}Na influx was to increase the rate and the magnitude of Na^+ influx (22). A very similar stimulation of Na^+ influx in isolated, resealed synaptic plasma membrane vesicles was induced by exposure of these membrane preparations to increasing concentrations of L-glutamic acid (Fig. 5B). The increases in Na^+ flux brought about by L-glutamate in both the synaptic plasma membrane preparation as well as in the synaptosomal preparation were found to be smaller at the high concentration range (10–100 μM) of this amino acid (Fig. 5A and 5B). In this respect the glutamate-stimulated Na^+ influx resembled the response of physiological receptors which showed

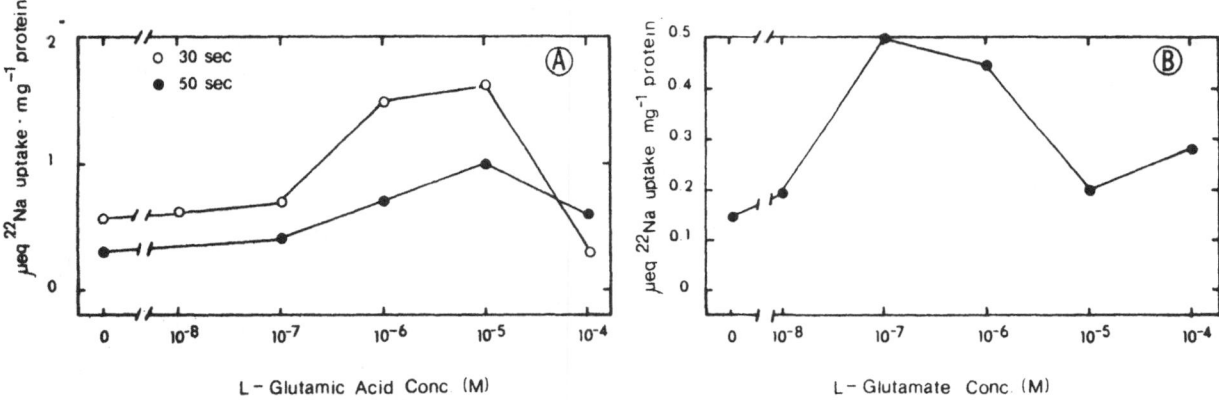

Fig. 5. Dose-response relationship of glutamate-induced Na^+ influx in synaptosomes (A) and synaptic plasma membrane vesicles (B). Aliquots (40 μl) of freshly prepared synaptosomes (0.88 mg protein/ml) were preincubated for 10 min with 10 μl of 7.5% ficoll, 0.32 M sucrose, 10 mM Tris · Cl in the presence or absence of the glutamate concentration shown. They were then transferred to a solution containing 100 mM NaCl, 0.05 μCi $^{22}NaCl$, 7.5% ficoll, 0.12 M sucrose, 20 mM Tris · Cl, and the ^{22}Na influx was determined by Millipore filtration after 30 and 50 s of incubation at 24 °C. (B) Synaptic membrane vesicles (20 μl, 2 mg protein/ml) were preincubated with various concentrations of L-glutamate, and Na influx was measured for incubation periods of 15 s to 2 min following addition of 70 μl of 142 mM NaCl, 0.05 μCi $^{22}NaCl$, 27 mM sucrose, 1 mM $MgSO_4$, 5 mM Tris · SO_4. The point of maximum influx (15 s to 30 s) for each condition was used to plot the data. Results taken from (22).

decrements in their response (desensitization) following repeated applications of high levels of this amino acid (28, 29).

Maximal enhancement of Na^+ influx into synaptosomes and synaptic membrane vesicles was obtained with 10^{-7} to 10^{-5} M concentrations of L-glutamate (Fig. 5A and 5B), which corresponded to 10^{-11} to 10^{-9} mol glutamate present in the assay medium. These amounts of L-glutamate are probably quite close to the levels necessary for maximal activation of its membrane receptor · ion channel complex since it has been shown that threshold physiological excitation is obtained with as little as 10^{-14} mol L-glutamate in the vicinity of its receptors (30). A further similarity between the glutamate-initiated Na^+ influx and the activation of physiological receptors was revealed when it was shown that the potent blocker of voltage-dependent Na^+ channels, tetrodotoxin, even at 1 μM concentration had no effect on the stimulation of Na^+ influx in synaptic membrane preparations (22). Electrical depolarization of neurons brought about by L-glutamic acid was also completely insensitive to the presence of tetrodotoxin (31, 32). In addition, the stimulation of Na^+ flux caused by L-glutamic acid was shown to be unrelated to any effects on the plasma membrane (Na^+–K^+)-ATPase, since L-glutamic acid at 0.1 and 1.0 μM concentrations had a small stimulatory rather than an inhibitory effect on the synaptosomal and synaptic plasma membrane (Na^+–K^+)-ATPase activity (22). On the basis of these observations, it would appear quite probable that the enhancement of Na^+ influx caused by L-glutamic acid was related to the activation of physiological receptor · ion channel complexes in these membrane preparations. Indeed, this type of

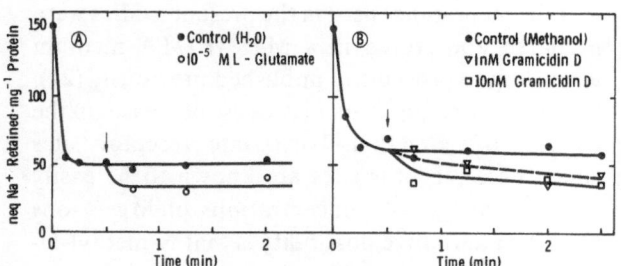

Fig. 6. Stimulation by L-glutamate (A) and gramicidin D (B) of ^{22}Na efflux from preloaded synaptic membrane vesicles. The vesicles were loaded at 37 °C for 5 min in the presence of 100 mM NaCl (15 μCi ^{22}NaCl), 5 mM Tris · SO_4, 1 mM $MgSO_4$, 120 mM sucrose (pH 7.4), and were stored in this medium at 4 °C for 24 h. The amount of ^{22}Na retained (zero time) was determined by direct filtration of 20 μl of loaded vesicles through Millipore filters (HA 0.45 μ). Efflux of ^{22}Na was initiated by diluting 20 μl of the vesicles into 100 mM choline-Cl, 5 mM Tris · SO_4, 1 mM $MgSO_4$, 125 mM sucrose (pH 7.4), and was stopped by filtering the incubation mixture through Millipore filters. All filters were washed with ice-cold choline-Cl medium. Efflux measurements were done at 24 °C. At the times indicated by the arrows, either 5 μl of H_2O or of L-glutamate (A), or 5 μl of methanol or of gramicidin D (B) were added to the incubation mixture. Each point is the mean of duplicate determinations.

Na^+ influx activation was also seen following exposure of the synaptic membrane vesicles to the excitatory amino acids L-aspartate and L-cysteine sulfinic acid but not following exposure to L-glutamine (Table 3). The amino acid L-glutamine does not have any neuroexcitatory activity and provides a useful control for the specificity of the effects of L-glutamic acid on Na^+ fluxes.

The increases in Na^+ flux brought about by L-glutamic acid were shown to be bidirectional in nature. When the resealed synaptic plasma membrane vesicles were internally loaded with ^{22}NaCl and then exposed to a Na^+-free medium (choline chloride replacing NaCl) which contained concentrations of L-glutamic acid in the range of 0.1–10 μM, they exhibited a more rapid and greater efflux of ^{22}Na than membrane vesicles incubated in Na^+-free medium without glutamate. In addition, if passive ^{22}Na efflux from preloaded vesicles was allowed to take place for 30 s and then L-glutamic acid was added to the incubation medium, a similar increase in the rate of ^{22}Na efflux was observed (Fig. 6A). The efflux of Na^+ brought about by L-glutamate was approximately equal to that which was produced by exposure of the loaded membrane vesicles to 1 nM or 10 nM concentration of the Na

Table 3. Effect of glutamate receptor agonists and of non-neuroactive amino acids on Na^+ influx into synaptic membrane vesicles. The influx studies were conducted at 24 °C for the period of 15 s to 2 min as described for Fig. 5B. Maximum influx produced by each agent was compared to the maximum influx of Na^+ in control samples (100%).

Amino acids	% of control Na^+ diffusion
1 μM L-glutamic acid	386
1 μM L-aspartic acid	218
1 μM L-cysteine sufinic acid	291
1 μM L-glutamine	110

ionophore gramicidin D (Fig. 6B). Exposure of the ^{22}NaCl-preloaded vesicles to 10 μM gramicidin D decreased the intravesicular ^{22}NaCl levels to those of osmotically ruptured membrane vesicles. These observations indicate that both L-glutamate and gramicidin D are capable of causing the efflux of Na$^+$ rather than simply bringing about inhibition of Na$^+$ binding to these membranes. Furthermore, it was determined that L-[^{3}H] glutamic acid applied to the extravesicular medium under the conditions of the Na$^+$-efflux measurements is not taken up at all by the NaCl-loaded vesicles. This finding negates the possibility that the glutamate-stimulated Na$^+$ efflux comes about as a result of Na$^+$ co-transport with glutamate. Also, unlike the dicarboxylic amino acid uptake process in the synaptosomes (15), the glutamate stimulation of Na$^+$ efflux appears to be temperature-independent. Exposure to a medium containing 10 μM L-glutamic acid either at 4°C or at 24°C produced approximately an equal magnitude of Na$^+$ efflux.

Both the bidirectionality of the L-glutamate-initiated Na$^+$ flux as well as the apparent temperature independence of this process are consistent with the function of an ion channel-activating system rather than with the activity of a carrier-mediated uptake process. When all of these observations are considered together, they are indicative of the presence of functional L-glutamate receptor · ion channel complexes in brain synaptic plasma membranes. They also suggest that the synaptic membrane vesicles provide a useful preparation for the study of both the glutamate receptor recognition and effector functions and for the exploration of the properties of the receptor macromolecular complex in central nervous system neurons.

Solubilization and purification of L-[^{3}H] glutamate binding sites from brain synaptic membranes

The characterization of the synaptic membrane sites to which glutamate binds has been pursued as the first step in the molecular exploration of the receptor complex (21). It was observed that the glutamate binding activity of isolated synaptic membranes was partially decreased following treatment of these membranes with the proteolytic enzyme pronase and was strongly inhibited by exposure of the membranes to the lectin con-

canavalin A (6). These observations were suggestive of the possible glycoprotein nature of the membrane sites to which L-[^{3}H] glutamic acid bound. Additionally, it was shown that treatment of the synaptic plasma membranes with the non-ionic detergent Triton X-100 under alkaline conditions could solubilize nearly all of the glutamate binding activity (6). The solubilized extract obtained after a 100 000 × g for 1 h centrifugation of the treated membranes exhibited L-glutamate binding with an affinity nearly identical to that of the membrane-attached site and its binding activity was strongly inhibited by both pronase and concanavalin A (6). The finding that the glutamate binding macromolecule was a membrane glycoprotein which could be solubilized with minimal effects on its glutamate and concanavalin A – binding activity led us to develop a scheme for the purification of this protein (21). The purification of the glutamate binding glycoprotein was accomplished through the use of two affinity chromatographic steps: an affinity batch separation of the binding protein on L-glutamate – loaded glass fiber which was followed by affinity chromatography through concanavalin A sepharose (21). The active binding fractions obtained following elution from the concanavalin A chromatographic step represented an approximately 200-fold purification of the glutamate-binding glycoprotein (21). More recent estimates are indicative of an even greater degree of purification of this binding protein which usually ranges from 500–1 000-fold purification.

The purified glutamate binding protein has repeatedly been found to have an estimated K_D for L-[^{3}H] glutamate of 0.65 to 0.85 μM (21). This K_D is higher than the dissociation constants which are determined for the synaptic plasma membranes, and it may be an indication of the changes in the microenvironment of the protein or of changes in the protein itself brought about by the extraction and purification procedures. However, despite the apparent decrease in the affinity of the protein for the ligand L-[^{3}H] glutamic acid, its sensitivity to the presence of various neuroexcitatory or neuroinhibitory amino acids remained almost identical to that which was described above for the glutamate binding process in synaptic membranes. The effects of some of these agents are summarized in Table 4. It is particularly important to mention that neither kainic acid nor N-methyl-D-aspartate caused any

Table 4. Inhibition of L-[³H] glutamate (0.4 μM) binding to the purified binding protein by various amino acids and amino acid analogs. All measurements of binding were obtained by Millipore filtration. Results are taken from Ref. 21.

Competitive ligand (1.0 μM)	% Inhibition	Competitive ligand (1.0 μM)	% Inhibition
Excitatory		*Inhibitory*	
L-aspartate	36.3 ± 2.6	Glycine	1.7 ± 1.6
D,L-homocysteic acid	17.7 ± 4.3	γ-aminobutyric acid	1.7 ± 1.2
Cysteine sulfinic acid	29.2 ± 3.5	β-alanine	1.9 ± 1.8
Antagonistic		*Non-neuroactive*	
Glutamate diethyl ester	29.7 ± 5.7	N-acetyl-L-aspartate	0.5 ± 0.3
		Amino oxyacetic acid	-6.1 ± 2.2*
		Glutamine	2.3 ± 2.0

* – sign denotes an increase in binding.

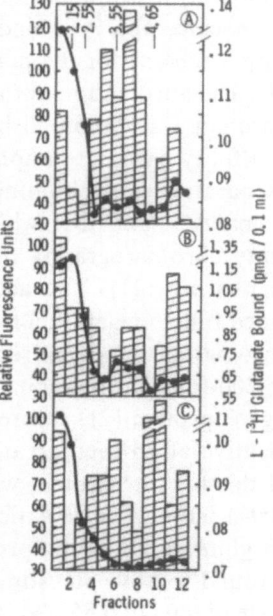

Fig. 7. Analysis of glutamate binding protein by centrifugation on 5 to 20% sucrose density gradients. Direction of centrifugation was from left to right. The samples placed on the gradient were: (A) glutamate binding protein, 200 μl, (B) binding protein pre-exposed to 1 μM L-glutamate, (C) binding protein treated with 0.1 mM 2-mercaptoethanol. The protein in (B) and (C) was incubated with the agents for 2.5 h at 4 °C before being loaded onto gradients which contained the same concentration of glutamate or mercaptoethanol. All sucrose gradients were made in 10 mM K-phosphate buffer which included 0.5% (v/v) Triton X-100. Centrifugation was at 189 000 × g for 8 h at 4 °C. Fractions were analyzed for protein (●) by the fluorescamine method of Bohlen *et al.* (40) and for L-[³H] glutamate binding by the method in (21). Proteins used as standards in centrifugation were dissolved in phosphate – Triton X-100 and were centrifuged under identical conditions. Their positions are indicated in (A): cytochrome C (2.1 S), ovalbumin (3.5 S), and bovine serum albumin (4.6 S).

inhibition of L-[³H] glutamate binding even when they were present in concentrations up to 10^{-4} M. These findings are again consonant with the level of activity exhibited by these agents on the L-[³H] glutamate binding process in the synaptic plasma membranes (Fig. 4 and Table 2). The similarity between the characteristics of the membrane-attached glutamate binding macromolecule and the purified glycoprotein is also apparent in the fact that L-aspartic acid was the most potent inhibitor of L-[³H] glutamate binding to the glycoprotein (Table 4), and this inhibition by aspartate was competitive in nature (Unpublished observations) just as the inhibition of glutamate interaction with the synaptic membrane was shown to be (6).

The molecular weight of this protein as estimated by sodium dodecyl sulfate (SDS) gel electrophoresis was found to be 13 800 (21). Sucrose density centrifugation studies have shown that the original estimate of M_r for this glycoprotein was probably accurate since most of the protein migrated to the same level in the sucrose density gradient as cytochrome C (sedimentation coefficient 2.1 S, M_r 12 750) (Fig. 7). All sucrose density centrifugation experiments were conducted in the presence of 0.5% (v/v) Triton X-100 in order to avoid the possible reaggregation of the isolated protein. However, despite such efforts, the protein tended to form aggregates which could best be demonstrated if the native protein was centrifuged on a sucrose gradient at high speeds for shorter periods of time (189 000 × g for 8 h) (Fig. 7).

It appeared that there were three major peaks of

protein concentration and of binding activity: one peak was centered near the top of the gradient with an estimated 2.1 S value, whereas the second peak was near the center of the gradient with an estimated 3.5 S value (Fig. 7A). The 3.5 S peak had the highest specific binding activity when low concentrations of ligand were used (78.8 nM L-glutamate). There was also a considerable amount of protein that formed larger aggregates and moved to a position in the gradient approximately equivalent to 5.2 S. This species of aggregated protein had a somewhat lower specific binding activity than the 3.5 S peak. Pre-exposure of the protein to 1 μM L-glutamate and inclusion of the same glutamate concentration in the sucrose gradient did not significantly alter the pattern of protein distribution but caused a marked decrease in the specific binding activity of the 3.5 S peak as compared to the other two peaks of binding activity (Fig. 7B). These observations suggest that the high affinity glutamate binding sites may be associated with the 3.5 S oligomer. The estimate of the sedimentation coefficients presented above is clearly imprecise in that it does not take into account the contribution of Triton X-100 to the hydrodynamic properties of the isolated protein.

It is not clear what controls the formation of the 3.5 S and 5.2 S species of this binding protein. Experiments in which the protein was pretreated with 2-mercaptoethanol (0.1 mM) and centrifuged in the presence of the same concentration of this agent have shown that there was a relative loss of protein associated with the 3.5 S peak and, to a lesser extent, with the 5.2 S peak. There was also an apparent shift of the protein to the smaller molecular weight species (Fig. 7C). The treatment with 2-mercaptoethanol brought about what appeared to be a selective decrease in the high specific activity of the 3.5 S peak (Fig. 7C). The effect of the reducing agent on this species might explain the previously described partial loss of binding activity of the purified binding protein following treatment with 0.1 mM 2-mercaptoethanol (21). Finally, the apparent decreases in the protein content of the 3.5 S and 5.2 S species following exposure to reducing conditions may indicate that the larger molecular weight species are formed through disulfide bond linkage of the smaller polypeptide chain. This might mean that the protein in its native state in the membrane is either a dimer or tetramer of the 2.1 S molecular species, and that during the purification

Table 5. Amino acid analysis of the glutamate binding glycoprotein from rat brain synaptic membranes. The values are the average of two determinations on a single sample hydrolyzed for 24 h at 110 °C in 6 N HCl.

Amino acid	Mean residue/serine
Aspartic acid	3.5
Threonine	2.5
Serine	1.0
Glutamic acid	4.9
Glycine	4.2
Alanine	4.4
Valine	8.3
Isoleucine	5.4
Leucine	7.4
Phenylalanine	6.3
Lysine	4.0
Histidine	2.5
Arginine	1.0
Proline	1.3
Tyrosine	2.1
Tryptophan	6.7
Half-Cystine	0.6
3-Methylhistidine	2.4
Total residues	68.5
Molecular weight (from summation)	9556

procedure there is a spontaneous reduction of the disulfide bonds leading to the formation of the M_r 13 000 protein subunit. This reduction of disulfide bonds could occur during the homogenization and solubilization steps and could be brought about by redox interaction between this protein and other SH-containing proteins in the membrane which are in close proximity to the glutamate binding glycoprotein.

A preliminary amino acid analysis of the purified glutamate binding protein from rat brain synaptic membranes is shown in Table 5. A minimum molecular weight of 9,556 was estimated assuming one serine residue per molecule. This value of 9,556 represents an underestimate of the actual M_r of the protein since it does not take into account the contribution by the carbohydrate residues to the M_r of the protein. Initial determinations have shown that carbohydrate residues constitute approximately 20% of the M_r of the protein. No definite conclusions can be reached at this stage about the precise identity of the subunits which make up the oligomers that are associated with the 3.5 S and 5.2 S glutamate binding protein peaks.

174

Studies which are currently in progress to determine the amino-and carboxyl-terminal amino acids of the isolated protein should provide a clearer picture of the subunit composition of this glycoprotein.

Evidence that the glutamate binding protein is an intrinsic membrane protein

It is known that some proteins which copurify with plasma membrane fractions are proteins which simply adhere to the membranes during the homogenization and subcellular fractionation steps (33). Such proteins are sometimes removed by treatment of the membranes with high ionic strength buffers or with chaotropic salt solutions (33). However, treatment of the synaptic plasma membrane with either high ionic strength media or with chaotropic salts such as KSCN, did not solubilize the glutamate binding protein. Even when the synaptic plasma membranes were treated with the ionic detergent Na-cholate at either 0.5 or 1% (w/v) concentrations, greater than 90% of the glutamate binding activity remained attached to the membrane fraction which was recovered after a $100\,000 \times g$ for 1 h centrifugation. However, the Na-cholate (0.5% w/v) treatment of the synaptic plasma membranes effectively solubilized 40–45% of the membrane-associated proteins and an approximately equal fraction of the membrane

Table 6. Cholate extraction of synaptic membrane protein, N-acetyl neuraminic acid, and organic phosphate. The synaptic plasma membranes were suspended in either 50 mM Tris · Cl (pH 7.4) or in the same buffer which contained 0.5% (w/v) Na-cholate (4.5 ml). After 45 min at 24 °C the suspensions were centrifuged at $100\,000 \times g$ for 1 h (4 °C). The supernatants were dialyzed against a 200-fold volume of 50 mM Tris · Cl and the membrane pellets were resuspended in 0.5 ml of the same buffer.

Membrane treatment		Protein (mg)	N-acetyl neuraminic acid content (μg)	Phosphate content (μmol)
Control	Pellet	4.60	145.1	5.52
	Supernatant	0.58	2.3	N.D.*
0.5% Cholate	Pellet	2.60	98.5	3.84
	Supernatant	2.21	19.3	N.D.*

* N.D. = not determined.

phospholipids, glycoproteins, and gangliosides (Table 6). Despite the fact that nearly one half of these membrane macromolecules were solubilized with this procedure, there was no loss of L-[³H] glutamate binding activity following this treatment of the membranes, and less than 3% of the glutamate binding activity was actually detected in the soluble fraction obtained after the Na-cholate extraction (Table 7). It is interesting to note that exposure of synaptic plasma membranes to Na-

Table 7. Effects of cholate treatment of synaptic membranes on [³H] kainic acid and [³H] glutamate binding. Binding of [³H] kainic acid (17 nM) to all fractions was measured by Millipore filtration and [³H] glutamate (92 nM) binding to membranes was measured by microfuge centrifugation and to the supernatants by Millipore filtration. All values are the mean (± S.E.) of the number of determinations in parentheses. Results are taken from (37).

Preparation	Protein content (mg)	[³H] kainic acid binding	[³H] glutamate binding
		(pmol · mg⁻¹ protein)	
Control membranes	3.15	0.173 ± 0.057 (7)	5.26 ± 0.9 (4)
0.5% Na cholate treated membranes	2.39	0.084 ± 0.055 (8)	17.08 ± 2.17 (4)
Control membrane supernatant	0.98	0	0
0.5% Na cholate soluble supernatant	1.93	0.065 ± 0.026 (7)	0.10 ± 0.02 (4)

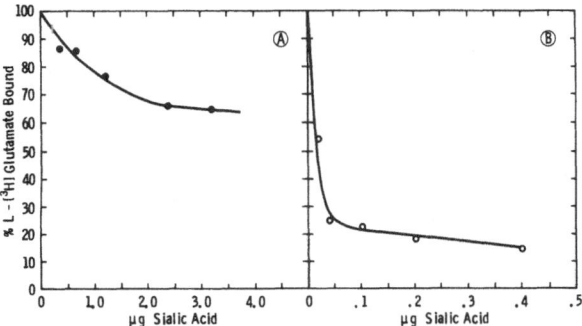

Fig. 8. Inhibition by whole brain ganglioside mixture (A) and by soluble cholate extract from synaptic membranes (B) of specific L-[³H] glutamate binding to the cholate-extracted membranes. Two different batches of synaptic plasma membranes were thawed out and treated with 0.5% (w/v) Na-cholate as described in Table 6. The final supernatant (cholate extract) was dialyzed against two changes of a 200-fold volume of H₂O, lyophilized, and resuspended in 0.8 ml H₂O. L-[³H] glutamate (92.4 nM) binding to 5 µl of cholate-extracted membranes (2.84 mg protein/ml) was determined in Tris · Cl buffer by the microfuge assay (19). All membranes were preincubated with gangliosides or extract for 5 min at 24 °C. Sialic acid content of gangliosides and extract were determined by the method in (36).

cholate (0.5% w/v) has consistently led to an enhancement of L-[³H] glutamate binding activity similar to that shown in Table 7. On the other hand, the same treatment of the synaptic membranes caused a 50% decrease in [³H] kainic acid (17 nM) binding to the membranes. Approximately 80% of the lost kainic acid binding activity was recovered in the supernatant obtained after a 100 000 × g for 1 h centrifugation of the cholate-extracted membranes (Table 7). The differential solubilization characteristics of the glutamate and of the kainic acid binding macromolecules are strongly suggestive of the distinct molecular nature of the two recognition sites. These findings also provide a possible explanation for the lack of inhibition by kainic acid of the high affinity glutamate binding activity in synaptic plasma membranes. The possibility that these two excitatory agents may interact with distinct recognition sites on the membrane is further strengthened by the fact that the purified glutamate binding glycoprotein does not bind [³H] kainic acid nor is its binding of L-[³H] glutamic acid affected by kainic acid concentrations as high as 100 µM.

The cause of the increase in L-[³H] glutamate binding to the cholate-extracted membranes is currently being investigated. It has been shown in initial studies that mixing of the cholate-extracted membranes with increasing amounts of the dialyzed soluble extract brought about a progressive inhibition of glutamate binding down to approximately the level of the untreated synaptic plasma membranes. This inhibition or modulation of glutamate binding was not reversed if the dialyzed soluble extract was heated to 100 °C for 10 min, or if this extract was pretreated with trypsin (0.5 µg/µl), phospholipase C (0.5 µg/µl), or deoxyribonuclease (0.5 µg/µl) for 1 h at 24 °C prior to boiling it at 100 °C for 10 min. It would appear, then, that the factor which modulates glutamate binding activity is a heat stable, non-dialyzable macromolecule or aggregate (Mr > 6–8 000) which is probably neither a peptide nor a phospholipid, nor a deoxyribonucleotide.

During the exploration of the possible nature of this factor which can modulate glutamate binding, we tested other components of the plasma membranes and found that commercially available gangliosides extracted from bovine brain tissue brought about a moderate decrease in glutamate binding activity of cholate-treated membranes (Fig. 8A). The inhibition of glutamate binding produced by the cholate extract of synaptic membranes appeared to be greater than that caused by the whole brain ganglioside mixture when the sialic acid content of these two preparations was considered (Fig. 8B). It is obvious that the supernatant obtained following cholate extraction contained not only gangliosides but also glycoproteins which contributed to the measured levels of sialic acid. However, a ganglioside preparation from rat brain synaptic membranes which we have prepared according to the method of Svennerholm & Fredman (38) also caused a strong inhibition of L-[³H] glutamate binding to the synaptic membranes.

The downward modulation of glutamate binding activity in these cholate-extracted membranes brought about by whole brain gangliosides was not completely reversible. When the membranes were preincubated with the whole brain ganglioside mixture, subsequently washed, and their L-[³H] glutamate binding activity measured, there was a definite concentration-dependent decrease in binding activity. Maximal inhibition (37.7%) of L-[³H] glutamate binding was obtained when the membranes were preincubated for 25 min at 24 °C in a ratio of 1 µg of protein to 3.8 µg of ganglioside prior to the washing step. These observations suggest incorporation of the gangliosides into the membrane matrix and the subsequent modulation of glutamate binding activity by these glycolipids. Indeed, such ganglioside incorporation into the cholate-extracted membranes has been shown through measurement of the increases in sialic acid content of the membranes following incubation with whole brain gangliosides and washing of the membrane pellet obtained after centrifugation at 39 000 $\times$ g for 30 min (Unpublished observations). An understanding of exactly how gangliosides may modulate the activity of the glutamate binding protein must await a more precise determination of which ganglioside species is the most active 'modulator' and, secondly, an analysis of the precise stoichiometry of the ganglioside-binding protein interaction or the ganglioside-membrane interaction. These issues are particularly important since the cholate treatment of synaptic membranes decreased the content of gangliosides but did not alter the ratio of gangliosides to protein. In spite of all the questions which remain to be answered, the studies performed to date have shed some light on the dependence of this putative L-glutamate receptor activity on its surrounding membrane environment.

Information regarding the influence of the lipid milieu on the function of an isolated membrane protein can also be obtained by studying changes in the activity of the protein upon its reconstitution into a well-defined lipid environment such as a liposome membrane. A number of different approaches have recently been explored for the reconstitution of the isolated glutamate binding protein into a liposomal structure. The method which has been found to give optimal results involved incubation of the protein with the liposomes at room temperature, followed by removal of protein or proteoliposome-associated Triton X-100 by treatment of this mixture with Bio-Beads SM-2 (Biorad). Under these conditions, 30 μg of the purified glutamate binding protein in 50 mM Tris · Cl buffer, without additional Triton X-100, were incubated at room temperature with liposomes formed from either phosphatidyl choline or phosphatidyl choline plus one or more phospholipids or glycolipids. When binary mixtures of lipids were used, they were present at molar ratios identical to those observed in synaptic membranes (39). The total amount of lipids was maintained constant at 20 mg/ml (≈ 25 μM). The lipids were dried under a nitrogen stream, then hydrated with 150 mM KCl, and the liposomes formed by sonicating the hydrated lipid suspension to a homogeneous opalescent state. The purified glutamate binding protein was incubated with these liposomes for 30 min at 24 °C prior to its transfer to a small column of Bio-Bead SM-2 where it was allowed to incubate for 4 h at 24 °C. This incubation step was found to remove approximately 80% of the Triton X-100 from standard buffer solutions which contained 0.5% Triton X-100. It also removed all of the soluble, non-reconstituted glutamate binding protein from solution. The eluate from Bio-Bead columns which received only the soluble glutamate binding protein exhibited negligible amounts of L-[^{3}H] glutamate binding activity and protein. Three different procedures (34, 40, 41) were used to measure the amount of protein reconstituted into phosphatidyl choline liposomes. The results from four different reconstitution experiments showed that the fraction of the total glutamate binding protein which was reconstituted into phosphatidyl choline liposomes that were obtained as a pellet following centrifugation at 39 000 $\times$ g for 30 min, was 26–30% of the protein added initially. The equilibrium binding kinetics of the protein reconstituted in phosphatidyl choline liposomes were almost identical to those of the soluble protein (Unpublished observations). The addition of Triton X-100 (10^{-5}–10^{-4} M) to phosphatidyl choline or to phosphatidyl choline-phosphatidyl serine liposomes led to a moderate increase in glutamate binding activity, whereas, larger concentrations of this detergent brought the binding activity back to its baseline levels (Fig. 9). These observations might be indicative of the fact that nearly all of the glutamate binding sites in the reconstituted protein must have been available for interaction with L-[^{3}H] glutamic acid since the treatment with high concentrations of the detergent Triton X-100 – a treatment that would be expected to disrupt the liposomes – did not lead to an enhancement of the glutamate binding activity (Fig. 9). No explanation can be offered at the present time for the increase in specific binding activity of the reconstituted protein brought about by the inclusion of small concentrations of Triton X-100 in the incubation medium. It is possible that this change in binding activity may be the result of

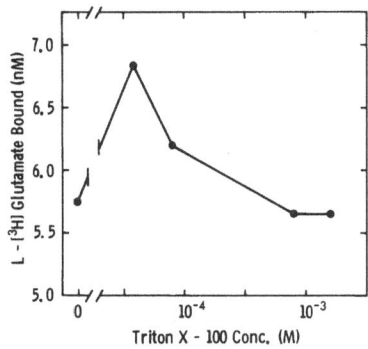

Fig. 9. Effect of increasing Triton X-100 concentrations on glutamate binding to the purified binding protein reconstituted into phosphatidyl choline-phosphatidyl serine liposomes. A 40 µl aliquot of the reconstituted preparation was diluted to 96 µl either with 50 mM Tris · Cl buffer or with Tris · Cl buffer which contained variable amounts of Triton X-100 to achieve the indicated detergent concentrations. After a 15 min room temperature preincubation, the binding assay was initiated by the addition of L-[³H]glutamate (4.6 nM). Glutamate binding was measured by Millipore filtration (21). Glutamate binding to liposomes without reconstituted binding protein functioned as blanks.

the direct interaction of the protein with this detergent. In general, these studies point to the fact that this protein can be successfully reconstituted into a liposomal structure and its properties can be determined under the conditions of a well-defined lipid environment.

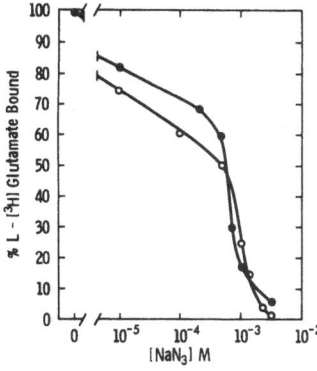

Fig. 10. Inhibition of L-[³H] glutamate binding to synaptic membranes and to the purified glutamate binding protein by NaN₃. All incubations were conducted at 24 °C for 25 min in the presence of 92.4 nM L-[³H] glutamate and of the indicated concentrations of NaN₃. Specific L-[³H] glutamate binding to synaptic membranes (●——●) was measured as described in (19) and to the purified protein (○——○) by the filtration procedure in (21).

Table 8. Effects of NaN_3 and *o*-phenanthroline on glutamate binding and uptake activities of synaptic membranes. Specific L-[³H] glutamate (92.4 nM) binding was measured at 24 °C for 25 min by microfuge centrifugation and L-glutamate (1 µM) uptake was determined at 24 °C for 2 min according to the method in (16).

Agent (1 mM)	% Control binding	% Control uptake
NaN_3	12.4 ± 3.9	90.3 ± 5.7
o-phenanthroline	16.4 ± 2.5	119.6 ± 7.8

Effects of iron ligands on the glutamate binding protein

The purified glutamate binding protein was shown to be strongly inhibited by the iron ligand NaN_3 (Fig. 10) (19). The effect of NaN_3 on the binding activity of the purified protein was not an artifact introduced through some change in the structure-function of the protein during the purification since the L-[³H] glutamate binding activity of synaptic plasma membranes was almost equally inhibited by NaN_3 (Fig. 10). An inhibition nearly identical to that observed with NaN_3 on both the membrane-attached and the purified binding protein was produced by other iron ligands such as KCN and metal chelators such as *o*-phenanthroline. The sensitivity of the binding activity of this protein to the effects of these iron ligands has been traced to the presence of 2 g atoms of Fe per mole of the binding protein (19). The activity of the glutamate recognition site is clearly dependent on the unobstructed availability of this metallic center in the protein. The inhibition of glutamate binding produced by the iron ligands was found to be that of a mixed type of inhibition (Unpublished observations). It would appear, then, that this glutamate binding protein which may function as the receptor site for this dicarboxylic amino acid in brain neurons is a metalloprotein whose response to L-glutamate depends on an intact metallic center at or near the binding site.

Unlike the sensitivity of the glutamate binding protein to these iron ligands, the high affinity, Na^+-dependent glutamate transport carrier which operates in the same synaptic plasma membrane preparations was quite insensitive to the presence of either NaN_3 or *o*-phenanthroline (Table 8). These

178

observations are suggestive of the differential importance of the metallic center in the activity of the glutamate receptor sites as opposed to the glutamate transport carriers. Furthermore, these findings indicate that the synaptic membrane glutamate binding sites which we have been studying are quite distinct from the high affinity glutamate transport carriers in these synaptic membranes.

The role of the metallic center in the function of this protein is presently unknown. It is important to note, however, that the agent 2,4,5-trihydroxyphenylalanine has been shown to be a strong and longlasting activator of physiologic glutamate receptors in spinal cord neurons, and its excitatory activity was postulated to be related to its interaction with a metallic center within the glutamate receptor macromolecule of neuronal membranes (42). When 2,4,5-trihydroxyphenylalanine was tested for its possible inhibitory activity, it was found to cause an inhibition of glutamate binding identical to that produced by NaN_3 and to have a very similar K_I: the K_I for competitive inhibition by NaN_3 was 0.8 mM and that for 2,4,5,-trihydroxyphenylalanine was 0.3 mM. Once again the inhibitory effects of this agent were confined to the high affinity glutamate binding process and did not affect the Na^+-dependent glutamate transport. This, of course, represents only presumptive evidence that 2,4,5,-trihydroxyphenylalanine may indeed be interacting with a metallic center in the physiologic receptor to produce its excitatory activity and, by extension, that such a metallic center is important in the function of these receptor sites. Whether this metallic center also participates in oxidation–reduction processes within the plane of the membrane matrix is not known. Such oxidation–reduction phenomena have been shown to take place in the plasma membranes of a number of cell types (43) and to be involved in the regulation of the cellular responses to hormones (44). It is intriguing to speculate that the glutamate receptor sites and, as a consequence, the excitability of neurons, may also be affected by the oxidation–reduction state of the neuronal membrane and of its environment.

Acknowledgement

This research was supported by grants GM 22357 from the National Institute of General Medical Sciences and DAAG 29-79-C-0156 from the Army Research Office.

References

1. Curtis, D. R. & Watkins, J. C., 1960. J. Neurochem. 6: 117–141.
2. Krnjevic, K., 1974. Physiol. Rev. 54: 418–540.
3. Curtis, D. R. & Johnston, G. A. R., 1974. Ergebn. Physiol. 69: 97–188.
4. Curtis, D. R. & Watkins, J. C., 1961. Nature 191: 1010–1011.
5. Coombs, J. S., Eccles, J. C. & Fatt, P., 1955. J. Physiol. (Lond.) 130: 326–373.
6. Michaelis, E. K., Michaelis, M. L. & Boyarsky, L. L., 1974. Biochim. Biophys. Acta 367: 338–348.
7. Roberts, P. J., 1974. Nature 252: 399–401.
8. Lunt, G. G., 1973. Comp. Gen. Pharmacol. 4: 75–79.
9. DeRobertis, E. & Fiszer dePlazas, S., 1976. J. Neurochem. 26: 1237–1243.
10. Simon, J. R., Contrera, J. F. & Kuhar, M. J., 1976. J. Neurochem. 26: 141–147.
11. Fiszer dePlazas, S. & DeRobertis, E., 1976. J. Neurochem. 27: 889–894.
12. Fonnum, F., 1968. Biochem. J. 106: 401–412.
13. Reyes, E. & Barela, T. D., 1980. Neurochem. Res. 5: 159–170.
14. Stephani, R. A., Rowe, W. B., Gass, J. D. & Meister, A., 1972. Biochemistry 11: 4094–4100.
15. Logan, W. J. & Snyder, S. H., 1972. Brain Res. 42: 413–421.
16. Kanner, B. I. & Sharon, I., Biochemistry 17: 3949–3953.
17. Takeuchi, A. & Onodera, K., 1973. Nature New Biol. 242: 124–126.
18. Onodera, K. & Takeuchi, A., 1976. J. Physiol. (Lond.) 252: 295–318.
19. Michaelis, E. K., 1979. Biochem. Biophys. Res. Commun. 87: 106–113.
20. Foster, A. C. & Roberts, P. J., 1978. J. Neurochem. 34: 1467–1477.
21. Michaelis, E. K., 1975. Biochem. Biophys. Res. Commun. 65: 1004–1012.
22. Chang, H. H. & Michaelis, E. K., 1980. J. Biol. Chem. 255: 2411–2417.
23. Williams, L. T. & Lefkowitz, R. J., 1977. J. Biol. Chem. 252: 7207–7213.
24. Shank, R. P. & Freeman, A. R., 1975. J. Neurobiol. 6: 289–303.
25. Freeman, A. R., 1976. Progr. Neurobiol. 6: 137–153.
26. Davies, J. & Watkins, J. C., 1979. J. Physiol. (Lond.) 297, 621–635.
27. Davies, J. & Watkins, J. C., 1977. Brain Res. 59: 311–322.
28. Takeuchi, A. & Takeuchi, N., 1965. J. Physiol. (Lond.) 177: 225–238.
29. Usherwood, P. N. R. & Machili, P., 1968. J. Exp. Biol. 49: 341–361.
30. Usherwood, P. N. R. & Machili, P., 1966. Nature 210: 634–636.

31. Ozeki, M., Freeman, A. R. & Grundfest, H., 1966. J. Gen. Physiol. 49: 1319–1334.
32. Curtis, D. R., Duggan, A. W., Felix, D., Johnston, G. A. R., Tebecis, A. K. & Watkins, J. C., 1972. Brain Res. 41: 283–301.
33. Kaplan, D. M. & Criddle, R. S., 1971. Physiol. Rev. 51: 249–272.
34. Lowry, O. H., Rosebrough, N. J., Farr, A. L. & Randall, R. J., 1951. J. Biol. Chem. 193: 265–275.
35. Bartlett, G. R., 1959. J. Biol. Chem. 234: 466–468.
36. Hammond, K. S. & Papermaster, D. S., 1976. Anal. Biochem. 74: 292–297.
37. Michaelis, E. K., Michaelis, M. L. & Grubbs, R. D., 1980. FEBS Lett. 118: 55–57.
38. Svennerholm, L. & Fredman, P., 1980. Biochem. Biophys. Acta 617: 97–109.
39. Smith, A. P. & Loh, H. H., 1979. Life Sciences 24: 1–20.
40. Bohlen, P., Stein, S., Dairman, W. & Udenfriend, S., 1973. Arch. Biochem. Biophys. 155: 213–220.
41. Bradford, M., 1976. Anal. Biochem. 72: 248–254.
42. Biscoe, T. J., Evans, R. H., Headly, P. M., Martin, M. R. & Watkins, J. C., 1976. Br. J. Pharmacol. 58: 373–382.
43. Crane, F. L., MacKellar, W. C., Morre, D. J., Ramasarma, T., Goldenberg, H., Grebing, C. & Löw, H., 1980. Biochem. Biophys. Res. Comm. 93: 746–754.
44. Crane, F. L. & Löw, H., 1976. FEBS Lett. 68: 153–156.

Received August 7, 1980.

Pyroglutamic acid

Non-metabolic formation, function in proteins and peptides, and characteristics of the enzymes effecting its removal

George N. Abraham and David N. Podell
Depts. of Medicine and Microbiology, and the Center for Interdisciplinary Research in Immunologic Diseases of the University of Rochester School of Medicine and Dentistry, Rochester, NY 14642, U.S.A.

Summary

The formation of pyrrolidone carboxylic acid (PCA, pGlu) during protein biosynthesis is discussed. Studies are summarized which demonstrate that PCA is formed during the later stages of biosynthesis at the terminal phases of translation or as a post-translational event, just prior to cellular secretion of protein with amino-terminal PCA. Of the studies cited, the most convincing evidence suggests that PCA is derived from glutamine. Enzymes which selectively remove PCA from the N-terminus, and of benefit in amino-acid sequence analysis, have been isolated and shown to have a ubiquitous distribution in various animal and plant cells. The investigations which lead to the isolation of these enzymes and the procedures for their use in removing amino-terminal PCA from proteins, are described. Finally, the biologic function of PCA and the effects of its chemical modification are discussed using the neuropeptide Thyrotropin Releasing Factor (TRF) as a specific example.

Introduction

Pyroglutamic acid (pGlu)*, also termed pyrrolidone carboxylic acid (PCA, pyr) or 5-oxo-L-proline, is an interesting cyclical amino acid. It may be formed either enzymatically as an intermediate in amino acid metabolic and transport pathways, or during protein biosynthesis during which it becomes the amino-terminal residue of many biologically significant peptides and proteins. Structurally, it may be considered to be internally cyclized glutamic acid. Although occasionally referred to as 5-oxo-L-proline, the designation may imply a possible derivation from this amino acid rather than from glutamic acid or glutamine and will not be utilized here.

In essence, the presence of the internal amide bond which forms between nitrogen -1 and carbon -5 produces unique properties for this common amino acid, and chemically defines PCA as 2-carboxy γ-butyrolactam. The interal linkage is neutral and functionally acts as an amide. The basic electron pair of nitrogen -1 is in resonance with and attracted toward carbon -5 by the presence of the double-bonded oxygen. Thus, unlike proline, PCA will not react with substances such as phenylisothiocyanate. Shown below are the formulas of PCA, and its two possible amino acid precursors, glutamine and glutamic acid.

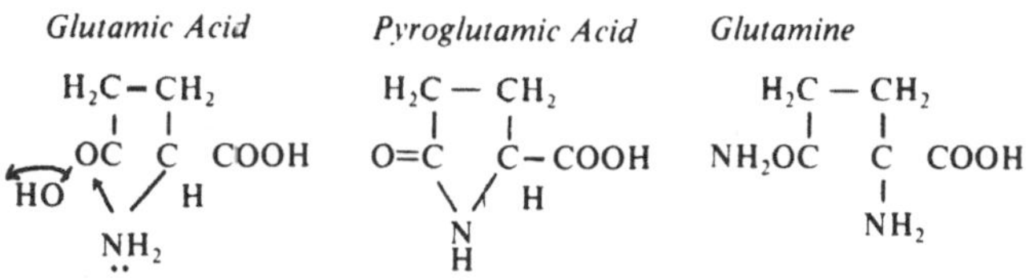

*The following terms and abbreviations are synonymous and will be utilized interchangeably throughout the text: pyroglutamic acid, pyrrolidonyl carboxylic acid, PCA, pGlu, pyr

Glutamic Acid	Pyroglutamic Acid	Glutamine
$H_2C - CH_2$	$H_2C - CH_2$	$H_2C - CH_2$
$HO \overset{OC}{} \quad C \quad COOH$ H	$O=C \quad C-COOH$ H	$NH_2OC \quad C \quad COOH$
NH_2	N H	NH_2

Molecular and Cellular Biochemistry 38, 181–190 (1981).   0300-8177/81/0381–0181/$ 2.00.

The purpose of this review will be to (a) summarize studies which demonstrate how and at what stage PCA is formed during protein biosynthesis, (b) summarize the characteristics of the non-energy dependent enzymes which remove pGlu from proteins or transport forms of amino acids, (c) mention the various methods in primary amino acid sequence analysis and some of the types of proteins on which the non-energy dependent enzyme may be used, and (d) show in the instances studied how this unusual amino acid may impart activity to an important and biologically active peptide.

Pyroglutamic acid formation

The metabolic formation and utilization of pyroglutamate as an intermediate in the gamma-glutamyl amino acid transport cycle has been superbly reviewed by Van der Werf & Meister (1). The biochemical relationship between pyrrolidone carboxylic acid derived from the energy-dependent, enzyme-catalyzed reactions of this metabolic pathway and PCA which is formed as the amino terminus of many proteins and peptides has not been established. Briefly, in the gamma-glutamyl cycle, pyroglutamic acid is formed after the enzymatic removal (see below) of the N-terminal gamma-glutamate residue bonded to any one of a number of amino acids by the cytoplasmic enzyme gamma-glutamyl cyclotransferase (GCT). The pyroglutamate formed is then converted to L-glutamic acid by 5-oxo-L-prolinase. This latter enzyme, originally isolated from rat kidney and other tissues by Van der Werf et al. (1971), is unusual in that it instigates reactions which involve the co-hydrolysis of both the ATP and internal amide bonds. The reactions may be summarized as follows:

(a) gamma-glutamyl amino acid $\xrightarrow{\text{GCT}}$ pyroglutamate + amino acid

(b) pyroglutamate $\xrightarrow[\text{L-glutamate}]{\text{5-oxo-prolinase}+Mg^{++}+k^{+}}$

$$ATP \searrow ADP + Pi$$

It has not been experimentally shown that the enzymes which catalyze the formation of pGlu in this pathway participate individually at some phase in biosynthesis of pGlu in proteins. It has been clearly demonstrated that ^{14}C-pyrrolidone carboxylic acid in culture medium is not utilized in protein biosynthesis. Kitos & Waymouth (5) added ^{14}C-pyrrolidone carboxylic acid (PCA) to culture media containing clone 929 mouse cells. After 4 days of culture the nutrient media, extracts of the cultured cells, and the atmosphere above the media were analyzed for ^{14}C. Nearly all of the radioactivity was recovered in the culture medium. This was then fractionated on cation exchange columns, and individual column fractions were subjected to paper chromatography in order to identify whether breakdown of (^{14}C) PCA had occurred. All radioactivity was obtained in a pool which migrated with an R_f identical to the pyrrolidone carboxylic acid standard. The authors concluded that the exogenous PCA was not taken up or utilized by murine L cells.

Subsequently, Moav & Harris (6) showed that addition of L-pyroglutamic acid (PCA) to cultures of rabbit lymph node cells did not affect the rate of cellular protein synthesis, nor was exogenous PCA incorporated into the rabbit immunoglobulin heavy chains which were synthesized and known to have this residue at the amino terminus. In an attempt to determine at what stage in protein synthesis PCA was incorporated, charged amino-acylated transfer RNAs were isolated from the lymph node cells and the acylated amino acids released and identified. The results suggested that PCA was bound to tRNA, and the authors speculated that the PCA-tRNA complex was most likely formed by cyclization of a glutamic-acid-tRNA-complex precursor.

Experimental support for this notion was provided by demonstrating that glutaminyl-tRNA can be converted in vitro to pyrrolidonyl carboxyl-tRNA. Bernfield & Nestor (7) isolated aminoacyl-tRNA synthetase and the pool of tRNAs from E. coli. Amino acids were then added to the tRNA pool using conditions which would acylate the tRNAs. Selectively labeled C^{14}-glutaminyl-tRNA was then isolated and treated with glutamine cyclo-transferase (GCT) obtained from papaya latex (8). The acyl-amino acid was removed from the tRNA complex and shown to be pyrrolidone carboxylic acid. While the investigators did not rule out the possibility that glutamine might be converted to glutamic acid as an intermediate in the conversion to pyrrolidonyl carboxyl-tRNA, they did provide some evidence which suggested that the action of GCT was specific for glutamine on the transfer RNA. Thus, it was not determined whether aminoterminal PCA was formed at the polypeptide or tRNA level.

Baglioni (9) extended these observations by using mouse myeloma cells whose predominant protein synthetic product was a monoclonal immunoglobulin with heavy chains containing aminoterminal PCA. Addition of radiolabeled glutamine, glutamic acid and PCA to culture media substantiated the earlier observations (5) that free PCA was not utilized or taken up by cells. Myeloma producing cells were incubated in the presence or (^{14}C) glutamine. Membrane bound polyribosomes from and immunoglobulin secreted by, these cells were isolated so that amino-terminal analysis could be performed on nascent and secreted radiolabeled proteins. The aminoterminal peptides were produced by pronase digestion and isolated by cation exchange chromatography of the digested proteins. Nascent protein was shown to contain predominantly N-terminal glutamic acid and secreted protein pyrrolidone carboxylic acid. Other data mentioned by the investigator were that (a) no PCA-tRNA was found in the cytoplasm of cells incubated with ^{14}C glutamine and (b) ^{14}C-PCA could not be charged to tRNAs extracted from these myeloma producing cells. Thus, the conclusion was reached that PCA must be formed by cyclization of an amino terminal glutamine most likely *after* conversion to glutamic acid on the polyribosome or just prior to secretion of the completed protein.

While the above data suggested that PCA could not be directly incorporated into protein, Rush & Starr (10) and Rush *et al.* (11) demonstrated that pyrrolidone carboxylic acid may nevertheless be converted into a form which could be utilized in protein synthesis by a 'decyclase' enzyme found in the human myeloma line which they studied. Murine plasmacytomas assayed simultaneously lacked the enzyme and were unable to utilize PCA directly in protein synthesis but nevertheless secreted immunoglobulin with PCA as the aminoterminal residue. Decyclase activity was, however, detected in murine-liver extracts.

Twardzik & Peterkofsky (12) attempted to determine whether glutamine or glutamic acid was the more direct precursor of pyroglutamic acid. By use of the mouse plasmacytoma RPC-20, which contained glutaminase but not glutamine synthetase, these investigators were able to obviate the conversion of glutamic acid to glutamine. When cultures of cells were incubated in media containing ^{3}H-glutamic acid and cold glutamine, only glutamic and pyroglutamic acid were detected in pronase hydrolysates of synthesized protein. When ^{14}C-glutamine and cold glutamic acid were utilized, amino-terminal peptides were shown to contain amino-terminal glutamic acid, glutamine, and pyrrolidonyl carboxylic acid, a result which suggested that PCA was derived from (^{14}C) glutamine after its conversion to glutamic acid. The investigators took care to utilize experimental conditions which prevented the spontaneous cyclization of glutamine to PCA which can occur at elevated temperatures in mildly acid or alkaline solutions.

Stott & Munro (13), building on previous studies, undertook a comprehensive approach toward determining the post-translational step in protein biosynthesis at which PCA is formed. Mouse-myeloma IgG was isolated as nascent protein on the polyribosome and as completed *intracellular* and mature secreted protein. When (^{3}H) nascent peptides and (^{14}C)-labeled intact heavy chains were co-digested with pronase and the amino terminal peptides isolated and analyzed, it was shown that less than 10% of the amino termini of the peptides contained PCA. When similar co-labeling and digestion experiments were performed to compare the ratio of amino-terminal PCA in intracellular to extracellular heavy chains, 60 to 70% of intracellular protein was shown to have N-terminal PCA. From these results, the investigators concluded that cyclization of the aminoterminal residue (i.e., glutamine or glutamic acid) to PCA occurs inside the cell prior to the secretion of the completed protein. In addition, they were unable to detect PCA-tRNA in cultures of rat liver cells incubated in the presence of radiolabeled glutamine, PCA, or glutamic acid.

Jones (14) examined the cell-free synthesis of immunoglobulin lambda light chains with aminoterminal PCA produced by the murine myeloma RPC-20. Microsomes, tRNA pools and appropriate initiating enzymes purified from the RPC-20 plasmacytoma were utilized to effect conditions of cell-free protein synthesis in which the incorporation of radiolabeled glutamic acid was maximized. The microsomal proteins were precipitated, reduced, digested with subtilisin, and the acidic subtilopeptides purified. These were subjected to high voltage electrophoresis and produced 2 major peaks of radioactivity which were abolished after treatment of the peptide pools with bacterial pyrrolidonyl carboxyl peptidase. The results demonstrated conclusively that in this system pyroglutamate can be formed while protein is still bound to microsomes. In order to determine if a specific glutamyl-tRNA was involved in pyroglutamate synthesis, the pool of RPC-20 tRNAs was subjected to reverse-phase chromatography, and 2 isoaccepting species of glutamyl-tRNAs were isolated. Addition of either to the cell-free system allowed synthesis of light chain-containing amino-terminal pyroglutamic acid. Finally, since the RPC-20 plasmacytoma line lacks the enzyme catalyzing glutamic acid to glutamine conversion, all pGlu synthesized must have been derived from glutamic acid. These results suggested that protein synthesis had been initiated prior to cyclization of glutamic to pyroglutamic acid.

Data which supported this notion were provided by Prasad & Peterkofsky (15), who synchronized RPC-20 plasmacytoma cells for initiation of protein synthesis. Light chain, produced at time intervals 2 and 60 min after protein synthesis was initiated, was immunoprecipitated with specific anti-lambda antiserum. By this method, it was shown the specific activity of methionine, but not other radiolabeled amino acids, was greatest in light chain isolated from the earliest (i.e., 2 min) cultures. This was interpreted as indicated the presence of a methionine-initiated peptide precursor on the light chain which required processing (i.e., removal prior to cyclization of amino terminal glutamate to pyroglutamate).

Burstein et al. (16) extended these studies and demonstrated conclusively that a short-lived precursor peptide of 19 residues is formed early in light chain synthesis. Cleavage of this extra peptide was necessary before the cyclization of amino-terminal glutamic acid or glutamine could occur to form the pyrrolidonyl carboxyl group. The experiments were performed using the mouse plasmacytoma MOPC-315 which produces type lamda light chains with an amino-terminal PCA. Light chain-specific mRNA

was prepared from the plasmacytoma polysome pool by immunoprecipitation with specific anti-murine light chain antibody, purified by oligo-DT chromatography, and the L chain-specific mRNAs translated in a wheat germ cell-free protein synthesis system. Protein was synthesized numerous times and in each instance (^{3}H)- or (S^{35})-labeled amino acid was added. By SDS polyacrylamide gel electrophoresis, an elongated light chain was found which in some instances contained amino-terminal ^{35}S-methionine. This was shown in other experiments to be a short-lived initiator residue. In addition to demonstrating the existence of a precursor molecule, the data assisted in defining the stage in biosynthesis at which pyroglutamic acid is formed and established that it could not be an initiator of protein synthesis.

Burstein & Schechter (17) extended these observations to 3 lambda light chain-producing mouse plasmacytomas utilizing similar conditions of cell-free mRNA translation. The focus of the study was to establish whether N-terminal glutamine or glutamic acid was the pyrrolidone carboxylic acid precursor. Light chains containing the octadecapeptide leader sequence (i.e., the precursor peptide less the cleaved initiator methionine) were subjected to automated sequence analysis for up to 40 residues. This allowed alignment of the identified residues after position 18 with those of mature light chain. When either (^{3}H) glutamic acid or (^{3}H) glutamine was utilized for protein synthesis, only glutamine was noted at position 19 (i.e., residue 1 of the mature light chain) and no redundancy was noted at any position. Identical results were noted for all 3 plasmacytoma lambda chains. Since no interconversions of glutamic acid to glutamine and vice versa are found in the cell-free system, the results clearly indicate that glutamine is the precursor for pyrrolidone carboxylic acid in this system.

Of some pertinence is the fact that of over 200 human and murine immunoglobulin heavy or light chains thus far subjected to amino terminal sequence analysis (18), only one human heavy chain isolated from a native protein contains an initial amino-terminal glutamine residue (19). Perhaps all amino terminal glutamine residues undergo enzymatic cyclization to form PCA prior to secretion from immunoglobulin-producing cells.

Pyrrolidonyl carboxy peptidase

Pyrrolidonyl carboxyl groups are present on numerous naturally occurring, biologically active proteins and peptides. In many instances, PCA inhibits the determination of primary structure at the amino terminus since one is unable to use biochemical methods, either automated or manual, which require a reactive primary amine group for sequential identification of amino acids carboxy distal to pGlu.

In some instances, chemical reduction of the pyrrolidone ring will permit sequence analysis. As one example, Takahaski & Cohen (20) have utilized diborane in tetrahydrofuran or tetramethylurea to reduce the pyrrolidone ring. Although this particular method allows simple and relatively rapid identification of PCA residues at the amino terminus of proteins, it is a qualitative technique, shows limited selectivity and only partially reduces carboxyl groups and peptide bonds. Further, there is less than 50% conversion of pyroglutamic acid into proline with simultaneous loss of peptide bonds by reduction. Thus, the procedure has restricted uses, especially when proteins or peptides are available in limited quantities.

Armentrout & Doolittle (21) noted that Pseudomonas fluorescens was able to maintain growth on media which contained pyrrolidone carboxylic acid as the only source of carbon and nitrogen. These investigators observed that an extract of the organism, instead of opening the pyrrolidone ring, quantitatively cleaved the dipeptide pyrrolidonyl-L-alanine into free PCA and L-alanine. They effected on 100-fold partial purification of the enzyme by 2-step $(NH_4)_2SO_4$ precipitation of a departiculated sonicate of bacteria, followed by DEAE-Sephadex chromatography. However, the partially purified enzyme was unstable in either a frozen or salt precipitated state, and it was rendered inactive by sulfhydryl inhibitors such as iodoacetamide and p-mercuriphenylsulfonate in low concentrations. That the enzyme was specific for the peptide bond joining the pyrrolidonyl group (pyr) to its neighboring carboxy-distal amino acid was demonstrated by its action on dipeptides such as pyr-L-valine and pyr-L-alanine, as well as on fibrinopeptides B from various mammalian species with amino termini of pyr-his, pyr-ser, and pyr-phe. While the rate of release of PCA was sometimes influenced by the neighboring amino acid, the enzyme was highly specific for the pyr-amino acid peptidyl bond only and showed no other non-specific protease activity. The reaction of this enzyme is thus:

pyrrolidonyl-amino acid   pyrrolidone carboxylic   amino acid
                                 acid

The same investigators then developed isolation methods which enhanced the enzyme's stability, activity, and purity (22). Additional purification steps involved precipitation of nucleic acids from the bacterial sonicate, addition of 2-mercaptoethanol, EDTA and 2-pyrrolidone to all buffers utilized, and preparative polyacrylamide gel electrophoresis. They observed that, while the enzyme was unstable in solution alone, hydrolysis of the pyr-L-alanine dipeptide was maintained for nearly a day. They reasoned that addition of 2-pyrrolidone to enzyme solutions would enhance enzyme stability. It was also noted that lyophilized preparations which has lost enzymatic activity could be reactivated by addition of sulfhydryl protective agents.

Uliana & Doolittle (23) studied the influence of the amino acid which was bonded to amino-terminal PCA on its cleavage by the enzyme. The cleavage rates of the dipeptides which were examined comprised 3 groups: L-pyr-L-alanine being hydrolized at twice the rate of pyr-L-isoleucine, which was hydrolyzed nearly twice as fast as pyr-L-valine, leucine, phenylalanine *or* tyrosine (in decreasing order of the rate of reaction with enzyme). L-pyrrolidonyl-L-proline and D-pyrrolidonyl-L-alanine were not hydrolyzed, nor did dipeptides containing D-pyrrolidonyl carboxylic acid or D-alanine inhibit cleavage of the L-pyr-L-alanine bond. This demonstrated the stringent requirements of pyrrolidonyl peptidase for the L-optical isomers of amino acids.

Armentrout (24) was able to isolate pyrrolidonyl carboxy peptidase from rat liver cells. The rat liver enzyme, while slightly more labile than the bacterial product, was also stabilized in solution by 2-pyrrolidone and was likewise activated by reducing agents. It was, however, of lower molecular weight, and while it hydrolyzed dipeptides in the same relative orders of structure as the bacterial product, there were minor differences in the relative rate relationships of peptide bond cleavage. The rat liver enzyme was more efficient in its removal of the pyrrolidonyl carboxyl group from fibrinopeptides B.

Almost concomitant with the above studies, Szewczuk & Mulczyk purified the peptidase activity from Bacillus subtilis (25) by use of a nearly identical purification procedure. The enzyme activity was assayed with the chromogenic substrate L-pyrrolidonyl-β naphthylamide, the percent of cleavage of the peptide bond being colorimetrically quantified by the amount of β-naphthylamide released. The bacillus enzyme was inactivated by mild heating (55 °C) and by the addition of Hg^{++} and Cu^{++}. Enzyme cleavage of the substrate was *competitively* inhibited by 2-pyrrolidone carboxylic acid. The ubiquitous nature of this enzyme was shown by finding peptidase activity in Streptococcus, Staphylococcus, Micrococcus, Sarcinia, and other Bacillus strains, as well as in several gram-negative bacterial strains such as Klebsiella, Neisseria, Enterobius and some strains of Escherichia.

Similar peptidase activity is also widely distributed in animal tissue and, remarkably, in plant cell extracts (26). Liver and kidney apparently contain the highest levels of this enzyme, but it is also found in spleen, lung, intestine, brain, heart and skeletal muscle of birds and mammals. Enzyme partially purified from pigeon liver, and with estimated molecular weights of 33 000 and 80 000 daltons, contained peptidase activity with nearly identical enzymatic and biochemical characteristics as that isolated from bacteria.

By use of the chromogenic L-pyr-β-naphthylamide substrate, Albert & Szewszuk (27) were able to determine the cellular localization of the pyrrolidonyl carboxy peptidase. Tissues which were snap-frozen immediately after sacrifice of the test animal were overlaid with L-pyrrolidone-β-naphthylamide at neutral pH, incubated at 37 °C, and then secondarily overlaid with tetraazotized O-dianizidine to colorimetrically localize free β-naphthylamide. Histochemical activity was assayed in numerous avian and rodent tissues. Since the kidney extracts and cells of all the species tested showed the greatest peptidase activity, cellular localization of the enzyme to the cytoplasm of endothelial cells of the proximal convoluted tubules was possible. Lesser amounts were histochemically detected in the cells of the distal convoluted tubules and no enzyme was detected in any cell nuclei or glomerular cells.

Curiously, pyrrolidonyl peptidase activity in bacteria is most likely membrane-associated. Exterkate (28) produced bacteria-burst spheroplasts by treatment of Streptococcus cremoris with lysozyme. The spheroplasts were lysed utilizing conditions which released intracellular marker enzymes and which allowed the conclusion that the pyrrolidonyl peptidase was associated with particulate cell structures. Further, since the enzyme was easily solubilized, it was inferred that it was weakly bonded by means of hydrophobic and/or electrostatic associations to the internal bacterial membrane.

Application of pyrrolidonyl carboxy peptidase (PCP) in protein sequencing

The knowledge that PCP is ubiquitous in its distribution and that it may be isolated from numerous sources to near homogeneity, as well as knowing the conditions for its storage with retention of enzyme activity (21, 22), were of considerable importance. With the advent of automated primary amino acid sequence technology which depends on a free amino terminal amino acid residue, it was apparent that a source of the enzyme would be required for the expeditious removal of amino-terminal amino acids blocked by the pyrrolindonyl group. Numerous attempts to effect large scale purifications of enzyme with retention of peptidase activity were, however, unsuccessful. By cell lysis combined with a gentle means of protein precipitation (presumed by the writer to be effected by either cold ethanol or 2-step ammonium sulfate), a preparation of enzyme has been obtained which may be stored in a lyophilized form at -70 °F with retention of activity for 3 years (29).

A general procedure for removal of pyrrolidone carboxylic acid from the amino terminus of proteins was devised by Podell & Abraham (30). The technique was influenced by obstacles encountered in previous studies, utilized portions of procedures devised by others (14, 21, 22, 25), and was successfully utilized on 3 immunoglobulin type lambda and 2 type gamma heavy chains. In brief, reduced and alkylated protein at 1 mg/ml concentrations (i.e., $2-4 \times 10^{-4}$ mM/mL) in 0.1 M phosphate buffer at pH 8.0, containing *freshly added* dithiothreitol (5 mM), disodium EDTA (10 mM), and glycerin (5% v/v), is incubated under a nitrogen atmosphere with crude calf liver pyrrolidonyl carboxy peptidase (30, 31, 32) at 4 °C for 8–10 h. After this time, an equivalent quantity of enzyme is again added and the digest is incubated at 37 °C for up to 14 h. Essentially, quantitative removal of amino-terminal pyrrolidonyl carboxylic acid from each of the above proteins was possible. Yields of greater than 80% of the neighboring amino acid residue, i.e., residue 1 of the enzyme-treated protein, was obtained by automated sequence analysis. The identical conditions have been utilized by Franklin *et al.* (31) with equivalent results on an immunoglobulin heavy chain disease protein and by Chiu *et al.* (32) with intact heavy chain and a heavy chain fragment obtained after cyanogen bromide digestion. The procedure was devised on the assumption that the peptide bond between amino-terminal PCA and its carboxy-distal amino acid will be in the group shown by Uliana & Doolittle (23) to be most resistant to peptidase treatment, i.e., peptide bond cleavage proceeds quantitatively but at a slow rate. Thus, reducing conditions, a stabilizing reagent (glycerin), a double addition of crude enzyme, a metallic ion chelating agent, and a low concentration of protein (to minimize aggregation) were utilized. These conditions are of some importance when one suspects that leucine, valine, methionine, phenylalanine or tyrosine are peptide-bonded to PCA.

With experiences gained from immunoglobulins (29), it is apparent that for proteins comprised of multiple polypeptide chains, separation of these constituent subunits is necessary before efficient removal of the N-terminal pyrrolidone ring is possible.

There are experimental data which suggest that deblocking of soluble and purified peptides occurs more readily. Reid & Thompson (33) isolated the subcomponent C1q from the first component of complement. This was oxidized, subjected to limited pepsin digestion and the shortened β chain isolated. This 97 amino acid long fragment was dissolved in 0.1 M phosphate, pH 7.4, peptidase added, and

incubated for 6 h at 37 °C without addition of reducing or chelating agents. Cleavage of the amino terminal pyrrolidonyl-leucine peptide bond was however effected. The conditions described will not render a similar bond in *intact* immunoglobulin heavy chains.

Bacterial enzyme (26) has been utilized by Gerber *et al.* (34) to cleave amino terminal PCA of a highly insoluble peptide derived from bacteriorhodopsin, a membrane protein. This 20-amino-acid-long peptide was produced by cyanogen bromide treatment of the parent protein, and after derivitization with 4-sulfophenylisothiocyanate, was treated with pyrrolidonyl peptidase under reducing conditions for 18 h, which effectively cleaved the amino terminal PCA-L-alanine bond.

Function of pyrrolidone carboxylic acid in proteins or peptides

The presence of an amino terminal pyroglutamic acid on a protein or peptide may in some instances enhance or be responsible for its biologic function or activity. A particularly well-studied example in the tripeptide thyrotropin releasing factor (TRF) which has the sequence pGlu-His-Pro. *In vivo*, this hypothalamic hormone mediates the release of thyrotropin by its action on the anterior pituitary gland (36) and *in vitro* has been shown to enhance prolactin synthesis and decrease growth hormone production in a cloned strain of rat pituitary cells (37, 38) possibly by its binding to cell-membrane receptors.

Hinkle *et al.* (37) have studied the effects of modification of each amino acid which comprises TRF, on its biologic activity, and affinity for the TRF receptor. They demonstrated that any structural substitution in the lactam ring of pyrrolidone carboxylic acid, effected both hormone synthesis and receptor binding. In instances simple modifications caused marked decreases in activity relative to parent TRF. As examples, shown below are TRF (a), and two analogs (b) and (c). In formula (b), carbon -4 is replaced by an oxygen linked both to carbon -3 and carbon -5. In formula (c) the oxygen of carbon -5 is replaced forming the amino acid proline, and producing the sequence Pro-His-Pro. These modifications produce compounds of diminished potency which show only 33% (b) and

0.8% (c) of the biologic activity of native TRF.

Of some interest was the finding that substitution of glutamic acid or glutamine for pGlu also causes a decrease in prolactin stimulating activity. However, because either residue may cyclize to pyroglutamate under the conditions of cell culture, any activity which was found was felt to be caused by the presence of native TRF.

Thyrotropin releasing factor (TRF) and 2 functional analogs

(a) TRF

(b)

(c)

PGlu   His   Pro

Similar modifications (39, 40) have also been shown to diminish the release of thyroid stimulating hormone from the anterior pituitary gland in an *in vivo* mouse model. As an example, substitution of the cyclopentane ring for the lactam ring caused greater than a 1000 fold decrease in TSH releasing activity.

The functional activity of pGlu on the amino terminus of immunoglobulins is less clear. The pyrrolidonyl group constitutes the amino-terminal residue of both the Mcg type lambda Bence-Jones dimer (41) and the heavy and light chain variable regions of the f(ab) fragment of IgG-New (32). The three-dimensional stucture of both molecules has been determined at the atomic level by x-ray crystallography (42, 43) and models constructed. Apparently the amino-terminal pGlu does not participate in binding of the antigen and no function has been ascribed to it by virtue of its three dimensional orientation which as shown, positions it away from the combining site cleft. The available data would suggest that the conversion of glutamine to pGlu in the immunoglobulin producing cell is a vestigial function.

Of particular interest are evolving but as yet preliminary data which suggest that free pyroglutamic acid may mediate particular neurobiologic functions. By use of paper chromatographic techniques, low levels of free pGlu were detected in normal human and guinea pig plasma (43) after treatment with perchloric acid to effect deproteination. By gas-liquid chromatography, micromolar concentrations of pGlu were determined for plasma, urine and cerebrospinal fluid (44). The pGlu found was assumed to be derived from the gamma glutamyl cycle (1, 2, 3) by the action of gamma-glutamylcyclotransferase on gamma-glutamyl-amino acids.

It is possible that PCA free in cerebral spinal fluid could exert some biologic effects. Lam *et al.* (45) demonstrated that free pyroglutamic acid in porcine hypothalamic tissue significantly inhibited prolactin release during prolactin purification. The mechanism of the inhibition was not determined. The study was well-controlled for spurious formation of PCA and its identification was accomplished by thin layer electrophoresis, and field desorption mass spectroscopy. Approximately 100 μg were detected in each 100 mg (dry weight) of hypothalamic tissue.

Conclusion

This review has focussed attention on aspects of pyroglutamic acid formation and function which have not been previously summarized. PCA is a crucial intermediate in the gamma-glutamyl metabolic cycle, and its function in this pathway has been very well delineated and reviewed by Meister and his colleagues (1, 2, 3).

The role of pyroglutamic acid in protein biosynthesis and in mediating the biologic function of proteins or peptides which contain it at the amino terminus, is less clear. This PCA is apparently not derived from that formed during the gamma-glutamyl cycle. As suggested by the above studies, PCA is most likely formed either late in protein translation by cyclization of N-terminal glutamine or may form just prior to secretion of completed protein from the cell. Regardless, all the experimental evidence cited conclusively shows that PCA formation occurs during the latter stages of protein biosynthesis and is apparently complete by the time mature, extracellular protein is noted either in culture media of cells, or in the fluid phase of cell-free synthesis systems.

Once formed, amino-terminal pyrrolidone carboxylic acid may at times be an impediment to protein sequence determination since reactions which require a free amino terminus are not possible. However, a non-energy dependent enzyme has been described which has been utilized to effect quantitative removal of pGlu of many previously blocked proteins.

Pyroglutamic acid is present on proteins and peptides of very diverse biologic function. Studies cited above show that in the hormone TRF, this amino acid is responsible for a major portion of hormone activity by its binding to a TRF membrane receptor. However, in other instances PCA may not confer any apparent function. An example is PCA which forms the amino terminal residue of many immunoglobulin heavy and light chains. Aside from functions as an incorporated amino acid, free pyrrolidone carboxylic acid may possibly have biologic function as an inhibitor of cellular hormone release possibly by blockade of specific hormone receptors. While this has only been noted during hormone isolation, it is presumed that an *in vivo* correlate of this phenomenon will be found.

In terms of future areas of research concerning this amino acid, it would be of interest to find the unique enzyme(s) which is responsible for conversion of glutamic acid or glutamine to pyroglutamic acid in protein biosynthesis or to unequivocally demonstrate if the enzymes of the gamma-glutamyl cycle can participate in this conversion. Finally, the experimental data mentioned which suggest that free pGlu may be inhibitory of hormone release and other studies (46, 47) which show that a substituted pyrrolidone ring may antagonize amino acid induced neuronal excitation, point to numerous other functions for this curious lactam at the internal or external cell membrane surface or cell-membrane receptor, levels.

Acknowledgements

The writing of this manuscript was performed utilizing facilities supported by U.S.P.H.S. research grant AI-11550, U.S.P.H.S. Training Grant 5 TO1 AI-00028, The David Welk Memorial Fund, Specialized Research Center Grant (CIRID) AI-15372, and the U.S.P.H.S. Medical Scientist Training Program (NIGMS).

The authors wish to thank Dr. Patricia Hinkle, Dept. Of Pharmacology, University of Rochester Medical Center for her helpful discussions concerning the role of PCA in TRF, and Dr. Kenneth Carle, Professor of Organic Chemistry, Hobart College, Geneva, New York for his elucidation of the resonant structure of PCA. Ms Nancy George edited and prepared this manuscript.

References

1. Van der Werf, P. & Meister, A., 1975. Adv. Enzymology 43: 519–566.
2. Meister, A., 1973. Science 180: 33–39.
3. Meister, A., 1974. Life Sciences 15: 177–190.
4. Van der Werf, P., Orlowski, M. & Meister, A., 1971. Proc. Natl. Acad. Sci. 68: 2982–2985.
5. Kitos, P. A. & Waymouth, C., 1966. J. Cell Physiology 67: 383–398.
6. Moav, B. & Harris, T. N., 1967. Biochem. Biophys. Res. Comm. 29: 773–776.
7. Bernfield, M. R. & Nestor, T., 1968. Biochem. Biophys. Res. Comm. 33: 843–848.
8. Messer, M. & Otteson, M., 1964. Biochem. Biophys. Acta 92: 409–412.
9. Baglioni, C., 1970. Biochem. Biophys. Res. Comm. 38: 212–219.
10. Rush, E. A. & Starr, J. L., 1970. Biochem. Biophys. Acta 199: 41–55.
11. Rush, E. A., McLaughlin, C. A. & Starr, J. L., 1971. Cancer Research 31: 1134–1139.
12. Twardzik, D. R. & Peterkofsky, A., 1972. Proc. Natl. Acad. Sci. 69: 274–277.
13. Stott, D. I. & Munro, A., 1972. Biochem. J. 128: 1221–1227.
14. Jones, G. H., 1974. Biochem. 13: 855–860.
15. Prasad, C. & Peterkofsky, A., 1975. J. Biol. Chem. 250: 171–179.
16. Burstein, Y., Kantor, F. & Schechter, I., 1976. Proc. Natl. Acad. Sci. 73: 2604–2608.
17. Burstein, Y. & Schechter, I., 1977. Biochem. J. 165: 347–354.
18. Kabat, E. A., Wu, T. T. & Bilofsky, H., 1979. In: Sequences of Immunoglobulin Heavy Chains. U.S. Department of Health, Education and Welfare, NIH publication No. 80–2008.
19. Kaplan, A. P., Hood, L., Terry, W. D. & Metzger, H., 1968. Immunochem. 8: 801–811.
20. Takahaski, S. & Cohen, L. A., 1966. Biochem. 5: 864–870.
21. Doolittle, R. F. & Armentrout, R. W., 1968. Biochem. 7: 516–521.
22. Armentrout, R. W. & Doolittle, R. F., 1969. Arch. Biochem. Biophys. 132: 80–90.

190

23. Uliana, J. A. & Doolittle, R. F., 1969. Arch. Biochem. Biophys. 131: 561–565.
24. Armentrout, R. W., 1969. Biochem. Biophys. Acta 191: 756–759.
25. Szewczuk, A. & Mulczyk, M., 1969. Eur. J. Biochem. 8: 63–67.
26. Szewczuk, A. & Kwiatkowska, J., 1970. Eur. J. Biochem. 15: 92–96.
27. Albert, Z. & Szewszuk, A., 1972. Acta Histochem. Bd. 44: 98–105.
28. Exterkate, F. A., 1977. J. Bacteriology 129: 1281–1288.
29. Abraham, G. N., unpublished data.
30. Podell, D. N. & Abraham, G. N., 1978. Biochem. Biophys. Res. Comm. 81: 176–185.
31. Franklin, E. C., Prelli, F., & Frangione, B., 1978. Proc. Natl. Acad. Sci. 76: 452–456.
32. Chiu, Y.-H., Lopez de Castro, J. A. & Poljak, R. J., 1979. Biochem. 18: 553–560.
33. Reid, K. B. M. & Thompson, E. O. P., 1978. Biochem. J. 173: 863–868.
34. Gerber, G., Anderegg, R. J., Herlihy, W. C., Gray, C. P., Biemann, K. & Khorana, H. G., 1979. Proc. Natl. Acad. Sci. 76: 227–231.
35. Jacobs, L. S., Snyder, P. J., Wilber, J. F., Utiger, R. D. & Daughaday, W. H., 1971. J. Clin. Endocrinol. 33: 996–998.
36. Hinkle, P. M. & Tashjian, A. H., Jr., 1973. J. Biol. Chem. 248: 6180–6186.
37. Dannies, P. S. & Tashjian, A. H., Jr., 1973. J. Biol. Chem. 248: 6174–6179.
38. Vale, W., Grant, G. & Guillemin, R., 1973. In: Frontiers in Neuroendocrinology (Ganong, W. F. & Martin, L., eds.), pp. 375–397. Oxford University Press, Toronto.
39. Goren, H. J., Baure, L. G. & Vale, W., 1977. Molecular Pharm. 13: 606–614.
40. Fett, J. W. & Deutsch, H. F., 1974. Biochem. 13: 4102–4114.
41. Schiffer, M., Girling, R. L., Ely, K. R., & Edmundson, A. B., 1973. Biochem. 12: 4620–4631.
42. Poljak, R. J., Amzel, L. M., Chen, B. L., Phizackerley, R. P. & Saul, F., 1974. Proc. Natl. Acad. Sci. 71: 3440.
43. Wolfersberger, M. G. & Tabachnik, J., 1973. Experientia 29: 346–347.
44. Wilk, S. & Orlowski, M., 1973. FEBS Letters 33: 157–160.
45. Lam, Y.-K., Knudsen, R., Folkers, K., Frick, W., Daves, G. D., Barofsky, D. F. & Bowers, C. Y., 1978. Biochem. Biophys. Res. Commun. 81: 680–683.
46. Stone, T. W., 1976. Experientia 32: 581–583.
47. Stone, T. W., 1976. J. Physiol. 257: 187–198.

Received January 30, 1981.

Gamma-carboxyglutamic acid

John P. Burnier, Marianne Borowski, Barbara C. Furie and Bruce Furie
Division of Hematology-Oncology, Dept. of Medicine and Dept. of Biochemistry and Pharmacology, Tufts-New England Medical Center and Tufts University School of Medicine, Boston, MA., U.S.A.

Summary

Gamma-carboxyglutamic acid is an amino acid with a dicarboxylic acid side chain. This amino acid, with unique metal binding properties, confers metal binding character to the proteins into which it is incorporated. This amino acid has been discovered in blood coagulation proteins (prothrombin, Factor X, Factor IX, and Factor VII), plasma proteins of unknown function (Protein C, Protein S, and Protein Z), and proteins from calcified tissue (osteocalcin and bone-Gla protein). It has also been observed in renal calculi, atherosclerotic plaque, and the egg chorioallantoic membrane, among other tissues. Gamma-carboxyglutamic acid is synthesized by the post-translational modification of glutamic acid residues. This reaction, catalyzed by a hepatic carboxylase, requires reduced vitamin K, oxygen, and carbon dioxide. The function of γ-carboxyglutamic acid is uncertain. In prothrombin γ-carboxyglutamic acid residues bound to metal ions participate as an intramolecular non-covalent bridge to maintain protein conformation. Additionally, these amino acids participate in the calcium-dependent molecular assembly of proteins on membrane surfaces through intermolecular bridges involving γ-carboxyglutamic acid and metal ions.

Introduction

γ-Carboxyglutamic acid is a naturally occurring amino acid with a dicarboxylic acid side chain. This amino acid has unique metal binding properties and confers these metal binding properties on the proteins into which it is incorporated. Because the biosynthesis of γ-carboxyglutamic acid requires vitamin K in the mammalian systems that have been investigated, the proteins which contain γ-carboxyglutamic acid have been known as the vitamin K-dependent proteins. In this article, we will review the chemical and biological properties of this amino acid and its role in the vitamin K-dependent proteins. Several detailed reviews on this subject with somewhat different emphasis have recently appeared (1–6).

History

As a result of the investigation of cholesterol metabolism in 1929, Dam observed that chickens fed a diet freed of sterols bled to death (7). The fat-soluble vitamin, vitamin K, was subsequently found to correct this hemorrhagic tendency and to relieve the prothrombin deficiency which this diet causes (8, 9). During this same period, the vitamin K antagonist dicoumarol was discovered to be the cause of a bleeding disorder in cattle fed moldy sweet clover which also rendered these animals deficient in prothrombin activity (10). Both the absence of vitamin K and the presence of the vitamin K antagonists had the same effects: A hemorrhagic syndrome due to low levels of prothrombin activity. With advances in the blood coagulation field, it became clear that this clotting abnormality was caused by the reduced activities of four blood clotting proteins – prothrombin, Factor IX, Factor X, and Factor VII – the vitamin K-dependent blood coagulation proteins.

The mechanism of vitamin K action was unclear. Numerous hypotheses were advanced suggesting

Molecular and Cellular Biochemistry 39, 191–199 (1981). 0300-8177/81/0391-0191/$03.40.
© 1981, Martinus Nijhoff/Dr W. Junk Publishers, The Hague.

that prothrombin biosynthesis was regulated by vitamin K at the transcriptional, translational, or post-translational level of protein synthesis. In 1968 Ganrot & Nilehn demonstrated that plasma from a patient treated with the vitamin K antagonist, sodium warfarin, contained low prothrombin *activity* but normal prothrombin *antigen* (11). A prothrombin-related protein, termed abnormal prothrombin, was identified which had impaired biological activity. This protein does not bind calcium or phospholipid vesicles in the presence of calcium (12-15). This is in contradistinction to prothrombin. Otherwise, the molecular weight, carbohydrate composition, and amino acid composition of the acid hydrolysates of prothrombin and abnormal prothrombin appeared to be identical (12, 13).

The extensive and protracted study of the role of vitamin K in the synthesis of the vitamin K-dependent blood clotting proteins culminated with the discovery of γ-carboxyglutamic acid in bovine prothrombin. A tryptic peptide of prothrombin behaved anomalously on electrophoretic analysis compared to that predicted from its amino acid analysis following acid hydrolysis (16). Structural investigation of these and similar fragments by Stenflo (17) and Nelsestuen *et al.* (18) identified γ-carboxyglutamic acid in these peptides. This structure was subsequently confirmed and a region of prothrombin sequenced to locate the position of γ-carboxyglutamic acid residues (19).

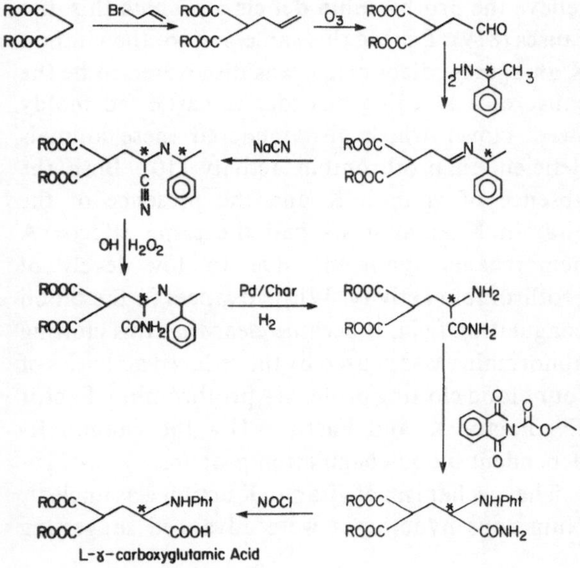

Chemical synthesis of γ-carboxyglutamic acid

Following the discovery of γ-carboxyglutamic acid many efforts have been made to synthesize this amino acid in the laboratory. Since γ-carboxyglutamic acid can not be obtained from natural sources in sufficient quantity for the preparation of derivatives which can can be used in the synthesis of peptides, these efforts play a crucial role in the investigation of the biological and chemical parameters of the vitamin K-dependent proteins.

There are two reported chiral syntheses of (L)-γ-carboxyglutamic acid. Starting with di-t-butylmalonate, Oppliger & Schwyzer (20) utilized a modified Strecker synthesis to prepare γ-γ'-di-t-butyl (L)-N-phthaloyl-γ-carboxyglutamic acid in an overall yield of 8% (Scheme I). Malonate was treated with allyl bromide to form the allymalonate which, upon ozonolysis, afforded the formylmethylmalonate. The formation of the Schiff's base with (-)-α-methylbenzylamine following by treatment with sodium cyanide resulted in the chiral nitrile. The nitrile was converted to the corresponding amide with alkaline hydrogen peroxide. The benzyl group was replaced by a phthaloyl group by hydrogenation over palladium on charcoal to give the amine and followed by treatment with N-ethoxycarboxyl-phthalimide. The amide was then converted to the acid by treatment with nitrosyl chloride.

Danishefsky *et al.* (21) used N-CBZ pyroglutamic acid as the starting material for the preparation of L-γ-carboxyglutamic acid. Conversion to the benzyl ester was accomplished with benzyl chloride and triethylamine. Treatment of this compound with Brederecks Reagent afforded the enamine. Upon addition of 2,2,2-trichlorothoxycarbonyl chloride in benzene, this material yielded the diastereomeric

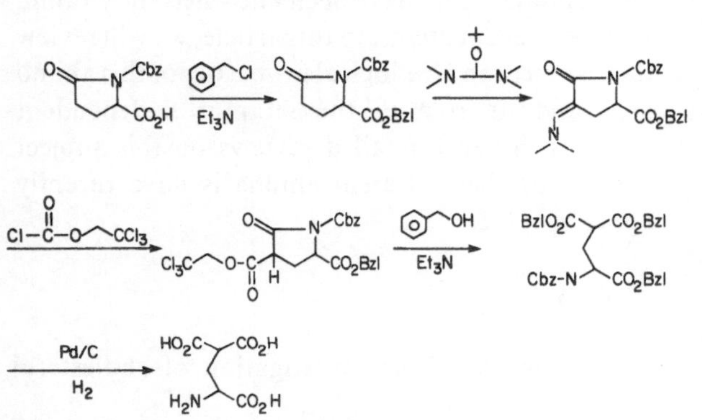

Scheme I

Scheme II

lactams. Conversion of the lactams to the tribenzyl ester of N-CBZ-(L)-γ-carboxyglutamic acid was accomplished with excess benzyl alcohol in the presence of triethylamine. Hydrogenation over palladium on charcoal afforded the free L-γ-carboxyglutamic acid. The overall yield for this synthesis is 20%. This synthesis exhibits promise for the preparation of a variety of L-γ-carboxyglutamic acid derivatives which can be used in both solution and solid phase peptide synthesis (Scheme II).

The majority of the syntheses of D,L-γ-carboxyglutamic acid have utilized serine as the starting material (22–27). A protected serine (Scheme III) is converted to the corresponding tosylate or halide. Subsequent treatment of these derivatives with a protected malonate using either sodium hydride or lithium diisopropylamide resulted in protected derivatives of γ-carboxyglutamic acid. Alternatively, acetamidoacrylic acid can be used as a starting material (28). Using this compound, a derivative of which is an intermediate in the serine-based synthetic schemes, shortens the synthetic transformations necessary to obtain D,L-γ-carboxyglutamic acid. When L-serine was used as the starting material the final product was optically inactive. This is due to the β-elimination which occurs when either the halo-alinate or serine tosylate is treated with the malonate salt.

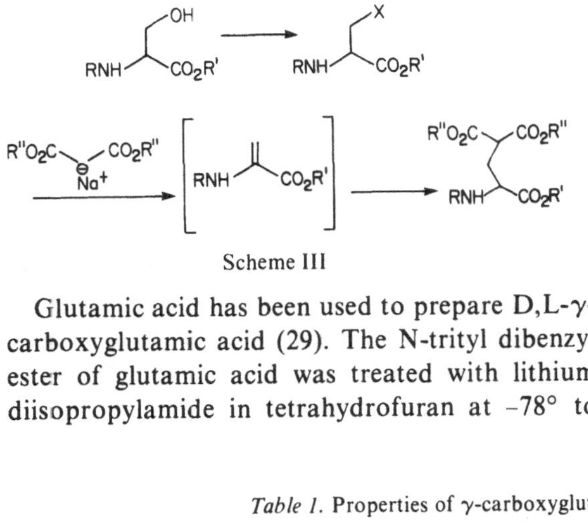

Scheme III

Glutamic acid has been used to prepare D,L-γ-carboxyglutamic acid (29). The N-trityl dibenzyl ester of glutamic acid was treated with lithium diisopropylamide in tetrahydrofuran at −78° to form the lithium salt at the gamma position. Treatment of this salt with benzyl chloroformate resulted in the n-trityl tribenzyl ester of γ-carboxyglutamic acid. Hydrogenation over palladium on charcoal removed the protecting groups.

The syntheses of racemic γ-carboxyglutamic acid require fewer synthetic transformations and the overall yields are much greater ($\cong$ 40%) than the chiral syntheses. As a result, the primary source of L-γ-carboxyglutamic acid has been through the resolution of racemic γ-carboxyglutamic acid derivatives. Marki et al. (30) has resolved DL-N-CBZ-γ, γ'-di-t-butyl-γ-carboxyglutamic acid to the L enantiomer (98% enantiomeric purity) through formation of the (−)quinine salt. Boggs et al. (25) resolved the same material by way of the tyrosine hydrazide salt. Overall yields for both of these resolutions was 15%.

L-γ-carboxyglutamic acid has a reported optical rotation of +35.3 (30). D-γ-carboxyglutamic acid has a reported optical rotation of −37.5 (30). The ^{13}C NMR chemical shift values of the carbon nuclei are pH dependent (31). At pH 5.4, resonances at 178.5, 178.0, 174.8, 54.3, 55.9, and 31.4 ppm downfield of tetramethylsilane have been assigned to the γ_1-carboxyl carbon, γ_2-carboxyl carbon, α-carboxyl carbon, Cα, Cγ, and Cβ respectively. The pKa values of titrating groups in the free amino acid include NH$_2$ (9.92), γ_1,γ_2-COOH (pK$_1$ 4.37, pK$_2$ 2.03), and α-COOH (2.08) (31). A summary of the chemical and physical parameters of γ-carboxyglutamic acid is listed in Table 1.

Detection and assay of γ-carboxyglutamic acid in proteins

γ-Carboxyglutamic acid readily decarboxylates to glutamic acid at high temperature in its protonated form. For this reason, amino acid analyses of γ-carboxyglutamic acid-containing

Table 1. Properties of γ-carboxyglutamic acid.

	Mp (°C)	α_D^{20}	pK, Carboxyls
D, L-γ-carboxyglutamic acid	90–92	0	pK$_1$ 4.37, pK$_2$ 2.03
D-γ-carboxyglutamic acid	157–159	−37.5	
L-γ-carboxyglutamic acid	167–167.5	+35.3	
	154–155	+33.9	

proteins following acid hydrolysis at 110° are negative for γ-carboxyglutamic acid. To quantitate γ-carboxyglutamic acid in proteins, alkaline hydrolysis has been widely applied (32, 33). Protein is dissolved in 2 M KOH, and the solution maintained for 22 hrs at 110° *in vacuo*. After neutralization and removal of salts, the hydrolysate is subjected to automated amino acid analysis on a cation exchange resin. Care must be taken to distinguish γ-carboxyglutamic acid from other highly acidic, ninhydrin positive components, including cysteic acid, taurine, methionine sulfoxide, phosphoserine, phosphothreonine, and amino malonic acid. In addition, dipeptides with elution profiles similar to γ-carboxyglutamic acid may be formed by partial hydrolysis. A variation of this method has been reported in which an anion exchange resin is employed (34). In this system γ-carboxyglutamic acid binds tightly to the resin and elutes late in the elution program.

Although these techniques are suitable for the quantitation of γ-carboxyglutamic acid in purified proteins or peptides, they do not work well for the identification and quantitation of γ-carboxyglutamic acid in tissue, biological fluids, or impure protein preparations. Major problems involve the limits of sensitivity of the ninhydrin detection system and confusion of γ-carboxyglutamic acid with other acidic amino acids or oligopeptides found in biological material. To circumvent these problems, Nelsestuen (35) has treated γ-carboxyglutamic acid-containing proteins with [³H] diborane. The γ-carboxyglutamic acid residues are reduced to 5,5′-[H]dihydroxyleucine, the protein hydrolyzed in acid, and the hydrolysate subjected to amino acid analysis. This method of analysis of [³H]-diborane-reduced protein provides a sensitive, albeit qualitative, method for identification of proteins which contain γ-carboxyglutamic acid.

More recently, Hauschka (36) has proposed a sensitive, quantitative, and specific assay for γ-carboxyglutamic acid in complex biological material. Tritium is exchanged with the proton of the γ-carbon in the γ-carboxyglutamate residues. This tritium is trapped during the thermal decarboxylation of γ-carboxyglutamic acid to glutamic acid since this tritium atom in glutamic acid is not exchangable. After removing other exchangable tritium atoms from the proteins by dialysis against water, the only remaining tritium is associated with glutamate residues in protein that had originally been γ-carboxyglutamate residues. This technique is highly specific for γ-carboxyglutamic acid and incorporates the high degree of sensitivity that radiolabeling allows. Furthermore, it is not necessary to prepare the amino acid hydrolysates of the proteins since this technique is highly specific, with only γ-carboxyglutamic acid residues labeled.

Direct automated sequence analysis of γ-carboxyglutamic acid containing proteins has suffered from low recoveries of the phenylthiohydantoin-γ-carboxyglutamic acid derivative because extraction of the thiazolinone derivative of the amino acid from the sequenator cup is poor. A procedure has been described in which n-butanol is substituted for chlorobutane in the Quadrol program (37), leading to quantitative recoveries.

Metal binding properties.

γ-Carboxyglutamic acid binds metal ions. Although direct evidence of the nature of this interaction has been made available recently (31, 38) the importance of metal ion binding to γ-carboxyglutamic acid was appreciated from indirect observations shortly after its discovery. Unlike prothrombin, abnormal prothrombin neither contains γ-carboxyglutamic acid nor binds metal ions. In light of its chemical structure, this amino acid was considered to be responsible for the metal binding properties of prothrombin.

The interaction of Ca(II) and γ-carboxyglutamic acid was first studied by Marki *et al.* (39). Evaluating the competition of H^+ and Ca^{++} for γ-carboxyglutamic acid using proton NMR, these authors suggested that the binding was characterized by a pK of 1.3. This corresponds to a dissociation constant, K_D, of 50 mM. Fundamental observations of the structure of the γ-carboxyglutamic acid-metal complex were made by Sperling *et al.* (31). At concentrations in solution in which the metal is limiting, the stoichiometry of the γ-carboxyglutamic acid-metal complex is 2:1. At higher concentrations, a 1:1 complex was observed.

The solution structure of the γ-carboxyglutamic acid-metal complex has been determined using paramagnetic Gd(III) and paramagnetic relaxation enhancement techniques (31). These studies have

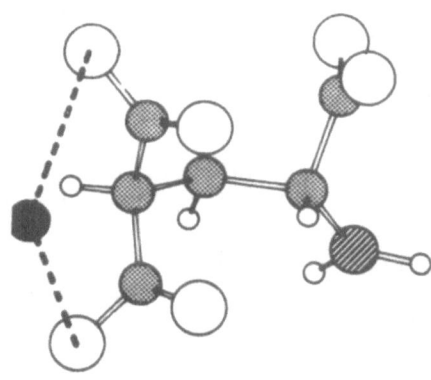

Fig. 1. Metal-γ-carboxyglutamate complex. This solution structure was determined by NMR paramagnetic-relaxation enhancement techniques. Metal (black), carbon (speckled), oxygen (white), nitrogen (lined). The smallest atoms are hydrogen. Coordination of the oxygen and the metal is indicated by the dashed line. [Modified from (31).]

revealed that the metal is bound symmetrically between the two γ-carboxyl groups (Fig. 1). The metal-γ-carboxyl carbon distance was defined as 3.2 Å. The precise orientation of the carboxyl oxygens and the Gd(III) were indeterminant by ^{13}C NMR relaxation techniques. Unidentate coordination was considered in which a single oxygen on each carboxyl group is a metal ligand. Alternatively, bidentate coordination was considered in which both oxygens on each carboxyl group are ligands of the metal. Based upon the preliminary report of the crystal structure of the D,L-γ-carboxyglutamic acid – Ca(II) complex in which the oxygen-Ca(II) distance is 2.4 Å (40), the unidentate structure is favored in complexes including the free amino acid.

A salient feature of the amino acid-metal complex is that the oxygen ligands are coordinated to one half of the primary coordination sphere of the metal (31). The other half of the metal coordination sphere is available to interact with other metal ligands. It would thus appear that the metal ion can serve as a bridge to link a γ-carboxyglutamic acid from one domain of the protein to another γ-carboxyglutamic acid in another domain. This type of intramolecular bridge represents one form of metal binding site seen in γ-carboxyglutamic acid-containing proteins (41). Alternatively, intermolecular bridges involving metal ions and γ-carboxyglutamic acid represent a structural mechanism for protein-protein or protein-membrane association.

The interaction of metal ions with γ-carboxy-

glutamic acid has provided insight into the nature of the metal binding sites of γ-carboxyglutamic acid-containing peptides and proteins. This approach has been extended by Hiskey and Schwyzer and their coworkers to the examination of the metal binding properties of model peptides containing γ-carboxyglutamic acid which have been prepared synthetically (38, 39).

The interaction of Ca(II) with L-Gla-L-Gla was studied via potentiometric titration, and yielded a K_D of 0.6 mM for the metal-peptide complex (39). The affinity of Ca(II) for N-CBZ-D-Gla-D-Gla-OMe was 0.6 mM, as measured by ^{43}Ca NMR in which the ^{43}Ca signal shift was monitored as a function of metal and peptide concentration (38). These values, by two independent methods, are in excellent agreement.

Peptides which contain a single γ-carboxyglutamic acid, including N-CBZ-Gly-Gla-Gly-OEt and N-CBZ-Gla-Ser-OMe, tend to form ternary complexes containing two mol of peptide per mol of metal. This is analogous to the free γ-carboxyglutamic acid-metal complex. Based upon measurements of the luminescence decay constants of bound Eu(III), it was found that the binding of Eu(III) by the peptide is associated with the displacement of about four water molecules from the inner coordination sphere of the metal (42). These results would suggest, as before, that each γ-carboxyglutamic acid residue contributes two oxygen ligands to the bound metal.

Other peptides do not appear to bind metal ions in this pattern. For instance, Phe-Leu-Gla-Gla-Leu-OMe and Phe-Leu-Gla-Glu-Leu-OMe bind metal ions in a 1:1 molar stoichiometry (42). More curiously, both of these peptides bind metal ions with about the same affinity. N-CBZ-Gla-Gla-OMe also binds two mol of Eu(III) with about the same affinity. These results raise questions as to the suitability of small peptides as models of domains of the vitamin K-dependent proteins.

The metal binding properites of the vitamin K-dependent blood coagulation proteins, specifically prothrombin, Factor X, and Factor IX, have been extensively studied. Detailed information about these studies is beyond the scope of this review. Interested readers are referred to Nemerson & Furie (3) for a current analysis. From the results of equilibrium and rate dialysis (43, 44), circular dichroism (45) and fluorescence spectroscopy

(46–48), and immunologic studies using conformation-specific antibodies (49–51), the following general comments can be made. These proteins contain multiple metal binding sites which fall into two classes: the high affinity metal binding sites and the lower affinity metal binding sites. These proteins contain two high affinity sites which bind calcium and many other ions. Occupancy of these sites by metal ions is associated with a conformational transition in those proteins examined. One high affinity site in prothrombin involves two γ-carboxyglutamic acid residues. A model has been proposed (41), based upon a natural abundance ^{13}C NMR study of a γ-carboxyglutamic acid-rich fragment of bovine prothrombin, in which two non-adjacent γ-carboxyglutamic acid residues in the polypeptide chain bind to a single metal ion (Fig. 2). This configuration is similar to that observed for the free γ-carboxyglutamic acid · metal complex. There are multiple lower affinity metal binding sites which also contain γ-carboxyglutamic acid. The precise structure of these sites is not known, but they may represent single γ-carboxyglutamic acid residues. Inasmuch as the high affinity sites represent intramolecular metal bridges, the lower affinity sites may represent intermolecular metal bridges from the protein to either other proteins or membanes containing metal ligands (46, 52, 53).

Recent studies on prothrombin fragment 1 (molecular weight 23 000) have emphasized that the metal binding properties of the functionally important proteins differ significantly from the peptide models containing γ-carboxyglutamic acid. It would appear from the luminescence decay of Eu(III) bound to fragment 1 that Eu(III) is highly coordinated to the protein (54). Only a single water molecule is bound to Eu(III) in the high affinity sites. This may be compared to 4 to 6 water ligands bound to Eu(III) in the lower affinity sites and 9 water ligands bound in the Eu(III) · aquo complex. The pH titration of the metal · protein complex further reveals a curious inflection at about pH 7 (55), suggesting that a group on prothrombin near the bound metal ion (e.g. histidine) may be involved in the binding site. These studies have focused upon the role of γ-carboxyglutamic acid in defining the metal binding properties of these proteins. The X-ray crystallographic studies currently underway on prothrombin fragment 1 should shed considerable light on the structure of these sites (56, 57).

Biosynthesis of γ-carboxyglutamic acid

The mechanism of γ-carboxyglutamic acid synthesis *in vivo* has not been fully elucidated. This amino acid is formed on the protein through a post-translational, vitamin K-dependent pathway in the hepatic microsomes. Although Ganrot & Nilehn had demonstrated the presence of an abnormal, inert form of prothrombin in humans treated with warfarin (11), conclusive demonstration of the existence of a protein precursor form of prothrombin was provided by Shah & Suttie (58) in 1971. Rats were placed on vitamin K-deficient diets and rendered deficient in prothrombin activity. Radiolabeled amino acids and, later, vitamin K were administered to the animals. The characteristic rise in the prothrombin activity was noted. The prothrombin synthesized was radioactive. If cycloheximide (an inhibitor of protein synthesis) was administered prior to infusion of vitamin K, prothrombin activity increased but the circulating

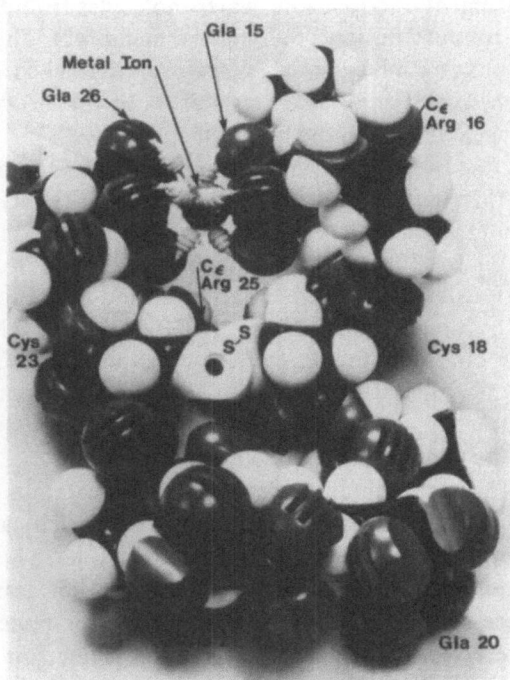

Fig. 2. Structure of the high affinity metal binding site of a prothrombin fragment. [From (41).]

prothrombin was not radioactive. These experiments indicated that vitamin K plays a role in the post-translational modification of a prothrombin precursor. This precursor was subsequently shown to be convertible to thrombin using Echis carinatus venom, but not with Factor Xa (59).

With the discovery of γ-carboxyglutamic acid in prothrombin (17, 18) and glutamic acid in equivalent positions in abnormal prothrombin, many laboratories have focused on the enzymatic reaction in which glutamic acid residues are converted to γ-carboxyglutamic acid residues. The experiments f Suttie (60), with later confirmation by Friedman (61), Johnson (62), and Olson (63), showed that ^{14}C-labeled bicarbonate was incorporated into prothrombin in an *in vitro* system which included the postmitochondrial supernates of livers from vitamin K-deficient rats and vitamin K.

The carboxylating system had requirements for the hydroquinone form of vitamin K and either bicarbonate or carbon dioxide (64). This system has now been studied in crude liver homogenates, hepatic microsomes, and partially purified microsomal preparations. Although initial assays of carboxylase activity evaluated the incorporation of ^{14}C bicarbonate into prothrombin, a synthetic peptide Phe-Leu-Glu-Glu-Leu has been used effectively as a substrate for ^{14}C bicarbonate incorporation (65).

The vitamin K-dependent carboxylating system is located on the rough endoplasmic reticulum in liver cells (66). A solubilized microsomal preparation contains carboxylase activity which is dependent upon molecular oxygen, carbon dioxide, and the reduced (hydroquinone) form of vitamin K (65, 67, 68, 69). If the quinone form of the vitamin is used, an additional requirement for NAPH or NADPH is present (62). Neither biotin nor ATP is necessary for carboxylase activity (70).

Three enzymatic activities appear to be closely related during γ-carboxyglutamic acid synthesis: (1) vitamin K-dependent carboxylation of glutamic acid by the carboxylase (2) vitamin K epoxide formation by an epoxidase (3) vitamin K reduction by a reductase. The relationship between these activities remains unclear since neither the carboxylase nor the epoxidase have been sufficiently purified and characterized. Molecular oxygen is required for both epoxidation and carboxylation. The hydroquinone form of vitamin K is the oxygen

Fig. 3. Vitamin K cycle.

acceptor, and is converted into vitamin K epoxide. Carbon dioxide or bicarbonate is required for carboxylation but not epoxidation. Based upon pharmacologic studies with carbonic anhydrase inhibitors, carbon dioxide may be the active species during carboxylation (67). However, definite proof is currently lacking.

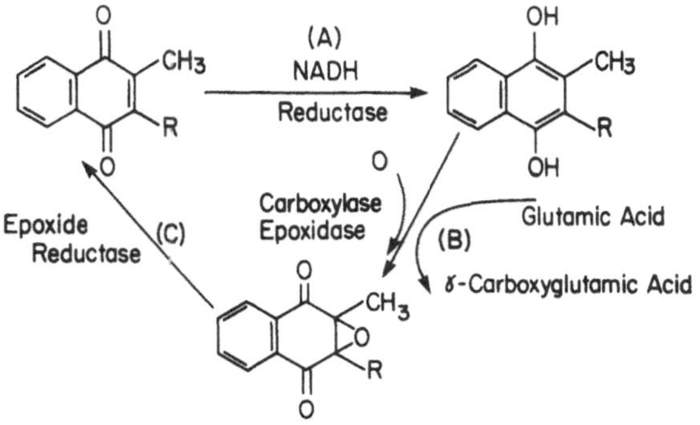

Warfarin inhibits the carboxylation process by preventing the recycling of vitamin K. At low doses it inhibits the epoxide-reductase conversion of the vitamin back to the oxidized form (71) (Fig. 3). At higher concentrations warfarin inhibits conversion of the vitamin to the epoxide by interfering with the reduction of the vitamin by NADH (step A) (1,72, 73). The anticoagulant tetrachloropyridinol inhibits vitamin K epoxidation by preventing the reduction and epoxidation (steps A and B) but has little effect on the epoxide reductase (73, 74). In contrast the principal site of action of the anticoagulant imidazopyridine is the epoxide reductase (74).

It is not known whether epoxidation and carboxylation are coupled. In the absence of purified, chemically defined systems, it has not been possible to determine the stoichiometry between carboxylation and epoxidation. Friedman *et al.* (75) elegantly demonstrated that the oxidation and epoxidation of reduced vitamin K are coupled to a cleavage of the γ-proton-γ-carbon bond in the glutamyl residue of the substrate without concurrent carboxylation. Using [^{3}H]-labeled glutamic acid residues in which tritium was incorporated into the β and γ position in the substrate Phe-Leu-Glu-Glu-Leu, [^{3}H] was released from the substrate in the presence of the microsomal system, oxygen, and reduced vitamin K even when the system was deprived of carbon dioxide or bicarbonate. These data indicate that

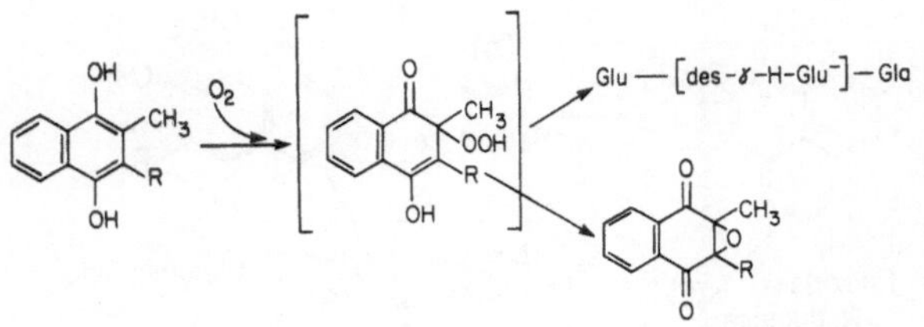

Fig. 4. Possible steps in vitamin K-dependent carboxylation.

vitamin K is involved in proton abstraction at the γ-carbon of the glutamyl residues and provides evidence against a concerted mechanism of which CO_2 fixation is part.

Evidence for a hydroperoxide intermediate of vitamin K has been provided by Larson & Suttie (76). Glutathione peroxidase, which reduces organic hydroperoxides as well as hydrogen peroxide, was shown to inhibit both carboxylation and epoxidation in an *in vitro* system. Catalase, which inhibits hydrogen peroxide but not organic hydroperoxides, exhibited no inhibition of either carboxylation or epoxidation. These data, along with those of Friedman (74), are consistent with the scheme outlined in Fig. 4. Hydroperoxide may arise from the reaction of the reduced vitamin K with superoxide (O_2^-). Esnouf has reported that superoxide dismutase, an inhibitor of superoxide, inhibits carboxylation (77). Other mechanisms involving free radicals have been proposed (74) but efforts to trap intermediates have so far proved unsuccessful.

γ-Carboxyglutamic acid in proteins

Plasma proteins

γ-Carboxyglutamic acid was first discovered in the vitamin K-dependent blood coagulation proteins, which include prothrombin, Factor X, Factor IX, and Factor VII. Because prothrombin is more abundant in plasma than these other proteins, most of the structural and functional studies concerning γ-carboxyglutamic acid have focused on prothrombin. As such, this protein is a model for the class of metal binding proteins which contain γ-carboxyglutamic acid. Unifying features of proteins within this class include (*1*) they contain γ-carboxyglutamic acid; (2) they require vitamin K for synthesis of the intact, functional protein; (3) they bind metal ions, although calcium ions may be the

most central and important of these ions; (4) these proteins may function in complex molecular assemblies on membrane surfaces.

1. Prothrombin

Prothrombin is the zymogen of the serine protease thrombin. It includes a single polypeptide chain of about 70 000 molecular weight. About 10% of the protein is carbohydrate. The sequence of the polypeptide and carbohydrate moiety is known. Prothrombin participates in the final stages of the blood coagulation cascade. Circulating in an inactive form in plasma, it is converted to its active form, thrombin, by a proteolytic mechanism by Factor Xa in the presence of Factor V, calcium ions, and membrane surfaces (for review, see (1)). Prothrombin contains ten γ-carboxyglutamic acid residues in the NH_2-terminal domain (19). The γ-carboxyglutamic acid residues occur in adjacent pairs (residues 7,8; 20,21; 26,27) or in close proximity (residues 15,17; 30,33). The amino terminal sequence of prothrombin is homologous to the other vitamin K-dependent plasma proteins (Fig. 5).

The metal binding properties of prothrombin have been extensively studied (3). Prothrombin has two classes of metal binding sites. The high affinity metal binding sites bind Ca(II) with a K_D of about 0.2 mM. Many different metal ions can occupy this site. It has been proposed that this site may be formed by two γ-carboxyglutamic acid residues in the polypeptide chain e.g. Gla 15 and Gla 26, which share a single bound metal ion (41). This site represents an intramolecular metal bridge which stabilizes the tertiary structure of the protein. Occupancy of this site by metal ions induces a conformational transition that can be monitored by spectroscopic and immunochemical techniques (45–51). Although metal-induced spectral perturbations may in part be due to dimerization (78), detection of structural transitions in the prothrombin-metal complex using conformation-specific antibodies emphasizes that metal ions stabilize a conformer of prothrombin. This structural transition has been localized to the amino terminal one-sixth of the polypeptide chain.

The lower affinity metal binding sites include γ-carboxyglutamic acid (41), but have not been

	1				5					10					15					20
Prothrombin	Ala	Asn	Lys	Gly	Phe	Leu	Gla	Gla	–	Val	Arg	Lys	Gly	Asn	Leu	Gla	Arg	Gla	Cys	Leu
Factor X (light chain)	Ala	Asn	Ser	–	Phe	Leu	Gla	Gla	–	Val	Lys	Gln	Gly	Asn	Leu	Gla	Arg	Gla	Cys	Leu
Factor VII	Ala	Asn	–	Gly	Phe	Leu	Gla	Gla	Leu	Leu	–	Pro	Gly	Ser	Leu					
Factor IX	Tyr	Asn	Ser	Gly	Lys	Leu	Gla	Gla	Phe	Val	Arg	–	Gly	Asn	Leu	Gla	Arg	Gla	Cys	Lys
Protein C	Ala	Asn	Ser	–	Phe	Leu	Gla	Gla	–	Leu	Arg	Pro	Gly	Asn	Val	Gla	Arg	Gla	Cys	Ser
Protein S	Ala	Asn	Ser	–	Phe	Leu	Gla	Gla												

				25					30					35					40
Prothrombin	Gla	Gla	Pro	Cys	Ser	Arg	Gla	Gla	Ala	Phe	Gla	Ala	Leu	Gla	Ser	Leu	Ser	Ala	Thr	Asp
Factor X (light chain)	Gla	Gla	Ala	Cys	Ser	Leu	Gla	Gla	Ala	Arg	Gla	Val	Phe	Gla	Asp	Ala	Gla	Gln	Thr	Asp
Factor IX																				
Protein C	Gla	Gla	Lys	Cys	Ser															
	₁Gla	Gla	Val	Cys	Gla	Phe	Gla	Gla	Ala	Arg	Gla	Ile	Phe	Gln	Asn	Ile	Ile	Asp	Thr	Met

				45					50
Prothrombin	Ala	Phe	Trp	Ala	Lys	Tyr	Thr	Ala	Cys	Glu
Factor X (light chain)	Phe	Trp	Ser	Lys	Tyr	Lys	Asp	Gly	Asp	
Protein C	Ala	Phe	Trp	Ser	Lys	Tyr	Ser	Asp	Gly	Asp

Fig. 5. Sequence homology of the γ-carboxyglutamic acid-containing regions of the vitamin K-dependent proteins from bovine plasma.

structurally characterized. Whether they involve just single γ-carboxyglutamic acid residues or a more complex organization is unknown. It is thought that these sites are involved in metal-dependent, intermolecular bridging from one protein to a membrane surface or another protein.

The isolation of abnormal prothrombin from cows treated with vitamin K antagonists also indicates the importance of γ-carboxyglutamic acid in metal binding and biological function. Abnormal prothrombin, with decreased or absent γ-carboxyglutamic acid, has impaired metal binding properties and almost absent coagulant activity (13, 14, 17). This protein does not bind to lipid surfaces and cannot be activated to thrombin by Factor Xa (15).

The uncarboxylated precursor forms have been characterized to a limited extent. Two forms have been prepared by Suttie *et al.* from liver isolated from warfarinized rats (80, 81). These forms have the same molecular weight as prothrombin. However, their isoelectric points (pI) are 7.2 and 5.8, compared to 5.0 for rat prothrombin. The study of prothrombin biosynthesis in rats has been greatly facilitated by the use of cultured rat hepatoma cells (82). Five distinct precursors of prothrombin, with pIs of 7.2, 6.7, 6.2, 5.8 and 5.5, were identified (83). Recently, specific antibodies have been isolated for bovine (79) and human (84) abnormal prothrombin. These antibodies do not cross-react with prothrombin. Abnormal prothrombin is not a component of normal plasma, but appears in plasma in the face of warfarin therapy, vitamin K deficiency, and liver disease (84).

2. Factor X

Factor X is a plasma glycoprotein that is the zymogen of the serine protease, Factor Xa. Factor X participates in an intermediate phase of the blood coagulation cascade. Factor X is converted to

Factor Xa by Factor IXa in the presence of Factor VIII, calcium and membrane surfaces or by Factor VIIa in the presence of tissue factor and calcium (for review, see (1)). Factor X is composed of two polypeptide chains linked by a single disulfide bond (85, 86). The heavy chain has a molecular weight of 38 000 and the light chain has a molecular weight of 18 000. Activation of Factor X to Factor Xa involves cleavage of a single peptide bond on the heavy chain (87) and modest changes in tertiary structure (88).

The amino terminal region of the light chain contains twelve γ-carboxyglutamic acid residues (89). This region retains considerable homology with the other vitamin K-dependent blood coagulation proteins (Fig. 5). Like prothrombin, Factor X has two high affinity metal binding sites and multiple lower affinity metal binding sites. A metal-induced structural transition has been postulated from fluorescence experiments (53). Factor X binds to phospholipid vesicles in the presence of metal ions. Factor Xa, but not Factor X, binds to a specific receptor on the platelet surface (91, 92).

In the absence of vitamin K or in the presence of vitamin K antagonists, abnormal Factor X circulates in the plasma (98). This species contains, on the average, less than one residue of γ-carboxyglutamic acid per molecule of Factor X (94). It has impaired metal binding properties and deficient coagulant activity (95).

3. Factor IX

Factor IX is a plasma glycoprotein of the serine protease, Factor IXa. This protein, inactive in one form of hemophilia (Hemophilia B), is a component of the intrinsic pathway of the blood coagulation cascade. It is converted proteolytically to Factor IXa by Factor XIa in the presence of calcium (for review, see (1)). Recently, it has also been clearly demonstrated that Factor IX may be activated by Factor VIIa in the presence of tissue factor and calcium (96). Factor IX is a single polypeptide chain with a molecular weight of 56 000 (97). During activation an inactive intermediate is formed which contains two polypeptide chains bound by a single disulfide bond (98). A second bond is then cleaved, yielding Factor IXa.

Factor IX contains twelve γ-carboxyglutamic acid residues near the NH$_2$-terminus (99). This region is homologous to the amino terminal se-

quences of the vitamin K-dependent proteins (100). Factor IX also has two high affinity metal binding sites and multiple lower affinity metal binding sites (101). Factor IXa and its intermediates have similar metal binding properties (102).

An abnormal Factor IX, with reduced coagulant activity, has been identified in plasma of patients treated with sodium warfarin (103–105). Since it had reduced affinity for barium salts, it was suggested that this protein lacks γ-carboxyglutamic acid.

4. Factor VII

Factor VII is a vitamin K-dependent plasma glycoprotein which participates in the extrinsic pathway of blood coagulation. In its zymogen form, it is a single polypeptide chain with a molecular weight of 56 000 (106). During activation, it is converted to a two chain serine protease (107). Factor VII contains γ-carboxyglutamic acid and has a primary structure near the NH$_2$-terminus homologous to the other vitamin K-dependent blood coagulation proteins (108) (Fig. 5). The structural features of this protein have not been extensively studied because it is present in blood at very low concentrations. However, like the other vitamin K-dependent blood coagulation proteins it has two high affinity metal binding sites and multiple lower affinity sites (109).

5. Protein C

Protein C is a plasma glycoprotein that contains γ-carboxyglutamic acid (110). With a molecular weight of 62 000, it consists of a heavy chain and a light chain connected by a disulfide bond. This protein is a zymogen of the serine esterase, activated Protein C (111, 112). Its light chain is homologous to those of the vitamin K-dependent blood coagulation proteins (111, 112) (Fig. 5).

The functional role of this protein is unknown. Because activated Protein C has anticoagulant activity (14) due to its degradation of Factor Va (115), is has been suggested that this protein may serve a regulatory role.

6. Protein S

Protein S is a plasma glycoprotein of unknown function. This protein is composed of a single polypeptide chain of 67 000 (116). Containing γ-carboxyglutamic acid, it has an amino terminal sequence homologous to the vitamin K-dependent blood coagulation proteins (117). Protein S binds to phospholipid vesicles in the presence of calcium (118).

7. Protein Z

Protein Z is a plasma glycoprotein of unknown function (119). It contains γ-carboxyglutamic acid, but its amino terminal sequence is not homologous to any of the vitamin K-dependent blood coagulation proteins. It has a molecular weight of 54 000.

Proteins in calcified tissues

The majority of the γ-carboxyglutamic acid-containing proteins occur in calcified tissues such as the organic matrix of bone or renal stones and ectopic calcifications including artherosclerotic plaque. The presence of γ-carboxyglutamic acid in these calcification proteins has stimulated investigation of their function in regulation of both normal and pathological mineralization.

8. Osteocalcin

Osteocalcin was the first γ-carboxyglutamic acid-containing protein to be identified in mineralized tissue (120). This abundant, calcium binding, acidic glycoprotein from chickens has a molecular weight of 6500. Similar proteins have been extracted from the decalcified bone of a variety of species. Its properties are listed in Table 2. It was apparent from the amino acid composition and sequence that the γ-carboxyglutamic acid-containing protein from bovine bone is a unique protein, not merely a proteolysis fragment of a vitamin K-dependent blood clotting factor with affinity for the calcium matrix of bone (121). Further proof has come from studies which showed that bone microsomes have the vitamin K-dependent carboxylation system for de novo synthesis of γ-carboxyglutamic acid (122). Bone culture cells are able to synthesize the γ-carboxyglutamic acid-containing bone protein and secrete it into the extracellular matrix in the same manner as that proposed for collagen (123).

The concentration of osteocalcin present in the bone matrix increases with the development of bone (124). The concentration of γ-carboxyglutamic acid in bone also varies with respect to tissue type, location and extent of mineralization, with the highest concentration occurring in the diaphysis (midshaft), an area less metabolically active than other regions. Recent investigations of the biosynthesis of osteocalcin indicate that various forms of the protein are present in developing bone. At least two isomeric forms of osteocalcin occur in embryonic bone and up to four or more species may be present in adult bone (124). Also, higher molecular weight γ-carboxyglutamic acid-containing proteins have been isolated in bone microsome cultures supplemented with warfarin (125). The isolated γ-carboxyglutamic acid-containing proteins of 75 000 molecular weight and 200 000 molecular weight have been proposed as osteocalcin precursers.

The physiological role of bone γ-carboxyglutamic acid-containing protein in calcified tissues is unknown, but it appears to have a complex function in the regulation of developing bone growth. This protein has a specificity for hydroxyapetite and not for amorphous calcium phosphate (126). It has been suggested that the three γ-carboxyglutamic acid residues in the bovine γ-carboxyglutamic acid-containing protein of bone bind selectively to three calcium ions arranged in an equilateral triangle within the ordered hydroxyapetite crystal lattice, an arrangement which does not exist in the disordered amorphous calcium phosphate (121). Elimination of the γ-carboxyglutamic results in a protein with no affinity for hydroxyapetite (126). This binding to hydroxyapetite appears to have an inhibitory effect on mineral deposition rather than a crystal nucleation role in promoting calcification (126). Such inhibition by a bone matrix component may play a role in the control of the rate and alignment of mineral deposition.

By comparison, chicken bone osteocalcin, with four γ-carboxyglutamic acid residues, has two metal binding sites with can be occupied by many cations, including calcium ions (127). The structural differences which characterize the bovine and chicken proteins have no known functional correlates.

The presence of γ-carboxyglutamic acid in cartilaginous regions in the shark (128) has further complicated understanding of the role of γ-carboxyglutamic acid in calcified tissues. The cartilage of chicks contains 10–25% of the γ-carboxyglutamic acid present in mineralized tissues. Surprisingly, shark skeletal tissues contain greater γ-carboxyglutamic acid in the uncalcified car-

Table 2. γ-carboxyglutamic acid-containing proteins.

	Molecular Wt.	mol Gla/mol Protein	Metal Binding Sites	Source	Function
Prothrombin (bovine)	70 000	10	Two classes	plasma	Zymogen of protease blood coagulation
Factor X (bovine)	56 000	12	Two classes	plasma	Zymogen of protease blood coagulation
Factor IX (bovine)	56 000	12	Two classes	plasma	Zymogen of protease blood coagulation
Factor VII (bovine)	56 000	9	Two classes	plasma	Zymogen of protease blood coagulation
Protein C (bovine)	56 000	11	?	plasma	Zymogen of esterase ? anticoagulant
Protein S (bovine)	67 000	10	?	plasma	Unknown
Protein Z (bovine)	55 000	6	?	plasma	Unknown
Bone-Gla protein (bovine)	5 700	3	One class	bone	Unknown; ? Inhibitor of hydroxyapeptite deposition
Bone-Gla protein (fish)	6 000	3	?	bone	
Osteocalcin (chicken)	6 500	4	Two classes	bone	
Atherocalcin (human)	80 000	12	?	Atherosclerotic plaque	Unknown
Gla-protein (rat)	6 000	3	?	Atherosclerotic plaque	Unknown
Gla-protein (human)	17 000	6	?	Renal Caculi	Unknown
Gla-protein (chicken)	100 000	2–10	Two classes	Chorioallantoic membrane of egg	Calcium transport

tilaginous bones than in the calcified regions such as skin or the calcified vertebral centrum (128). These results indicate that these are not exclusively associated with mineralization but they may inhibit crystal deposition or perhaps serve to regulate calcium movements throughout skeletal tissues.

Recently, a radioimmunoassay for the bovine γ-carboxyglutamic acid-containing bone protein has been developed (129, 130). A specific antiserum, directed against the bone protein, has been used to detect a cross-reacting plasma protein of similar molecular weight. This protein circulates in plasma from 200 ng/ml in fetal calves to 26 ng/ml in adult cows.

9. γ-Carboxyglutamic acid containing protein of atherosclerotic plaque and other ectopic calcifications

γ-Carboxyglutamic acid-containing proteins have been isolated from the atherosclerotic plaque of rat (130) and human (131) tissues, and their properties are listed in Table 2. The quantity of the human protein, atherocalcin, present is proportional to the pathological severity of the vascular disease: least in the fatty streak lesions, increasing in fibrous plaque and the greatest in calcified plaques (131). The function of the γ-carboxyglutamic acid-containing protein from atherosclerotic tissue has not been determined. It may mediate calcification via interactions with the lipid-rich plaque in an analogous manner to the γ-carboxyglutamic acid-Ca^{++}-phospholipid interaction occurring with prothrombin.

In addition to atherosclerotic plaques, γ-carboxyglutamic acid-containing protein has been isolated from ectopic calcifications (132). These include subcutaneous plaques and calcified skin which form in dermatomyositis and calcium-containing material from the skin of patients with scleroderma. This material is composed primarily of hydroxyapetite. Since γ-carboxyglutamic acid is absent from the normal aorta or skin tissues, ectopic mineralization provides further evidence for the role of this amino acid in calcification processes.

10. γ-Carboxyglutamic acid-containing protein of renal calculi

γ-Carboxyglutamic acid has been identified in matrix protein from calcified renal stones (133). This protein appears to be unique, differing in size and amino acid composition from the blood coagulation proteins and osteocalcin (Table 1). In analyses of renal stones with varying compositions, this protein was present only in those composed of hydroxyapeptite or calcium oxalate, and it was absent from those which did not contain calcium such as pure struvite ($MgNH_4PO_4$), uric acid or cystine stones. Calculi composed of a mixture of both hydroxyapetite and struvite contained γ-carboxyglutamic in proportion to the amount of hydroxyapetite.

The kidney is actively involved in calcium homeostasis and has a vitamin K-dependent carboxylation system for γ-carboxyglutamic acid synthesis (134). It is not certain, however, whether the kidney stone protein is produced *de novo* by kidney tissue or if it accumulates from the glomerular filtrate.

The presence of γ-carboxyglutamic acid in other mineralized tissues

Organic matrix proteins from calcified tissues which contain mineral phases of calcite, aragonite or fluorapetite have been analyzed for the presence of γ-carboxyglutamic acid (135). These proteins were obtained from various invertebrates such as aragonitic mollusc shells, calcitic sea urchin spines, crab carapace or foraminifera tests, and calcitic and hydoxyapetite-containing brachiopod shells. Vertebrate mineralizations including the calcitic hen egg shell, aragonitic fish otolith or fluorapetite-containing shark tooth have also been investigated. The results from these analyses indicate that the non-collagenous invertebrate tissues, regardless of mineral phase deposited, do not contain γ-carboxyglutamic acid. In vertebrates, all collagenous matrices contain γ-carboxyglutamic acid. However, the noncollagenous aragonite from fish otolith also contained this amino acid. Furthermore, the organic matrix from fluorapetite shark tooth contained a substantial quantity of γ-carboxyglutamic acid. This indicates that γ-carboxyglutamic acid is not uniquely associated with collagen containing matrices and is not specific for the hydroxyapetite mineral phase.

The studies of the distribution of γ-carboxyglutamic acid in animals provides insight into the evolution of vitamin K-dependent carboxylation. On the basis of current data, such systems have evolved only in vertebrates. The presence of γ-carboxyglutamic acid in the plasma of the lamprey eel, a 'living fossil' (136), in shark cartilage (128), and in the fossils of mammoth bone and 48 000 yr old whale bone (137) indicates an early appearance of a carboxylation system in vertebrate tissues.

γ-Carboxyglutamic acid-containing proteins not associated with calcification

Recent reports have identified γ-carboxyglutamic acid and vitamin K-dependent carboxylation systems from a wide distribution of species and tissues. As a result speculations have been made concerning a possible role of γ-carboxyglutamic acid in calcium transport, ribosome structure, growth regulation and calcium homeostasis. Such functions indicate a vast diversity of roles for this specialized amino acid. However, identification of this amino acid can be difficult. Some of these preliminary observations have not been confirmed by laboratories with special expertise in this field (138).

A γ-carboxyglutamic acid-containing protein has been found in chick chlorioallantoic membrane (139), a calcium-transporting placenta-like tissue which separates the calcium-rich eggshell from the embryonic circulation. This protein appears concurrently with the onset of calcium transport function and is synthesized by a vitamin K-dependent carboxylation system located within the membrane (140). A vitamin K-dependent carboxylation system has been found in human placenta, but it is unknown whether the protein formed is also involved in calcium transport (141).

γ-Carboxyglutamic acid has been reported in ribosomes of mammals, wheat germ and *E. coli* (142, 143), but not confirmed (138). γ-Carboxyglutamic acid has also been identified in lung microsomes, kidney (134), spleen, pancreas, and cultured fibroblasts. The zymogen of the activator of the clottable protein in the horseshoe crab, L. polyphemus, has been reported to contain γ-carboxyglutamic acid (144). However, this observation has not been confirmed in other laboratories that have studied this protein.

Metabolism of γ-carboxyglutamic acid

The excretion of free γ-carboxyglutamic acid and γ-carboxyglutamic acid containing peptides represents the final catabolic pathway of the vitamin K-dependent proteins. The free amino acid is not metabolized (145, 146) and less than 5% of γ-carboxyglutamic acid in the urine is bound to protein. Consequently, monitoring urinary γ-carboxyglutamic acid excretion can be a method for the determination of pathological conditions of vitamin K-dependent pocesses such as blood coagulation, bone metabolism and ectopic calcifications. Normal 5 yr old children excrete approximately 100 μmole of γ-carboxyglutamic acid per gram of creatinine (147). This value decreases with age until at 15 years the normal adult value of 44 μmoles of γ-carboxyglutamic acid per gram of creatinine is obtained.

A change in the dynamic state of either mineralization or coagulation can lead to detectable changes in the urinary excretion rate of γ-carboxyglutamic acid (148). Warfarin therapy, through partial inhibition of γ-carboxyglutamic acid synthesis, reduced the urinary γ-carboxyglutamic acid excretion to approximately 50% of normal (148). About 25% of the normal excretion rate of γ-carboxyglutamic acid is not affected by anticoagulation. This is attributed to dietary sources and γ-carboxyglutamic acid-containing proteins of extrahepatic origin. Increased γ-carboxyglutamic acid excretion of 69 μmole per gram of creatinine occurs in patients with osteoporosis (149). Given the contribution of osteocalcin to γ-carboxyglutamic acid excretion, this corresponds to a three-fold increase in bone turnover. Also, excretion rates doubled in patients with scleroderma and severe calcification (149) and were significantly elevated in patients with juvenile dermatolmyositis, including those with ectopic calcifications (150).

Conclusion

Since the discovery of γ-carboxyglutamic acid six years ago, significant progress has been made in determining its unique biological function. To date it has been clearly implicated in the blood coagulation mechanism and in processes related to mineralization. Its special metal binding properties indicate that it may play a special role in calcium or magnesium homeostasis, metal ion transport, and physiologic mechanisms regulated by metal ions. The importance of calcium in the regulation of biochemical pathways, stabilization of enzyme and protein structure, and control of physiologic events may suggest a structural role for γ-carboxyglutamic acid in these systems. Improved understanding of the function γ-carboxyglutamic acid and γ-carboxyglutamic acid-containing proteins should shed considerable light on this class of calcium-binding proteins in the future.

Acknowledgements

J.P.B. was supported by an Institutional National Research Service Award T32 HL-07437 from the National Institutes of Health. B.C.F. is the recipient of a Research Career Development Award from the National Institutes of Health. B.F. is an Established Investigator of the American Heart Association and its Massachusetts Affiliate. The work described from this laboratory has been supported by grants HL-18834 and HL-21543 from the National Institutes of Health.

References

1. Davie, E. W. & Hanahan, D. J., 1977. The Plasma Proteins (Putnam, F. W., ed.) 3: 421–544.
2. Jackson, C. M. & Nemerson, Y., 1980. Ann. Rev. Biochem. 49: 765–811.
3. Nemerson, Y. & Furie, B., 1980. CRC Crit. Rev. Biochem., 9: 45–85.
4. Suttie, J. W., 1980. CRC Crit. Rev. Biochem. 8: 191–223.
5. Suttie, J. W. & Jackson, C. M., 1977. Physiol. Rev. 57: 1–70.
6. Stenflo, J. & Suttie, J. W., 1977. Ann. Rev. Biochem. 46: 157–172.
7. Dam, H., 1929. Biochem. Z. 215, 475–492.
8. Dam, H., 1935. Nature 135: 652–653.
9. Dam, H., Schonheyder, F. & Tage-Hansen, E., 1936. Biochem. J. 30: 1075–1079.
10. Campbell, H. A. & Link, K. P., 1941. J. Biol. Chem. 138: 21–33.
11. Ganrot, P. O. & Nilehn, J. E., 1968. Scand. J. Clin. Lab. Invest. 22: 23–28.
12. Stenflo, J. & Ganrot, P. O., 1972. J. Biol. Chem. 247: 8160–8166.
13. Nelsestuen, G. L. & Suttie, J. W., 1972. J. Biol. Chem. 247: 8176–8182.
14. Stenflo, J. & Ganrot, P. O., 1973. Biochem. Biophys. Res. Comm. 50: 98–104.

15. Esmon, C. T., Suttie, J. W. & Jackson, C. M., 1975. J. Biol. Chem. 250: 4095–4099.

16. Nelsestuen, G. L. & Suttie, J. W., 1973. Proc. Natl. Acad. Sci. U.S.A. 70: 3366–3370.

17. Stenflo, J., 1974. Proc. Natl. Acad. Sci., U.S.A. 71: 2730–2733.

18. Nelsestuen, G. L., Zytkovicz, T. H. & Howard, J. B., 1974. J. Biol. Chem. 249: 6347–6350.

19. Magnusson, S., Sottrup-Jensen, L., Petersen, T. E., Morris, H. R. & Dell, A., 1974. FEBS Lett. 44: 189–193.

20. Oppliger, M. & Schwyzer, R., 1977. Helv. Chim. Acta. 60: 43–47.

21. Danishefsky, S., Berman, E., Clizbe, L. & Hirama, M., 1979. J. Am. Chem. Soc. 101: 4385–4386.

22. Marki, W. & Schwyzer, R., 1975. Helv. Chim. Acta 58: 1471–1477.

23. Weinstein, B., Watrin, K. G., Loie, H. J. & Martin, J. C., 1976. J. Org. Chem. 41, 3634–3635.

24. Boggs, N. T., III, Gawley, R. E., Koehler, K. A. & Hiskey, R. G., 1975. J. Org. Chem. 40: 2850–2851.

25. Boggs, N. T., III, Goldsmith, B., Gawley, R. E., Koehler, K. A. & Hiskey, R. G., 1979. J. Org. Chem. 44: 2262–2269.

26. Morris, H. R., Thompson, R. & Dell, A., 1975. Biochem. Biophys. Res. Comm. 62: 856–861.

27. Juhasz, A. and Bajusz, S., 1980. Int. J. Peptide Protein Res. 15: 154–158.

28. Fernlund, P., Stenflo, J., Roepstorff, P. & Thomsen, J., 1975. J. Biol. Chem. 250: 6125–6133.

29. Zee-Cheng, R. K. Y. & Olson, R. E., 1979. In: Vitamin K Metabolism and Vitamin K-dependent Proteins (Suttie, J. W., ed.). Baltimore: University Park Press, 157–160.

30. Marki, W., Oppliger, M., Thanei, P. & Schwyzer, R., 1977. Helv. Chim. Acta. 60: 798–806.

31. Sperling, R., Furie, B. C., Blumenstein, M., Keyt, B. & Furie, B., 1978. J. Biol. Chem. 253: 3893–3906.

32. Hauschka, P. V., 1977. Anal. Biochem. 80: 212–223.

33. Madar, D. A., Willis, R. A., Koehler, K. A. & Hiskey, R. G., 1979. Anal. Biochem. 92: 466–472.

34. Tabor, H. & Tabor, C. W., 1977. Anal. Biochem. 78: 554–556.

35. Zytkovicz, T. H. & Nelsestuen, G. L., 1975. J. Biol. Chem. 250: 2968–2972.

36. Hauschka, P. V., 1979. Biochemistry 18: 4992–4999.

37. Fernlund, P. & Stenflo, J., 1979. In: Vitamin K Metabolism and Vitamin K-dependent proteins (Suttie, J. W., ed.). Baltimore: University Park Press, pp 161–165.

38. Robertson, P., Jr., Hiskey, R. G. & Koehler, K. A., 1978. J. Biol. Chem. 253: 5880–5883.

39. Marki, W., Oppliger, M. & Schwyzer, R., 1977. Helv. Chim. Acta 60: 807–815.

40. Satyshur, K. A., 1978. Structural studies of modified amino acids by x-ray crystallography: γ-carboxyglutamic acid and methylated amino acids. Ph. D. Thesis. University of Wisconsin (Madison).

41. Furie, B. C., Blumenstein, M. & Furie, B., 1979. J. Biol. Chem. 254: 12521–12530.

42. Sarasua, M. M., Scott, M. E., Helpern, J. A., Ten Kortenaar, P. B. W., Boggs, N. T., III, Pedersen, L. G., Koehler, K. A., and Hiskey, R. G., 1980. J. Am. Chem. Soc. 102: 3404–3412.

43. Bajaj, S. P., Butkowski, R. J. & Mann, K. G., 1975. J. Biol. Chem. 250: 2150–2156.

44. Furie, B. C., Mann, K. G. & Furie, B., 1976. J. Biol. Chem. 251: 3235–3241.

45. Bloom, J. W. & Mann, K. G., 1978. Biochemistry 17: 4430–4438.

46. Nelsestuen, G. L., 1976. J. Biol. Chem. 251: 5648–5656.

47. Pendergast, F. G. & Mann, K. G., 1977. J. Biol. Chem. 252: 840–850.

48. Marsh, H. C., Robertson, P., Scott, M. E., Koehler, K. A. & Hiskey, R. G., 1979. J. Biol. Chem. 254: 10268–10275.

49. Furie, B., Provost, K. L., Blanchard, R. A. & Furie, B. C., 1978. J. Biol. Chem. 253: 8980–8987.

50. Furie, B. & Furie, B. C., 1979. J. Biol. Chem. 254: 9766–9771.

51. Tai, M. M., Furie, B. C. & Furie, B., 1980. J. Biol. Chem. 255: 2790–2795.

52. Lim, T. K., Bloomfield, V. A. & Nelsestuen, G. L., 1977. Biochemistry 16: 4177–4181.

53. Nelsestuen, G. L. & Broderius, M., 1977. Biochemistry 16: 4172–4177.

54. Scott, M. E., Sarasua, M. M., Marsh, H. C., Harris, D. L., Hiskey, R. G. & Koehler, K. A., 1980. J. Am. Chem. Soc. 102: 3413–3419.

55. Scott, M. E., Koehler, K. A. & Hiskey, R. G., 1979. Biochem. J. 177: 879–886.

56. Aschaffenburg, R., Blake, C. C. F., Burridge, J. M. & Esnouf, M. P., 1977. J. Mol. Biol. 114: 575–579.

57. Hu Kung, W. J. & Tulinsky, A. Regulation of Coagulation (Mann, K. G. & Taylor, F. B., Jr., eds.) New York: Elsevier/North Holland, pp. 81–88.

58. Shah, D. V. & Suttie, J. W., 1971. Proc. Natl. Acad. Sci., U.S.A. 68: 1653–1657.

59. Suttie, J. W. Mechanism of action of vitamin K: 1973. Science 179: 192–194.

60. Esmon, C. T., Sadowski, J. A. & Suttie, J. W., 1975. J. Biol. Chem. 250: 4744–4748.

61. Friedman, P. A. & Shia, M. A., 1976. Biochem. Biophys. Res. Comm. 70; 647–654.

62. Girardot, J. M., Mack, D. O., Floyd, R. A. and Johnson, B. C., 1976. Biochem. Biophys. Res. Comm. 70: 655–662.

63. Jones, J. P., Fausto, A., Houser, R. M., Gardner, E. J. & Olsen, R. E., 1976. Biochem. Biophys. Res. Comm. 72: 589–597.

64. Esmon, C. T. & Suttie, J. W., 1976. J. Biol. Chem. 251: 6238–6243.

65. Suttie, J. W., Hageman, J. M., Lehrman, S. R. & Rich, D. H., 1976. J. Biol. Chem. 251: 5827–5830.

66. Helgeland, L., 1977. Biochim. Biophys. Acta 499: 181–193.

67. Jones, J. P., Gardner, E. J., Cooper, T. G. & Olson, R. E., 1977. J. Biol. Chem. 252: 7738–7742.

68. Mack, D. O., Suen, E. T., Girardot, J. M., Miller, J. A., Delaney, R. & Johnson, B. C., 1976. J. Biol. Chem. 251: 3269–3276.

69. Sadowski, J. A., Esmon, C. T. & Suttie, J. W., 1976. J. Biol. Chem. 251: 2770–2776.

70. Friedman, P. A. & Shia, M. A., 1977. Biochem. J. 163: 39–43.

71. Whitlon, R., D. S., Sadowski, J. A. & Suttie, J. W., 1978. Biochemistry 17: 1371–1377.

206

72. Bell, R. G. & Galdwell, P. T., 1973. Biochemistry 12: 1759–1762.

73. Willingham, A. K. & Matschiner, J. T., 1974. Biochem. J. 140: 435–441.

74. Friedman, P. A. & Griep, A. E., 1980. Biochemistry 19: 3381–3386.

75. Friedman, P. A., Shia, M. A., Gallop, P. M. & Griep, A. E., 1979. Proc. Natl. Acad. Sci., U.S.A. 76: 3126–3129.

76. Larson, A. E. & Suttie, J. W., 1978. Proc. Natl. Acad. Sci., U.S.A. 75: 5413–5416.

77. Esnouf, M. P., Green, M. R., Hill, H. A. O., Irvine, G. B. & Walter, S. J., 1978. Biochem. J. 174: 345–348.

78. Jackson, C. M., Peng, C. W., Brueckle, G. M., Jonas, A. & Stenflo, J., 1979. J. Biol. Chem. 254: 5020–5026.

79. Blanchard, R. A., Furie, B. C. & Furie, B., 1980. J. Biol. Chem. 255: 2790–2795.

80. Esmon, C. T., Grant, G. A. & Suttie, J. W., 1975. Biochemistry 14: 1595–1600.

81. Grant, G. A. & Suttie, J. W., 1976. Biochemistry 15: 5387–5393.

82. Munns, T. W., Johnston, M. F. M., Liszewski, M. K., & Olson, R. E., 1976. Proc. Natl. Acad. Sci., U.S.A. 73: 2803–2807.

83. Graves, C. B., Grabau, G. G., Olson, R. E. & Munns, T. W., 1980. Biochemistry 19: 266–272.

84 Blanchard, R. A., Furie, B. C., Jorgenson, M., Kruger, S. & Furie, B., 1981. N. Engl. J. Med. 305 (in press).

85. Jackson, C. M., 1972. Biochemistry 11: 4873–4881.

86. Fujikawa, K., Legaz, M. E. & Davie, E. W., 1972. Biochemistry 11: 4882–4891.

87. Titani, K., Fujikawa, K., Enfield, D. L., Ericson, L. H., Walsh, K. A. & Neurath, H., 1975. Proc. Natl. Acad. Sci., U.S.A. 72: 3082–3086.

88. Furie, B. & Furie, B. C., 1976. J. Biol. Chem. 251: 6807–6814.

89. Thogersen, H. C., Petersen, T. E., Sottrup-Jensen, L., Magnusson, S. & Morris, H. R., 1978. Biochem. J. 175: 613–627.

90. Magnusson, S., Petersen, T. E., Sottrup-Jensen, L. & Claeys, H., 1975. In: Proteases and Biological Control (Reich, E. et al., eds.). Cold Spring Harbor, pp. 123–149.

91. Miletich, J. P., Jackson, C. M. & Majerus, P. W., 1978. J. Biol. Chem. 253: 6908–6916.

92. Dahlback, B. & Stenflo, J., 1978. Biochemistry 17: 4938–4945.

93. Gaudernack, G., Berre, A. G., Osterud, B. & Prydz, H., 174. Thromb. Diath. Haemorrh. 31: 40–51.

94. Lindhout, M. J., Kop-Klaasen, B. H. M., Kop, J. M. M. & Hemker, H. C., 1978. Biochim. Biophys. Acta 533: 302–317.

95. Lindhout, M. J. & Hemker, H. C., 1978. Biochim. Biophys. Acta 533: 318–326.

96. Osterud, B. & Rapaport, S. I., 1977. Proc. Natl. Acad. Sci., U.S.A. 74: 5260–5264.

97. Fujikawa, K., Thompson, A. R., Legaz, M. E., Meyer, R. G. & Davie, E. W., 1973. Biochemistry 12: 4938–4945.

98. Fujikawa, K., Legaz, M. E. & Davie, E. W., 1974. Biochemistry 13: 4508–4516.

99. DiScipio, R. G. & Davie, E. W., 1979. Biochemistry 18: 899–904.

100. Katayama, K., Ericsson, L. H., Enfield, D. L., Walsh, K. A., Neurath, H., Davie, E. W. & Titani, K., 1979. Proc. Natl. Acad. Sci., U.S.A. 76: 4990–4994.

101. Amphlett, G. W., Byrne, R. & Castellino, F. J., 1978. J. Biol. Chem. 253: 6774–6779.

102. Amphlett, G. W., Byrne, R. & Castellino, F. J., 1979. J. Biol. Chem. 254: 6333–6336.

103. Larrieu, M. J. & Meyer, D., 1970. Lancet ii, 1085.

104. Thompson, A. R., 1977. J. Clin. Invest. 59: 900–910.

105. Orstavik, K. H. & Laake, K., 1978. Thromb. Res. 13: 207–218.

106. Radcliffe, R. & Nemerson, Y., 1975. J. Biol. Chem. 250: 388.

107. Radcliffe, R. & Nemerson, Y., 1976. J. Biol. Chem. 251: 4797–4802.

108. Kisiel, W., Fujikawa, K. & Davie, E. W., 1977. Biochemistry 16: 4189–4194.

109. Strickland, D. K. & Castellino, F. J., 1980. Arch. Biochem. Biophys. 199: 61–66.

110. Stenflo, J. 1976. J. Biol. Chem. 251: 355–363.

111. Kisiel, W., Ericsson, L. H. & Davie, E. W., 1976. Biochemistry 15: 4893–4900.

112. Esmon, C. T., Stenflo, J., Suttie, J. W. & Jackson, C. M., 1976. J. Biol. Chem. 251: 3052–3056.

113. Fernlund, P., Stenflo, J. & Tufvesson, A., 1978. Proc. Natl. Acad. Sci., U.S.A. 75: 5889–5892.

114. Kisiel, W., Canfield, W. M., Ericsson, L. H. & Davie, E. W., 1977. Biochemistry 16: 5824–5831.

115. Walker, F. J., Sexton, P. W. & Esmon, C. T., 1979. Biochim. Biophys. Acta 571: 333–342.

116. DiScipio, R. G., Hermodson, M. A., Yates, S. G. & Davie, E. W., 1977. Biochemistry 16: 698–706.

117. DiScipio, R. G. & Davie, E. W., 1979. Biochemistry 18: 899–904.

118. Nelsestuen, G. L., Kisiel, W. & DiScipio, R. G., 1978. Biochemistry 17: 2134–2138.

119. Prowse, C. V. & Esnouf, M. P., 1977. Biochem. Soc. Trans. 5: 255–256.

120. Hauschka, P. V., Lian, J. B. & Gallop, P. M., 1975. Proc. Natl. Acad. Sci., U.S.A. 72: 3925–3929.

121. Price, P. A., Poser, J. W. & Raman, N., 1976. Proc. Natl. Acad. Sci., U.S.A. 73: 3374–3375.

122. Lian, J. B. & Friedman, P. A., 1978. J. Biol. Chem. 253: 6623–6626.

123. Nishimoto, S. K. & Price, P. A., 1979. J. Biol. Chem. 254: 437–441.

124. Hauschka, P. V., 1979. In: Vitamin K Metabolism and Vitamin K-dependent proteins (Suttie, J. W., ed.) University Park Press, Baltimore, 227–236.

125. Lian, J. B. & Heroux, K. M., 1979. In: Vitamin K Metabolism and Vitamin K-dependent proteins (Suttie, J. W., ed.). Baltimore: University Park Press, pp. 245–254.

126. Poser, J. W. & Price, P. A., 1979. J. Biol. Chem. 254: 431–436.

127. Hauschka, P. V. & Gallop, P. M., 1978. In: Calcium binding proteins and Calcium function (Wasserman, R. H. et al., eds.), Amsterdam: North Holland, pp. 338–347.

128. Lian, J. B., Glowacki, J. A. & Glimcher, M. J., 1979. In: Vitamin K Metabolism and Vitamin K-dependent proteins

(Suttie, J. W., ed.). Baltimore: University Park Press, pp. 263–268.

129. Price, P. A. & Nishimoto, S. K., 1980. Proc. Natl. Acad. Sci., U.S.A. 77: 2234–2238.

130. Deyl, Z., Macek, K., Vancikova, O. & Adam, M., 1979. Biochim. Biophys. Acta 581: 307–315.

131. Levy, R. J., Lian, J. B. & Gallop, P. M., 1979. Biochem. Biophys. Res. Comm. 91: 41–49.

132. Lian, J. B., Skinner, M., Glimcher, M. J. & Gallop, P. M., 1976. Biochem. Biophys. Res. Comm. 73: 349–355.

133. Lian, J. B., Prien, E. L., Jr., Glimcher, M. J. & Gallop, P. M., 1977. J. Clin. Invest. 59: 1151–1157.

134. Hauschka, P. V., Friedman, P. A., Traverso, H. P. & Gallop, P. M., 1976. Biochem. Biophys. Res. Comm. 71: 1207–1213.

135. King, K., Jr., 1978. Biochim. Biophys. Acta 542: 542–546.

136. Zytkovicz, T. H. & Nelsestuen, G. L., 1976. Biochim. Biophys. Acta 444: 344–348.

137. King, K., Jr., 1978. Nature 273: 41–43.

138. Petersen, T. E., Thogersen, H. C., Magnusson, S. & Sottrup-Jensen, L., 1979. In: Vitamin K Metabolism and Vitamin K-dependent proteins (Suttie, J. W., ed.). Baltimore: University Park Press, pp. 171–174.

139. Tuan, R. S., Scott, W. S. & Cohn, Z. A., 1978. J. Biol. Chem. 253: 1011–1016.

140. Tuan, R. S., 1979. J. Biol. Chem. 254: 1356–1364.

141. Friedman, P. A., Hauschka, P. V., Shia, M. A. & Wallace, J. K., 1979. Biochim. Biophys. Acta 583: 261–265.

142. Van Buskirk, J. J. & Kirsch, W. M., 1978. Biochem. Biophys. Res. Comm. 82: 1329–1331.

143. Van Buskirk, J. J. & Kirsch, W. M., 1978. Biochem. Biophys. Res. Comm. 80: 1033–1038.

144. Tai, J. Y. & Liv, T. Y., 1977. J. Biol. Chem. 252: 2178–2181.

145. Fernlund, P., 1976. Clin. Chim. Acta 72: 147–155.

146. Shah, D. V., Tews, J. K., Harper, A. E. & Suttie, J. W., 1978. Biochim. Biophys. Acta 539: 209–217.

147. Gundberg, C. M., Lian, J. B. & Gallop, P. M., 1979. Anal. Biochem 98: 219–225.

148. Levy, R. J. & Lian, J. B., 1979. Clin. Pharmacol. Ther. 25: 562–570.

149. Gallop, P. M., Lian, J. B. & Hauschka, P. V., 1980. New Engl. J. Med. 302: 1460–1466.

150. Lian, J. B., Pachman, L., Partridge, N. E. H., Gundberg, C. & Gallop, P. M., 1979. Arthritis. Rheum. 22: 634–635.

Received August 14, 1980.

Folylpoly-γ-glutamate synthesis by bacteria and mammalian cells

David J. Cichowicz, Siang K. Foo and Barry Shane[1]
Dept. of Biochemistry, School of Hygiene and Public Health, The Johns Hopkins University, 615 North Wolfe Street, Baltimore, MD 21205, U.S.A.

Summary

The purification and properties of folylpolyglutamate synthetase from *Corynebacterium sp,* and some properties of partially purified enzyme from *Lactobacillus casei, Streptococcus faecalis, Neurospora crassa,* pig liver, and Chinese hamster ovary cells, are described.

The *Corynebacterium* enzyme catalyzes a MgATP-dependent addition of glutamate to a variety of reduced pteroate and pteroylmono-, di-, and triglutamate substrates, with the concomitant production of MgADP and phosphate. Although glutamate moieties are added in a sequential fashion, the kinetic mechanism, which is Ordered Ter Ter, precludes the sequential addition of glutamate moieties to enzyme-bound folate. It is suggested that catalysis precedes via the formation of a pteroyl-γ-glutamyl phosphate intermediate.

The *in vivo* distribution of folylpolyglutamates in bacteria and mammalian cells, which differ from source to source, appear to be a reflection of the ability of folylpolyglutamates to act as substrates for folylpolyglutamate synthetases from different sources.

Only one enzyme appears to be involved in the conversion of pteroylmonoglutamates to polyglutamate forms in both bacteria and mammalian cells. Bacterial folylpolyglutamate synthetases use a variety of pteroylmonoglutamates as their preferred monoglutamate substrate, but use 5,10-methylenetetrahydropteroylpolyglutamates as their preferred, and sometimes only, polyglutamate substrate. Mono- and polyglutamyl forms of tetrahydrofolate are the preferred substrates of mammalian folylpolyglutamate synthetases.

Abbreviations used

PteGlu, pteroylmonoglutamic acid, folic acid; $H_4PteGlu_n$, 5,6,7,8-tetrahydropteroylpoly-γ-glutamate, n indicating the number of glutamate moieties; $pABAglu_n$, p-aminobenzoylpoly-γ-glutamate. The symbols (*l*) and (*d*) are used to denote the natural and unnatural diastereoisomers of $H_4PteGlu_n$, respectively, due to the asymmetric center at position C-6, Unless indicated otherwise, all reduced folates used in this study were a mixture of the (*l*) and (*d*) isomers.

[1] *To whom reprint requests should be addressed.*

Introduction

Folate coenzymes act as acceptors or donors of one carbon units in a variety of reactions involved in amino acid and nucleotide metabolism (1). The one carbon units, which are derived principally from the β carbon of serine can be at the oxidation levels of formaldehyde, formate, or methanol, and excess one carbon units are removed from the one carbon pool by their oxidation to CO_2. Most of these reactions, known as one carbon metabolism, have been studied using reduced pteroylmonoglutamates as substrates (2). However, it has been known for many years that folates exist naturally primarily as

Molecular and Cellular Biochemistry 39, 209–228 (1981).   0300–8177/81/0391–0209/$04.00.

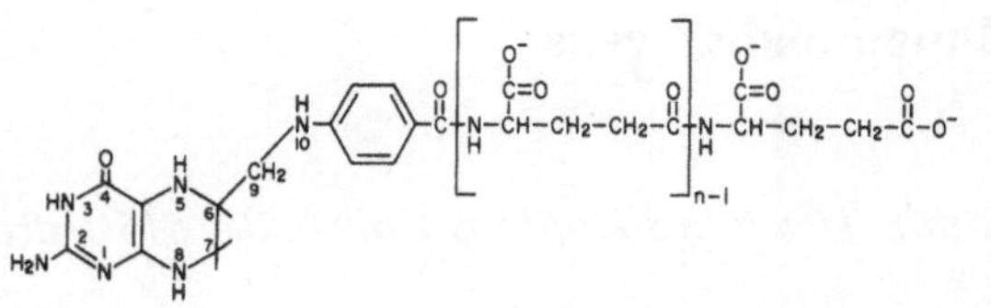

Fig. 1. Structure of 5,6,7,8-etrahydropteroylpoly-γ-glutamate (H₄PteGluₙ). One carbon moieties are attached at the N-5 and/or N-10 positions.

polyglutamate derivatives with the glutamate moieties linked via γ-carboxyl peptide bonds (Fig. 1).

Some of the physiological roles of folyl-polyglutamates have been recently reviewed (3). Folylpolyglutamates do not cross, or are only poorly transported across, cell membranes (4, 5). Consequently, metabolism of pteroylmonoglutamates to polyglutamate forms allows the cell to concentrate folates at much higher levels than in the external medium. Folylpolyglutamates are as effective as, and in many cases more effective than, pteroylmonoglutamates as substrates for the enzymes of one carbon metabolism (2, 3, 6–17). Many of these enzyme activities are associated in the cell, either as protein complexes or as multi-functional polypeptides (18–22). Preliminary studies suggest that folylpolyglutamate substrates are channelled from active site to active site in these complexes without release of the intermediate products, a phenomenum that is not observed with monoglutamate substrates (23, 24). An important regulatory role of folylpolyglutamates is also suggested by the observations that these compounds are effective inhibitors of a number of enzymes involved in one carbon metabolism while the corresponding monoglutamate derivatives are ineffective or poor inhibitors of the same enzymes (6, 11, 13, 25, 26).

The importance of folylpolyglutamate formation has been demonstrated in cultured Chinese hamster ovary (CHO) cell mutants which lack folylpolyglu-tamate synthetase activity (27–29). Although folate transport by these cells is unimpaired, intracellular folate levels are reduced due to an inability to synthesize folylpolyglutamates, and the mutant cells require exogenous methionine, glycine, purines, and thymidine for growth while the wild type will grow in the absence of these compounds provided sufficient folate, vitamin B12, and homocysteine are supplied

in the medium (27, 30).

Different glutamate chain length folates are found in different tissues and it has been suggested that the one carbon flux through various folate-dependent metabolic reactions may be regulated under different growth conditions by varying the glutamate chain length of folates (31). A major interest of our laboratory is to understand the mechanisms by which folylpolyglutamates of specific glutamate chain length are synthesized by different tissues and organisms, and whether regulation of this process serves as a means of regulating one carbon metabolism. The properties of some folylpolyglutamate synthetases are des-cribed in this report. These enzymes catalyze the general reaction

$$H_4PteGlu_n + glutamate + ATP \rightarrow H_4PteGlu_{n+1} + ADP + Pi$$

Materials and methods

Materials

[³H]PteGlu, labelled in the 3′,5′, and 9 positions (20–50 Ci/mmol), [U-¹⁴C]glutamate (10 mCi/mmol), [8-¹⁴C]ATP (50 mCi/mmol), and [γ-³²P]ATP were obtained from Amersham Corp., and [carboxy-¹⁴C]pABA (35.6 mCi/mmol) from ICN. Nucleotide and amino acid derivatives were obtained from Sigma Chem. Co., P-L Biochemicals, and Vega-Fox.

Folic acid (PteGlu) and (dl)H₄PteGlu were obtained from Sigma Chem. Co. and methotrexate from Aldrich Chem. Co. Folic acid polyglutamates PteGlu₂₋₇ and PteGluₙ-[¹⁴C]Glu-Glu (n = 1–3, 0.5 mCi/mmol) were synthesized by the method of Baugh et al. (32). Pteroylamino acid analogs were synthesized by a modification of the method of Plante et al. (33). Reduced one-carbon forms of folate were synthesized as described previously (5, 6). (l)-H₄PteGluₙ was prepared by enzymatic reduction of PteGluₙ using dihydrofolate reductase purified from methotrexate-resistant *Lactobacillus casei* as described by Whiteley et al. (34). (l)-10-formyl-H₄PteGlu was prepared from (l)-H₄PteGlu using purified *Clostridium* 10-formyltetrahydrofo-late synthetase (5, 6). All folate derivatives were purified by chromatography on DEAE cellulose and were stored in K phosphate buffer, pH 7, containing 0.2 M β-mercaptoethanol at –196°C. The identity of each compound was confirmed by its chromatographic behavior on DEAE-cellulose and BioGel P4, by its absorption spectrum, and, in some cases, by differential microbiological assay. The concentration of each compound was calculated from its absorbance (35).

Cell culture conditions

Corynebacterium sp, Lactobacillus casei, and *Streptococcus faecalis* were cultured as described previously (4, 36). CHO cells were cultured in α-minimal essential medium (MEM) supplemented with 10% dialyzed fetal calf serum as described by Taylor & Hanna (30). Crude extracts of the bacterial and mammalian cells were prepared by sonication.

Labelling of cellular folates

Corynebacterium folates were labelled by culturing the bacteria for 4 days in the presence of [^{14}C]pABA (0.1 μCi/ml) as described previously (37,38). *L. casei* and *S. faecalis* were cultured for 22 h in the presence of 20 nM [^{3}H]PteGlu. CHO cells were cultured for 2 days in α-MEM containing 2 μM[^{3}H]PteGlu.

The cells were centrifuged, washed with 0.9% NaCl, resuspended in 20 mM K phosphate buffer, pH 7, containing 100 mM mercaptoethanol. Intracellular folates were extracted by heating at 100° for 5 min, and the residue removed by centrifugation.

Male McCollum rats were injected intraperitoneally with [^{3}H]PteGlu and were sacrificed by decapitation after 24 h. Livers were perfused with ice-cold 0.9% NaCl, excised, and an aliquot was homogenized with 3 vol. 6.7% trichloroacetic acid and centrifuged. The supernatant was extracted with peroxide-free diethyl ether (3 × 4 vol) to remove the bulk of the trichloroacetic acid.

Identification of folylpolyglutamate chain length

Folates in bacterial and cell culture extracts were cleaved to pABAglu$_n$ and a pterin derivative as described previously (39). The procedure involved acidification in the presence of mercaptoethanol to convert 10-formyl- and 5-formyl-H$_4$PteGlu$_n$ to 5,10-methenyl-H$_4$PteGlu$_n$, NaBH$_4$ reduction to

convert 5,10-methenyl-H$_4$PteGlu$_n$ to 5-methyl-H$_4$PteGlu$_n$, treatment with HgCl$_2$ to remove mercaptoethanol, base treatment to convert 5-methyl-H$_4$PteGlu$_n$ to 5-methyl-H$_2$PteGlu$_n$ and 10-formyl-PteGlu$_n$ to PteGlu$_n$, acidification to convert 5-methyl-H$_2$PteGlu$_n$ to pABAglu$_n$, and Zn treatment to cleave PteGlu$_n$ to pABAglu$_n$. The overall procedure allows the quantitative conversion of all naturally occurring folates to pABAglu$_n$.

Labelled and unlabelled pABAglu$_n$ in the extracts were converted to azodyes of naphthylethylene diamine which were purified and separated from the pterin derivative by chromatography on BioGel P2 (40). The azo dyes of pABAglu$_n$ were separated, according to glutamate chain length, by chromatography on BioGel P4. (40). Alternatively, the purified azo dyes were reconverted to pABAglu$_n$, by treatment with Zn under acid conditions, and the pABAglu$_n$ compounds were separated by high performance liquid chromatography (HPLC) on a strong anionic exchanger (Whatman SAX).

Folylpolyglutamate synthetase assay

Enzyme activity was routinely measured by the incorporation of [^{14}C]glutamate into folylpolyglutamates using unlabelled H$_4$PteGlu as the folate substrate (41).

Reaction mixtures for bacterial enzyme, unless indicated otherwise, contained: 100 mM tris-50 mM glycine buffer, pH 10, (dl)H$_4$PteGlu (100 μM), L-[^{14}C]glutamate (250 μM), ATP (5 mM), MgCl$_2$ (10 mM), KCl (200 mM), dithiothreitol (5 mM), β-mercaptoethanol (10 mM; derived from folate solution), bovine serum albumin (50 μg), DMSO (50 μl), and enzyme preparation in a total volume of 0.5 ml. The tubes were capped and incubated for 2 h at 37°C. The reaction was stopped by the addition of ice-cold 30 mM β-mercaptoethanol (1.5 ml) containing 10 mM glutamate.

The assay mixture for the mammalian enzyme was similar except tris buffer, pH 8.5 (200 mM), KCl (30 mM), and (dl)H$_4$PteGlu (50 μM) were used. Bovine serum albumin and DMSO were omitted.

Folate product was separated from unreacted labelled glutamate by a modification of the procedure of McGuire et al (42). The reaction mixture was applied to a DEAE cellulose column (2 × 0.7 cm) protected by a 3 mm layer of nonionic cellulose, and allowed to drain in. The column was

212

washed with 10 mM tris buffer, pH 7.5 containing 80 mM NaCl (3×5 ml) to remove [^{14}C]glutamate, and the labelled folate product eluted with 0.1 N HCl (3 ml).

Results

Identification of folylpolyglutamate chain length

The identification of intracellular folate derivatives is complicated by the large number of possible derivatives arising from different combinations of one carbon moieties, oxidation levels, and glutamate chain lengths, and by the lability of these compounds. A number of simplified procedures have been described for the elucidation of the glutamate chain lengths of these compounds, based on the cleavage of folates at the C,9-N,10 bond to yield the corresponding p-aminobenzoylpoly-γ-glutamates (pABAglu$_n$) (43–45). Although the initial applications of these methods have been criticized as some folates were resistant to the procedures or were converted to N-substituted pABAglu$_n$ (46–48), the method has recently been modified to allow the quantitative conversion of all naturally occurring folates to unsubstituted pABAglu (39). The modified method is compared to the original Zn/HCl cleavage procedure in Table 1. pABAglu$_n$ can be separated, according to glutamate chain length, by chromatography on anionic resins or, after conversion to the azo-dyes of naphthylethylenediamine, by gel chromotography on BioGel P4. Alternatively, the azo-dyes of pABAglu$_n$ can be purified by chromatography on BioGel P2, reconverted to pABAglu$_n$ by Zn/HCl treatment, and then separated by ion-exchange chromatography. The latter procedure allows the removal of the pterin derivative obtained after cleavage of folates and also removes nonspecific A$_{280 \text{ nm}}$ absorbing material, allowing the detection of unlabelled pABAglu$_n$ derived from endogeneous folates.

In vivo synthesis of folylpolyglutamates by bacteria

(i) Corynebacterium species

Initial studies were carried with *Corynebacterium sp,* as this organism has been reported to overproduce pteroyltriglutamates (49), making it a potentially good candidate for the purification and characterization of folylpolyglutamate synthetase. After 4 days of culture, *Corynebacterium sp* metabolized [^{14}C]pABA to pteroyltri- and tetraglutamate derivatives (Fig. 2). Practically all the intracellular folates were tetraglutamate derivatives while tri- and tetraglutamates predominated in the culture medium. At earlier time periods, the proportion of extracellular pteroyltriglutamate to pteroyltetraglutamate was increased while the small amounts of pteroylmono- and diglutamate present were decreased (38). In the absence of added [^{14}C]pABA, similar folates were excreted into the

Table 1. Conversion of cellular folates to pABAglu$_n$.

Labelled folates from a variety of bacterial and mammalian sources were subjected to a Zn/HCl cleavage procedure (40) or the modified cleavage procedure described in the Methods section. Cleavage of folates to unsubstituted pABAglu$_n$ was assessed as described previously (39).

Folate source	pABAglu$_n$ formed (%)	
	Zn/HCl procedure	Modified procedure
L. casei	45.1	97.1
S. faecalis	37.3	96.2
Corynebacterium sp.	60.9	90.4
Rat liver	54.2	95.7
CHO cells	23.2	91.7

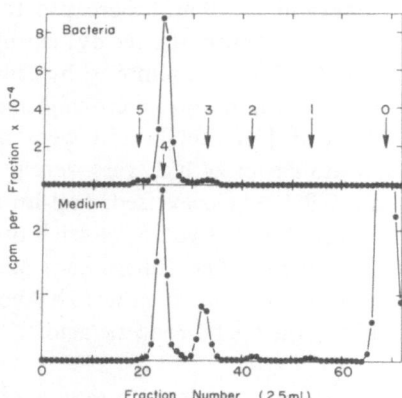

Fig. 2. BioGel P4 elution profile of labelled azo dyes of pABAglu derived from *Corynebacterium* folates. *Corynebacterium* wa cultured for 4 days in medium containing [^{14}C]pABA, an labelled bacterial folates were cleaved to pABAglu$_n$, converted t azodyes of naphthylethylene diamine, and chromatographed o BioGel P4. The numbers 0 to 5 indicate the elution positions c azodyes of pABAglu$_{0-5}$ chromatographed under identica conditions.

medium together with fairly large amounts of pABA. These data suggest at least two rate-limiting steps in the biosynthesis of folylpolyglutamates by *Corynebacterium*. One step appears to be the conversion of pABA to a pteroate derivative. The pteroate derivative(s) is rapidly metabolized to pteroyltriglutamate derivatives without any appreciable build up of pteroylmono- and diglutamates. Pteroyltriglutamate is converted to pteroyl-tetraglutamate at a slower rate and further elongation of the glutamate chain does not take place to any observable extent.

The major intracellular folates in *Corynebacterium* have been identified as 10-formyl-H_4PteGlu$_4$ and 10-formyl-PteGlu$_4$ with lesser amounts of 5-formyl-H_4PteGlu$_4$ and H_4PteGlu$_4$. 10-formyl-PteGlu$_{3,4}$ and pABAglu$_{3,4}$ predominate in the medium due to the aerobic culture conditions (38).

(ii) Lactobacillus casei and Streptococcus faecalis

L. casei and *S. faecalis* require exogenous folate primarily for the synthesis of purines and thymidylate (16). *L. casei* cultured in the absence of purines and thymine metabolized [³H]PteGlu to polyglutamates of chain length up to eleven with the octa- and nonaglutamates predominating (Fig. 3). The major one carbon form was H_4PteGlu$_n$ with lesser amounts of 10- and 5-formyl H_4PteGlu$_n$.

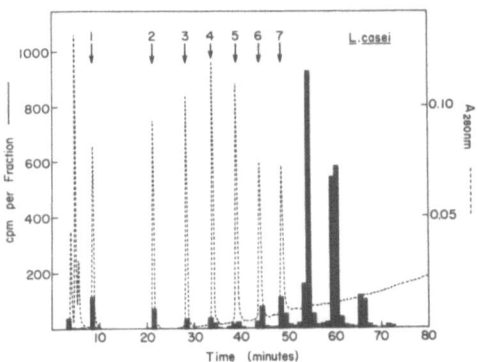

Fig. 3. HPLC elution profile of labelled pABAglu$_n$ derived from *L. casei* folates. *L. casei* was cultured for 22 h in medium containing [³H]PteGlu and intracellular folates were cleaved to pABAglu$_n$, purified, and chromatographed, together with pABAglu$_{1-7}$ standards, on a strong anionic exchanger at a flow rate of 1 ml/min. The numbers 1 to 7 indicate the elution positions of the standards which were detected by A_{280nm}. The small labelled peak eluting at 4 min is the labelled pterin derivative obtained after cleavage of labelled folates. Most of the labelled pterin derivative is removed in the purification procedure.

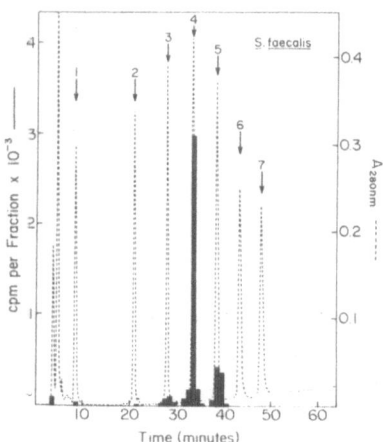

Fig. 4. HPLC elution profile of labelled pABAglu$_n$ derived from *S. faecalis* folates. The experimental conditions were as described in the legend to Fig. 3.

Under the same culture conditions, *S. faecalis* metabolized [³H]PteGlu to polyglutamates of chain length up to five, with the tetraglutamate predominating (Fig. 4). The major one carbon forms in *S. faecalis* were 5- and 10-formyl-H_4PteGlu$_n$ with lesser amounts of H_4PteGlu$_n$.

In vivo synthesis of folylpolyglutamates by mammalian cells

(i) Chinese hamster ovary cells

The distribution of labelled folylpolyglutamates in CHO cells cultured for 2 days in α-minimal essential medium containing 10% dialyzed fetal calf serum and 2 μM [³H]PteGlu is shown in Table 2. Only traces of pteroylmono- to tetraglutamate were detected. Longer glutamate chain length folates up to the nonaglutamate built up with pteroylhexa- and heptaglutamates predominating.

(ii) McCollum rat liver

The distribution of labelled folates in rat liver 24 h following a labelled dose of [³H]PteGlu is shown in Table 2. Also shown is the endogeneous distribution of unlabelled folylpolyglutamates detected by the A_{280nm} of pABAglu$_n$ following HPLC analysis of these derivatives. Folates of glutamate chain length up to seven were detected in rat liver with pteroylpentaglutamate predominating in both the labelled and unlabelled distributions. Rat liver also contains significant amounts of pteroyltetra- and hexaglutamates.

Table 2. Distribution of labelled and endogenous folyl-polyglutamates in CHO cells and rat liver.

CHO cells were cultured in medium containing 2 μM [^{3}H]PteGlu for 48 h. Rats were injected with [^{3}H]PteGlu (200 ng) and sacrificed 24 h following the dose. Folates were cleaved to pABAglu$_n$ and separated by HPLC. Endogenous folates in rat liver was detected by A$_{280nm}$.

Polyglutamate chain length	CHO cell folates	Rat liver folates	
	Labelled	Labelled	Endogenous
	distribution (%)		
1	0.5	2.6	1.0
2	0.1	0.8	0.3
3	0.1	3.1	1.9
4	0.7	23.4	11.0
5	11.5	65.6	68.8
6	42.1	4.3	16.5
7	33.5	0.3	0.5
8	9.7	0	0
9	0.8	0	0

Corynebacterium sp. folylpolyglutamate synthetase

(i) *Enzyme purification*

The purification of *Corynebacterium* folyl-polyglutamate synthetase is summarized in Table 3. Enzyme in crude extracts was labile at 4 °C unless stored in the presence of K + and phosphate (41). As a result, 50 mM K phosphate buffer, pH 7–50 mM KCl was used as the basal buffer throughout most of the purification procedure. The enzyme bound tightly to DEAE cellulose and butylagarose and was eluted later than the bulk of the protein by increasing the KCl concentration. Final purification was achieved by chromatography on AMP-hexyl-agarose. Binding of enzyme required low ionic strength (5 mM K phosphate, pH 7) and the enzyme was eluted by increasing the ionic strength.

MgATP^{2-} did not elute the enzyme from the column.

SDS gel electrophoresis of the purified protein demonstrated one major band (M$_r$ = 53 000) and two very faint bands. By this criterion the enzyme was greater than 95% pure. The purified preparation was extremely labile at 4 °C and –20 °C. However, it was stable when stored in 50 mM K phosphate buffer, pH 7–50 mM KCl–30% DMSO at –20 °C or –196 °C.

(ii) *General properties*

Enzyme activity was absolutely dependent on a folate substrate, ATP, Mg^{2+}, K$^+$, and enzyme preparation. The pH optimum was 9.5 to 10.0 in a variety of buffer systems with approximately 15% maximal activity at pH 8. Borate and phosphate buffers were inhibitory.

Maximal activity was observed with 200 mM K$^+$ with reduced activity at higher concentrations. NH$_4^+$ stimulated activity to a lesser extent while Na$^+$ and Li$^+$ were ineffective. The optimal Mg^{2+} concentration was dependent on the ATP concentration, as Mg^{2+} was required to convert ATP^{4-} to MgATP^{2-}, the substrate form of the nucleotide. Free ATP^{4-} was a potent inhibitor of the reaction and excess Mg^{2+} was inhibitory. Mn^{2+} and Co^{2+} were ineffective substitutes for Mg^{2+} in the pH range 7–10.

The relative molecular mass of the synthetase as judged by chromatography on Sephadex G-150 (M$_r$ = 51 000) was similar to that observed after SDS gel electrophoresis (M$_r$ = 53 000). Although the native enzyme eluted primarily as a monomer, some anomalous behavior on Sephadex G-150, in particular a skewing of the activity profile towards the higher molecular weight side, which was more

Table 3. Purification of *Corynebacterium sp.* folylpolyglutamate synthetase.

Fraction	Specific activity	Purification	Yield
	μmol H$_4$PteGlu$_2$/h/mg	-fold	%
1. Sonicate	0.0049	1.0	100
2. 0–50% ammonium sulfate	0.0058	1.2	94
3. DEAE cellulose	0.846	173	74
4. Sephadex G-150	5.76	1176	51
5. Butyl-agarose	24.4	4970	35
6. AMP-agarose	34.3	6994	15

pronounced in buffers containing high K^+ and phosphate concentrations, and a requirement for bovine serum albumin in the assay mixture when low protein concentrations were used, suggests that the active form of the protein may be a multimer.

(iii) Folate substrate specificity

The effectiveness of a variety of pteroate and pteroylamino acid derivatives as substrates of the *Corynebacterium* folylpolyglutamate synthetase are shown in Table 4. The enzyme exhibited a wide substrate specificity. At low concentrations (10 μM), H_4PteGlu and 5,10-methylene-H_4PteGlu were the most effective substrates and appeared to have high affinity for the enzyme. Other reduced pteroylmonoglutamates had lower affinity for the enzyme but were effective substrates at higher concentrations. Their order of substrate effectiveness was 10-formyl-H_4PteGlu > 5-methyl-H_4PteGlu > 5-formyl-H_4PteGlu. H_2PteGlu was also a substrate for the enzyme demonstrating reasonable apparent affinity but with a lower V_{max} than H_4PteGlu. Substrate inhibition was noted with some of the folate substrates, making a comparison of maximum catalytic rates difficult. Although PteGlu did not appear to be a substrate, some activity was observed with high concentrations of aminopterin and methotrexate.

H_2Pte and H_4Pte were also effective substrates for the enzyme demonstrating high apparent affinities but a lower V_{max} than H_4PteGlu. The copurification of activity with H_2Pte and H_4PteGlu as substrates suggests that dihydrofolate synthetase and folylpolyglutamate synthetase activities are associated on a single polypeptide in *Corynebacterium*. Whether both activities are associated with a single catalytic site has not been ascertained.

The affinity of the various folate analogs for the enzyme was indirectly assessed by measuring the effect of 1 mM analog on the activity obtained with 10 μM H_4PteGlu as substrate (Table 4) (41). In general, the analogs affected activity in a manner

Table 4. Folate substrates and inhibitors of *Corynebacterium* folylpolyglutamate synthetase.

Folate analogs were tested as substrates at 10 μM, 100 μM, and 1 mM concentrations as indicated. Activities are expressed relative to that obtained with 10 μM H_4PteGlu. In the inhibition study, 1 mM analog was added to complete reaction mixtures containing 10 μM H_4PteGlu, and the total amount of labelled product measured.

Analog	Substrate concentration			Inhibition study
	10 μM	100 μM	1 mM	
	Relative activity			
None	_[a]	–	–	100
H_4PteGlu	100	248	137	120
H_2PteGlu	7	38	18	20
PteGlu	0	1	1	92
5-formyl-H_4PteGlu	1	6	51	115
10-formyl-H_4PteGlu	4	42	100	150
5,10-methylene-H_4PteGlu	67	327	159	150
5-methyl-H_4PteGlu	2	21	97	120
H_4Pte	40	40	45	69
H_2Pte	48	36	22	31
pABAglu	0	0	1	91
aminopterin	0	1	14	79
methotrexate	0	1	5	88
H_4Pte-aspartate	–	0	–	99

[a] Not applicable or not determined.

Table 5. Pteroylamino acids as substrates and inhibitors of *Coryne-bacterium* folylpolyglutamate synthetase.

Amino acid	Substrate (50 μM)	
	(l)-H$_4$Pte-	(l)-5,10-methylene-H$_4$Pte-
	Relative activity[a]	
L-aspartate	0	0
L-glutamate	100	47
D,L-aminoadipate	0	0
D,L-aminopimelate	0	0
L-glu + L-aspartate	95	44
L-glu + D,L-aminoadipate	96	44
L-glu + D,L-aminopimelate	98	50

[a] Activity relative to that obtained with 50 μM (l)H$_4$PteGlu.

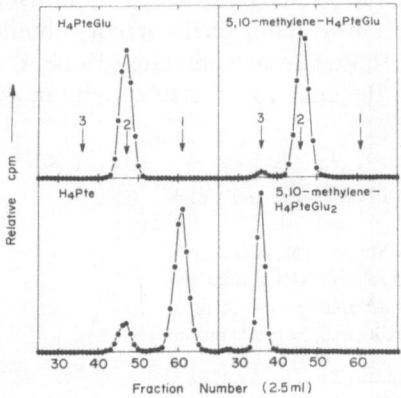

Fig. 5. BioGel P4 elution profiles of labelled azo dyes of pABAglu$_n$ derived from labelled products of the *Coryne-bacterium* folylpolyglutamate synthetase reaction with various folate substrates. Assay conditions, using the indicated substrates (100 μM), were as described in the Methods section. The elution positions of azo dyes of pABAglu$_{1-3}$ are indicated.

predicted by their ability to serve as substrates for the reaction. For instance, 5-methyl-H$_4$PteGlu, a good substrate with poor apparent affinity, increased the amount of labelled product, while H$_4$Pte, a substrate with high affinity but a low V$_{max}$, decreased the amount of labelled product. Marked inhibition was observed with the dihydro-derivatives, H$_2$Pte and H$_2$PteGlu, again presumably reflecting the high affinity and low V$_{max}$ of these compounds suggested by the substrate data.

H$_4$Pte-aspartate, H$_4$Pte-aminoadipate, and H$_4$Pte-aminopimelate were not substrates for the *Corynebacterium* enzyme and had no apparent

affinity as judged by their inability to inhibit activity with H$_4$PteGlu as substrate (Table 5).

The products of the reactions with most of the substrates shown in table 4 contained one additional glutamate moiety (Fig. 5). The only exceptions were H$_4$Pte, which was converted to a mixture of H$_4$PteGlu and H$_4$PteGlu$_2$, and 5,10-methylene-H$_4$PteGlu, which was converted predominantly to 5,10-methylene-H$_4$PteGlu$_2$ with lesser amounts of 5,10-methylene-H$_4$PteGlu$_3$ (Fig. 5).

The substrate effectiveness of different glutamate chain length folates is shown in Table 6. Although H$_4$PteGlu was the most effective monoglutamate substrate, H$_4$PteGlu$_2$ was a very poor substrate, and no activity was observed with H$_4$PteGlu$_3$. 5,10-Methylene-H$_4$PteGlu$_2$ was the only effective diglutamate substrate and a small amount of activity was detected with 5,10-methylene-H$_4$PteGlu$_3$. With di- and triglutamate substrates, the only products detected contained one additional glutamate moiety. These data are consistent with the observed rapid *in vivo* biosynthesis of pteroyltriglutamates and the slower *in vivo* conversion of pteroyl-triglutamate to tetraglutamate forms. Tetraglu-tamates did not inhibit the activity obtained with pteroylmonoglutamate substrates (Table 6) and had no apparent affinity for the enzyme. The types of folylpolyglutamates synthesized by *Corynebac-terium* reflect the specificity of folate substrates for the organism's folylpolyglutamate synthetase rather than end product inhibition of the enzyme.

Table 6. Folylpolyglutamate substrates of *Corynebacterium* folylpolyglutamate synthetase.

Glutamate chain length	Substrate (50 μM)		
	(l)-H$_4$PteGlu$_n$	(l)-5,10-methylene-H$_4$PteGlu$_n$	(l)-10-formyl-H$_4$PteGlu$_n$
	Relative activity[a]		
1	100	46.3	11.5
2	1.5	33.3	0.4
3	0	0.2	0
4	0	0	0
5	0	0	0
1 + 4	98.1	54.2	12.4

[a] Activity relative to that obtained with 50 μM (l)-H$_4$PteGlu.

Table 7. Nucleotide analogs as substrates and inhibitors of *Corynebacterium* folylpolyglutamate synthetase.

The magnesium salts of nucleotide analogs were tested as substrates at 100 μM and 5 mM concentrations, as indicated. Activities are expressed relative to that obtained with 100 μM ATP. In the inhibition study, 5 mM analog (unless indicated otherwise) was added to complete reaction mixtures containing 100 μM ATP.

Analog	Substrate concentration		Inhibition study
	100 μM	5 mM	
	Relative activity		
None	–[a]	–	100
ATP	100	125	125
GTP	0.8	4.4	93
dATP	80	92	86
UTP	4.7	49	87
CTP	1.1	13	94
dTTP	0.4	0.3	96
β,γ-Methylene-ATP	0.3	0.8	0.3
ADP	–	–	7.9
AMP	–	–	6.4
P$_i$ (10 mM)	–	–	53
P$_i$ (50 mM)	–	–	3.2

[a] Not applicable or not measured.

(iv) Nucleotide substrates and inhibitors

The effectiveness of the magnesium salts of various nucleotides as substrates for the *Corynebacterium* enzyme are shown in Table 7. At 100 μM concentrations, which is above the Km for MgATP^{2-}, dATP was almost as effective as ATP as a substrate, UTP acted as a poor substrate, and other analogs were ineffective. At 5 mM concentrations, ATP, dATP, and UTP were effective substrates while CTP and GTP were poor substrates. Binding of analogs to the enzyme was assessed by comparing the effect of 5 mM analog on the activity obtained in the presence of 100 μM ATP (Table 7). In each case, each of the naturally occuring nucleotide analogs affected activity in a manner predicted by its ability to act as a substrate suggesting that the ability of naturally occurring nucleotides to act as substrates for the enzyme is defined primarily by the ability of these compounds to bind to the nucleotide site.

On the other hand, β,γ-methylene-ATP, the phosphonate derivative of ATP, was not a substrate but had high affinity for the nucleotide site and was a very effective inhibitor of the reaction. ADP, AMP, phosphate, and free ATP^{4-} were also effective inhibitors. The large degree of inhibition observed with 50 mM phosphate was primarily due to precipitation of Mg phosphate at pH 10.

(v) Amino acid substrates and inhibitors

The affinity of glutamate analogs for the enzyme was assessed by the ability of unlabelled analogs (5 mM) to inhibit the incorporation of L-[14C]glutamate (250 μM) into $H_4PteGlu_2$. Unlabelled L-glutamate inhibited the incorporation by 93%. No inhibition was observed with 5 mM D-glutamate, L-aspartate, D,L-aminoadipate, D,L-aminopimelate, glutarate, L-2-hydroxyglutarate, L-glutamine, L-α-aminobutyrate, γ-aminobutyrate, N-acetylglutamate, L-methionine, L-methionine sulfoxide, L-methionine sulfoximine, L-lysine, glycine, acetyl CoA, CoA, or glutathione. Weak inhibition was observed with L-glutamate γ-methylester. This compound was not tested as a substrate and the possibility that the preparation may be been contaminated with a small amount of L-glutamate could not be completely excluded.

(vi) Products and stoichiometry of the reaction

The stoichiometry of the reaction was investigated using $H_4PteGlu$ as the folate substrate and L-[14C]glutamate, [14C]ATP, or [γ-32P]ATP as the labelled cosubstrate (41, 50). [14C]ADP formation required the presence of all substrates and enzyme while the small amount of [14C]AMP formed was unaffected by ommission of individual substrates or enzyme. The stoichiometry of ADP synthesis: $H_4PteGlu_2$ synthesis was 0.95:1.

Considerable ATPase activity was detected with [γ-32P]ATP as substrate, even in the absence of $H_4PteGlu$, glutamate, and enzyme. This activity, which was stimulated by phosphate, appeared to be due to a nonenzymatic transphosphorylation which is catalyzed by bivalent metal ions (51). Addition of

enzyme alone stimulated 32Pi release to an extent that could be mimicked by phosphate at a concentration similar to that present as a stabilizer in the enzyme preparation. Additional 32Pi release over that observed in the presence of enzyme alone required the presence of all three substrates and displayed the same pH optimum as $H_4PteGlu_2$ synthesis. The stoichiometry of the additional 32Pi release: $H_4PteGlu_2$ synthesis was 0.99:1.

(vii) Kinetic mechanism

The requirement for all three substrates for ATP hydrolysis suggested that the mechanism was sequential. The kinetic mechanism was further investigated using $H_4PteGlu$, MgATP, and glutamate as the substrates using procedures described by Fromm (52). Initial velocity studies (50) were consistant with an Ordered Ter Ter sequential mechanism. Kinetic constants for substrates of the enzyme are shown in Table 8. The maximum catalytic rate with (dl)$H_4PteGlu$ as the folate substrate was 45 μmol of $H_4PteGlu_2$ formed/h/mg protein which is equivalent to a turnover number of 40 molecules of product formed/min/molecule of enzyme monomer. Product inhibition and competitive inhibition studies (50) were also consistent with an Ordered Ter Ter mechanism with the following order of substrate addition:

MgATP $\quad$ $H_4PteGlu$ $\quad$ glutamate $\quad$ MgADP $\quad$ $H_4PteGlu_2$ $\quad$ phosphate

$\downarrow$ $\qquad$ $\downarrow$ $\qquad\quad$ $\downarrow$ $\qquad\quad$ $\uparrow$ $\qquad\quad$ $\uparrow$ $\qquad\quad$ $\uparrow$

β,γ-Methylene-ATP, a competitive inhibitor of MgATP, demonstrated an affinity for the enzyme approximately one order of magnitude greater than that shown by MgATP (Table 8).

Table 8. Kinetic constants of substrates, products, and inhibitors of *Corynebacterium* folylpolyglutamate synthetase.

Compound	K_m	K_I	V^{max}
	μM	μM	μmol/h/mg
MgATP	18	10	45.1
$H_4PteGlu$	2.1	12.7	45.4
Glutamate	160	–	41.2
Phosphate	–	750	–
β,γ-Methylene-ATP	–	0.58	–

Lactobacillus casei and Streptococcus faecalis folylpolyglutamate synthetases

Preliminary studies have been carried out on the substrate specificities of folylpolyglutamate synthetases from *L. casei* and *S. faecalis* (Table 9). *L. casei* preferentially utilizes 5,10-methylene-H_4PteGlu$_n$ as its mono- and polyglutamate substrates. *S. faecalis* preferentially utilizes 10-formyl-H_4PteGlu as the monoglutamate substrate but the most effective polyglutamate substrate is 5,10-methylene-H_4PteGlu$_n$.

The level of enzyme activity in crude extracts from both organisms was unaffected by culturing the bacteria in the presence or absence of adenine, thymine, or by varying the folate concentration in the medium.

The low levels of *L. casei* enzyme activity with folylpolyglutamate substrates of glutamate chain length greater than five is consistent with the build up of folylpolyglutamates observed in the *in vivo* metabolism studies (Fig. 3). Unfortunately, we do not have pteroylocta- or nonaglutamate standards available to test as substrates. With the *S. faecalis* enzyme, 5,10-methylene-H_4PteGlu$_3$ was the longest glutamate chain length folate that acted as an effective substrate (Table 9) which is consistent with the build up of pteroyltetraglutamates in this organism (Fig. 4).

CHO folylpolyglutamate synthetase

Previous studies by Taylor & Hanna (28) have shown that partially purified folylpolyglutamate synthetase from CHO cells preferentially uses H_4PteGlu as the pteroylmonoglutamate substrate.

The folylpolyglutamate substrate specificity of the CHO enzyme is shown in Table 10. H_4PteGlu$_n$ is also the preferred polyglutamate substrate. Although pteroylpentaglutamates are poor substrates for the enzyme, these compounds inhibit activity with pteroylmonoglutamate substrates. This apparent affinity by pteroylpentaglutamates which is not reflected by the substrate abilities of these

Table 9. Folylpolyglutamate substrates of bacterial folylpolyglutamate synthetases.

Glutamate chain length	Substrate (50 μM)		
	(l)-H_4PteGlu$_n$	(l)-5,10-methylene-H_4PteGlu$_n$	(l)-10 formyl-H_4PteGlu$_n$
	Relative activity[a]		
Lactobacillus casei			
1	30	100	9
2	48	303	27
3	17	81	17
4	8	10	7
5	2	6	1
6	0	7	0
7	0	3	0
Streptococcus faecalis			
1	21	20	100
2	14	197	27
3	1	20	0
4	0	1	0
5	0	0	0
6	0	0	0
7	0	0	0

[a] Activity relative to that obtained with the preferred pteroylmonoglutamate substrate.

Table 10. Folylpolyglutamate substrates of CHO cell folylpolyglutamate synthetase.

Glutamate chain length	Substrate (20 μM)		
	(l)-H$_4$PteGlu$_n$	(l)-5,10-methylene-H$_4$PteGlu$_n$	(l)-10-formyl-H$_4$PteGlu$_n$
	Relative activity[a]		
1	100	49	34
2	99	19	20
3	69	27	6
4	20	9	0
5	8	4	0
6	1	6	0
7	0	3	0
1 + 5	66	37	14
1 + 6	96	51	23
1 + 7	99	46	37

[a] Activity relative to that obtained with 20 μM (l)-H$_4$PteGlu as substrate.

compounds suggests the possibility that the final distribution of folylpolyglutamates in CHO cells is regulated in part by end product inhibition.

A similar phenomenum has been reported by McGuire *et al.* (42) who have extensively characterized partially purified folylpolyglutamate synthetase from rat liver. These investigators have reported that H$_4$PteGlu$_5$ is a poor substrate for the rat liver enzyme but is an effective inhibitor of activity with H$_4$PteGlu as substrate.

However, data on the *in vivo* metabolism of [^{3}H]PteGlu by CHO cells (Table 2) suggests that pteroylmonoglutamates are rapidly metabolized to pentaglutamates and that further glutamate chain elongation procedes at a slower rate. This pattern of metabolism is reflected by the substrate effectiveness of the various polyglutamate derivatives shown in Table 10, and suggests that the final distribution of folylpolyglutamates in CHO cells primarily reflects the ability of the different folylpolyglutamates to act as substrates for folylpolyglutamate synthetase, and that end product inhibition plays only a minor role in determining the final distribution. Similar, the distribution of folates in rat liver (Table 2) with pentaglutamates predominating can be explained by the relatively poor substrate effectiveness of H$_4$PteGlu$_5$.

The relative effectiveness of the polyglutamate substrates for the CHO enzyme, compared to

(l)H$_4$PteGlu, was increased at higher substrate concentrations (100 μM). At 100 μM concentrations, (l)H$_4$PteGlu$_{1,4,5}$ were converted to products containing one additional glutamate moiety. At a 10 μM concentration, (l)H$_4$PteGlu was converted to a mixture of H$_4$PteGlu$_{2,3}$.

Hog liver folylpolyglutamate synthetase

(i) Enzyme purification

The partial purification of folylpolyglutamate synthetase from hog liver is summarized in Table 11. Enzyme was purified approximately 200 fold with the resulting removal of contaminating γ-glutamylhydrolase (conjugase) activity. Attempts at further purification of the enzyme have, thus far, been unsuccessful due to the lability of the preparation. A similar phenomenum has been observed with partially purified enzyme from rat liver (42).

(ii) Substrate specificity

Preliminary studies on the pteroylmonoglutamate substrate specificity of partially purified hog liver folylpolyglutamate synthetase are summarized in Table 12. H$_4$PteGlu was the most effective monoglutamate substrate followed by 10-formyl-H$_4$PteGlu. At a 50 μM concentration, 5-methyl-H$_4$PteGlu was approximately 25 per cent as effec-

Table 11. Partial purification of folylpolyglutamate synthetase from hog liver.

Fraction	Folylpolyglutamate synthetase			γ-Glutamylhydrolase
	Specific activity	Purification	Yield	Specific activity
	units/mg protein	-fold	%	units/mg protein
crude extract	0.045	1	100	5.4
pH 5.8 supernatant	0.31	6.9	96	8.0
0–40% ammonium sulfate	1.07	24	90	0.32
phosphocellulose	8.06	179	74	0.01

1 unit = 1 nmol product/h.

Table 12. Pteroylmonoglutamate substrates of hog liver folylpolyglutamate synthetase.

Folate (50 μM)	Relative activity
H_4PteGlu	100
H_2PteGlu	12
5-formyl-H_4PteGlu	43
10-formyl-H_4PteGlu	61
5,10-methylene-H_4PteGlu	19
5-methyl-H_4PteGlu	25

Table 13. Ammonium sulphate fractionation of N. Crassa folylpolyglutamate synthetase.

Ammonium sulphate fraction	Substrate	
	H_4PteGlu	H_4PteGlu$_3$
%	Specificity activity, nmol/h/mg	
crude extract	0.44	0.16
0–30	0.06	0.01
30–40	0.02	0.01
40–50	0.08	0.05
50–60	1.23	0.77
60–100	0.31	0.12

tive a substrate as H_4PteGlu. The substrate specificities shown in Table 13 are similar to those reported for partially purified enzyme from CHO cells (28) and rat liver (42). The reduced activity with 5-methyl-H_4PteGlu reflected a lowered affinity of this compound for the enzyme as its relative effectiveness was decreased at lower substrate concentrations and increased at higher substrate concentrations.

Neurospora crassa folylpolyglutamate synthetase

N. crassa has been reported to possess two folylpolyglutamate synthetases, one specific for the conversion of H_4PteGlu to H_4PteGlu$_2$, and the other for the conversion of H_4PteGlu$_2$ to longer glutamate chain length derivatives (53). The two enzymes were differentiated by ammonium sulfate fractionation and by unpublished genetic means.

However, we have been unable to confirm this observation. The distribution of enzyme activity in various ammonium sulfate fractions is shown in Table 13. Protein catalyzing the addition of glutamate to both H_4PteGlu and H_4PteGlu$_3$ was found in the 50–60% ammonium sulfate precipitate. The products of the reaction with H_4PteGlu as substrate contained a mixture of H_4PteGlu$_{2-4}$ while H_4PteGlu$_3$ was converted to H_4PteGlu$_{4,5}$.

Discussion

Although the physiological role of folylpolyglutamates as cofactors in one carbon metabolism is now well established, the mechanism by which these compounds are synthesized has, until recently, received little attention. In the last few years, folylpolyglutamate synthetases from E. coli (54), CHO cells (28), and rat liver (42) have been partially purified and characterized, and the Corynebacterium enzyme (41) has been purified to homogeneity. The properties of the Corynebacterium enzyme are described in this report, together with preliminary characterizations of

222

folylpolyglutamate synthetases from a number of other bacterial and mammalian sources, and the factors governing the *in vivo* distribution of folylpolyglutamates in different tissues and cell lines are assessed.

The properties of the *Corynebacterium* folylpolyglutamate synthetase are similar to those reported for partially purified enzyme from *E. coli* (54) in that there is a requirement for a monovalent cation, of which K^+ is the most effective, and an energy source, and both $H_4PteGlu$ and 10-formyl-$H_4PteGlu$ are substrates. However, the *E. coli* enzyme utilized 10-formyl-$H_4PteGlu$ more effectively than $H_4PteGlu$, and H_2Pte, $H_2PteGlu$, and 5-formyl-$H_4PteGlu$ were not substrates, while $H_4PteGlu$, H_2Pte, and H_4Pte are effective substrates for the *Corynebacterium* enzyme. The co-purification of activity with H_2Pte and $H_4PteGlu$ as substrates suggests that dihydrofolate synthetase and folylpolyglutamate synthetase activities are associated with a single protein in *Corynebacterium sp.* These activities are thought to reside on separate proteins in *E. coli*.

Two folylpolyglutamate synthetases have been reported in *N crassa* (53), one specific for the synthesis of $H_4PteGlu_2$ and the other specific for the synthesis of longer glutamate chain length folate homologues. The activities were differentiated by ammonium sulfate fractionation. Similarly, the *E. coli* enzyme catalyzes the conversion of 10-formyl-$H_4PteGlu$ to the diglutamate form only (54). On the other hand, mammalian enzyme from CHO cells (28) and rat liver (42) catalyze the sequential addition of glutamate to $H_4PteGlu$, provided that low levels of the monoglutamate substrate are used. These data have lead to the postulate that two enzymes are required for the synthesis of folylpolyglutamates by bacteria and lower eukaryotes, while a single enzyme carries out this function in mammalian cells. Studies by Taylor & Hanna (29) on a variety of CHO cell mutants with defective folylpolyglutamate synthetases have confirmed that a single enzyme is involved in this process in mammalian cells.

We have been unable to confirm the presence of two synthetases in *N. crassa*. In addition, although $H_4PteGlu$, the most effective monoglutamate substrate, is only converted to the diglutamate derivative by *Corynebacterium* enzyme, and $H_4PteGlu_2$ is a very poor substrate for the enzyme, 5,10-methylene-$H_4PteGlu_2$ is an effective substrate. The preferred pteroylmono- and polyglutamate substrates for a number of folylpolyglutamate synthetases are summarized in Table 14. Although the preferred pteroylmonoglutamate substrate for bacterial folylpolyglutamate synthetases varies depending on the source of the enzyme, in each case studied 5,10-methylene-$H_4PteGlu_n$ was the preferred, and sometimes only, polyglutamate substrate. The evidence strongly supports the view that only one enzyme is involved in the polymerization of the glutamate chain of folates in bacteria, and that the failure to detect folates of glutamate chain length greater than two in previous studies with *E. coli* (54) and *Corynebacterium* (37, 41) enzyme was due to the change in one carbon form of the folate

Table 14. Preferred substrates of folylpolyglutamate synthetases.

Source	Monoglutamate	Polyglutamate
Corynebacterium	$H_4PteGlu$	5,10-methylene-$H_4PteGlu$
L. casei	5,10-methylene-$H_4PteGlu$	5,10-methylene-$H_4PteGlu$
S. faecalis	10-formyl-$H_4PteGlu$	5,10-methylene-$H_4PteGlu$
E. coli[a]	10-formyl-$H_4PteGlu$	?
N. crassa[b]	$H_4PteGlu$	$H_4PteGlu$
rat liver[c]	$H_4PteGlu$	$H_4PteGlu$
hog liver	$H_4PteGlu$	$H_4PteGlu$
CHO cells[d]	$H_4PteGlu$	$H_4PteGlu$

[a] From ref. (54).
[b] From ref. (53) and this report.
[c] From ref. (42).
[d] From ref. (28) and this report.

substrate required for further polymerization of the glutamate chain.

In previous studies (41), we reported variable activity with 5,10-methylene-$H_4PteGlu_n$ as substrate and suggested that the optimum assay conditions for polyglutamate substrates may be different from monoglutamate substrates. The variability was due primarily to removal of formaldehyde by dithiothreitol and mercaptoethanol in the assay mixture. In addition, large excesses of formaldehyde inhibited the activity of the *Corynebacterium* enzyme. As a result of these effects, little activity is seen at low concentrations of 5,10-methylene-$H_4PteGlu_2$ and then a cooperative effect is observed as the substrate concentration is increased. This cooperative effect can be eliminated if the formaldehyde concentration is kept fixed (usually 5 mM) while the substrate concentration is varied. The pH optimum and ionic requirements of the enzyme with 5,10-methylene-$H_4PteGlu_2$ as substrate were identical to those described for $H_4PteGlu$.

Folylpolyglutamate synthetases recognize folate substrates which vary considerably in size. For instance, the *Corynebacterium* enzyme will bind to various degrees of efficiency, substrates ranging from pteroate derivatives to pteroyltriglutamates while the *L. casei* enzyme catalyzes the formation of polyglutamates of chain length up to eleven from pteroylmonoglutamates.

A reduced pterin moiety appears to be essential for effective analog binding to the *Corynebacterium* enzyme, as PteGlu, which was not a substrate, did not inhibit activity with $H_4PteGlu$ as substrate. In fact, in the limited studies carried out, analog binding to the enzyme correlated well with the substrate effectiveness of the analog, and varied considerably depending on the state of reduction and the one carbon group of the pterin moiety. pABAglu, which is not a substrate, did not inhibit activity, which is consistent with the importance of the pterin moiety in substrate binding. However, H_4Pte-aspartate, H_4Pte-aminoadipate, and H_4Pte-aminopimelate and their 5,10-methylene-derivatives, were not substrates or inhibitors of the enzyme, demonstrating that a reduced pterin moiety is not a sufficient condition for analog binding. Although these data might be interpreted to indicate a requirement for both a reduced pterin moiety and a glutamate residue for effective binding, the high

affinity of H_2Pte and H_4Pte would argue otherwise. It should be noted that we have not demonstrated that the dihydrofolate synthetase and folylpolyglutamate synthetase activities, which are associated on a single polypeptide in *Corynebacterium*, share a common catalytic site. However, it is interesting that H_2Pte and $H_2PteGlu$ are effective inhibitors of the *E. coli* enzyme (54) but are not substrates for this enzyme.

The poor activity observed with $H_4PteGlu_2$ and 10-formyl-$H_4PteGlu_2$ as substrates for the *Corynebacterium* enzyme may reflect that only 5,10-methylene-$H_4PteGlu_2$ has the conformational ability to bind both at a pterin site and keep the terminal glutamate moiety in the active site. By extension, the poor activity of 5,10-methylene-$H_4PteGlu_3$ and the lack of activity with 5,10-methylene-$H_4PteGlu_4$ may be explained by an inability to fit the terminal glutamate into the active site. However, it this is so, it is difficult to understand why pteroyltetraglutamates are not inhibitors of the reaction. The affinity of folate compounds for the enzyme may reflect a cooperative effect resulting from two low affinity binding sites, for instance a pteridine and a terminal glutamate site, in which case compounds which fail to interact at both sites would not be expected to be substrates or inhibitors of the reaction. Although the high affinities of H_2Pte and H_4Pte may suggest other mechanisms, it is noteworthy that we have, thus far, been unable to find a folate analog that will bind to the enzyme, as measured by inhibition, and not act as a substrate. It may be that H_2Pte or H_4Pte binding to a pteroate binding site impairs the ability of folates to bind to a separate pteroylglutamate site. With H_4Pte as the substrate, considerable amounts of $H_4PteGlu_2$ product were formed in addition to $H_4PteGlu$, even at fairly high substrate concentrations (100 μM). One might expect only small amounts of $H_4PteGlu_2$ to be formed under these conditions, due to competition between H_4Pte and the relatively low amounts of $H_4PteGlu$ product for the enzyme. This competition was very apparent with 5,10-methylene-$H_4PteGlu$ as substrate where only trace amounts of 5,10-methylene-$H_4PteGlu_3$ were formed, and in mammalian systems where polyglutamates of chain length greater than two are only formed from $H_4PteGlu$ when very low substrate concentrations are used (28, 42). The relatively high amounts of $H_4PteGlu_2$ detected with

H_4Pte as substrate may reflect substrate channelling from a dihydrofolate synthetase active site to the folylpolyglutamate synthetase active site. It is clear, however, that further studies will be required before definitive conclusions can be made concerning the factors controlling the folate substrate specificity of this enzyme.

The folate substrate specificities of mammalian folylpolyglutamate synthetases are less clearly defined. In all cases studied, $H_4PteGlu_n$ appear to be the preferred polyglutamate substrates although other one carbon forms will function as substrates. Pentaglutamate derivatives appear to bind well to the rat liver (42) and CHO enzymes, as judged by their ability to inhibit the incorporation of glutamate into $H_4PteGlu_2$. However, in vivo and in vitro studies clearly demonstrate these compounds to be substrates for the enzyme. Their ability to bind to the enzymes appear to be greater than suggested by their substrate effectiveness, which suggests that folylpolyglutamates may play a role in determining the final distribution of folylpolyglutamates in mammalian tissues, by end product inhibition of folylpolyglutamate synthetase. However, such a role for these compounds must await more detailed kinetic studies. Such studies have been hampered by the inability to purify mammalian folylpolyglutamate synthetases to homogeneity, due to their extreme lability during attempted purification procedures. It is possible that the pentaglutamate derivatives bind well to the enzyme but have low V_{max} values due to difficulty in positioning the terminal glutamate residues in the catalytic site.

$H_4PteGlu$ and 10-formyl-$H_4PteGlu$ are the most effective pteroyl monoglutamate substrates for the mammalian enzymes (28, 42). Although PteGlu did not appear to be a substrate for the partially purified CHO enzyme (28), McGuire et al. (42) have demonstrated that PteGlu and methotrexate are reasonable substrates for the rat liver enzyme provided high levels of mercaptoethanol are added to the assay mixture. The activity of 5-methyl-$H_4PteGlu$ is of particular interest due to current theories on the interrelationship between vitamin B12 and folate metabolism (55). In brief, the 'methyl trap' hypothesis states that under conditions of vitamin B12 deficiency, the activity of the B12-dependent methionine synthetase is reduced and folates build up as the 5-methyl-$H_4PteGlu_n$ derivative. This leads to a functional folate deficiency and impaired DNA synthesis due to the reduced levels of other folate coenzyme forms. In addition, cellular folate levels are reduced due to an inability to convert monoglutamates to poly-glutamates, as a result of 5-methyl-$H_4PteGlu$ being a poor substrate for folylpolyglutamate synthetase. This latter contention has now been supported by experimental evidence. Studies on folylpolyglu-tamate synthetases in crude extracts of mammalian tissues have shown that 5-methyl-$H_4PteGlu$ was utilized approximately 50 per cent as well as $H_4PteGlu$ by the sheep liver enzyme (56) and was inactive for the rat liver enzyme (57) However, these data are open to dispute, due to the low levels of activity being measured and the possibility of nonspecificity due to the use of crude extracts. More recent studies with partially purified enzyme from CHO cells (28), rat liver (24), and hog liver indicate that 5-methyl-$H_4PteGlu$ is 10–20% as active as $H_4PteGlu$ when low substrate concentrations are used (5–10 μM), and the relative effectiveness of 5-methyl-$H_4PteGlu$ increases with increased sub-strate concentrations, indicating a lowered affinity for 5-methyl-$H_4PteGlu$. The K_m values of $H_4PteGlu$ for mammalian folylpolyglutamate synthetases have not been determined, as yet, as the enzyme has not been purified. Apparent K_m values for partially purified rat liver enzyme are in the range of 5–10 μM (42). This range is considerably higher than the concentrations of pteroylmonoglutamates norm-ally found in mammalian tissues, Consequently, the trapping of folate as 5-methyl-$H_4PteGlu$ under conditions of vitamin B12 deficiency would be expected to severely impair the rate of poly-glutamate synthesis and lead to decreased folate tissue stores.

The specificity of the glutamate binding site of bacterial and mammalian folylpolyglutamate syn-thetases have been assessed by the ability of unlabelled glutamate analogs to inhibit the incorporation of [^{14}C]glutamate into $H_4PteGlu$ (41, 42, 54). The glutamate binding site demonstrates remarkable specificity for L-glutamate, which is consistent with the failure to detect any pteroyl-amino acids other than the L-glutamate derivatives in biological extracts. A wide variety of glutamate analogs, homologs, and isomers showed no affinity for the enzyme. γ-Glutamylglutamate did not inhib-it activity, which is consistent with in vivo studies suggesting that the polyglutamate chain is extended by addition of glutamate moieties one at a time.

The nucleotide specificities of different folyl-polyglutamate synthetases are quite wide. The magnesium salts of ATP and dATP are effective substrates for both bacterial and mammalian enzymes. Other purine nucleotide triphosphates will function as substrates but exhibit lower affinities for the enzymes. Surprisingly, MgUTP and MgCTP were effective substrates for the *Corynebacterium* enzyme (41) when present at high concentrations. Naturally occurring nucleotide triphosphates bind to the *Corynebacterium* enzyme in a manner predicted by their ability to act as substrates, so it would appear that the substrate effectiveness of these compounds is defined primarily by their ability to bind to the nucleotide site. β,γ-Methylene-ATP was a very effective inhibitor of the reaction but did not act as a substrate. The high affinity of this compound for the *Corynebacterium* enzyme can be explained in terms of the mechanism discussed below.

Kinetic analyses of the folylpolyglutamate synthetase catalyzed reaction are complicated by the potential conversion of substrate to more than one product, a phenomenum that is more likely to happen at low substrate concentrations. This problem has been avoided with the *Corynebacterium* enzyme by using $H_4PteGlu$ as the folate substrate (50). Under initial rate conditions and with low substrate concentrations, $H_4PteGlu$ is converted to a single product, $H_4PteGlu_2$. Initial rate, product inhibition, and inhibitor studies indicated that the kinetic mechanism of the *Corynebacterium* enzyme was sequential and of the Ordered Ter Ter type. The order of substrate addition was MgATP, $H_4PteGlu$, and glutamate and the order of product release was MgADP, $H_4PteGlu_2$, and phosphate. It is apparent that the enzyme cannot catalyze the sequential addition of glutamate to enzyme-bound folate. The folate product has to be released and then rebind to the enzyme before an additional glutamate moiety can be added. A sequential mechanism was also demonstrated by ATP hydrolysis studies.

The kinetic analyses do not distinguish between a concerted mechanism or one involving a tightly bound intermediate, although a dissociable intermediate can be excluded. The pH profile of the enzyme, with an optimum around pH 9.5–10, resembles the titration curve of the amino group of glutamate. It is possible that the reaction proceeds via the formation of a $H_4Pte-\gamma$-glutamylphosphate intermediate followed by a nucleophilic attack by the free amine of glutamate on the mixed anhydride intermediate. This would be consistent with the order of addition of the substrates and the high affinity and lack of catalytic activity of β,γ-methylene-ATP. Other mechanisms cannot, however, be excluded.

The mechanism of the mammalian enzyme has not been ascertained as yet. Most mammalian folylpolyglutamate synthetases exhibit maximum activity at about pH 8.5. With enzyme from CHO cells (28) and hog liver, at least, broad pH optima have been observed over the pH range 8.5–9.5. It seems likely that the catalytic mechanism of the mammalian enzyme will be similar to that suggested for the bacterial enzyme. Mammalian folyl-polyglutamate synthetases will only catalyze the conversion of $H_4PteGlu$ to polyglutamates of chain length greater than two if low substrate concentrations are used. This implies that the diglutamate product competes with the monoglutamate substrate, and suggests that the mammalian enzyme cannot catalyze the sequential addition of glutamate to enzyme bound folate.

Inhibitors of folylpolyglutamate synthetase would be expected to increase the cellular requirements for folate and/or products of one carbon metabolism in much the same way that mammalian cells lacking this enzyme activity have higher requirements for these compounds. Selective inhibition of this enzyme would require a folate analog rather than a inhibitor of glutamate or nucleotide binding. Two potential candidates, assuming the catalytic mechanism described above, are H_4Pte-methionine sulfoximine and $H_4Pte-\gamma$-glutamylphosphonate. Preliminary studies on the synthesis of the latter compound have been recently described (58).

In this report, the distribution of folylpoly-glutamates in a variety of bacterial and mammalian cells have been described. The methodologies used will be described in greater detail elsewhere. However, the data presented allows the question of why different folylpolyglutamates predominate in different tissues and cells to be answered. Although end product inhibition may play a role in defining the distribution of polyglutamates in mammalian tissues, it is clear that the ability of different glutamate chain length folylpolyglutamates to act as substrates for the enzymes from different sources can entirely explain the *in vivo* distribution of folylpolyglutamates in the different biological samples. For instance, under the culture conditions used, *Corynebacterium* reached a bacterium concentration of approx. 4 mg dry weight per ml after 4 days of culture, and the bacterial suspension contained approx. 4 nmol folate per ml, of which about 25% was intracellular. Total folate synthesized was about 3.5 nmol per mg protein (38). The bacterium reached late log phase after about 2 days but folate biosynthesis continued for at least 6 days. The specific activity of folylpolyglutamate synthetase in sonicates of *Corynebacterium*, using $H_4PteGlu$ as substrate and saturating levels of glutamate, was about 10 nmol of $H_4PteGlu_2$ formed per h per mg protein. Thus, the activity demonstrated with H_2Pte, $H_4PteGlu$, and 5,10-methylene-$H_4PteGlu_2$ as substrates is considerably in excess of that required for the demonstrated *in vivo* synthesis of folylpolyglutamates. These data are consistent with the build up of pteroyltriglutamate in this organism without any appreciable build up of mono- and diglutamate derivatives, which is particularly pronounced in early stages of bacterial culture (38). The low activity of 5,10-methylene-$H_4PteGlu_3$ is consistent with the slower rate of conversion of pteroyltriglutamate to tetraglutamate observed *in vivo*. The maximal rate with this substrate, equivalent to 20 pmol product per h per mg protein or approximately 2 nmol product per 100 h per mg protein, is just sufficient to account for the observed *in vivo* synthesis of pteroyltetraglutamate. Only preliminary studies have been carried out with the triglutamate substrates and further studies are required to establish the maximal catalytic rates with these compounds more precisely.

Preliminary data are also presented on the *in vivo* distribution of folylpolyglutamates in *L. casei, S. faecalis,* CHO cells, and rat liver and the polyglutamate substrate specificity of enzyme from the first three sources. The substrate specificity of rat liver enzyme has been reported by McGuire *et al.* (42). In all of these cases, the predominant folylpolyglutamates found *in vivo* are poor substrates for the organism's or tissue's folylpolyglutamate synthetase, while shorter glutamate chain length folates that do not build up *in vivo* are effective substrates for the enzyme.

Although the final distribution of folylpolyglutamates in tissues appears to be a function of the properties of the tissue's folylpolyglutamate synthetase, it is not clear that the final distribution is the optimum one for the enzymes of one carbon metabolism. For instance, it is not known whether pteroyltetraglutamates are the optimal substrates for one carbon metabolism in *S. faecalis* or whether octa- and nonaglutamates are optimal in *L. casei*. Also, in cases where substrate channelling may occur, as has been reported for some multifunctional enzymes of folate metabolism, it has not been been demonstrated that differences exist in the optimal glutamate chain length of substrates for enzymes from different tissues which can be correlated with the type of folylpolyglutamate that predominates in that particular tissue. MacKenzie & Baugh (24) have reported that pteroylpentaglutamates are channelled more effectively than mono-, tri-, and heptaglutamates by pig liver formiminotransferase-cyclodeaminase. However, comparative studies on this bifunctional protein from different sources have not been carried out.

It has been suggested that one carbon metabolism may be regulated by changing the glutamate chain length of folates under different conditions of growth and nutritional requirements (31). However, Taylor & Hanna (28) have reported that the levels of folylpolyglutamate synthetase in CHO cells are unaffected by variations in the growth medium or culture conditions. Similar results are reported here for enzyme from *L. casei* and *S. faecalis*. Preliminary results from our laboratory indicate no differences in the distribution of folylpolyglutamates in CHO cells cultured in medium containing or lacking products of one carbon metabolism. The presence of adenine, but not thymine, in the culture medium of *L. casei* and *S. faecalis* caused a small decrease in the average glutamate chain length of folylpolyglutamates. However, this was due to a redistribution of folate one carbon forms favouring formyl derivatives rather than regulation of folylpolyglutamate synthetase per se. This redistribution lead to a slower rate of folylpolyglutamate synthesis as 10-formyl-$H_4PteGlu_n$ are very poor substrates for bacterial folylpolyglutamate synthetases. Although folylpolyglutamates are the preferred substrates for the individual enzymes of one carbon metabolism, and probably also serve a regulatory role in modifying the one carbon flux through the various metabolic cycles of one carbon metabolism, it appears unlikely that these metabolic cycles are regulated by changing the glutamate chain length of folates under different growth and nutritional conditions.

Acknowledgements

The expert technical assistance of Edward Bolgiano is gratefully acknowledged. We would also like to thank Dr. Jesse Rabinowitz (U. C. Berkeley) for the gift of purified *Clostridium* 10-formyl-tetrahydrofolate synthetase, and Dr. Gary Henderson (Scripps Clinic and Research Foundation, La Jolla) and Dr. Roy Kisliuk (Tufts Medical School, Boston) for gifts of methotrexate-resistant *L. casei* strains.

This work was supported in part by Grant CA 22717 from the National Cancer Institute, Department of Health and Human Services, and by Grant 543 from the Nutrition Foundation. DJC is a predoctoral trainee supported by NIH Research Service Award 5T32 ESO7067.

References

1. Blakley, R. L., 1969. The Biochemistry of Folic Acid and Related Pteridines (Neuberger, A. & Tatum, E. L., eds.), pp. 219–358. North Holland, Amsterdam.
2. Brody, T., Shane, B. & Stokstad, E. L. R., 1981. The Handbook of the Vitamins (Machlin, J. L., ed.), Marcel Dekker, New York, in press.
3. Covey, J. M., 1980. Life Sci. 26: 665–678.
4. Shane, B. & Stokstad, E. L. R., 1975. J. Biol. Chem. 250: 2243–2253.
5. Shane, B. & Stokstad, E. L. R., 1976. J. Biol. Chem. 251: 3405–3410.
6. Cheng, F. W., Shane, B. & Stokstad, E. L. R., 1975. Can. J. Biochem. 53: 1020–1027.
7. Coward, J. K., Paraswaran, N. K., Cashmore, A. R. & Bertino, J. R., 1974. Biochemistry 13: 3899–3903.
8. Coward, J. K., Chello, P. L., Cashmore, A. R., Parameswaran, N. K., DeAngelis, L. M. & Bertino, J. R., 1975. Biochemistry 14: 1548–1552.
9. Curthoys, N. P. & Rabinowitz, J. C., 1972. J. Biol. Chem. 247: 1965–1971.
10. Burton, E. G. & Metzenberg, R. L., 1975. Arch. Biochem. Biophys. 168: 219–229.
11. Colnick, B. J. & Cheng, V.-C., 1978. J. Biol. Chem. 253: 3563–3567.
12. Baggott, J. E. & Krumdieck, C. L., 1979. Biochemistry 18: 1036–1041.
13. Kisliuk, R. L., Gaumont, Y. & Baugh, C. M., 1974. J. Biol. Chem. 249: 4100–4103.
14. Powers, S. G. & Snell, E. E., 1976. J. Biol. Chem. 251: 3786–3793.
15. Salem, A. R., Pattison, J. R. & Foster, M. A., 1972. Biochem. J. 126: 993–1004.
16. Shane, B. & Stokstad, E. L. R., 1977. J. Gen. Microbiol. 103: 261–270.
17. Whitfield, C. D., Steers, E. J. & Weissbach, H., 1970. J. Biol. Chem. 245: 390–401.
18. Paukert, J. L., Straus, L. D. & Rabinowitz, J. C., 1976. J. Biol. Chem. 251: 5104–5111.
19. MacKenzie, R. E., 1979. Chemistry and Biology of Pteridines (Kisliuk, R. L. & Brown, G. M., eds.), pp. 443–446. Elsevier, New York.
20. Rowe, P. B., McCairns, E., Madsen, G., Sauer, D. & Elliot, H., 1978. J. Biol. Chem. 253: 7711–7721.
21. Smith, G. K., Mueller, W. T., Wasserman, G. F., Taylor, W. D. & Benkovic, S. J., 1980. Biochemistry 19: 4313–4321.
22. Ferone, R. & Roland, S., 1980. Proc. Natl. Acad. Sci. USA 77: 5802–5806.
23. MacKenzie, R. E., Aldridge, M. & Paquin, J., 1980. J. Biol. Chem. 255: 9474–9478.
24. MacKenzie, R. E. & Baugh, C. M., 1980. Biochim. Biophys. Acta 611: 187–195.
25. Matthews, R. G. & Baugh, C. M., 1980. Biochemistry 19: 2040–2045.
26. Friedkin, M., Plante, L. T., Crawford, E. J. & Crumm, M., 1975. J. Biol. Chem. 250: 5614–5621.
27. McBurney, M. W. & Whitmore, G. F., 1974. Cell 2: 173–182.
28. Taylor, R. T. & Hanna, M. L., 1977. Arch. Biochem. Biophys. 181: 331–344.
29. Taylor, R. T. & Hanna, M. L., 1979. Arch. Biochem. Biophys. 197: 36–43.
30. Taylor, R. T. & Hanna, M. L., 1975. Arch. Biochem. Biophys. 171: 507–520.
31. Baggott, J. E. & Krumdieck, C. L., 1979. Chemistry and Biology of Pteridines (Kisliuk, R. L. & Brown, G. M. ed.), pp. 347–351. Elsevier, New York.
32. Baugh, C. M., Stevens, J. C. & Krumdieck, C. L., 1970. Biochim. Biophys. Acta 212: 116–125.
33. Plante, L. T., Crawford, E. J. & Friedkin, M., 1967. J. Biol. Chem. 242: 1466–1476,
34. Whiteley, J. M., Henderson, G. B., Russell, A., Singh, P. & Zeverly, E. M., 1977. Anal. Biochem. 79: 42–51.
35. Blakley, R. L., 1969. The Biochemistry of Folic Acid and Related Pteridines (Neuberger, A. & Tatum, E. L., ed.) pp. 92–94. North Holland, Amsterdam.
36. Shane, B. & Stokstad, E. L. R., 1977. J. Gen. Microbiol. 103: 249–259.
37. Shane, B., Brody, T. & Stokstad, E. L. R., 1979. Chemistry and Biology of Pteridines (Kisliuk, R. L. & Brown, G. M. ed.) pp. 341–346, Elsevier, New York.
38. Shane, B., 1980. J. Biol. Chem. 255: 5649–5654.
39. Foo, S. K., Cichowicz, D. J. & Shane, B., 1980. Anal. Biochem. 107: 109–115.
40. Brody, T., Shane, B. & Stokstad, E. L. R., 1979. Anal. Biochem. 92: 501–509.
41. Shane, B., 1980. J. Biol. Chem. 255: 5655–5662.
42. McGuire, J. J., Hsieh, P., Coward, J. K. & Bertino, J. R., 1980. J. Biol. Chem. 255: 5776–5788.

228

43. Houlihan, C. M. & Scott, J. M., 1972. Biochem. Biophys. Res. Comm. 48: 1675–1681.
44. Baugh, C. M., Braverman, E. & Nair, M. G., 1974. Biochemistry 13: 4952–4957.
45. Tyerman, M. J., Watson, J. E., Shane, B., Schutz, D. E. & Stokstad, E. L. R., 1977. Biochim. Biophys. Acta 497: 234–240.
46. Mariyuma, T., Shiota, T. & Krumdieck, C. L., 1978. Anal. Biochem. 84: 277–295.
47. Baugh, C. M., Braverman, E. B., Nair, M. G., Horne, D. W., Briggs, W. T. & Wagner, C., 1979. Anal. Biochem. 92: 366–369.
48. Lewis, G. P. & Rowe, P. B., 1979. Anal. Biochem. 93: 91–97.
49. Hutchins, B. L., Stokstad, E. L. R., Bohonos, N., Sloane, N. H. & SubbaRow, Y., 1948. J. Am. Chem. Soc. 70: 1–3.
50. Shane, B., 1980. J. Biol. Chem. 255: 5663–5667.
51. Lowenstein, J. M., 1958. Biochem. J. 70: 222–230.
52. Fromm, H. J., 1975. Mol. Biol. Biochem. Biophys. 22: 41–160.
53. Sakami, W., Ritari, S. J., Black, C. W. & Rzepka, J., 1973. Fed. Proc. 32: 471.
54. Mansurekar, M. & Brown, G. M., 1975. Biochemistry 14: 2424–2430.
55. Shane, B. & Stokstad, E. L. R., 1981. Advances in Nutrition Research (Draper, H. H., ed.) Plenum Press, New York, in press.
56. Gawthorne, J. M. & Smith, R. M., 1973. Biochem. J. 136: 295–301.
57. Spronk, A. M., 1973. Fed. Proc. 34: 471.
58. Coward, J. K., 1979. Drug Actions and Design: Mechanism-Based Enzyme Inhibitors (Kalman, ed.) pp. 13–21, Elsevier, New York.

Received January 14, 1981.

Immunocytochemical and autoradiographic localization of GABA system in the vertebrate retina

Jang-Yen Wu[1], Christopher Brandon[1], Y. Y. Thomas Su[2], and Dominic M. K. Lam[2]
Dept. of Cell Biology[1] and Cullen Eye Institute[2], Baylor College of Medicine, Texas Medical Center, Houston, TX 77030, U.S.A.

Summary

The localization of γ-aminobutyric acid (GABA) neurons in the goldfish and the rabbit retina has been studied by immunocytochemical localization of the GABA-synthesizing enzyme L-glutamate decarboxylase (GAD, L-glutamate 1-carboxy-lase, EC 4.1.1.15) and by [³H] GABA uptake autoradiography. In the goldfish retina, GAD is localized in some horizontal cells (H1 type), a few amacrine cells and sublamina b of the inner plexiform layer. Results from immunocytochemical studies of GAD-containing neurons and autoradiographic studies of GABA uptake reveals a marked similarity in the labeling pattern suggesting that in goldfish retina, the neurons which possess a high-affinity system for GABA uptake also contain significant levels of GAD. In the rabbit retina, when Triton X-100 was included in immunocytochemical incubations with a modified protein A-peroxidase-antiperoxidase method, reaction product was found in four broad, evenly spaced laminae within the inner plexiform layer. In the absence of the detergent, these laminae were seen to be composed of small, punctate deposits. When colchicine was injected intravitreally before glutamate decarboxylase staining, cell bodies with the characteristic shape and location of amacrine cells were found to be immunochemically labeled. Electron microscopic examination showed that these processes were presynaptic to ganglion cell dendrites (infrequently), amacrine cell telodendrons, and bipolar cell terminals. Often, bipolar cell terminals were found which were densely innervated by several GAD-positive processes. No definite synapses were observed in which a GAD-positive process represented the postsynaptic element. In autoradiographic studies by intravitreal injection of [³H] GABA a diffuse labeling of the inner plexiform layer and a dense labeling of certain amacrine cell bodies in the inner nuclear layer was observed. Both immunocytochemical and autoradiographic results support the notion that certain, if not all, amacrine cells use GABA as their neurotransmitter.

Introduction

The presence of γ-aminobutyric acid (GABA) in uniquely high concentrations in the vertebrate central nervous system was first reported in 1950 (1, 2). Since that time, this substance has also fulfilled most of the conventional criteria for the identification of a neurotransmitter. It now appears established that GABA is an inhibitory neurotransmitter at the crustacean neuromuscular junction and that it probably also is the major inhibitory neuro-transmitter in the vertebrate retina and other parts of the central nervous system (3–7).

Several approaches have been extensively used in the past to identify GABAergic neurons in retina-including microchemical measurements of GABA (8–10) and ³H-GABA autoradiography (11–14). Both GABA and its rate-limiting synthetic enzyme L-glutamate decarboxylase, (EC 4.1.1.15) have been measured after microdissection of the retina and shown to be concentrated in the inner plexi-form layer (8, 9). Autoradiographic studies with

Molecular and Cellular Biochemistry 39, 229–238 (1981).   0300–8177/81/0391–0229/$02.00.

intravitreal injection of ³-H-GABA into intact animals have led to the labeling of certain amacrine cell bodies and to the diffuse labeling of IPL due probably to the presence of both sodium-dependent and sodium-independent high affinity binding (11–14). Not all amacrine cells were labeled, and the interesting suggestion was made that GABA neurons represent at most a subgroup of amacrine cells (15).

The approach that we have been using in the identification of GABA-ergic pathways in the vertebrate central nervous system is to purify the GABA-synthesizing enzyme to homogeneity, to prepare monospecific antibody against GAD and to visualize its cellular and subcellular locations by indirect immunocytochemical techniques (11, 12, 16–26). The rational for our approach is that there is a good correlation between GABA levels and GAD activity in the nervous system of vertebrates (27–29). Hence GAD is a better marker for GABA-ergic neurons than GABA *per se,* which may redistribute or be metabolized during the preparation of the tissue (27, 30).

This review is intended to summarize some of the results that have been obtained with the vertebrate retina using immunocytochemical and autoradiographic techniques and to present evidence supporting the notion that some types of horizontal and amacrine cells in the vertebrate retina use GABA as their transmitter.

Materials and methods

Purification of L-glutamate decarboxylase

GAD was purified from mouse brain to homogeneity by the initial extraction of GAD from the crude mitochondrial fraction, followed by ammonium sulfate fractionation and a series of column chromatography on Sephadex G-200, calcium phosphate gel, and DEAE-Sephadex. The criteria of purity have been established by several different methods, e.g., polyacrylamide gel electrophoresis, high speed sedimentation equilibrium, immunodiffusion and immunoelectrophoresis (16, 17, 19). Similar procedures were used for the purification of GAD from catfish brain (18, 19).

Production and characterization of L-glutamate decarboxylase antibodies

Antibodies against the purified GAD were produced in rabbits by biweekly injection of a total of 50–600 μg of proteins over a period of 8 weeks. The specifications of the antibodies thus obtained were characterized by immunodiffusion, enzyme inhibition test, immunoelectrophoresis, and microcomplement fixation test (31–33).

Immunocytochemistry

(a) Tissue fixation and sectioning

Some animals were injected with colchicine (0.25 mg in 0.1 ml of sterile 0.15 M NaCl) intravitreally, under ether anesthesia, 36–48 h before enucleation (11, 26). Eyes were removed from light-adapted goldfish (Carissius auratus), or pentobarbital-anaesthetized rabbits. After removal of the cornea, the lens and vitreous were gently removed and the entire eye cup was immersed in fixative and agitated on an orbital rotator. The rabbit fixative was 2% formaldehyde (from paraformaldehyde) + 0.1% acrolein (17 μM) + 0.002% $CaCl_2$ in 155 mM sodium phosphate buffer, pH 7.3. For the goldfish, the fixative was 4% paraformaldehyde in 100 mM NaCl and 25 mM sodium phosphate, pH 7.2 (12). Phosphate-buffered saline (PBS) was 25 mM sodium phosphate/130 mM NaCl (rabbit) or 25 mM sodium phosphate/100 mM NaCl (goldfish), pH 7.2. After 1.5–2 h at room temperature, the tissue was transferred to fresh fixative without acrolein and stored overnight at 4 °C.

After overnight fixative, the retina is cut into rectangular pieces while still attached to the sclera. The position of each piece within the retinal field is recorded before its removal. Retina and pigment epithelium are separated from the sclera and embedded in molten low-gelling temperature agarose (4% in PBS) at 34 °C. After 1 h at 4 °C, small blocks of agarose containing the retinal pieces are cut into 60 μm-thick Vibratome sections into PBS.

(b) Staining

For staining, sections are incubated in 20 mm × 60 mm plastic petri dishes on an orbital rotator at room temperature, in the following sequence:
(i) 20% dimethylsulfoxide in PBS, 1 h *OR*; 0.025% digitonin in PBS, 2 h (aids antibody penetration) *OR*;

0.2% Triton X-100 in PBS (solubilizes membrane lipids extensively).

(ii) 10% normal goat serum in PBS, 2 h (blocks 'non-specific' IgG binding).

(iii) PBS, 30 min (wash).

(iv) Anti-GAD serum (anti-mouse brain GAD for mammalian retina; anti-catfish GAD for goldfish retina) or control (preimmune) serum dilutions of 1:250 to 1:500, in PBS containing 0.1% normal goat serum. 16 h, 4 °C with orbital agitation.

(v) PBS, 2 × 60 min (wash).

(vi) Protein A solution (50 μg/ml), 1.5 h.

(vii) PBS, 2 × 60 min (wash).

(viii) Peroxidase-antiperoxidase complex (34) (1:100 dilution or 45 μg/ml), 1.5 h.

(ix) PBS, 2 × 60 min (wash).

(x) 30 mg diaminobenzidine tetrahydrochloride in 50 ml PBS + 0.015% H_2O_2 5–8 min to develop reaction product.

The stained sections were briefly washed in PBS, post-fixed for 1 h with 1% glutaraldehyde in PBS, treated with 1% OsO_4 in PBS for 2–3 h, stained *en bloc* with 1% uranyl acetate in 0.1 M sodium acetate, dehydrated with graded ethanols, and infiltrated with Epon. For embedding, sections were placed in small drops of resin at intervals on a smooth sheet of aluminum foil, then covered with a weighted microscope slide that had been treated with dichlorodimethylsilane to prevent epoxy from adhering to it. After polymerization, the foil was easily peeled off to yield a 50 μm sheet of epoxy containing the sections mounted with the stained face upward. Sections could be coverslipped with oil or glycerol for examination and photography. For microtomy, small pieces of the stained sections were cut out with a razor blade, glued to smooth epoxy blocks with cyano-acrylate glue and sectioned *en face*.

Autoradiography

An *in vivo* administration technique was used, since this procedure has been shown to minimize glial uptake of GABA (35, 36).

[³H]-GABA, 45.3 Ci/mmol, 100 μl in 50 μl of isotonic saline, was injected under ether anesthesia into the vitreous body of a rabbit eye. After 2 h the animal was deeply anesthetized with pentobarbital and the eye removed. The dissected eyecup was immersed in 2.5–3% glutaraldehyde in 0.1–0.15 M sodium phosphate, pH 7.2–7.4 for 2 h at room temperature and overnight at 4 °C. Pieces of dissected retina are then osmicated, dehydrated in graded ethanols, and embedded in Epon. Three-micron-thick sections, on glass slides, are coated by dipping with a 50% aqueous solution of Kodak NTB-2 autoradiographic emulsion under dim red light. Slides are stored desiccated at −70 °C and developed at roughly three-day intervals with Dektol developer (35).

Experimental and discussion

(a) Goldfish retina

We chose the goldfish retina for immunocytochemical studies of GAD because the GABergic pathways in the goldfish retina have been extensively studied by autoradiographic and biochemical methods (10, 12, 35, 37). Using the antibody against GAD purified from catfish brain, our immunocytochemical study (12) shows that GAD is localized in some horizontal cells, a few amacrine cells and sublamina b of the inner plexiform layer (Fig. 1). In the goldfish retina, different types of horizontal cells can be classified physiologically and morphologically according to their functional contacts with photoreceptors (38). Thus, rod horizontal cells receive input exclusively from rods, and cone horizontal cells can be subdivided into H1, H2 and H3 cells, which receive input predominantly from red, green and blue-sensitive cones, respectively. The positions of the GAD-positive horizontal cells in the inner nuclear layer indicate that these are the perikarya of H1 horizontal cells. To enhance GAD-positive staining in cell bodies and axons of GAD-containing cells, 50 μm sections were incubated with 0.1% Triton X-100 and the anti-GAD serum (a 1:4000 dilution was used for most Triton X-100 treated tissue) overnight before the normal immunocytochemical procedure (39). With this treatment, both the perikarya and axons of some horizontal cells are heavily stained (Fig. 1). Again, the positions of the GAD-positive cell bodies indicate that these are H1 horizontal cells. It follows that the GAD-positive axons are most probably axons of H1 cells. H2, H3 and rod horizontal cells, photoreceptors, bipolar cells and Müller (glial) cells do not show detectable GAD-positive reaction product.

232

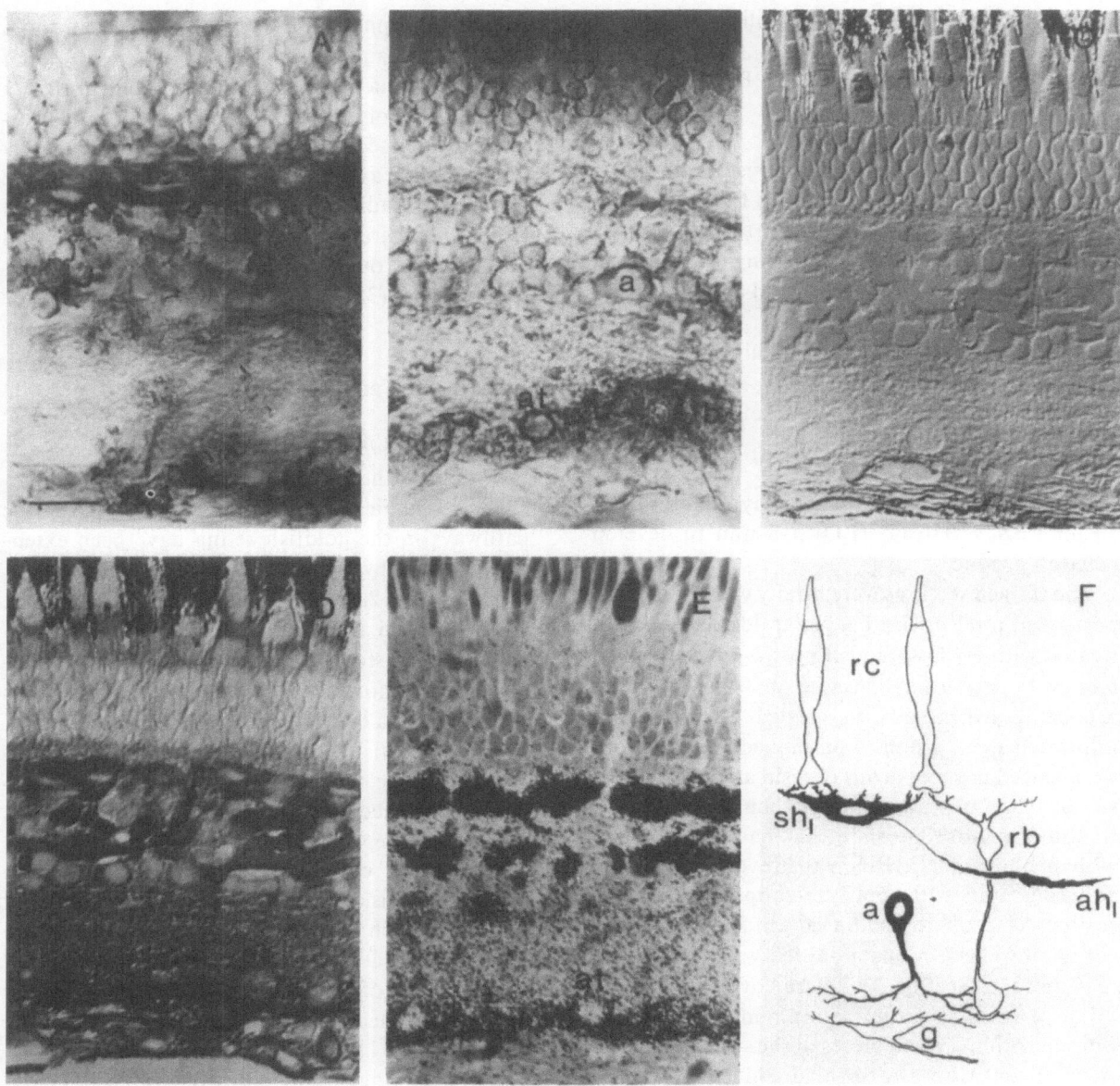

Fig. 1a, b. Immunocytochemical localization of GAD in 50 μm section of goldfish retina. Focusing on the outer retina A, GAD-positive reaction product is seen over the somata of some cone horizontal cells (h). Note that the nuclei of these cells are not stained and therefore probably do not contain GAD. Scale bar 20 μm. Focusing on the inner retina B, GAD-positive reaction product is seen over some amacrine cells (a, the nucleus is not stained) and in sublamina b of the inner plexiform layer, indicating that GABAergic terminals are probably concentrated in this sublamina b. Note dense reaction product around the axon terminal (at) of a type b bipolar cell. C, Control experiment, where a section treated with non-immunized serum shows very little GAD-positive reaction product. The dark structures between photoreceptors are melanin granules in pigment epithelial cells. D, Staining of GAD in 5 μm section shows that some somata and axons of cone horizontal cells, probably H1 cells are stained. Sublamina b of the inner plexiform layer is also stained, especially around the axon terminal of some type b bipolar cells. E, Autoradiographic section of a goldfish retina incubated with 10^{-6} M ^{3}H-GABA. As shown earlier (35, 37) high-affinity GABA uptake is localized in the somata and axons of H1 horizontal cells, and in some Ab pyriform amacrine cells which make synaptic connections in sublamina b of the inner plexiform layer. F, Schematic diagram of probable GABAergic neurons (H1 horizontal cells and some Ab amacrine cells) and their functional connections in the goldfish retina as revealed by our immunocytochemical and autoradiographic studies, re: red-sensitive cones; sh_l and ah_l:soma and axon of a H1 cell; rb:red-sensitive centre-depolarizing bipolar cell (type b); a: pyriform amacrine cell which makes contact with rb; g:retinal ganglion cell.

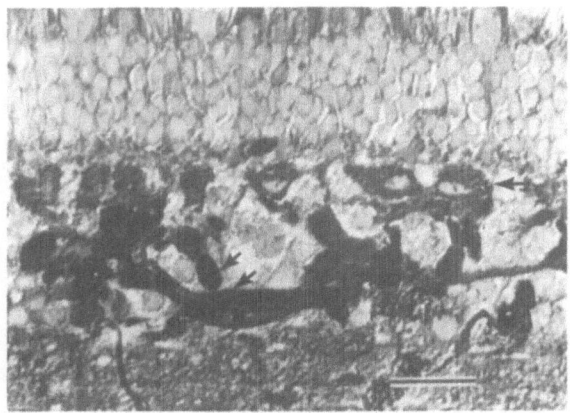

Fig. 2. A 3 μm section of a goldfish retina treated with 0.1% Triton X-100 and anti-GAD serum (1:4000 dilution) overnight and processed for immunocytochemistry. Because this treatment enchanced the penetration of the antiserum and conjugate into the tissue, GAD-positive reaction product is much more intense than that shown in Fig. 1. In particular, both the somata (horizontal arrow) and axons (oblique arrows) of the H1 horizontal cells are clearly stained. Scale bar 20 μm.

The identities of the GAD-positive amacrine cells cannot be determined without serial reconstruction and electron microscopic studies. The presence of GAD in sublamina b of the inner plexiform layer, especially around the axon terminals of some centre-depolarizing bipolar cells (type b) (40, 41), suggests that GAD-containing amacrine cells make synaptic contacts with these bipolar cells. This result and those of autoradiographic studies of ³H-GABA uptake in the inner plexiform layer, indicate that at least some GABAergic amacrine cells are Ab pyriform cells which make contact with red-sensitive centredepolarizing bipolar cells in the goldfish retina (40-42).

Comparison between the immunocytochemical studies of GAD-containing neurones and autoradiographic studies of GABA uptake reveals a marked similarity in the labeling patterns (Figs. 1, 2). Our findings therefore demonstrate that in goldfish retina, the neurones which possess a high-affinity system for GABA uptake also contain significant levels of GAD. In addition, this study confirms earlier biochemical results showing that at least some isolated axons of cone horizontal cells in the goldfish retina synthesize GABA and contain high specific activities of GAD (10). These findings, and those of autoradiographic (10, 43) and electrophysiological (44) studies of the GABA system in

the teleost retina, point to GABA as being the transmitter used by H1 horizontal cells of the goldfish retina. The absence of GABA uptake and GAD in all other horizontal cell types (H2, H3 and rod) indicates that they are not GABAergic. This raises the possibility that horizontal cells which are in contact with different types of photoreceptors may use different neurotransmitters.

(b) Rabbit retina

The rabbit was chosen as a suitable species for analysis of the retinal GAD system for several reasons. The rabbit retina has been extensively characterized anatomically, electrophysiologically, and pharmacologically (45–52). Moreover, a suitable *in vitro* preparation has been developed which permits biochemical manipulation of the intact but isolated retina (53), as, for example, for autoradiographic studies. In addition, GABA neurons specifically mediate complex receptive field properties and enhance Y-cell center-surround antagonism (45). Finally, according to Dubin's classification, the synaptic organization of the rabbit retina is less complex than that of other popular experimental animals such as goldfish and frog (54).

In autoradiographic studies using [³H] GABA, silver grains were observed in a broad band over the full depth of the inner plexiform layer (Fig. 3); there was little if any apparent lamination within this band. In addition, numerous cell bodies within the inner half of the inner nuclear layer showed heavy labeling. Occasional cell bodies in the ganglion cell layer were also labeled, although many were clearly devoid of grains. The outer plexiform layer and horizontal cell layer were relatively free of label. The different grain densities of the areas shown in Fig. 3 probably reflect the different distances of these areas from the site of injection of [³H] GABA.

Similar silver grains labeling has been reported by Ehinger (14) in the same system. However, in the rat (55, 56), guinea pig, goat, and cat (57), uptake of [³H] GABA was almost exclusively into Müller (glial) cells. In lower vertebrates, such as the goldfish (35), frog (36), pigeon, and chicken (58), [³H] GABA uptake occurred exclusively into neuronal elements. It is of interest that most of the above experiments, except those of Ehinger (14), were carried out *in vitro*. Following our own *in vitro* studies of [³H] GABA uptake in the rabbit retina (data not shown), autoradiographs showed ac-

234

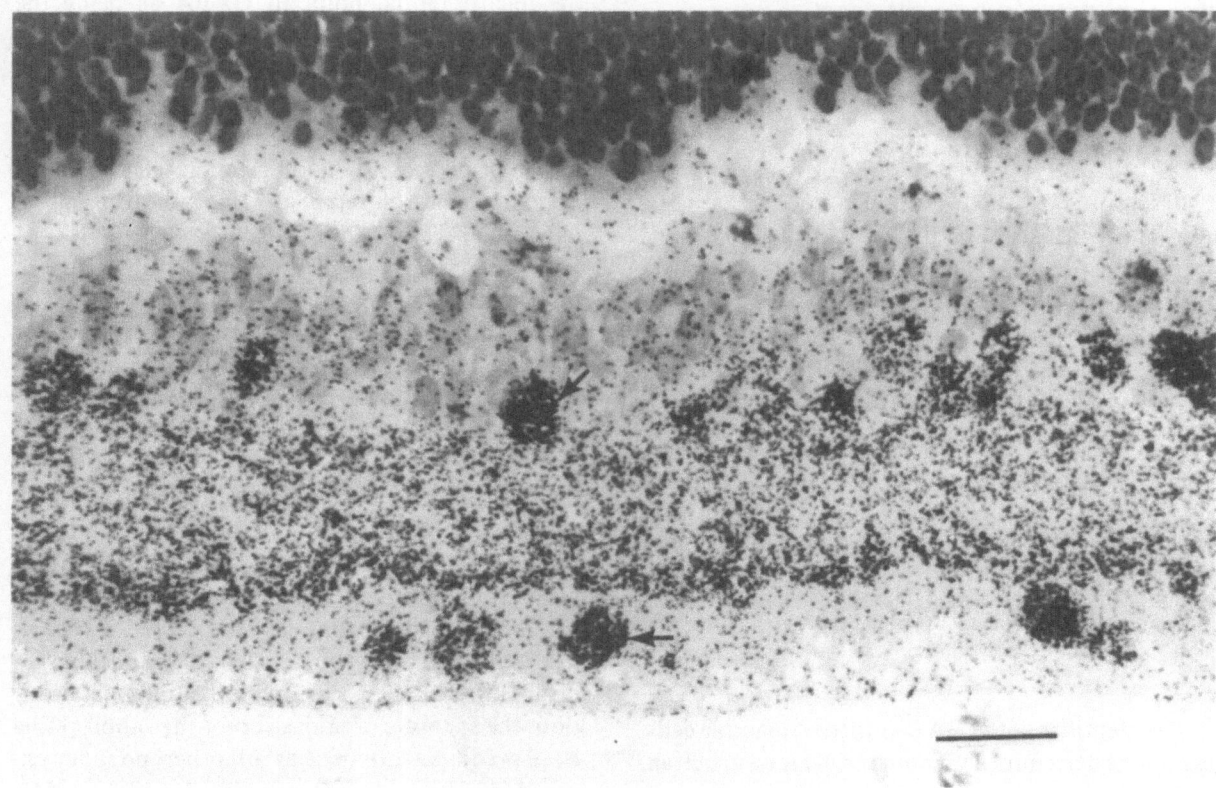

Fig. 3. Bright-field micrographs of autoradiograms of rabbit retina incubated *in vivo* with [³H] GABA. Silver grains appear diffusely over the IPL (inner plexiform layer) over amacrine cell bodies in the INL (inner nuclear layer) and over some cell bodies in the GC (ganglion cell layer). The outer plexiform layer is unlabeled (×725).

cumulation of grains principally over Müller cells rather than neurons, in a pattern similar to that reported for the rat and other species. We interpret such a pattern as that of a lower-affinity uptake system for GABA which is operational, or at least detectable, only when the neuronal transport system has been impaired or has ceased to function due to neuronal death or damage. Such damage would be more likely to occur *in vitro* for mammalian retinas than those of the more resilient lower vertebrates and would be much less likely under the *in vivo* conditions used here for the rabbit retina.

GAD immunocytochemistry was first carried out in the presence of 0.25% Triton X-100 to eliminate membrane barriers to antibody penetration (11, 26). Specific immunochemical reaction deposit formed four discrete laminae within the inner plexiform layer (Fig. 4a). The laminae were approximately equal in intensity and were evenly spaced throughout the layer. Control sections showed no reaction product (Fig. 4b). This pattern bears a striking resemblance to the lamination of amacrine cell processes in Golgi-impregnated retinas, and of dopaminergic (59) and cholinergic (60) inner plexiform layer processes.

When Triton treatment was omitted, and dimethylsulfoxide used to increase antibody penetration without the complete destruction of cell membranes, GAD-positive reaction product was observed in much smaller, more discrete deposits (Fig. 4c-e); lamination was less distinct under these conditons because the limited antibody penetration led to less superposition of stained structures. Some lamination was still discernible, however, even in 1 µm plastic sections (Fig. 4d). When sections were viewed *en face,* stained processes sometimes formed long strings of varicosities that were interspersed with individual punctate deposits (Fig. 4e).

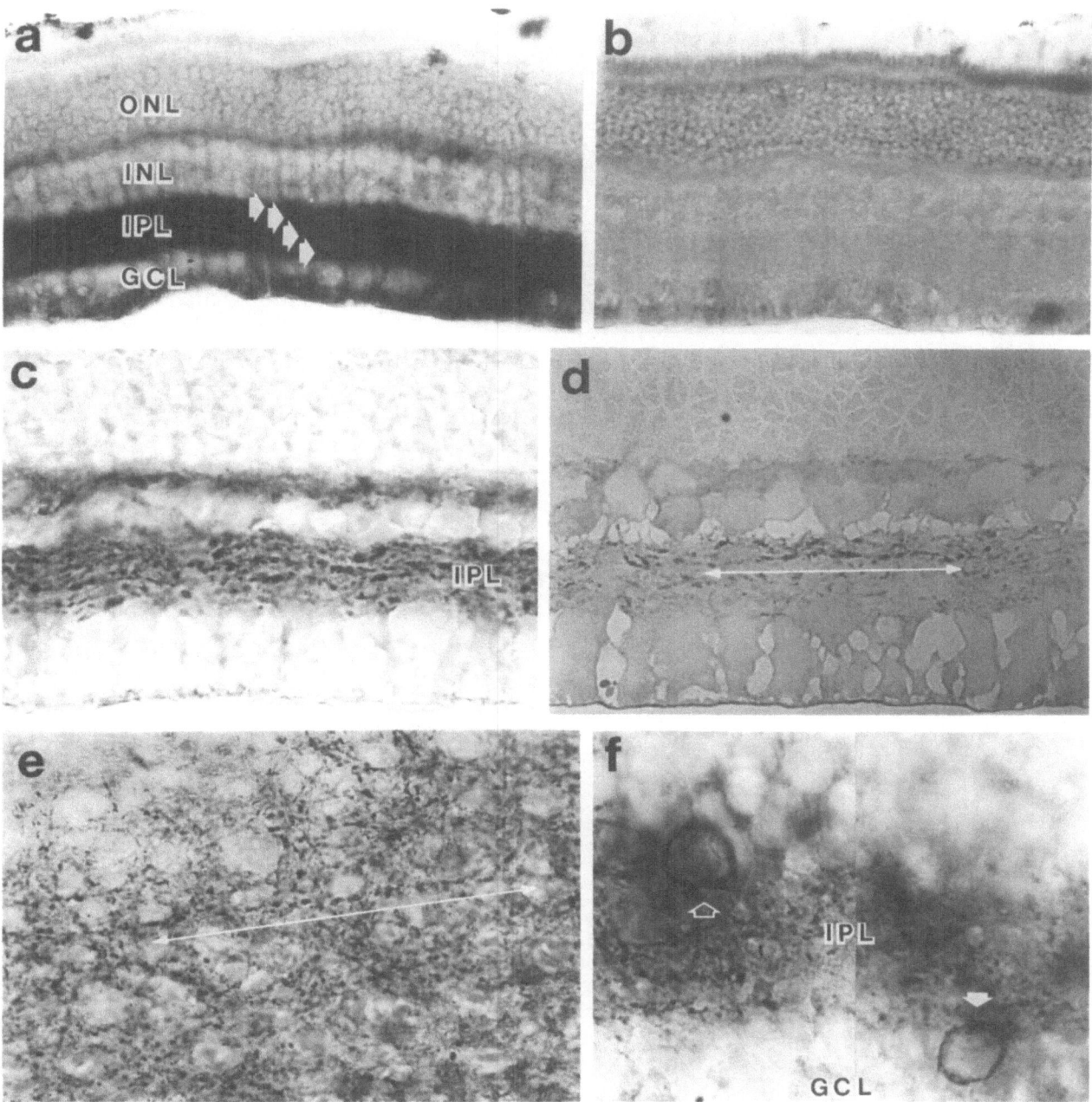

Fig. 4. Immunocytochemical localization of GAD in rabbit retina. (a) Fifty-micron cross-section of retina stained for GAD in the presence of 0.2% Triton X-100. Reaction product is visible as four dense bands, or laminae, within the inner plexiform layer (IPL) (×400). No reaction product is observed in other layers of the retina, or in the section treated with control (non-immune) serum (×400) (b). (c) A similar section, treated with GAD antiserum in the absence of Triton. Lamination is less apparent because of limited antibody penetration, but reaction product is more clearly discernible as discrete, punctate structures in the IPL (×1000). (d) A one-micron semithin section shows that long laminated processes show GAD immunoreactivity (double-headed arrow) (×1000). (e) A fifty-micron section through the IPL in the plane of the retina. Long, very straight strings of beaded varicosities are often observed when viewed in this plane (double-headed arrow) (×750). (f) An immunoreactive amacrine cell body (open arrow) and a presumed misplaced amacrine cell body (closed arrow), rendered visible by intravitreal injection of colchicine 36 h before fixation of the retina (×1250). The misplaced type of cell is rarely found.

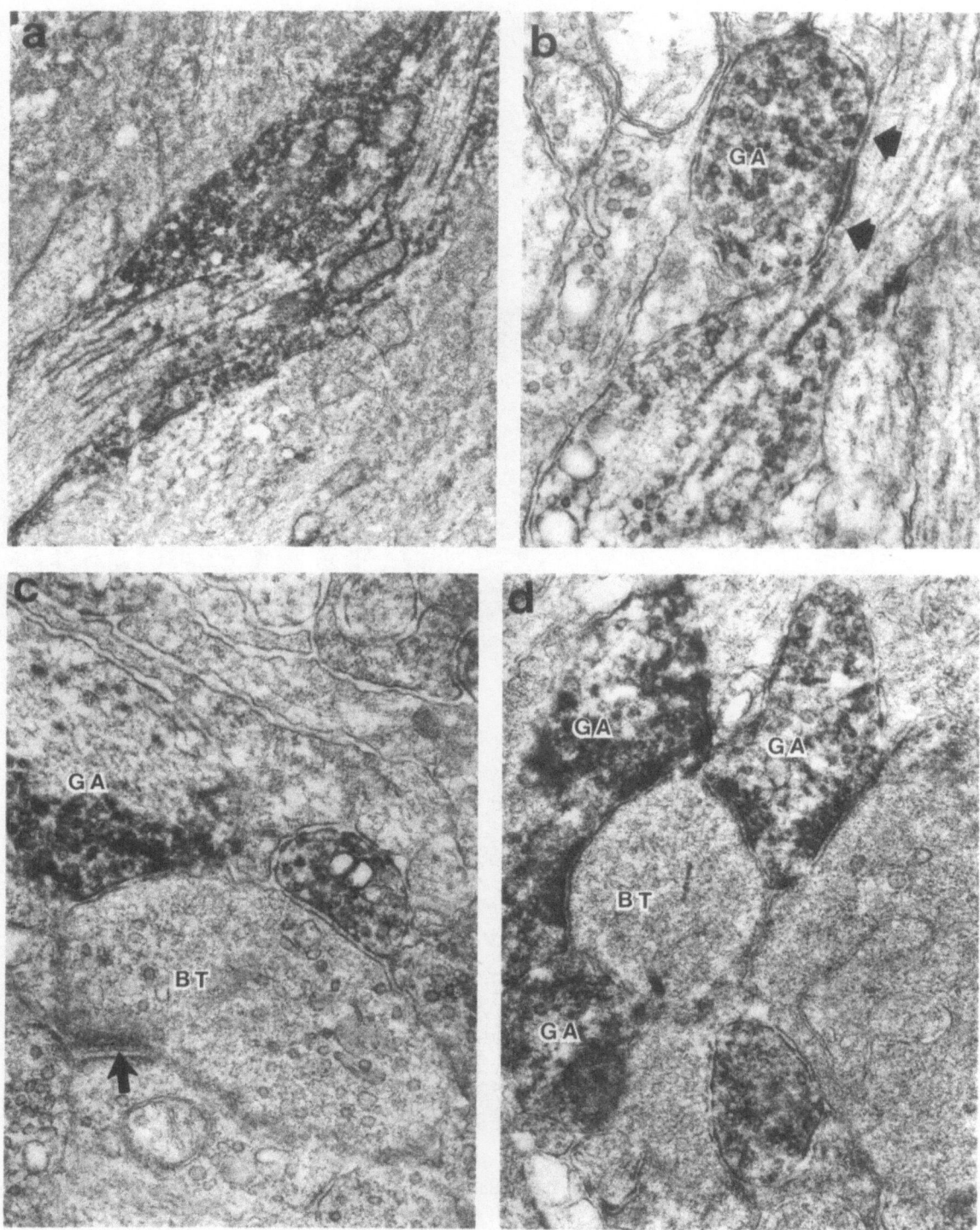

Fig. 5. Montage of electron micrographs of GAD-positive processes in the IPL of the rabbit retina. (a) Amacrine cell varicosity containing numerous stained synaptic vesicles and microtubules (× 28 200). (b) Amacrine-to-amacrine synapses in the rabbit retina; in these examples the presynaptic processes are GAD-labeled. Occasionally, the postsynaptic element may be identified as a second GAD-stained process, as indicated by the presence of a weakly staining varicosity; otherwise, postsynaptic elements are free of reaction product (× 52 300). (c) Amacrine-to-bipolar synapses in the rabbit retina. BT, bipolar terminal. GAD-stained terminals were often seen surrounding bipolar terminals, which were usually identified by their characteristic ribbons (arrowheads) (× 39 250). (d) Bipolar cell terminals in the rabbit retina. Bipolar terminals were profusely innervated by GAD-containing processes. The postsynaptic element is involved in the dyadic relationship characteristic of bipolar terminals (arrowheads) (× 39 250).

The high concentration of GAD within axon terminal permitted its ready visualization there by antibody staining, even at 1:1000 dilutions of the primary antiserum. However, in cell bodies and axons, normal GAD levels were apparently too low for reliable localization. *In vivo* administration of colchicine before fixation causes GAD to accumulate within cell bodies and axons due to a blockage of axon transport; the accumulated enzyme can then be visualized immunocytochemically (61). Localization experiments were therefore carried out using retinas from rabbits that had received intravitreal injections 36 hr before enucleation. Under these conditions, stained cell bodies were routinely observed in the inner third of the inner nuclear layer (Fig. 4f); they had the general unipolar morphology of amacrine cells, the labeled processes were sometimes traced from them into the IPL (Fig. 4f).

GAD-stained processes, when sectioned longitudinally, often appeared in the electron microscope as dense varicosities characterized by accretions of stained synaptic vesicles and microtubules (Fig. 5a). Since colchicine was not used in these experiments, regions between varicosities were generally not stained.

In principle, an amacrine cell may be presynaptic to any of three cell types (ganglion, bipolar, amacrine), or postsynaptic to two (bipolar, amacrine). Among the first group, GABA-amacrine:ganglion cell synapses were observed the least often (not shown); GABA-amacrine:bipolar and GABA-amacrine:amacrine synapses were far more numerous (Fig. 5b-d). Post-synaptic amacrine processes were identified by their small size and relatively low vesicle density, by the presence of membranous tubular structures, and sometimes by the presence of varicosities containing synaptic vesicles (Fig. 5b).

GABA-amacrine:bipolar synapses were identified most easily when the postsynaptic process contained a synaptic ribbon (Fig. 5c-d). Often, bipolar terminals were strikingly surrounded by a dense plexus of GAD-positive amacrine boutons (Fig. 5d). This arrangement provides a morphological substrate for a potent GABA-mediated inhibition of a certain type of bipolar cell. In summary, the results from autoradiographic experiments agreed well with the pattern of GAD immunocytochemical staining showing uptake into neuronal cell bodies and into structures within the inner plexiform layer. Similar studies in frog, cat and primate retina are in progress.

Acknowledgment

This work was supported in part by grants from National Institute of Health (NS 13224 and EY 02423).

References

1. Awapara, J., 1950. Federation Proc. 9: 148.
2. Roberts, E. & Frankel, S., 1950. Federation Proc. 9: 219.
3. Davidson, M., 1976. Neurotransmitter Amino Acids. New York: Academic Press, pp. 57.
4. Krnjevic, K., 1974. Physiol. Rev. 54: 418–540.
5. Bonting, S. L., 1976. Transmitter in the Visual Process (ed.). New York: Pergamon Press.
6. Graham, Jr., L. T., 1974. The Eye (Davson, H. & Graham, L. T., Jr., eds.). New York: Academic Press, pp. 283–342.
7. Neal, M. J., 1976. Gen. Pharmac. 7: 321–332.
8. Kuriyama, K., Sisken, B., Haber, B. & Roberts, E., 1968. Brain Res. 9: 165–168.
9. Graham, L. T., Jr., 1972. Brain Res. 36: 476–479.
10. Lam, D. M. K., 1975. Cold Spring Harb. Symp. Quant. Biol. 40: 571–579.
11. Brandon, C., Lam, D. M. K. & Wu, J.-Y., 1979. Proc. Nat. Acad. Sci. USA 76: 3557–3561.
12. Lam, D. M. K., Su, Y. Y. T., Swain, L., Marc, R. E., Brandon, C. & Wu, J.-Y., 1979. Nature (London) 278: 565–567.
13. Bruun, A. & Ehinger, B., 1974. Exptl. Eye Res. 19: 435–447.
14. Ehinger, B., 1970. Exper. 26: 1063–1064.
15. Ehinger, B. & Falck, B., 1971. Brain Res. 33: 157–172.
16. Wu, J.-Y., Matsuda, T. & Roberts, E., 1973. J. Biol. Chem. 248: 3029–3034.
17. Wu, J.-Y., 1976. GABA in Nervous System Function (Roberts, E., Chase, T. & Tower, D., eds.). New York, Raven Press: pp. 7–55.
18. Su, Y. Y. T., Wu, J.-Y. & Lam, D. M. K., 1979. J. Neurochem. 33: 169–179.
19. Wu, J.-Y., Su, Y. Y. T., Lam, D. M. K., Brandon, C. & Denner, L., 1980. Brain Res. Bull. 5 (2): 63–70.
20. Wu, J.-Y., 1978. Physiol. Rev. 58 (4), 863–904.
21. Saito, K., Barber, R., Wu, J.-Y., Matsuda, T., Roberts, E. & Vaughn, J. E., 1974. Proc. Nat. Acad. Sci. USA 71: 269–273.
22. McLaughlin, B. J., Wood, J. G., Saito, K., Barber, R., Vaugh, J. E., Roberts, E. & Wu, J.-Y., 1974. Brain Res. 76: 377–391.
23. McLaughlin, B. J., Wood, J. G., Saito, K., Roberts, E. & Wu, J.-Y., 1975. Brain Res. 85: 355–371.
24. McLaughlin, B. J., Barber, R., Saito, K., Roberts, E. & Wu, J.-Y., 1975. J. Comp. Neur. 164: 305–322.

238

25. Gottesfeld, Z. Brandon, C., Jacobowitz, D. M. & Wu, J.-Y., 1980. Brain Res. Bull. 5 (2): 1-6.

26. Brandon, C., Su, Y. Y. T., Lam, D. M. K. & Wu, J.-Y., 1980. Brain Res. Bull. 5(2): 21-29.

27. Baxter, C. F., 1970. Handbook of Neurochemistry, (Lajtha, A., ed.) New York: Plenum Press, vol. 3: pp. 289-353.

28. Kuriyama, K., Haber, B., Sisken, T. & Roberts, E., 1966. Proc. Nat. Acad. Sci. USA 55: 846-849.

29. Kravitz, E. A. & Potter, D. D., 1965. J. Neurochem. 12: 323-328.

30. Fonnum, F., 1975. Metabolic Compartmentation and Neurotransmission (Berl, S., Clarke, D. D. & Schneider, D., eds.). New York: Plenum, pp. 99-122.

31. Saito, K., Wu, J.-Y. & Roberts, E., 1974. Brain Res. 65: 277-285.

32. Wong, E., Schousboe, A., Saito, K., Wu, J.-Y. & Roberts, E., 1974. Brain Res. 68: 133-142.

33. Su, Y. Y. T., Wu, J.-Y. & Lam, D. M. K., 1979. Soc. for Neuroscience, abstract, vol. 5: 599.

34. Petrali, J. P., Hinton, D. M., Moriaty, G. C. & Sternberger, L. A., 1974. J. Histochem. Cytochem. 22: 782-801.

35. Lam, D. M. K. & Steinman, L., 1971. Proc. Nat. Acad. Sci. USA. 68: 2777-2781.

36. Voaden, M. J., Marshall, J. & Murani, N., 1974. Brain Res. 67: 115-132.

37. Marc, R. E., Stell, W. K., Bok, D. & Lam, D. M. K., 1978. J. Comp. Neurol. 182: 221-246.

38. Stell, W. K. & Lightfoot, D. O., 1975. J. Comp. Neurol. 159: 473-502.

39. Grzanna, R., Moliver, M. E. & Coyle, J. T., 1978. Proc. Nat. Acad. Sci. USA 75: 2502-2506.

40. Famiglietti, E. V., Kaneko, A. & Tachibana, M., 1977. Science 198: 1267-1269.

41. Stell, W. K., Ishida, A. T. & Lightfoot, D. O., 1977. Science 198: 1269-1271.

42. Lam, D. M. K., Marc, R. E., Sarthy, P. V., Chin, C. A., Su, Y. Y. T., Brandon, C. & Wu, J.-Y., 1980. Neurochemistry 1: 183-190.

43. Lam, D. M. K., 1975. Nature 254: 345-347.

44. Lam, D. M. K., Lasater, E. M. & Naka, K., 1978. Proc. Nat. Acad. Sci. USA 75: 6310-6313.

45. Caldwell, J. H. & Daw, N. W., 1978. J. Physiology 276: 257-276.

46. Caldwell, J. H. & Daw, N. W., 1978. J. Physiology 276: 299-310.

47. Caldwell, J. H. & Daw, N. W., 1978. J. Physiology 276: 277-298.

48. Barlow, H. B., Hill, R. W. & Levick, W. R. 1964. J. Physiol. (London) 173: 377-407.

49. Miller, R. F., 1979. The Neurosciences, 4th Study Program, (Schmitt, F. O. & Worden, F. G., eds.) MIT Press, pp. 227-245.

50. Masland, R. H., 1977. J. Comp. Neurol. 175: 275-285.

51. Ames, A., III & Pollen, D. A., 1969. J. Neurophysiol. 32: 424-442.

52. Parks, J. M., Ames, A., III & Nesbett, F. B., 1977. J. Neurochem. 27: 987-997.

53. Masland, R. H. & Ames, A., III, 1975. J. Neurobiol. 6: 305-312.

54. Dubin, M. W., 1970. J. Comp. Neurol. 140: 479-506.

55. Neal, M. J. & Iversen, L. L., 1972. Nature (London) New Biol. 235: 217-218.

56. Marshall, J. & Voaden, M. J., 1974. Exp. Eye Res. 18: 367-370.

57. Marshall, J. & Voaden, M. J., 1975. J. Neurochem. 15: 459-461.

58. Marshall, J. & Voaden, M. J., 1974. Invest. Ophthalmol. 13: 602-607.

59. Ehinger, B., 1966. Z. Zellforsch. Mikrosk. Anat. 71: 146-152.

60. Nichols, C. W. & Koelle, G. B., 1968. J. Comp. Neurol. 133: 1-16.

61. Ribak, C. E., Vaughn, J. E. & Roberts, E., 1978. Brain Res. 140: 315-332.

Received September 17, 1980.

L-glutamate transport in renal plasma membrane vesicles

Bertram Sacktor
Laboratory of Molecular Aging, Gerontology Research Center, National Institute on Aging, National Institutes of Health, Baltimore City Hospitals, Baltimore, MD 21224 U.S.A.

Summary

This review describes the uptake of L-glutamate by well-characterized preparations of renal brush border (luminal) and baso-lateral membrane vesicles derived from the plasma membrane of the polar proximal tubular cell. L-glutamate is taken up against its concentration gradient, from both sides, by co-transport systems in which the movement of the amino acid into the cell is coupled to the influx of Na^+ and efflux of K^+ down their respective electrochemical gradients. The presence of these ion gradient-energized systems, specific for L-glutamate, may account for the exceedingly high intracellular concentration of this metabolically important amino acid in the renal tubule.

Introduction

L-glutamate has a central role in renal tubular metabolism (1). Consequently, the uptake of the acidic amino acid by the kidney cell is of crucial importance. Previous studies at various levels of tissue organization, ranging from normal human subjects and patients with autosomal recessive dicarboxylic aminoaciduria to animal renal cortical slices, individual nephrons perfused in vivo and in vitro, and cells grown in culture, indicate that the kidney has a specific acidic amino transport system (2,3). These studies also show that L-glutamate is reabsorbed in the proximal region of the nephron and suggest that the uptake is mediated by a saturable, energy-dependent, uphill system. Additionally, it was found that the transtubular flux of L-glutamate in microperfused tubules is stimulated by Na^+ (4). However, until recently, direct information on the mechanisms by which the acidic amino acid crosses the plasma membrane of the renal cell was limited. Interpretation of the findings was difficult because of the partial metabolism of the amino acid, the failure to dissociate metabolic

from transport processes, the uncertainties in distinguishing uptake across the luminal segment of the plasma membrane of the polar tubular cell from uptake via the baso-lateral segment, and the inability to establish defined ionic gradients to drive the transport. Recent studies with well-characterized preparations of luminal (brush border) and baso-lateral membrane vesicles obviate many of these difficulties.

Although, in general, the renal tubule carries out uphill transport of all amino acids, the uptake of L-glutamate (L-aspartate) is unique in that the intracellular concentration of the dicarboxylic amino acid reaches levels at least 20 times its respective plasma concentration (5, 6). As illustrated schematically in Fig. 1 this impressive accumulation by the polar tubular cell may be mediated by uptake from the glomerular filtrate across the luminal (brush border) membrane, from the interstitial fluid across the baso-lateral membrane, or from both. In serum and, thus, in the filtrate, the concentration of L-glutamate is approximately 0.15–0.20 mM. In the cortex, the intracellular L-glutamate concentration is about

Molecular and Cellular Biochemistry 39, 239–251 (1981). 0300-8177/81/0391-0239/$02.60.

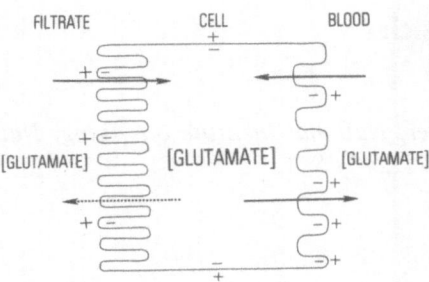

Fig. 1. Schematic model of the renal tubular cell showing the relative distribution of L-glutamate in the glomerular filtrate, peritubular fluid and cell, and indicating the requirement for active transport systems to effect the accumulation of the amino acid.

6 mM (5); and when the nephron is given an amino acid load, the concentration of L-glutamate in the proximal convoluted tubular cell may reach 35 mM (6). In addition, as shown in Fig. 1, L-glutamate which bears a negative charge at physiological pH, in contrast to net neutrally charged amino acids and D-glucose, must enter the cell against a membrane potential. Thus, the transport mechanisms for L-glutamate may be different from the mechanisms of uptake for the previously studied neutral compounds (7, 8). This question and the characteristics of L-glutamate transport in membrane vesicles derived from either the brush border or baso-lateral segment on the plasma membrane will be discussed in this review.

Experimental methods

Preparation of membrane vesicles

Two kinds of renal plasma membrane vesicles were used in these studies. One, the brush border (microvillus) membrane vesicle, was derived from that segment of the plasma membrane of the polar cell that abuts the glomerular filtrate in the lumen of the proximal tubule. The other, the baso-lateral membrane vesicle, represents that segment of the plasma membrane that is in direct contact with the interstitial fluid and the blood. Unless noted otherwise, the brush border membrane vesicles were isolated by a $CaCl_2$ precipitation technique (9). The quality of the preparations was evaluated randomly by enrichment of enzyme markers; specific activities of the brush border enzymes trehalase and γ-glutamyltranspeptidase were increased approximately 10- to 12-fold relative to the cortex homogenate (10). In contrast, (Na + K)ATPase, a marker enzyme for baso-lateral membranes, was either not detectable or of extremely low activity (11). The baso-lateral membrane vesicles were prepared by a newly developed Percoll gradient technique (12). The enrichment factor for (Na + K)ATPase in this membrane preparation was about 11, and there were no increases in the specific activities of γ-glutamyltranspeptidase or maltase, relative to the cortex homogenate. In experiments in which the intravesicular medium was varied, the vesicles were preloaded by carrying out the entire washing procedures in the described medium.

Transport measurements

Uptakes of L-[^{3}H]glutamate, L-[^{3}H]aspartate, L-[^{3}H]proline, and D-[^{14}C]glucose were measured by a Millipore filtration technique (13), at 20 °C. The radioactive substrates taken up by the membrane vesicles, and then extracted, had R_f values in thin layer chromatographic systems identical with authentic compounds, demonstrating that they were not metabolized.

Results

The Na$^+$ gradient-dependent L-glutamate uptake system in brush border membrane vesicles

Fig. 2 shows several general properties of the L-glutamate uptake system in microvillar mem-

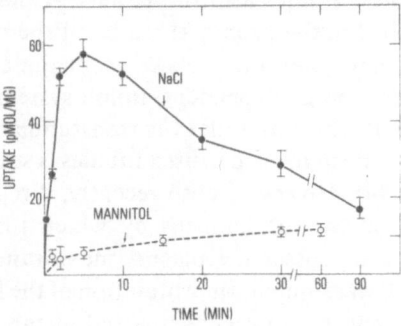

Fig. 2. The effect of a Na$^+$ gradient (extravesicular > intravesicular) on L-glutamate uptake in brush border membrane vesicles. From Schneider, Hammerman and Sacktor (16).

brane vesicles. When both the intravesicular and extravesicular media were isotonic mannitol, the initial rate of uptake was low and steady state levels were reached in about 1 h. However, when 100 mM NaCl isosmotically replaced mannitol in the extravesicular medium and a Na^+ gradient ($[Na^+]_o >$ $[Na^-]_i$) was imposed on the system, the uptake of L-glutamate was markedly stimulated (14–16). Initial rates (15 s) were increased approximately 5 to 10 times. Accumulation of L-glutamate in the membrane vesicles was maximal in about 5 min. Thereafter, the amount of amino acid in the vesicles decreased, indicating efflux. The final level of uptake of L-glutamate in the presence and absence of the Na^+ gradient was the same, suggesting that equilibrium had been established.

At the peak of the 'overshoot', the accumulation of L-glutamate reached 4 to 5 times the final equilibrium value. This finding suggests that the imposition of a large extravesicular to intravesicular Na^+ gradient provided the driving force to effect the transient movement of the amino acid into brush border membrane vesicles against its concentration gradient. The overshoot was transient with these vesicular preparations because of the limited energy inherent in the salt gradient present at the initiation of the incubation and its dissipation with time (8). When the membrane vesicles were preloaded with NaCl so that the extravesicular and intravesicular concentrations of Na^+ were equal, the overshoot was abolished (16). It was noted, however, that the initial rate of L-glutamate uptake in the presence of Na^+, but in the absence of a Na^+ gradient, i.e. $[Na^+]_o = [Na^+]_i$, was three times greater than in the absence of Na^+. These results indicate that it was not the concentration of Na^+ per se but the Na^+ gradient that was crucial in energizing uphill transport. This view was supported by the finding that gramicidin, an ionophore that increased permeability of the brush border membrane and electrogenically dissipated the Na^+ gradient in mannitol-loaded vesicles (17), precluded the concentrative transport of L-glutamate (16).

Na^+ specificity

The specificity of the Na^+ gradient in stimulating the initial rate of L-glutamate uptake was evident from the finding that the rate in the presence of a NaCl gradient was about ten times greater than with the chloride salts of K^+ or choline$^+$ (16). A small (two-fold), but statistically significant, enhancement in uptake was found with a Li^+ gradient, relative to that with a K^+ gradient or mannitol. The weak substitution of Li^+ for Na^+ in the uptake of L-proline and D-glucose was previously seen (13, 18). The initial rate of L-glutamate uptake in the presence of Na^+, but in the absence of a Na^+ gradient, was also greater than in the presence of K^+, Li^+, choline$^+$, or Tris$^+$ in the nongradient mode (16). At equilibrium (90 min), the uptake of L-glutamate was independent of the nature of the salt gradient, thus precluding the possibility of osmotically induced changes as a cause for the enhanced uptake with Na^+.

Amino acid specificity

The specificity of the Na^+ gradient-dependent glutamate transport system for acidic amino acids was evident from findings that the uptake of 25 μM L-[^{3}H]glutamate in brush border membrane vesicles was competitively inhibited by 5 mM unlabeled L-glutamate and L-aspartate but it was not decreased by 5 mM neutral amino acids, imino acids, nor basic amino acids (16). In the absence of Na^+, neither of the acidic amino acids inhibited the uptake of L-[^{3}H]glutamate. In addition, mono- and dicarboxylic compounds, including glutarate, succinate, and acetate, failed to effect the uptake of L-glutamate. Also, the butyric acid analogs α-amino-isobutyrate, β-aminoisobutyrate, and γ-aminobutyrate did not inhibit.

Table 1. Effects of other amino acids and analogs of L-glutamate on the transport of L-[^{3}H]glutamate[a].

Test compound	Relative uptake of L-[^{3}H]glutamate
	%
None	100
L-glutamate	12 ± 1
D-glutamate	96 ± 3
L-aspartate	13 ± 1
D-aspartate	13 ± 1
L-α-Aminoadipate	102 ± 4
L-glutamine	100 ± 5
L-asparagine	103 ± 2
L-cysteate	11 ± 1

[a] Data are from Schneider, Hammerman & Sacktor (16).

242

Table 1 describes the specificity of the Na⁺ gradient-dependent L-glutamate system in further detail. The system was selectively stereospecific, in that L-glutamate competitively inhibited whereas D-glutamate did not. In contrast, both L-aspartate and D-aspartate were potent inhibitors of L-glutamate uptake. Substitutions on the α-amino, α-carboxyl, or γ-carboxyl group of L-glutamate resulted in loss of inhibitory activity. Thus, the L-glutamate transport system differed from the L-glutamine transport system. A very strict requirement for side chain length extending from the α-carbon was found (16). The addition of a methylene group to L-glutamate, i.e. L-aminoadipate, resulted in an inactive compound, whereas L-aspartate, which differs from L-glutamate by having one less methylene group, was a strong inhibitor. L-Cysteate was a very effective inhibitor, but L-homocysteate as well as L-cysteine were inactive.

The inhibition of L-[³H]glutamate uptake by L-aspartate, D-aspartate, and L-cysteate suggests that these compounds share the L-glutamate carrier. This suggestion is consistent with other studies in which their efficacy to accelerate exchange diffusion was examined (16). For example, it was found that preloading the vesicles with unlabeled L-glutamate, but not with D-glutamate, stimulated the uptakes of both L-[³H]-glutamate and L-[³H]aspartate. Preloading the vesicles with L-aspartate, D-aspartate and L-cysteate accelerated the exchange diffusion of L-[³H]glutamate and L-[³H]aspartate. These findings are in accord with earlier studies on the specificity of the L-glutamate transport system in more physiologically intact preparations (3). Moreover, these results, together with earlier reports on the specificities of the Na⁺ gradient-dependent uptakes of other classes of amino acids (14), suggest that the ability of the kidney to transport amino acids selectively can be ascribed to an intrinsic property of the proximal tubule luminal membrane.

The kinetics of the Na⁺ gradient-dependent L-glutamate uptake system

The initial rate of L-glutamate uptake into the brush border membrane vesicles, in the presence or absence of a Na⁺ gradient, was dependent on the concentration of the amino acid (16). In the absence of Na⁺, the uptake of L-glutamate uptake increased

linearly with increasing substrate concentration throughout the range from 5 μM to 5 mM. Thus, the Na⁺ gradient-independent transport system for L-glutamate appeared not to saturate. The simplest interpretation of this finding suggests that the Na⁺-free system represents passive diffusion, although the possibility that this system was comprised of a passive diffusion component and a carrier-mediated process saturable at extremely high concentrations of the amino acid was not ruled out. In contrast, in the presence of a Na⁺ gradient, the rate of L-glutamate uptake decreased at higher L-glutamate concentrations, providing evidence for saturability. If at each concentration the Na⁺-free uptake was subtracted from the uptake measured in the presence of the Na⁺ gradient, the data exhibited a Michaelis-Menton relationship and described a saturable Na⁺ gradient-dependent L-glutamate transport process. The apparent Km was about 25 μM, indicating a high affinity uptake system. At L-glutamate concentrations of 100 μM to 5 mM, however, a plot of uptake versus amino acid concentration was biphasic. At least one low affinity Na⁺ gradient-dependent system that had an apparent Km of several millimolar was evident. The finding of both high and low affinity Na⁺ gradient-dependent L-glutamate uptake systems in brush border membrane vesicles was consistent with the suggestion of a two-component system in the rat kidney (15). The high affinity system saturated at a level approximating the concentration of L-glutamate in human plasma (19). Also, the apparent Km of the high affinity uptake system in the isolated membrane vesicles agreed with the values reported for the Na⁺-dependent transport processes in the microperfused proximal tubule (4) and in a cultured kidney cell line (20).

The effect of the concentration of extravesicular Na⁺ on the initial rate of L-glutamate uptake was also examined (16). Stimulation of uptake was seen with a concentration as low as 10 mM Na⁺. The rate increased with increasing concentrations, with no evidence for saturation with respect to Na⁺ at a concentration as high as 100 mM.

The energetics of the Na⁺ gradient-dependent L-glutamate uptake system

The specific effect of the Na⁺ gradient in energizing the uphill transport of L-glutamate suggests that the translocation of the amino acid was coupled to the flux of Na$^+$. An important aspect of the co-transport system was the question whether the coupling mechanism was electroneutral or electrogenic, since both types of Na$^+$ co-transport mechanisms were found in the renal brush border membrane (8). If electroneutral, then the charge associated with Na$^+$ was compensated by co-transport of anion, e.g. glutamate and/or other anions, or the countertransport of a cation via the same carrier. In this case, transport across the membrane would be electrically silent and, therefore, independent of membrane potential. If, on the other hand, the mechanism was electrogenic, then the charge associated with Na$^+$ was not compensated via the carrier. Instead, the co-transport process resulted in the net transfer of charge across the membrane that must be compensated subsequently at a different site. In this case, co-transport would be influenced by the membrane potential.

Three different experimental strategies were used to determine whether Na$^+$-L-glutamate co-transport was electroneutral or electrogenic (16). These were studies with (a) specific ionophores, i.e. valinomycin and trifluoromethoxyphenylhydrazone (FCCP), that generate K$^+$ and H$^+$ diffusion

potentials; (b) Na$^+$ salts comprised of anions of different conductances; and (c) membrane potential-sensitive optical probes.

The effect of the membrane potential on the Na$^+$ gradient-dependent uptake of L-glutamate was determined in membrane vesicles in which K$^+$ diffusion potentials was induced predictably by valinomycin. In an experiment, shown in Fig. 3A, membrane vesicles were preloaded with K$^+$. The valinomycin-induced K$^+$ diffusion potential (interior negative) had no effect on Na$^+$-L-glutamate co-transport. In contrast, in control experiments (not illustrated), valinomycin greatly enhanced the Na$^+$ coupled D-glucose uptake. Presumably, the ionophore induced the efflux of K$^+$ down its electrochemical gradient with concomitant generation of a hyperpolarized membrane. The development of this potential accelerated the influx of Na$^+$ coupled electrogenically to the transport of the sugar, as reported earlier (17). On the other hand, the uptake of a solute whose co-transport with Na$^+$ resulted in the net transfer of a positive charge should be inhibited by a membrane potential (interior positive). In an experiment, shown in Fig. 3B, a K$^+$ gradient was established, extravesicular > intravesicular. Here, valinomycin induced the inward movement of the ion, resulting in a depolarized membrane. The uptake of L-glutamate was relatively unaffected. In contrast, the uptake of D-glucose was markedly inhibited (16).

Fig. 3C illustrates how a membrane potential (interior negative) generated by a H$^+$ diffusion potential, rather than by a K$^+$ diffusion potential, affected the uptake of L-glutamate. In this experiment, the diffusion potential was induced by the mitochondrial uncoupler, FCCP. Again, Na$^+$-L-glutamate co-transport was not appreciably affected, but Na$^+$-D-glucose co-transport was greatly stimulated by the interior negative potential (16).

The role of the membrane potential on Na$^+$-L-glutamate co-transport was studied additionally by examining the effect of Na$^+$ gradients using Na$^+$ salts comprised of anions of different conductances. Since the permeability coefficient for Cl$^-$ was greater than that for SO$_4^{2-}$ (17), it was reasonable to assume that Cl$^-$ entered the intravesicular space more rapidly than SO$_4^{2-}$ and developed a membrane potential, relatively more negative on the

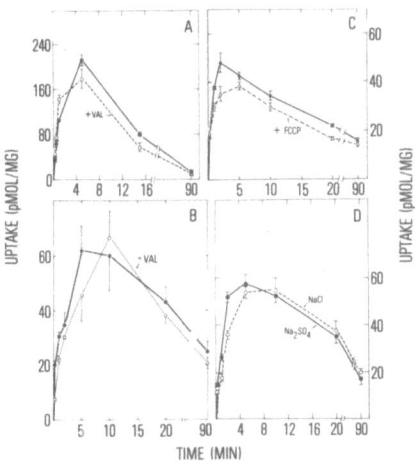

Fig. 3. The effect of a membrane potential on the Na$^+$-L-glutamate co-transport system. (A) and (B) show the effect of valinomycin-induced K$^+$ diffusion potentials, inside negative and positive, respectively. (C) shows the effect of a FCCP-induced H$^+$ diffusion potential, inside negative. (D) shows the effect of the membrane potential generated by anions of differing conductances on the uptake of L-glutamate. From Schneider, Hammerman and Sacktor (16).

inside. Accordingly, if the Na^+ gradient-dependent uptake of a solute was electrogenic, its transport would be increased by Cl^- and decreased by SO_4^{2-}. If the Na^+ gradient-dependent uptake was electroneutral, however, transport would be unaffected. Fig. 3D shows that the uptake of L-glutamate was not altered significantly when a Na_2SO_4 gradient was substituted for a NaCl gradient. In contrast, the uptake of D-glucose was strongly inhibited when the relatively impermeant SO_4^{2-} anion was used (16). Essentially identical results were obtained in comparing Cl^- with a second relatively impermeant anion, isethionate (16). When the transports of L-glutamate and D-glucose were determined in the presence of a $NaNO_3$ gradient, it was found that the initial rate of uptake of the sugar and the transient overshoot was greater than that with NaCl. The uptake of the acidic amino acid, however, was not affected appreciably (16). Since the conductance of NO_3^- was greater than that of Cl^-, one would predict enhanced development of membrane hyperpolarity with a $NaNO_3$ gradient, and, if the Na^+ gradient-dependent transport was electrogenic, uptake would be stimulated, whereas, if electroneutral, uptake would be unaffected. These results with various anions together with the findings that K^+ and H^+ diffusion potentials affected L-glutamate and D-glucose uptakes differently, strongly suggested that the Na^+ gradient-energized uphill translocation of L-glutamate was electroneutral, i.e. the co-transport across the microvillus membrane was not associated with the net transfer of electrical charge.

Studies of membrane potential-sensitive fluorescence of the probe 3,3'-dipropyl thiocarbocyanine iodide (DiS-C_3-(5)) strengthened the view that the co-transport of Na^+ and L-glutamate carried no net charge, i.e. did not depolarize the membrane, as was found for the co-transport of Na^+ with either D-glucose or L-proline (21). With L-glutamate, deviation, if any, from base-line fluorescence was not specific for the L-isomer, not dependent on Na^+, nor inhibited by the combined presence of valinomycin and nigericin, ionophores that would short-circuit K^+ and Na^+ gradient-dependent potentials (16). In contrast, with D-glucose there was a rapid transient increase in fluorescence, dependent on the D-isomer and Na^+, and inhibitable by the ionophores and phlorizin (21). In the case of the sugar, the increase in fluorescence was explainable by the entrance into the vesicles of Na^+ being co-transported with D-glucose, the inside of the vesicle becoming more positive, depolarizing the membrane.

These studies provided strong evidence that the Na^+ gradient-dependent uptake of L-glutamate in renal brush border membrane vesicles was mediated by an electroneutral mechanism. This was in contrast to the Na^+ gradient-dependent transports of neutral amino acids and D-glucose, which were found to be electrogenic (22–25), but similar to Na^+ gradient-dependent transport of phosphate, which was reported to be electroneutral (26, 27). The simplest stoichiometry consistent with an electroneutral Na^+ gradient-dependent L-glutamate uptake in these membrane vesicles would be the co-transport of one Na^+ with one glutamate anion.

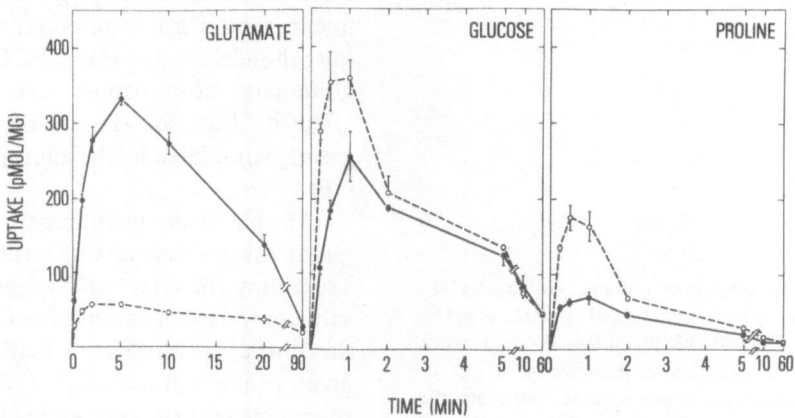

Fig. 4. The effects of intravesicular K^+ on the Na^+ gradient-dependent uptakes of L-glutamate, D-glucose, and L-proline. From Schneider & Sacktor (29).

The effect of an intravesicular > extravesicular K^+ gradient on the Na^+ gradient-dependent uptake of L-glutamate

In the experiments illustrated in Fig. 3 it was observed that a K^+ gradient ($[K^+]_i > [K^+]_o$) stimulated the Na^+ gradient-dependent uptake of L-glutamate. This effect of K^+ was explored further. Fig. 4 compares the Na^+ gradient-dependent transport of L-glutamate with those of L-proline and D-glucose when the membrane vesicles were preloaded with either KCl or mannitol. It was found that L-glutamate transport was increased several-fold when the vesicles were preloaded with K^+ (28). In contrast, uptakes of L-proline and D-glucose were relatively decreased in the KCl-preloaded membrane vesicles, due, in part, to the absence of a Cl^- electrochemical gradient that would contribute to the driving force in the electrogenic Na^+-D-glucose and the Na^+-L-proline co-transports (17, 24).

The effect of intravesicular K^+ in increasing the uptake of L-glutamate was relatively specific for that cation, only Rb^+ could substitute (29). L-glutamate uptake in membrane vesicles preloaded with the chloride salts of Li^+, $Tris^+$, choline$^+$, or tetraethylammonium$^+$ did not enhance uptake and were identical with that found with mannitol.

The effect of intravesicular K^+ in stimulating the Na^+ gradient-dependent uptake of L-glutamate was dependent on the presence of a K^+ gradient ($[K^+]_i > [K^+]_o$) (29). When the intravesicular concentration of K^+ was kept constant, but the $[K^+]_i/[K^+]_o$ ratio was decreased by increasing the

$[K^+]_o$, uptake of L-glutamate was diminished. At a constant $[K^+]_i/[K^+]_o$ ratio, L-glutamate transport increased with higher $[K^+]_i$. An enhancement of the uptake was found with an $[K^+]_i$ as low as 0.1 mM. A concentration of 1 mM gave half-maximal stimulation, and an intravesicular concentration of 10 mM saturated the system (29). These findings indicated that the Na^+ gradient-dependent L-glutamate transport exhibited marked sensitivity to K^+.

Fig. 5 shows that the action of the extravesicular > intravesicular K^+ gradient in stimulating the uptake of L-glutamate had an absolute requirement for Na^+. Importantly, this experiment also demonstrated that when Na^+ was present in both the extravesicular and intravesicular media. i.e. in the absence of a Na^+ gradient, the K^+ gradient ($[K^+]_i > [K^+]_o$) effected the transient accumulation of the amino acid to a level greater than the final equilibrium value. Therefore, the K^+ gradient ($[K^+]_i > [K^+]_o$) was able to energize the uphill transport of L-glutamate. When K^+ and Na^+ were present in both the intravesicular and extravesicular media, and $[K^+]_i = [K^+]_o$ and $[Na^+]_o = [Na^+]_i$, i.e. in the absence of ionic gradients, there was no overshoot or transient uphill transport of L-glutamate.

These findings demonstrated that the concentrative uptake of the acidic amino acid could be energized either by a K^+ gradient ($[K^+]_i > [K^+]_o$) (29) or by a Na^+ gradient ($[Na^+]_o > [Na^+]_i$) (16). The effect of the K^+ gradient was not attributable to an alteration of the membrane potential, since it was found that inside negative or positive K^+ diffusion potentials, induced by valinomycin; H^+ diffusion potentials, induced by uncouplers; or anion gradients had no significant affect on Na^+ gradient-dependent L-glutamate uptake (16). Therefore, these findings suggested a direct interaction of K^+ with the Na^+-L-glutamate carrier. In addition, from the results that the K^+ gradient energized the concentrative uptake of L-glutamate in the absence of membrane potential or Na^+ driving forces, it was hypothesized that the co-transport of Na^+-L-glutamate was coupled to the transmembrane flux of K^+ (29).

Although efflux of K^+ from the membrane vesicle coupled to the uptakes of L-glutamate and Na^+ was not demonstrated directly, recent experiments demonstrating that the action of K^+ on Na^+-

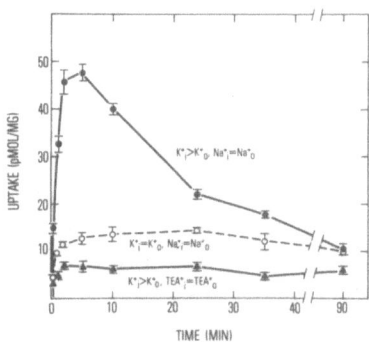

Fig. 5. Demonstration that the K^+ gradient-dependent stimulation of L-glutamate uptake had an absolute requirement for Na^+ and the K^+ gradient energized the uphill transport of the amino acid. From Schneider & Sacktor (29).

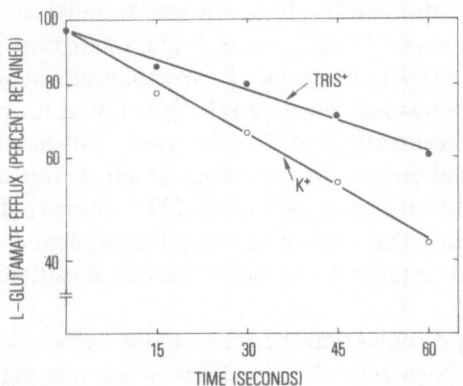

Fig. 6. The effect of extravesicular K^+ on the efflux of L-glutamate (Sacktor, Lepor & Schneider, unpublished data).

L-glutamate transport was reversible strongly supported this hypothesis. Fig. 6 shows that efflux of L-glutamate from brush border membrane vesicles followed first-order kinetics and that the rate of efflux was increased by an extravesicular > intravesicular K^+ gradient. In this experiment, the $t_{1/2}$ in the absence of K^+ was 85 s. In the presence of K^+ in the extravesicular medium, $t_{1/2}$ was decreased to about 50 s. The effect of K^+ on the efflux of L-glutamate was specific for that cation, only Rb^+ could substitute whereas neither Li^+, choline$^+$, nor $Tris^+$ had any effect.

The energetics of the K^+ and Na^+ gradient-dependent transport of L-glutamate

Since a K^+ gradient ($[K^+]_i > [K^+]_o$) provided the driving force for the concentrative uptake of L-glutamate in the absence of a Na^+ gradient ($[Na^+]_o = [Na^+]_i$) and a K^+ gradient ($[K^+]_o > [K^+]_i$) stimulated the rate at which the acidic amino acid effluxed from the membrane vesicle, findings which would imply a coupled transmembrane flux of K^+; and since the substrate specificities and affinities for the Na^+ and Na^+ plus K^+ gradient-dependent systems were identical (29), findings which would be consistent with the hypothesis that the same carrier was involved, the question was posed as to whether the uptake of L-glutamate co-transported with both cations remained an electroneutral system or was converted from an electroneutral to an electrogenic process in the presence of K^+. This question remains the subject of considerable controversy.

It was found that a valinomycin-generated membrane potential (interior negative) had no affect on the K^+ gradient-dependent co-transport of Na^+-L-glutamate (29). Furthermore, when inside negative membrane potentials were established by an extravesicular > intravesicular SCN^- gradient, the anion gradient had only an exceedingly small affect on the uptake of L-glutamate, energized by a K^+ gradient (29). In contrast, the conductance of the anion was sufficient to drive uphill the electrogenic transport of D-glucose, even though the Na^+ concentrations in the intravesicular and extravesicular media were initially identical (29). Since neither anion-induced nor valinomycin-generated membrane potentials significantly affected L-glutamate uptake, an electroneutral K^+ gradient-dependent Na^+-L-glutamate co-transport system was suggested, thus indicating that the energetic mechanism did not change from that found for the Na^+ gradient-dependent L-glutamate transport system (28, 29).

But, in other studies it was claimed that K^+ altered the uptake process from one being electroneutral in the absence of the cation to one being electrogenic (carrying in a net positive charge) in its presence (30). Contrary to this suggestion, however, was the observation, in agreement with the earlier reports (16, 28, 29), that valinomycin had no effect on L-glutamate uptake when measured with an inwardly-directed K^+ gradient ($[K^+]_o > [K^+]_i$), whereas the electrogenic uptake of D-glucose was inhibited by the inside positive membrane potential (30). With an outwardly-directed K^+ gradient ($[K^+]_i > [K^+]_o$), that induced a membrane potential (inside negative), a small stimulation at a single time-point, the 20 s uptake value, was reported. The lack of an effect at 1 min and, indeed, the decreased uptake at 2 min were not satisfactorily explained. The influence of the membrane potential on L-glutamate uptake was also examined under conditions of an outwardly-directed H^+ gradient, the intravesicular pH being 6.25 and the extravesicular pH being 7.4. In the absence of K^+, FCCP had no effect, confirming previous observations (16). When K^+ was present in the intravesicular space, FCCP slightly increased the 20 s uptake of the amino acid. Again, no differences were found after incubations of 1 and 2 min (30). Finally, when the membrane vesicles were preloaded with K^+ gluconate, uptake of L-glutamate was enhanced when a more permeant anion, such as Cl^-, NO_3^-, or SCN^-, was

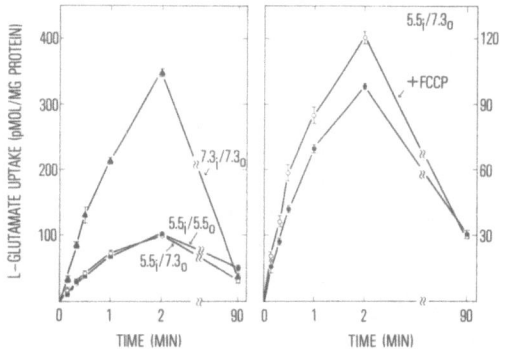

Fig. 7. The inhibition of the K^+ plus Na^+ gradient-dependent uptake of L-glutamate by a low intravesicular pH and the effect of FCCP. *Left.* Membrane vesicles were preloaded with 50 mM K gluconate, 225 mM mannitol, and either 75 mM Hepes/Tris, pH 7.3 (▲) or 75 mM Mes/Tris, pH 5.5 (●, ○). The uptake media contained 100 mM Na gluconate, 125 mM mannitol, and either 75 mM Hepes/Tris, pH 7.3 (▲, ○) or 75 mM Mes/Tris, pH 5.5 (●). *Right.* Membrane vesicles were loaded with the pH 5.5 medium and uptake was measured at pH 7.3. FCCP (20 μM) was added, as indicated. The concentration of L-[³H]glutamate was 25 μM. (Sacktor & Cheng, unpublished data).

added as Na^+ and K^+ salts to the extravesicular medium (30). These observations, plus changes, perhaps of questionable specificity (16), in the fluorescence of the dye DiS-C₃-(5) led these workers to conclude that L-glutamate uptake in the presence of K^+ and Na^+ gradients was electrogenic (30).

Since the findings from the two studies led to opposite conclusions, and this difference in proposed mechanism has considerable theoretical implications, the question was recently re-investigated. Two apparent discrepant observations seemed paramount, namely: (a) the effects of a H^+ diffusion gradient (inside negative) generated by FCCP on the initial rate of L-glutamate uptake; and (b) the effects of anions of relatively high conductance of K^+ plus Na^+ gradient-dependent L-glutamate transport. The new experiments described below may resolve some of the dilemma.

It was found previously that although the Na^+ gradient-dependent uptake of L-glutamate had a broad pH optimum, being essentially constant from pH 5.5 to 7.5 (16), L-glutamate uptake in the presence of K^+ plus Na^+ gradients was very sensitive to pH, being markedly decreased at pH 5.5 relative to that at 7.5 (29). Fig. 7 now shows that it was the intravesicular pH that was crucial. An intravesicular pH of 5.5 inhibited, relative to an intravesicular pH of 7.3, independent of whether

the extravesicular pH was 5.5 or 7.3. Thus, when a H^+ diffusion gradient was established to test the effect of a FCCP-induced inside negative membrane potential on the K^+ plus Na^+ gradient-dependent uptake of L-glutamate, the system was strongly inhibited by the low intravesicular pH. The addition of FCCP would not only generate the potential, but by accelerating the efflux of H^+ down its electrochemical gradient would tend to relieve the inhibition. This could result in a slight stimulation in the rate of L-glutamate uptake, as shown in Fig. 7. It should be recalled, moreover, that the enhancement due to a FCCP-induced H^+ diffusion potential on the Na^+-D-glucose uptake system, an electrogenic process, was manifold greater (17).

Similarly, the effect of anion replacement in causing a transient and relatively small increase in L-glutamate uptake might be due to factors other than the generation of a membrane potential (inside negative). It was reported previously that the isosmotic replacement of an intravesicular solute by a solute with a lower reflection coefficient caused the enlargement of the intravesicular space resulting in the non-specific stimulation in the rate of D-glucose uptake (13). An analogous non-specific stimulation could account for the enhanced uptake

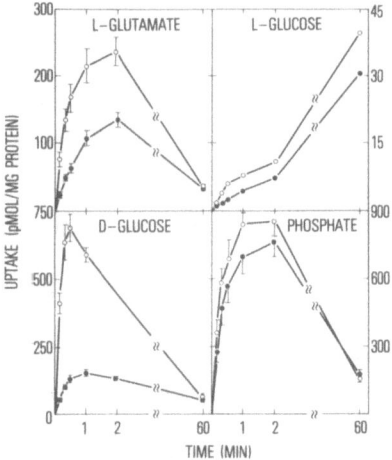

Fig. 8. Effects on anion displacement on the uptakes of L-glutamate, L- and D-glucose, and phosphate. Membrane vesicles were preloaded with 33.3 mM K_2SO_4, 66.6 mM Tris sulfate and 5 mM Hepes/Tris, pH 7.5. The uptake medium was 33.3 mM K_2SO_4, 5 mM Tris sulfate, pH 7.5, and either 100 mM NaSCN (○) or 50 mM Na_2SO_4 and 16.7 mM Tris sulfate (●). The concentrations of L-[³H]glutamate and [³²P]-K_2HPO_4 were 25 μM and the concentrations of L-[³H]glucose and D-[³H]glucose was 50 μM. (Sacktor & Cheng, unpublished data).

seen with L-glutamate. Fig. 8 illustrates experiments in which membrane vesicles preloaded with a relatively impermeant anion, i.e. sulfate, was incubated, in a Na^+ gradient ($[Na^+]_o > [Na^+]_i$), $[K^+]_i = [K^+]_o$ mode, in media containing an anion of greater conductance, i.e. SCN^-. The initial rate of uptake of L-glutamate approximately doubled. However, the initial rate of L-glucose was increased by about the same magnitude, and the uptake of the L-sugar was known to be completely independent of Na^+, K^+ and membrane potential (13). The Na^+ gradient-dependent uptake of phosphate was also enhanced, even though the Na^+-phosphate co-transport system was found to be mediated by an electroneutral mechanism (26, 27). On the other hand, the electrogenic uptake of Na^+-D-glucose was greatly stimulated by the anion replacement, more than ten-fold. This increase would be due primarily to the generated inside negative membrane potential but also, in part, to the transient enlargement of the intravesicular volume.

These recent findings pointed out some of the complexities of the membrane vesicle system and the cautions that must be observed in the interpretation of experimental findings. On the basis of this new evidence, the previous suggestion that the K^+ plus Na^+ gradient-dependent transport of L-glutamate was mediated by an electroneutral mechanism (29) was strengthened. Therefore, the view that the basic energetics of the system was not altered by the presence of K^+ was supported. Since as found previously the Na^+ gradient-dependent uptake of L-glutamate (in the absence of K^+) was electroneutral (8, 16), leading to the proposal that the simplest stoichiometry consistent with such a mechanism would be the co-transport of one Na^+ with one glutamate anion (16), the finding that the K^+ plus Na^+ gradient-energized uptake of the amino acid was electroneutral, too, prompted two other possible stoichiometric relationships to be hypothesized, if a transmembrane flux of K^+ was assumed (29). These were: (a) the influx of two Na^+ and one L-glutamate anion/efflux of one K^+; or (b) the influx of one Na^+, one L-glutamate anion, and one H^+/efflux of one K^+. With the latter alternative stoichiometry it should be noted that the influx of a H^+ was not distinguished from the efflux of a OH^-. The experiments in Fig. 7 showing the marked inhibition of the K^+ plus Na^+ gradient-dependent L-glutamate uptake by a low intra-

vesicular pH might provide some evidence favoring the second hypothesis.

Interestingly, the controversy as to whether L-glutamate transport in the membrane vesicle system was electroneutral or electrogenic also appeared in studies in which more physiologically intact preparations were used. The finding of an electroneutral L-glutamate transport system in brush border membrane vesicles agreed completely with the results of direct electrophysiological measurements in the microperfused *Triturus* proximal tubule. In the newt kidney, the Na^+-dependent transports of D-glucose and L-alanine caused depolarization of the tubule luminal membrane, whereas the transports of L-glutamate and L-aspartate were found to be entirely nonelectrogenic (31, 32). In a preliminary report, however, a slight drop in the peritubular cell membrane potential was noted in the L-glutamate microperfused rat tubule (33). In view of the possibility that other ion movements across either the luminal or baso-lateral membrane might occur during the transepithelial transport of L-glutamate small shifts in membrane potential in the intact tissue would sometimes be difficult to interpret. Another possibility would be the species difference. Perhaps the same could account for the apparent discrepancy in the membrane vesicle studies, since one study was carried out with preparations from the rabbit (29), whereas the other used membranes from the rat (30).

The effect of an intravesicular > extravesicular OH^- gradient on the uptake of L-glutamate

As described in Fig. 7, when the intravesicular pH was low the uptake of L-glutamate was significantly decreased. The low pH value, however, was indicative not only of a high concentration of H^+ but also of a low concentration of OH^-. This effect of pH on L-glutamate uptake was examined further in recent preliminary experiments. Fig. 9 shows that a OH^- gradient ($[OH^-]_i > [OH^-]_o$) or H^+ gradient ($[H^+]_o > [H^+]_i$), in the absence of Na^+ and K^+ driving forces, i.e. $[Na^+]_o = [Na^+]_i$ and $[K^+]_i = [K^+]_o$, increased the initial rate of L-glutamate uptake. When the pH of the intravesicular and extravesicular media were identical, 7.5, uptake reached the equilibrium level in about 10 min. However, in the presence of the OH^- gradient (intravesicular pH 7.5 versus extravesicular pH 5.5) the uptake of L-

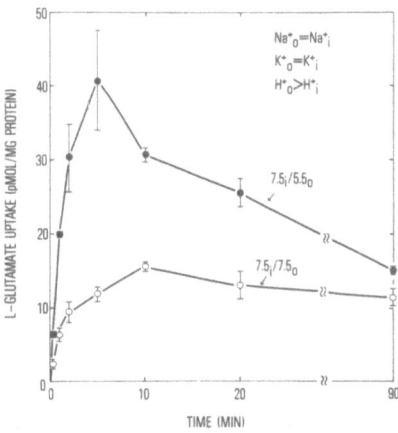

Fig. 9. The effect of a OH$^-$ gradient [OH$^-$]$_i$ > [OH$^-$]$_o$) on the uptake of L-glutamate. Membrane vesicles were preloaded with 12.5 mM Na$_2$SO$_4$, 62.5 mM K$_2$SO$_4$, and 37.5 mM Hepes/Tris, pH 7.5. The uptake medium was the same (O) or the buffer replaced by 65 mM Mes/Tris, pH 5.5 (●). The concentration of L-[^{3}H]glutamate was 25 μM. (Sacktor & Cheng, unpublished data).

glutamate reached a maximum at 5 min at which time the accumulated level was greater than at equilibrium. Then the amino acid effluxed and its intravesicular concentration fell to about the equilibrium value. This apparent transient uphill uptake could be attributed to several mechanisms. First, it was possible that the H$^+$ gradient ([H$^+$]$_o$ > [H$^+$]$_i$), energizing the H$^+$-Na$^+$ exchange reaction in these membranes (34, 35), caused a disequilibrium of Na$^+$ so that, although no Na$^+$ gradient was initially imposed on the system, a Na$^+$ gradient ([Na$^+$]$_o$ > [Na$^+$]$_i$) was, in fact, created. This possibility was largely ruled out by the finding that amiloride, a relatively specific inhibitor of the exchange reaction (35), did not alter the OH$^-$-driven overshoot. A second explanation for the uphill transport stems from the stoichiometric relationships proposed for the K$^+$ plus Na$^+$ gradient-dependent L-glutamate transport system. It was hypothesized that the influx of one glutamate anion and one Na$^+$ was coupled to the efflux of one K$^+$ and one OH$^-$. If this be the case, then the OH$^-$ gradient ([OH$^-$]$_i$ > [OH$^-$]$_o$) could provide the ionic force to drive the concentrative uptake of L-glutamate, despite the absence of Na$^+$ and K$^+$ gradients. Although this second mechanism still remains feasible, a third possible mechanism was discovered (Sacktor & Cheng, unpublished obser-

vations). It was found that a OH$^-$ gradient ([OH$^-$]$_i$ > [OH$^-$]$_o$) effected the transient uphill uptake of L-glutamate, even when K$^+$ and Na$^+$ were deleted from the incubation media. This finding suggests a OH$^-$-L-glutamate exchange system in the renal brush border membrane. Further studies are needed to verify the presence of this anion-anion anti-port mechanism.

The L-glutamate uptake system in baso-lateral membrane vesicles

Previous studies of the uptake of amino acids (L-phenylalanine, L-proline) as well as sugars by baso-lateral membrane vesicles showed that their transports were neither concentrative nor Na$^+$ gradient-dependent (23, 36). In contrast, a recent investigation of the uptake of L-glutamate by the membrane vesicles revealed that the transport of the acidic amino acid was different.

It was found that a Na$^+$ gradient ([Na$^+$]$_o$ > [Na$^+$]$_i$) stimulated the uptake of L-glutamate by baso-lateral membrane vesicles and, in fact, the gradient provided the ionic driving force for the uphill transport of the acidic amino acid (12). This concentrative uptake by the baso-lateral membrane preparations could not be attributed to contamination by brush border membranes, as shown by the low activities of brush border marker enzymes in the baso-lateral preparation and by the absence from the preparation of Na$^+$ gradient-dependent D-glucose uptake. Like with brush border membrane vesicles (29), a K$^+$ gradient ([K$^+$]$_i$ > [K$^+$]$_o$) increased the uptake of L-glutamate with the baso-lateral membrane vesicles (12). This effect was specific for K$^+$, only Rb$^+$ could substitute. The action of the K$^+$ gradient in enhancing the uptake of L-glutamate had an absolute requirement for Na$^+$. Nevertheless, in the presence of Na$^+$, but in the absence of a Na$^+$ gradient, i.e. [Na$^+$]$_o$ = [Na$^+$]$_i$, the K$^+$ gradient could energize the concentrative uptake of L-glutamate. This effect of the K$^+$ gradient was not the consequence of an alteration in membrane potential, suggesting that the K$^+$ plus Na$^+$ gradient-dependent transport system in baso-lateral membrane was electroneutral, as was the case in brush border membranes.

250

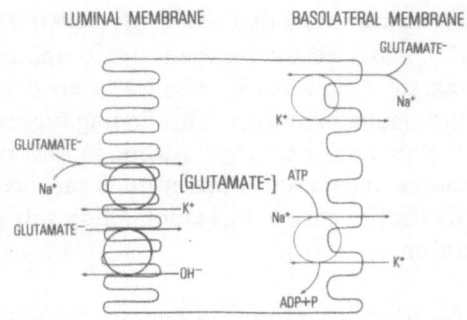

LUMINAL MEMBRANE BASOLATERAL MEMBRANE

Fig. 10. A schematic model for L-glutamate uptake and intracellular accumulation by the renal tubular cell.

Discussion

The findings that an inwardly directed Na^+ gradient and an outwardly directed K^+ gradient provide the ionic driving forces to energize the concentrative uptake of L-glutamate across both the luminal membrane and the baso-lateral membrane suggest a mechanism whereby the acidic amino acid may be accumulated to high levels in the renal tubular cell. This hypothetical model is illustrated schematically in Fig. 10. In the cell in situ it would be the ouabain-sensitive ATPase localized in the baso-lateral membrane and catalyzing the extrusion of Na^+ coupled to the intake of K^+ that maintains the Na^+ electrochemical gradient (extracellular > intracellular) and the K^+ electrochemical gradient (intracellular > extracellular). L-glutamate in the glomerular filtrate will be taken up at the luminal membrane against its concentration gradient by a brush border membrane co-transport system that is coupled to the influx of Na^+ and efflux of K^+ moving down their respective electrochemical gradients. An additional system, an anion-anion exchange, in which the L-glutamate anion enters the cell in exchange for OH^-, may also contribute to the uptake across the luminal membrane. At the baso-lateral membrane, an analogous mechanism exists, in which L-glutamate in the peritubular fluid is transported uphill into the cell, presumably likewise co-transported with Na^+ and K^+ down their respective electrochemical gradients. Whether an anion-anion anti-port system can also contribute to the uptake of L-glutamate from the blood side is not known. Nevertheless, the concentrative uptakes of L-glutamate energized by a Na^+

gradient, augmented by a K^+ gradient, at both sides of the polar tubular cell is unique. These systems may account for the exceedingly high intracellular concentration of this metabolically important amino acid in the renal tubule.

References

1. Cohen, J. J. & Kamm, D. E., 1976. In: The Kidney Eds. Brenner, B. M. & Rector, F. C., Vol. I, W. B. Saunders, Co., Philadelphia, pp. 126–214.
2. Segal, S. and Thier, S. O., 1973. In: Handbook of Physiology Eds. Berliner, R. W. & Orloff, J., Sect. 8, American Physiological Society, Washington, D. C., pp. 653–676.
3. Silbernagl, S., Foulkes, E. C. & Deetjen, P., 1975. Rev. Physiol. Biochem. Pharmacol 74: 106–167.
4. Ullrich, K. J., Rumrich, G. & Kloss, S., 1974. Pfluegers Arch. 351: 35–48.
5. Blazer-Yost, B., Reynolds, R. & Segal, S., 1979. Am. J. Physiol. 236: F398–F404.
6. Burch, H. B., Chan, A. W. K. & Lowry, O. H., 1976. In: Current Problems in Clinical Biochemistry Eds. (Schmidt, U. & Dubach, U. C., Vol. VI, Hans Huber Publishers, Bern, Switzerland, pp. 394–402.
7. Kinne, R., Murer, H., Kinne-Saffran, E., Thees, M. & Sachs, G., 1975. J. Membr. Biol. 21: 375–395.
8. Sacktor, B., 1980. Curr. Top. Membranes Transp. 13: 291–300.
9. Beck, J. C. & Sacktor, B., 1978. J. Biol. Chem. 253: 5531–5535.
10. Sacktor, B., 1977. In: Mammalian Cell Membranes Eds. Jamieson, G. A. & Robinson, D. M., Vol. IV, Butterworth, London, pp. 221–254.
11. Malathi, P., Preiser, H., Fairclough, P., Mallett, P. & Crane, R. K., 1979. Biochim. Biophys. Acta 554: 259–263.
12. Sacktor, B., Rosenbloom, I. L., Liang, C. T. & Cheng, L., 1981. J. Membr. Biol. 60: 63–71.
13. Aronson, P. S. & Sacktor, B., 1975. J. Biol. Chem. 250: 6032–6039.
14. Sacktor, B., 1978. In: Renal Function Eds. Giebisch, G. H. & Purcell, E. F., Josiah Macy, Jr. Foundation, New York, pp. 221–229.
15. Weiss, S. D., McNamara, P. D., Pepe, L. M. & Segal, S., 1978. J. Membr. Biol. 43: 91–105.
16. Schneider, E. G., Hammerman, M. R. & Sacktor, B., 1980. J. Biol. Chem. 255: 7650–7656.
17. Beck, J. C. & Sacktor, B., 1975. J. Biol. Chem. 250: 8674–8680.
18. Hammerman, M. & Sacktor, B., 1978. Biochim. Biophys. Acta 509: 338–347.
19. Melancon, S. B., Dallaire, L., Lemieux, B., Robitaille, P. & Potier, M., 1977. J. Pediatr. 91: 422–427.
20. Scott, D. M. & Pateman, J. A., 1978. Biochim. Biophys. Acta 508: 379–388.
21. Beck, J. C. & Sacktor, B., 1978. J. Biol. Chem. 253: 7158–7162.
22. Fass, S. J., Hammerman, M. R. & Sacktor, B., 1977. J. Biol. Chem. 252: 583–590.

23. Evers, J., Murer, H. & Kinne, R., 1976. Biochim. Biophys. Acta 426: 598–615.
24. Hammerman, M. R. & Sacktor, B., 1977. J. Biol. Chem. 252, 591–595.
25. Hammerman, M. R. & Sacktor, B., 1978. Biochim. Biophys. Acta 509: 338–347.
26. Hoffmann, N., Thees, M. & Kinne, R., 1976. Pfluegers Arch. Eur. J. Physiol. 362: 147–156.
27. Cheng, L. & Sacktor, B., 1981. J. Biol. Chem. 256: 1556–1564.
28. Sacktor, B. & Schneider, E. G., 1980. Int. J. Biochem. 12: 229–234.
29. Schneider, E. G. & Sacktor, B., 1980. J. Biol. Chem. 255: 7645–7649.
30. Burckhardt, G., Kinne, R., Stange, G. & Murer, H., 1980. Biochim. Biophys. Acta 599: 191–201.
31. Maruyama, T. & Hoshi, T., 1972. Biochem. Biophys. Acta 282: 214–225.
32. Hoshi, T., Sudo, K. & Suzuki, Y., 1976. Biochim. Biophys. Acta 448: 492–504.
33. Frömter, E., 1979. J. Physiol. (Lond.) 288: 1–31.
34. Murer, H., Hopfer, U. & Kinne, R., 1976. Biochem. J. 154: 596–604.
35. Kinsella, J. L. & Aronson, P. S., 1980. Am. J. Physiol. 238: F461–F469.
36. Slack, E. N., Liang, C.-C. T. & Sacktor, B., 1977. Biochem. Biophys. Res. Commun. 77: 891–897.

Received May 5, 1981.

Glutamate as a precursor of GABA in rat brain and peripheral tissues

Helen L. White

Dept. of Pharmacology, Wellcome Research Laboratories, Research Triangle Park, N.C. 27709, U.S.A.

Summary

The formation of GABA from L-glutamate was investigated in homogenates of rat brain, liver, and kidney, using highly purified $[^{14}C]$-L-glutamic acid as substrate and a thin-layer chromatographic separation of products. In agreement with other workers, liberation of $[^{14}C]$-CO_2 was found to be stoichiometric with GABA formation in brain homogenates, but not in liver or kidney extracts. Subcellular fractionation and dialysis experiments suggested that most of the GABA synthesis in these peripheral tissues, unlike brain, does not occur via a direct decarboxylation of glutamate and requires one or more cofactors other than pyridoxal phosphate. NAD stimulated GABA formation in dialyzed extracts, and inhibition of GABA-transaminase, both *in vitro* and *in vivo*, caused marked inhibition of GABA formation from glutamate in peripheral extracts. Although a very low GAD activity in liver and kidney cannot be excluded, these experiments suggest a major pathway from glutamate to GABA in these homogenates which includes (1) conversion of glutamate to α-ketoglutarate by glutamate dehydrogenase or transaminases, (2) conversion of α-ketoglutarate to succinic semialdehyde, and (3) formation of GABA from succinic semialdehyde and glutamate by GABA-transaminase.

Introduction

Glutamic acid is the immediate precursor of the major inhibitory transmitter, γ-aminobutyric acid (GABA), in the central nervous systems of all species that have been studied thus far, and the enzyme glutamate decarboxylase (GAD) (4.1.1.15) is known to catalyse this reaction in brain (1). There are, however, few published studies relating to the relatively low capacities for GABA synthesis in peripheral tissues such as kidney and liver, and there remains considerable confusion with respect to the enzymatic pathway involved.

Haber *et al.* (2), finding differences between GABA synthesizing systems in brain and peripheral tissues, introduced the concept of GAD II, a different glutamate decarboxylase. Others (3, 4, 5) have clearly refuted this concept by showing that it was based on artifactual results, apparently caused by impurities in the radioactive substrate. Drummond & Phillips (4) reported that GAD of mouse kidney appeared similar to that of brain, based on its response to the inhibitor aminooxyacetic acid. They suggested that the low GAD activities they observed in kidney (about 5% of that in brain) and the even lower activities in liver and pancreas, might be associated with nerve endings in these tissues. More recently, Wu & co-workers (5) have reported that GAD of mouse brain does not cross-react with crude mouse peripheral tissue extracts, in support of the idea that peripheral tissues may contain a different form of GAD.

An alternative enzymatic pathway from glutamate to GABA has been suggested by Seiler & Wagner (6), who found that GABA synthesis in a crude nuclear fraction of rat liver was markedly stimulated by the cofactor NAD^+. Their proposed pathway involves a very speculative conversion of

Molecular and Cellular Biochemistry 39, 253–259 (1981).   0300–8177/81/0391–0253/$01.40.
© 1981, Martinus Nijhoff/Dr W. Junk Publishers, The Hague.

glutamate to an α-imino derivative, subsequent decarboxylation to succinic semialdehyde, and then transamination of this compound to GABA.

The aim of the present study was to determine whether, using highly purified glutamate as substrate, a direct decarboxylation of this compound to GABA can be demonstrated in peripheral tissues of rat and, if so, whether this enzyme resembles the GAD of brain in its kinetic and molecular properties.

Materials and methods

Purification of substrate

^{14}C-L-Glutamic acid (New England Nuclear Corp., uniformly labeled, 292 Ci/mol) was mixed with unlabeled glutamic acid to give the desired specific radioactivity (generally 1 to 5 Ci/mol) and chromatographed on silica gel (Whatman LK5D precoated plates with preadsorbent layer), using the eluting solvent, 1-butanol:water:glacial acetic acid (70:40:5; vols; top layer after rapid shaking for 5 min). In this system glutamic acid is well separated from GABA, γ-guanidino butyric acid, α-ketoglutaric acid, succinic acid, and succinic semialdehyde, but not from putrescine. Various batches of [^{14}C]-L-glutamic acid contained, before purification, as much as 2% of a material that co-chromatographed with α-ketoglutarate. The glutamic acid region was scraped from the TLC plate and extracted from the silica gel with 2 small volumes of water ($\sim$2 ml total). The water extract was then washed with 10 ml diethyl ether to remove traces of butanol.

Homogenate preparations

Sprague-Dawley male rats were sacrificed by decapitation. Brains, livers, and kidneys were removed and frozen immediately on dry ice. Tissues were weighed while frozen, and homogenates were prepared, using a Teflon/glass motorized tissue grinder, in 10-fold (tissue wt/buffer vol) buffer consisting of 50 mM potassium phosphate, 0.1 mM pyridoxal phosphate, 0.5 mM dithiothreitol, 0.1 mM EDTA, pH 7.6. Homogenates were stored at -70 °C until assayed. Protein was determined using the Lowry procedure (7) with bovine albumin

as standard. In some experiments rats were pretreated orally with 500 mg/kg ethanolamine O-sulfate 4 h prior to sacrifice.

Partially purified brain extracts were prepared by homogenizing whole rat brains in a 4-fold tissue wt/buffer volume of 0.1 M potassium phosphate (pH 6.9), 1 mM dithiothreitol, 1 mM pyridoxal phosphate, 0.5% Triton X-100. After centrifugation at 16 000 g for 30 min at 4 °C, the fraction precipitated from the supernatant by ammonium sulfate between 20 and 45% saturation was resuspended in a small volume of the above buffer and dialyzed for 4 h against a 3000-fold volume of the same buffer. The extract was stored at -70 °C. GABA-transaminase was purified as described in an earlier publication (8).

Assay procedures

[^{14}C]-CO$_2$ liberation from [^{14}C]L-glutamic acid was routinely measured by incubation of 50 μl tissue extract (containing 4.5 mg wet tissue) in the presence of 1 mM [^{14}C]L-glutamic acid (uniformly labeled), 0.1 mM pyridoxal phosphate, 0.1 mM dithiothreitol, 0.02 mM EDTA, 20 mM potassium phosphate, pH 6.8 (unless indicated otherwise) in a total volume of 0.30 ml. Blanks either contained no extract or included 0.1 mM hydrazinopropionate to inhibit all GAD and GABA-T activity. Assay mixtures were incubated at 37 °C in disposable glass cultures tubes (15 $\times$ 85 mm, Becton Dickinson) topped with Parafilm-covered corks, each of which was equipped with a small hook. Suspended from each hook was a 3 $\times$ 0.5 cm strip of Whatman #2 filter paper, which was impregnated with 10 μl of Hyamine hydroxide (New England Nuclear Corp.). After 30 min incubation, the tubes were placed in an ice-water bath and acidified with 0.1 ml of 0.1 N HCl. Liberated [^{14}C]-CO$_2$ was quantitatively trapped on the Hyamine-saturated filter paper by incubating for an additional hour at 37 °C. Filter strips were then transferred to scintillation vials containing 15 ml of scintillator [made by dissolving 4 g of Ominifluor (New England Nuclear Corp.) in 1 l toluene and then adding 40 ml Triton X-100]. Samples were chilled for at least 2 h before counting in order to allow for decay of chemiluminescence caused by Hyamine. Precision among triplicate assays was within 5%.

GABA synthesis from [^{14}C]-glutamate was measured by thin-layer chromatography of the above acidified incubation mixtures after the filter paper strips were removed. In an alternative method, designed to facilitate the thin-layer procedure, the total assay volume was reduced to 55 μl, with concentrations of all components as above, except that the equivalent of 2.2 mg of wet tissue was present in each assay. Incubation mixtures were applied to the pre-adsorbent layer of Whatman LK5D pre-scored 20 × 20 cm silica gel G plates and allowed to dry thoroughly at room temperature before development with 1-butanol:water:glacial acetic acid (70:40:5; top layer after 5 min rapid shaking). In this system the Rf value for GABA was 0.2; for glutamic acid, 0.12; and for α-keto-glutarate, 0.5. After chromatography, plates were dried at room temperature for at least 2 h and then exposed to Kodak SB-5 X-ray film for 3 or 4 days in order to prepare autoradiograms. Areas of the plate corresponding to radioactive GABA were scraped and counted in Aquasol II scintillator.

GABA-transaminase was assayed as described earlier (8).

Materials

[^{14}C]L-glutamic acid (uniformly labeled) was purchased from New England Nuclear Corp. Aminooxyacetic acid was from Aldrich Chemical Co., and 3-mercaptopropionic acid was from Sigma. Ethanolamine O-sulfate was obtained from B. F. Goodrich Chemical Co. and recrystallized before use. The sodium salt of hydrazinopropionic acid was supplied by Dr. K. Ingold of Wellcome Research Laboratories.

Experimental

After purification, the [^{14}C]-L-glutamic acid used in these experiments was at least 99.99% radio-chemically pure, as determined by thin-layer chromatography. This substrate was incubated with crude extracts of rat brain, kidney, and liver, and both GABA formation and CO_2 liberation estimated. L-glutamate was used at a concentration of 1 mM in this experiment, since this was its K_m concentration for rat brain GAD. The formation of GABA from glutamate was found to be stoichiometrically equivalent to liberation of CO_2 only when brain extracts were assayed, as shown in Table 1. With rat kidney, and especially with rat

Table 1. GABA and CO_2 formation from L-glutamic acid in crude extracts.

Tissue	nmol/hr/mg tissue	
	CO_2	GABA
Brain	10.1	9.03 ± 0.05
Kidney	4.6	1.49 ± 0.05
Liver	2.6	0.38 ± 0.04

GABA and CO_2 produced from [^{14}C]-L-glutamate (1 mM) were determined in the same assays, at pH 6.8, using freshly prepared crude homogenates of brain, liver, and kidney from the same rats.

Table 2. Subcellular distribution of GABA synthesizing activity in rat tissues*.

	Brain	Kidney	Liver
Total activity in crude extract (nmol/hr)	2575	97.1	40.8
Specific activity in crude extract (nmol/hr/mg tissue at 1 mM substrate)	10.8	1.8	0.47
% Recovered in subcellular fractions:			
P_1	77.1	<10	<10
P_2	10.1	<10	<10
P_3	3.0	0	0
S_3	10.4	0	0
Total % recovered	100.6	<20	<20

* A portion of each tissue was homogenized in a 4-fold volume of 50 mM potassium phosphate, 0.1 mM EDTA, 0.5 mM dithiothreitol, 0.1 mM pyridoxal phosphate, pH 7.4, and fractionated by successive centrifugations at 4 °C. A 10 min spin at 120 g gave membrane fractions, P_1. Supernatants were then centrifuged at 10 000 g for 30 min to give mitochondrial fractions, P_2. Supernatants of this spin were then centrifuged at 100 000 g for 60 min to give microsomal fractions, P_3, and soluble fractions, S_3. After resuspension of pellets in homogenate buffer, aliquots of each fraction were incubated with 1 mM [^{14}C]-L-glutamic acid, and GABA formation was determined by the autoradiographic procedure. Results are means of triplicate assays.

liver extracts, CO_2 liberation exceeded GABA formation.

Subcellular fractionation of crude extracts by differential centrifugation demonstrated another marked difference between brain and peripheral GABA synthesis. As shown in Table 2, GAD activity in rat brain crude extracts was completely recovered in membrane, mitochondrial, and soluble fractions. However, when kidney and liver extracts were carried through the same separation procedures, very little GABA production was detected in any of the separated fractions. This suggested that GABA formation observed in the original crude extracts of these peripheral tissues may have depended on a soluble cofactor or on multiple enzymes that were separated from one another during centrifugation.

Further evidence for a cofactor requirement was

Table 3. Effect of dialysis on GABA synthesizing activities in crude extracts.

Tissue	Activity (nmol/h per mg wet tissue)		
	Before Dialysis	Dialyzed	
			+NAD
Brain	9.2	10.6	12.3
Kidney	0.81	0.21	0.39
Liver	0.23	0.061	0.17

Crude extracts were dialyzed for 20 h against 160 volumes of buffer consisting of 50 mM potassium phosphate, 0.1 mM EDTA, 0.5 mM dithiothreitol, and 0.1 mM pyridoxal phosphate, pH 7.6. GABA formation from 1 mM [^{14}C]-L-glutamic acid was assayed using the autoradiographic method in the absence and presence of 1 mM NAD (nicotinamide-adenine dinucleotide). Activities are means of triplicate determinations expressed as nmol/hr/mg wet tissue.

obtained by dialysis of crude extracts against buffer containing pyridoxal phosphate and then assaying for GABA production from L-glutamic acid in the absence and presence of the cofactor, nicotinamide-adenine dinucleotide (NAD). The results in Table 3 (obtained at pH 7.6 rather than pH 6.8 as in Table 1) show that, although GABA formation in brain extracts was slightly stimulated by dialysis and by NAD addition, only about 26% of the GABA synthesizing activity remained in kidney and liver extracts. Dialysis apparently caused removal of one or more soluble factors, since activity was at least partially restored by the addition of 1 mM NAD to assay mixtures. The further addition of 0.1 mM coenzyme A had little effect on GABA formation, but markedly increased CO_2 liberation in peripheral extracts.

The apparent requirement by liver and kidney extracts for a cofactor other than pyridoxal phosphate indicated that GABA synthesis from glutamic acid in these tissues might depend on one or more enzymes other than glutamate decarboxylase. A radioactive product in addition to GABA, co-chromatographing with α-ketoglutarate, was observed in experiments with these homogenates.

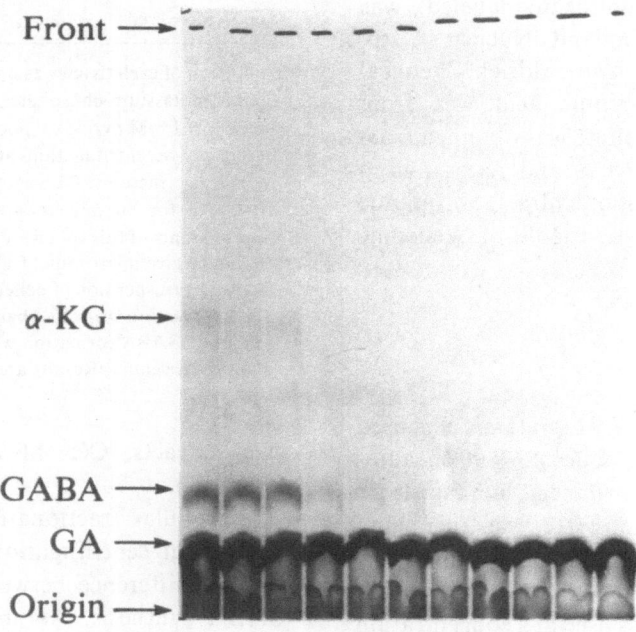

Fig. 1. Autoradiogram showing thin-layer chromatographic separation of incubation mixtures after reaction of [^{14}C]-L-glutamate with crude kidney extracts. Lanes 1–3 include homogenates from 3 different untreated rats; lanes 4–6, homogenates from 3 pre-treated rats in which GABA-T of kidney was >90% inhibited; lanes 7–9, control rat homogenates preincubated for 5 min at 37 °C with 0.1 mM hydrazinopropionic acid; and lanes 10–11 reagent blanks.

Table 4. Specificity of inhibitors.

Inhibitor	I_{50}(GABA-T)	I_{50}(GAD)	Ratio I_{50}(GAD)/I_{50}(GABA-T)
	(μM)	(μM)	
Hydrazinopropionic acid	0.003	0.6	200
Ethanolamine O-sulfate	300	~20 000	67
Aminooxyacetic acid	0.06	0.75	12
3-Mercaptopropionic acid	100	6.5	0.065

I_{50} concentrations were determined *in vitro* using partially purified brain glutamate decarboxylase and GABA-transaminase. Enzymes were preincubated with inhibitors in buffer for 5 min at 37 °C prior to substrate addition.

This can be seen in Fig. 1 in the case of kidney homogenate. Thus it is possible that α-ketoglutarate might be an intermediate in the enzymatic conversion from glutamate to GABA in these experiments, most probably via the action of glutamate dehydrogenase, which requires either NAD or NADP as cofactor. The possible participation of GABA-transaminase (GABA-T; aminobutyrate-aminotransferase; EC 2.6.1.19) was investigated by preincubating extracts with the GABA-T inhibitor, ethanolamine O-sulfate, and the GAD inhibitor, 3-mercaptopropionic acid. Although neither of these compounds is completely selective in its inhibition (Table 4), their use at appropriate concentrations can help to distinguish GAD and GABA-T activities. At a concentration of 5 mM, ethanolamine O-sulfate inhibited GABA-T activity in crude extracts of liver and kidney by 90% and 80% respectively. Rat brain GAD was inhibited only 7% at the same concentration. 3-Mercaptopropionic acid at 0.1 mM exhibited the reverse selectivity *in vitro,* being more inhibitory toward GAD than GABA-T. Results of experiments with these inhibitors, given in Table 5, show that 3-mercaptopropionic acid was a more potent inhibitor of GABA synthesis from glutamate in brain homogenates than in kidney or liver homogenates. On the other hand, the GABA-T inhibitor, ethanolamine O-sulfate, was a much more potent inhibitor of GABA synthesis in the peripheral tissue homogenates. Hydrazinopropionic acid and aminooxyacetic acid at concentrations that inhibit both GAD and GABA-T, strongly inhibited all GABA synthesis in these experiments.

GABA-T, measured by the conversion of GABA to succinate or succinic semialdehyde, was inhibited by over 94% in rat kidneys and livers after *in vivo* pre-treatment orally with ethanolamine O-sulfate at 500 mg/kg, 4 h prior to sacrifice. In the same homogenates, GABA synthesis from L-glutamic acid was also strongly inhibited, as shown in Table 6. Fig. 1 is a copy of an autoradiogram

Table 5. Effects of inhibitors on GABA synthesis from L-glutamic acid in crude homogenates of different tissues.

Inhibitor	Percent inhibition		
	Brain	Liver	Kidney
Ethanolamine O-sulfate (5 mM)	7.4	43	54
3-Mercaptopropionic acid (10^{-4} M)	75	50	52
Aminooxyacetic acid (10^{-5} M)	88	87	82
Hydrazinopropionic acid (10^{-4} M)	100	100	100

Crude homogenates were preincubated with inhibitors for 5 min at 37 °C before addition of glutamate. Percent inhibitions are means from duplicate or triplicate assays performed by the autoradiographic method. Maximum variation among replicate determinations was ±5%.

Table 6. Effect of *in vivo*[a] GABA-T inhibition on GABA synthesizing capacity of rat peripheral tissues.

Activity	Percent inhibition	
	Liver	Kidney
GABA-T	94.7 ± 4.2	99.0 ± 0.8
GABA synthesis	80.9 ± 10.6	82.0 ± 5.4

[a] Sprague-Dawley male rats were pre-treated orally with 500 mg/kg ethanolamine O-sulfate 4 h prior to sacrifice. Activities of GABA-transaminase (GABA-T) and enzymatic synthesis of GABA from L-glutamate were assayed in portions of the same crude homogenates. Results are expressed as the mean and S.E. (N = 3) based on activities obtained with an untreated control group in the same experiment.

258

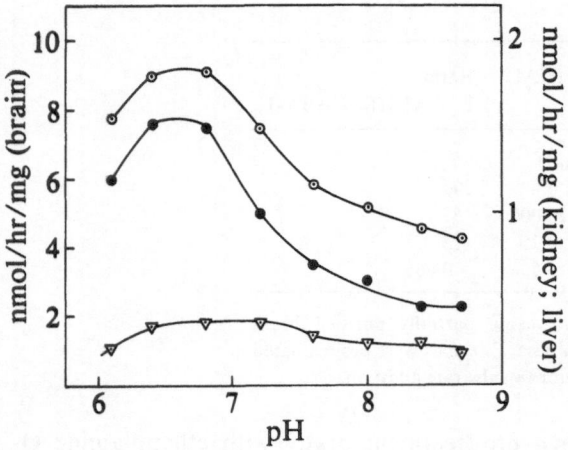

Fig. 2. pH profile for GABA synthesis as determined by the thin-layer procedure, using crude homogenates of brain ○, left-hand ordinate; kidney, ● and liver ▽, right-hand ordinate.

obtained with kidney homogenate after *in vivo* GABA-T inhibition.

The pH-activity profiles for GABA synthesis in brain and kidney homogenates appeared similar (Fig. 2), with pH optima between 6.4 and 6.8. The pH optimum found with liver extract was, however, quite different, with maximal activity occurring between pH 6.5 and 7.2.

Discussion

Estimates of maximal GAD activity in' crude extracts of rat or mouse brain range from 10 to 48 nmol of GABA formed per h per mg of wet tissue (4, 5, 9–15). Since the data in Table 1 of the present study was obtained using L-glutamate at its K_m concentration with rat brain GAD, the maximal activity for the brain enzyme would be 18 to 20 nmol per h per mg tissue, well within the range of published values.

The lack of stoichiometry between CO_2 liberation and GABA formation in liver and kidney extracts agrees with earlier work of Drummond & Phillips (4), who showed that the measurement of [^{14}C]-CO_2 liberated from [^{14}C]-glutamate does not necessarily correspond with GABA formation in peripheral tissues of mice, and with MacDonnell & Greengard (9) who, using a fluorometric assay involving ninhydrin, reported a similar finding with rat tissues. The indiscriminate application of the simple decarboxylation assay by earlier workers (2, 16) has apparently contributed to the conflicting

data in the literature concerning GAD in peripheral tissues.

It has also been reported (9) that treatment of crude homogenates with 0.5% Triton X-100 activates GAD, while inhibiting other interfering decarboxylases which could produce CO_2. An attempt to replicate this finding was not successful, since pretreatment of crude brain extracts with Triton X-100 caused about 25% inhibition of both GABA and CO_2 formation (data not shown). It appears that Triton could be an aid in homogenization to insure cell breakage and release of enzyme from membrane structures, but it probably does not directly stimulate GAD activity.

The effects of dialysis and attempts to obtain subcellular fractions (Tables 2 and 3) strongly suggest that GABA synthesis in rat liver and kidney is not catalyzed by a direct decarboxylation of glutamic acid, as in brain, but depends on at least one cofactor other than pyridoxal phosphate and may involve multiple enzymes. Seiler & Wagner (6) observed that NAD stimulated GABA synthesis in a crude rat liver preparation, and therefore the same cofactor was added to dialyzed extracts in the present study. The resulting stimulation shown in Table 3 points to a possible participation by glutamate dehydrogenase, which would convert glutamate to α-ketoglutarate. It is also conceivable that the same conversion could be catalyzed by transaminations with ketoacids which would be present in undialyzed extracts. α-Ketoglutarate might then be converted by decarboxylation, perhaps by pyruvate decarboxylase (EC 4.1.1.1), to succinic semialdehyde, which, together with glutamic acid, could serve as a substrate for GABA-transaminase (EC 2.6.1.19; aminobutyrate-amino-transferase) in the reverse direction. This sequence of reactions is outlined in Fig. 3, the last step of which is identical to the final step in the scheme proposed by Seiler & Wagner (6).

Evidence in support of this pathway was provided by the use of known inhibitors of GAD and GABA-T. Aminooxyacetic acid and hydrazino-propionic acid, as expected (15, 17), strongly inhibited enzyme activity in all homogenates at the high, non-selective concentrations employed in this study. A concentration of 3-mercaptopropionic acid which inhibited GABA-T activity by about 50% also inhibited GABA synthesis from L-glutamate to the same extent in crude homogenates of liver and kidney, while it inhibited brain GAD activity to

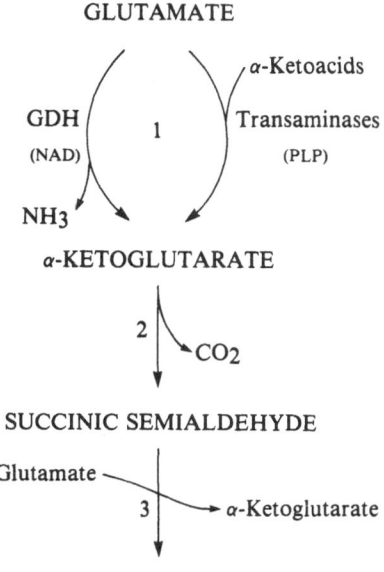

GLUTAMATE

α-KETOGLUTARATE

SUCCINIC SEMIALDEHYDE

GABA

Fig. 3. Possible pathway for GABA synthesis from glutamate in peripheral tissues. Step 1 represents conversion of glutamate to α-ketoglutarate via glutamate dehydrogenase (GDH) or various α-amino acid transaminases; step 2 may be catalyzed by a decarboxylase such as pyruvate decarboxylase; and step 3, by GABA-transaminase.

a greater extent. On the other hand, ethanolamine O-sulfate, a known GABA-T inhibitor (18), caused greater inhibition in peripheral extracts than in brain. Pre-treatment of rats with a single dose of this compound resulted in more than 90% inhibition of peripheral GABA-T activity and, at the same time, at least 80% inhibition of GABA synthesis from glutamic acid. These results indicate that GABA-T in crude homogenates may play a predominant role in formation of GABA, especially when one considers the relatively high concentrations of GABA-T that are found in liver and kidney (8).

The relevance of these findings to actual GABA synthesizing activities *in vivo* is somewhat obscure. These experiments do not exclude the possibility that a very low activity of a true glutamate decarboxylase may also occur in peripheral tissues, and it could be that the pathway in Fig. 3 does not represent a normal *in vivo* route to GABA, except perhaps under certain conditions. Although, significant amounts of GABA can be detected in these tissues (4), it may be derived from dietary sources as well as *in vivo* synthesis.

A biological role for GABA in peripheral tissues has not yet been well defined. However, the results of this study imply that pharmacological or clinical use of GABA-T inhibitors may not elevate GABA in kidney or liver as markedly as in brain, since GABA synthesis and catabolism would both be strongly inhibited in these tissues. Likewise, *in vivo* use of a glutamate decarboxylase inhibitor might selectively block GABA synthesis only in the central nervous system.

Acknowledgements

I thank L. D. Faison for expert technical assistance; Dr. K. Ingold for purification of ethanolamine O-sulfate and synthesis of sodium hydrazinopropionate; and K. Rohrbach for assistance in dosing animals.

References

1. Baxter, C. F., 1976. In: GABA in Nervous System Function (Roberts, E., Chase, T. N. and Tower, D. B., eds.) pp. 61–87. Raven Press, New York.
2. Haber, B., Kuriyama, K. & Roberts, E., 1970. Biochem. Pharmacol. 19: 1119–1136.
3. Miller, L. P. & Martin, D. L., 1973. Life Sci. 13: 1023–1032.
4. Drummond, R. J. & Phillips, A. T., 1974. J. Neurochem. 23: 1207–1213.
5. Wu, J.-Y., Chude, O., Wein, J., Roberts, E., Saito, K. & Wong, E., 1978. J. Neurochem. 30: 849–857.
6. Seiler, N. & Wagner, G., 1976. Neurochemical Res. 1: 113–131.
7. Lowry, O. H., Rosebrough, N. J., Farr, A. L. & Randall, R. J., 1951. J. Biol. Chem. 193: 265–275.
8. White, H. L. & Sato, T. L., 1978. J. Neurochem. 31: 41–47.
9. MacDonnell, P. & Greengard, O., 1975. J. Neurochem. 24: 615–618.
10. Morin, A. M. & Wasterlain, C. G., 1978. J. Neurochem. 31: 371–373.
11. Wu, J.-Y., Matsuda, T. & Roberts, E., 1973. J. Biol. Chem. 248: 3029–3034.
12. Tappaz, M. L., Brownstein, M. J. & Kopin, I. J., 1977. Brain Res. 125: 109–121.
13. Sims, K. L. & Pitts, F. N., 1970. J. Neurochem. 17: 1607–1612.
14. Salganicoff, L. & de Robertis, E., 1965. J. Neurochem. 12: 287–309.
15. Roberts, E. & Simonsen, D. G., 1963. Biochem. Pharmacol. 12: 113–134.
16. Lancaster, G., Mohyuddin, F., Scriver, C. R. & Whelan, D. T., 1973. Biochim. Biophys. Acta 297: 229–240.
17. van Gelder, N. M., 1968. J. Neurochem. 15: 747–757.
18. Fowler, L. J. and John, R. A., 1972. Biochem. J. 130: 569–573.

Received August 11, 1980.

The GABA postsynaptic membrane receptor-ionophore complex
Site of action of convulsant and anticonvulsant drugs

Richard W. Olsen

Division of Biomedical Sciences and Dept. of Biochemistry Univ. of California, Riverside, CA 92521, U.S.A.

Summary

The function of the inhibitory neurotransmitter, γ-aminobutyric acid (GABA), has been implicated in the mode of action of many drugs which excite or depress the central nervous system. Many convulsant agents appear to block GABA action whereas anticonvulsants enhance GABA action. Some of these drug effects involve altered GABA-mediated synaptic transmission at the level of GABA biosynthesis, release from nerve endings, uptake into cells, and metabolic degradation. A greater number of agents of diverse classes appear to affect GABA action at the postsynaptic membrane, as determined from both electrophysiological and biochemical studies. The recently developed *in vitro* radioactive receptor binding assays have led to a wealth of new information about GABA action and its alteration by drugs. GABA inhibitory transmission involves the regulation, by GABA binding to its receptor site, of chloride ion channels. In this GABA receptor-ionophore system, other drug receptor sites, one for benzodiazepines and one for barbiturates/picrotoxinin (and related agents) appear to form a multicomponent complex. In this complex, the drugs binding to any of the three receptor categories are visualized to have an effect on GABA-associated chloride channel regulation. Available evidence suggests that the complex mediates many of the actions of numerous excitatory and depressant drugs showing a variety of pharmacological effects.

Abbreviations

THIP, 4, 5, 6, 7-tetrahydroisoxazolo [5, 4-*c*] pyridin-3-ol; TETS, tetramethylene disulfotetramine; DMBB, 5-ethyl-5-(1, 3-dimethylbutyl) barbituric acid; CHEB, 5-ethyl-5-(2-cyclohexylidene-ethyl) barbituric acid; GABA, γ-amino-*n*-butyric acid; DABA, L-2, 4-diaminobutyric acid.

Introduction

γ-Aminobutyric acid (GABA), the major inhibitory neurotransmitter in the central nervous system (CNS), has become increasingly implicated for a role in maintaining the overall electrical activity of the CNS at a level below that associated with epilepsy. Thus, any interference with inhibitory synaptic transmission mediated by GABA leads to seizures, while the enhancement of GABAergic synaptic transmission prevents seizures (1). Many drugs with convulsant and anticonvulsant activity appear to act at the level of GABA synapses, principally at the postsynaptic cell membrane.

The action of GABA involves a rapid and reversible binding to a chemically specific recognition site in the postsynaptic cell membrane surface, the receptor protein (2, 3). GABA occupancy of the receptor regulates the opening and closing of membrane chloride ion channels (4–6). Since the equilibrium Nernst potential for Cl^- is near the cell resting potential, activation of Cl^- channels by GABA stabilizes the postsynaptic cell membrane potential near the resting level and inhibits the cell by preventing any significant depolarization during any simultaneous excitatory input.

Molecular and Cellular Biochemistry 39, 261–279 (1981). 0300-8177/81/0391-0261/$03.80.

Radioactive ligand binding assays have recently made possible the *in vitro* study of the GABA receptor-chloride ion channel complex. Numerous convulsant and anticonvulsant drugs interact with this system *in vitro,* providing clues to their possible site and mechanism of action. The GABA receptor-chloride ion channel appears to involve a complex of at least three drug receptor classes: the GABA receptor site, the picrotoxinin/barbiturate receptor site, and the benzodiazepine receptor site. Drugs which mimic or inhibit the pharmacological actions of the prototypic substances inhibit the binding of the radiolabeled ligands to their respective receptor sites. *In vitro* interactions between the various receptors are also observable, consistent with the convergence of the three categories of drugs at their common physiological level, the GABA-regulated chloride ion channel.

GABA binding sites with receptor-like specificity can be studied with tritiated GABA or biologically active analogues under appropriate assay conditions. These include employment of sodium ion-free assay solutions (3, 7) and thoroughly disrupted and washed brain membrane fractions (2, 3, 7, 8) in order to minimize association of the labeled GABA with nonreceptor binding sites (3, 7) and to remove endogenous GABA from the preparations (8, 9). Sodium-independent GABA binding sites have been shown to meet numerous criteria for receptor identification, such as low number, reasonable affinity, tissue and subcellular location (10–12), inhibition by appropriate concentrations of GABA analogues, and only those analogues, shown to be active as agonists or antagonists on physiological measurements of GABA receptors (2, 11, 13–15), and interaction with other drug receptors known to affect GABAergic synaptic transmission (16).

Radiolabeled benzodiazepines bind to sites in CNS membranes which meet similar criteria for specificity including quantities and location (17, 18). Inhibition by a series of analogues of diazepam suggest that the binding sites are related to the anxiolytic, anticonvulsant, sedative, and muscle relaxant actions of the benzodiazepines (17, 18). These receptor binding sites appear to be physically coupled to GABA receptor sites on the basis of *in vitro* interactions between the two types of binding (16). Anion effects on benzodiazepine binding also suggest a possible coupling to chloride ion channels (19). These *in vitro* (cell-free) studies are consistent with physiological experiments in intact

animals or in nervous system tissue preparations showing an enhancement of GABAergic synaptic transmission by benzodiazepines, acting at post-synaptic sites distinct from the GABA recognition site (20).

Picrotoxin is a small molecular weight convulsant drug of plant origin which universally blocks GABAergic synaptic transmission (21), without blocking GBA binding to its recognition site (11, 22). Studies in my laboratory have employed a radiolabeled biologically active analogue of picrotoxin, [³H] α-dihydropicrotoxinin (DHP), to assay CNS membrane sites related to the convulsant actions of the drug (2, 11, 23, 24). DHP binding sites are similar in quantity and location to GABA and benzodiazepine receptors (25–27). These sites are inhibited by appropriate concentrations of numerous convulsant drugs known to inhibit GABA synapses (2), including convulsant barbiturates (28) and a convulsant benzodiazepine substance (26, 27, 29). Many CNS depressant substances including anesthetic, hypnotic, and anticonvulsant barbiturates (28) and diphenylhydantion (24) inhibit DHP binding at relevant concentrations. Furthermore, at least some DHP

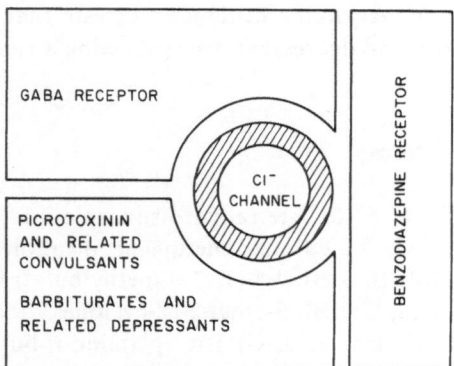

Fig. 1. Theoretical model of the GABA receptor-ionophore complex, including receptor sites for convulsant and anti-convulsant drugs. The complex is envisioned as containing three drug receptor sites, the GABA receptor, the benzodiazepine receptor, and the picrotoxinin-barbiturate receptor. Associated with, or part of, these receptors is the chloride ion channel whose opening is regulated by GABA agonists binding to the GABA receptor. The activity of the chloride ion channel may also be modulated in a positive manner (depressant drugs) to potentiate the inhibitory chloride ion permeability, or in a negative manner (excitatory agents), to block the chloride ion channel. Modulatory agents may be exogenous or endogenous substances. The presence of all these components in all GABA receptor systems in all parts of the brain is not obligatory, and some of the components may also exist in an uncoupled state.

binding sites are coupled to benzodiazepine receptors and GABA rceptors, as shown by *in vitro* interactions in which drugs binding to picrotox-inin/barbiturate receptor sites show allosteric perturbations of the GABA (30–32) and benzo-diazepine receptor sites (33–39); these interactions are strictly dependent on the presence of anions which can permeate the GABA receptor-regulated chloride ion channels (31, 36, 40).

This article will review briefly the evidence for a role of GABA in seizures and in the mode of action of convulsant and anticonvulsant drugs (my apologies for the omission of many possible refer-ences). A summary of *in vitro* binding studies on the GABA, benzodiazepine, picrotoxinin/barbiturate receptor-chloride ion channel complex will focus on the interactions of convulsant and anticon-vulsant drugs with this complex, and the relevance of these biochemical observations to pharmaco-logical actions *in vivo*.

Table 1 summarizes the interaction of convulsant and anticonvulsant drugs with various levels of the GABA system and may be referred to throughout the following discussion. Fig. 1 provides a schematic model of the postsynaptic GABA receptor iono-phore complex, (26, 39) indicating the three classes of drug receptor involved.

Pharmacological evidence for the involvement of GABA in seizures

Any impairment of GABAergic transmission results in seizures (1, 21, 41). Such interference may be at the level of GABA synthesis, release from nerve endings, or action on postsynaptic membrane receptor-ionophores.

The activity of L-glutamic acid decarboxylase (GAD), the enzyme catalyzing the biosynthesis of GABA in CNS, can be inhibited specifically by substrate analogues, e.g., mercaptopropionic acid and allylglycine (or a metabolite), or nonspecifically by carbonyl reagents, such as hydrazides, which react with the pyridoxal phosphate cofactor of GAD (1, 42); all of these GAD inhibitors have convulsant activity. Seizures also accompany a deficiency of the vitamin pyridoxine (B$_6$), apparent-ly due to an impaired synthesis of GABA in CNS (41). The convulsant action of tetanus toxin may be related to its inhibition of release of GABA from nerve terminals (21). Furthermore, anatomical evi-dence for a decrease in GABAergic nerve terminals in animal focal epilepsy has been obtained (43).

Drugs which antagonize GABAergic synaptic transmission are convulsants (1, 21, 44–50). These include agents which block GABA binding to its receptor site or agents which prevent the response to GABA at the level of the chloride ionophore. The convulsants bicuculline and picrotoxin are well known antagonists of GABA synapses (21, 51). Subconvulsant doses of picrotoxin also potentiate the seizures accompanying ethanol withdrawal (52, 53) and in some of the kindling animal models of epilepsy (M. Kalichman, unpublished).

Drugs which enhance GABAergic transmission at the level of metabolism, uptake, or receptor-ionophores generally have anticonvulsant activity (1, 20, 54–71).

Raising CNS GABA levels by inhibiting the enzyme which degrades GABA, GABA transminase (GABA-T), appears to be a useful anticonvulsant strategy (1, 56, 62, 63). Examples of compounds which inhibit GABA-T are amino-oxyacetic acid, gabaculine, γ-vinyl GABA, or γ-acetylenic GABA. The action of valproic acid (Di-*n*-propyl acetate) may involve an inhibition of GABA metabolism (56) (although postsynaptic effects may be involved as well).

Potentiation of GABA synaptic action by in-hibitors of GABA transport has remained a theoretically important strategy for anticonvulsant therapy. However, this approach has been hampered by the inability of most substances which inhibit GABA uptake *in vitro* to pass the blood-brain-barrier (21, 64). At least one such compound, nipecotic acid methylester, has anticonvulsant ac-tivity (64–66).

GABA itself does not pass the blood-brain-barrier very well at all (56, 57, 64), and GABA analogues which mimic GABA action on receptors generally share this property (56, 65), although homotaurine (3-aminopropane sulfonic acid) has been reported to show anticonvulsant activity (67). Inhibition of GABA-T may allow higher and therapeutic levels of GABA agonists to enter the brain (63). GABA therapy for seizure (or other) disorders generally has proved unsuccessful (1, 65) (if the compound does not enter the brain), or even harmful. This is perhaps due to metabolites with undesired side effects (1), or to the inappropriate flooding of all brain GABA synapses when only a few selected synapses could show beneficial effects

264

Table 1. Interaction of convulsant and anticonvulsant drugs with GABA-mediated inhibitory synapses.

Drug	GABA system affected				
	Metabolism	Synaptic Transmission	Receptor-Ionophore Binding		
			GABA	P/B	BZ
I. *Depressants*					
A. *GABA-related*					
1. GABA	(1, 56, 57,	(4–6, 21)	10^{-8}; 10^{-7} (2, 3, 121)	–	↑ 10^{-6} (16, 176–182)
2. Muscimol	64, 65)	(21)	10^{-9}; 10^{-8} (2, 15)	–	↑ 10^{-7}
3. THIP	(64,68, 69)	(68)	10^{-8}; 10^{-7} (2,68)	–	n.a. (183, 184)
4. 3-Aminopropane sulfonic acid	(1, 65, 67)	(21)	10^{-8}; 10^{-7} (2, 3)	–	↑ 10^{-6} (184–186)
5. Cetyl GABA	(70)	–	–	–	–
6. Progabamide	(71)	–	10^{-6} (71)	–	–
7. DABA	(64)	(64)	n.a. (2,7)	–	n.a. (184)
8. Nipecotic acid (and esters)	(64–66)	(64)	n.a. (2, 13)	–	–
9. Baclofen	–	n.a. (21)	10^{-4} (2,209)	–	–
10. Amino-oxyacetic acid	(1, 56, 57, 62)	–	–	–	–
11. Gabaculine	–	–	–	–	–
12. γ-Vinyl GABA	–	–	–	–	–
13. γ-Acetylenic GABA	–	–	–	–	–
14. Valproic acid (Also IC)		Potentiates (81–83)	n.a.(*)	10^{-3}(**)	n.a.(*)
IB. *Benzodiazepine-related*					
1. Diazepam	–	Potentiates (20, 58	↑ 10^{-7} (189)	10^{-6} (27, 29)	10^{-8} (17, 18)
2. Chlordiazepoxide	–	59, 104–120)	–	10^{-5} (27, 29)	10^{-7} (17, 18)
3. Flunitrazepam	–	Potentiates (20, 58,	–	10^{-5} (27, 19)	10^{-8} (17, 18)
4. Clonazepam	–	59, 104–120)	–	10^{-5} (27, 29)	10^{-8} (17, 18)
5. CL 218, 872	–	–	–	–	10^{-8} (166)
6. β-carboline-3-carboxylic acid ethyl ester	–	–	–	–	10^{-8} (173)
7. Nicotinamide	–	–	–	–	10^{-3} (171)
8. Hypoxanthine (also IC)	–	–	10^{-3} (214)	10^{-4} (29, 172)	10^{-3} (167, 169)
9. Adenosine	–	–	10^{-3} (214)	n.a. (172)	10^{-3} (167, 169)
10. Methaqualone	–	(88)	–	–	10^{-4}(***)
11. Meprobamate	–	–	–	10^{-3}(*)	10^{-3}(*)
IC. *Barbiturate-related*					
1. Pentobarbital	–	Potentiates (20, 54, 55,	↑ 10^{-4} (31)	10^{-4} (28, 212)	↑ 10^{-4} (36)
2. Phenobarbital	–	59, 60, 72, 89–99)	n.a.(*)	10^{-4} (28)	n.a. (36)
3. Diphenylhydantoin (also IB)	–	Potentiates (84–86)	n.a. (22)	10^{-4} (24)	10^{-4}(***)
4. Etazolate (SQ 20009)	–	–	↑ 10^{-5} (30)	10^{-5} (26, 39)	↑ 10^{-5} (33, 34)
5. Chlormethiazole	–	–	n.a.(*)	10^{-4} (146)	10^{-3}(*)
6. Carbamazepine	–	–	n.a.(*)	10^{-4} (146)	10^{-3}(*)
7. Ethanol	?	Potentiates (80)	–	10^{-2}(**)	↑ 10^{-2} (205)
8. Allantoin	–	–	–	10^{-4} (172)	–
9. Ethosuximide	–	–	–	?	?
10. Trimethadione	–	–	–	?	?
II. *Excitants*					
A. *Gaba-related*		(Antagonist)			
1. Bicuculline	–	(21)	10^{-6} (2, 7)	10^{-4} (24)	n.a. (177)
2. Benzyl penicillin (also IIB)	–	(45, 73, 74)	10^{-4} (2)	10^{-4} (24)	–
3. Strychnine	–	n.a. (21)	10^{-5} (122)	10^{-4} (24)	n.a. (17, 18)

Table 1. Interaction of convulsant and anticonvulsant drugs with GABA-mediated inhibitory synapses *(continued)*

Drug	GABA system affected				
	Metabolism	Synaptic Transmission	Receptor-Ionophore Binding		
			GABA	P/B	BZ
4. Mercaptopropionic acid	(1, 42)	–	–	–	–
5. Allyglycine	(1, 42)	–	–	–	–
6. Hydrazides	(1, 42)	–	–	–	–
7. Tetanus toxin	(1, 21, 42)	–	–	–	–
II.					
B. *Picrotoxin-related*		(Antagonist)			
1. Picrotoxinin	–	(21, 51, 72, 143, 144)	n.a. (2)	10^{-6} (24)	n.a. (17, 18)
2. Tutin	–	(21)	n.a. (2)	10^{-6} (24)	–
3. α-dihydropicrotoxinin	–	(23, 24)	n.a. (2)	10^{-6} (24)	–
4. Isopropyl bicyclophosphate	–	(49)	n.a. (2)	10^{-5} (145)	10^{-4}(*)
5. TETS	–	(50)	n.a. (2)	10^{-5} (145)	10^{-4}(*)
6. DMBB	–	(79)	n.a. (2)	10^{-7} (28)	$\uparrow 10^{-4}$ (36)
7. CHEB	–	(79)	n.a. (2)	10^{-6} (28)	n.a. (36)
8. Benzodiazepine RO5-3663		(47, 48)	n.a.(*)	10^{-7} (27, 29)	10^{-4}(*)
9. Pentylenetetrazole[+]	–	(45, 76–78)	n.a. (22)	10^{-5}(*)	10^{-4}(167)
10. Bemegride	–	–	–	?	?

The numbers in parentheses are the references. In the case of receptor binding studies, the effective concentrations for inhibition (IC_{50} values) are given to the nearest order of magnitude, or the concentrations effective in allosteric modulation of binding, when indicated by an $\uparrow$. In the binding columns, P/B refers to the picrotoxinin/barbiturate receptor; BZ refers to the benzodiazepine receptor. n.a. means the compound was not active at a high concentration (10^{-5}-10^{-3} M); (–) means the compound was not tested (or at least the results not reported here). (*) signifies unpublished observations of the author. (+) signifies that this compound (pentylenetetrazole), which inhibits BZ binding at 10^{-4} M, should also be in a third subclass of category II. ** signifies unpublished observations by M. K. Ticku, *** by M. Karobath.

of enhanced activity, or to an excitatory effect (65), probably resulting from disinhibition of tonically inhibited neural circuits. However, hydrophobic analogues of GABA which enter the brain and there show either GABA-mimetic activity (such as THIP (68, 69)) or become metabolized to GABA (such as cetyl-GABA (70), or SL76002 = Progabamide (71)) show promise as anticonvulsants.

Evidence is accumulating that many CNS depressant drugs with anticonvulsant activity potentiate GABAergic inhibitory synaptic transmission and/or interact with the GABA system *in vitro,* implying *in vivo* effects.

Physiological evidence for a role of GABA in the action of convulsant and anticonvulsant drugs

GABA-mediated inhibitory synaptic transmission is antagonized by a variety of substances which possess convulsant action. Bicuculline is the best known specific GABA antagonist (21), and this compound appears to block GABA binding to the receptor site (7, 8). Numerous other convulsants inhibit GABAergic synapses at a site distinct from the GABA receptor *sensu stricto,* perhaps at the chloride ion channel. Examples of these convulsant agents are picrotoxin (21, 46, 51, 72), bicyclophosphate cage convulsants (49, 55), benzyl penicillin (45, 73–75), tetramethylene disulfotetramine (50), pentylenetetrazol (45, 75–78), convulsant barbiturates (79), and a convulsant benzodiazepine (47, 48). All of these agents interact in some way with biochemical assays of the GABA receptor-ionophore complex, as studied with radioactive picrotoxinin and benzodiazepine binding *in vitro* (see below).

The activity of GABAergic synapses is potentiated by anticonvulsant drugs such as benzodiazepines and barbiturates, and perhaps also by diphenylhydantoin, valproic acid, and ethanol. One report of ethanol enhancement of GABAergic transmission has appeared (80), and several observations of valproic acid augmentation of GABAergic synaptic inhibition (81–83), at least one of them at the level of the postsynaptic membrane response to GABA (81). This effect could not be due to inhibition of GABA metabolism. At least one observation of diphenylhydantoin enhancement of CNS inhibition has been reported (84), and potentiation of GABA responses has been well documented in invertebrate CNS (85, 86); some GABAergic synapses in mammalian CNS are not potentiated (71, 87). The anticonvulsant action of methaqualone has also been reported to involve GABA (88).

Barbiturates potentiate GABAergic transmission at numerous regions of the CNS (20, 21, 54, 55, 59, 60, 72, 89–98). This activity also results in an effective reversal of the antagonism of GABA synapses by drugs such as bicuculline (55, 99) and, especially, picrotoxin (54, 72, 99). Barbiturate potentiation of GABA responses at the postsynaptic level has been demonstrated with cultured spinal neurons (90, 91); pentobarbital mimicked the action of GABA in activating chloride ion channels (91), whereas phenobarbital prolonged the lifetime of GABA-activated chloride ion channels (90). These observations provide an important step closer to a molecular understanding of barbiturate action on GABA synapses. This action may be related to anticonvulsant activity of the barbiturates, although these drugs also inhibit excitatory post-synaptic potentials and nerve firing (100, 101) and modify neurotransmitter release (102, 103).

The 'GABA hypothesis' of benzodiazepine action has been accumulating support for several years (20, 21, 59, 104). *In vivo*, benzodiazepines decrease both neuronal electrical activity and levels of cyclic GMP in cerebellum, an effect blocked by GABA antagonists such as picrotoxin or bicuculline, and mimicked by drugs which increase GABA activity (104). The anticonvulsant effects (58, 59) and perhaps also the antianxiety effects (105, 106) of benzodiazepines appear to be mediated by an augmentation of GABA action. Benzodiazepines potentiate GABA synapses throughout the CNS (20, 47, 54, 59, 93, 107–120), as measured by many different techniques including brain tissue slices (114). This enhancement has been

shown to be at the postsynaptic membrane in many cases, such as those involving cultured neurons (119–120).

Receptor binding studies *in vitro* indicate a physical coupling between both benzodiazepine and barbiturate receptors with GABA receptors in a multi-receptor, chloride ion channel protein complex in the postsynaptic membrane.

Biochemical evidence for convulsant and anticonvulsant drug receptor sites in the GABA post-synaptic receptor-ionophore complex

The GABA receptor-ionophore in mammalian brain appears to involve a protein complex containing receptor sites for GABA, benzodiazepines, and picrotoxinin/barbiturates (Fig. 1), as well as a chloride ion channel. The three receptor sites can be assayed *in vitro* by suitable radioactive ligand binding techniques, as described in references (2, 3, 8, 9, 24, 27, 28, 29, 36, 39, 121, 122).

A. GABA receptor binding

GABA receptor binding to mammalian brain homogenates was first described with [³H] GABA, using disrupted membrane fractions and sodium ion-free assay conditions, in order to minimize association of GABA with sodium-dependent uptake sites found in neuron and glia cell membranes (7). Subsequent characterization of these sodium-independent GABA binding sites revealed that they met numerous criteria for identification as receptor sites. These GABA binding sites showed a subcellular distribution consistent with a synaptic location (2, 3, 8) and a tissue (within CNS) specificity (10, 11) expected from physiological measurements of GABAergic function. Furthermore, these binding sites were depleted in a variety of lesions and mutations known to decrease GABA-sensitive neurons, including the human disorders of Parkinson's disease (123) and Huntington's chorea (123, 124), virus infections (125) or mutations (12) affecting cerebellum granule cells, and chemical or knife lesions of the striatum (126) or other brain regions (127). The same binding sites appear to be increased in number in the substantia nigra of animals with lesions of the GABAergic striatonigral tract (128, 129) or in the corresponding human situation, Huntington's chorea (128, 130). This effect may be similar to the 'denervation supersensitivity' well-known for other receptor systems (131).

More importantly, the chemical specificity of sodium-independent binding sites (2, 3, 7, 11, 13–15) shows a perfect correlation with properties expected of GABA receptors from electrophysiological studies (4, 5, 21). All compounds which inhibit GABA receptor binding have been found to mimic or inhibit the action of GABA at synapses (11, 13, 22). We now know that certain drugs may affect GABA postsynaptic responses at sites distinct from the GABA receptor (recognition) site, but the activity of a long series of GABA analogues of restricted configuration correlates very well between sodium-independent binding and synaptic activity (13, 15), but not with activity on GABA transport sites (15, 64). In particular, 'GABA receptor sites' are those (the sodium-independent sites) which are inhibited by appropriate concentrations of receptor-specific analogues such as muscimol, THIP (see Table 1), isoguvacine, 3-aminopropane sulfonic acid, and piperidine-4-sulfonic acid (13, 15), compounds which can also be used as radioactive ligands for GABA receptor sites (132–134). These binding sites are also inhibited by the GABA antagonist bicuculline (2, 7, 8), an analogue of which has also been used for GABA-sensitive receptor binding assays (135). GABA receptor binding is not inhibited by GABA analogues such as L-2, 4, diaminobutyric acid (DABA) and nipecotic acid (15) which specifically inhibit GABA uptake but have no postsynaptic agonist or antagonist activity (21, 64).

Original studies suggested one apparent population of GABA receptor binding sites with K_D of about 300 nM (3), although physiological measurements suggest that GABA concentrations on the order of at least 100 times higher are needed for chloride channel activation (4–6). The number of these binding sites (B_{max}) was appropriately low, roughly 1 pmol/mg membrane protein in dense regions of brain such as cerebellar or cerebral cortex (3), assayed at 0° in 50 mM Tris-citrate buffer, pH 7.1. Subsequent work on either Triton X-100 washed (136–138) or frozen-thawed, multiple buffer-washed membranes (8) (to remove endogenous GABA (9) or other inhibitors of GABA binding (138–140)) revealed two apparent populations of binding sites, with a high affinity population ($K_D = 20$ nM, $B_{max} = 0.3$ pmol/mg in

cerebellum or cortex (2, 9, 121, 122, 124)) becoming detectable in addition to (not instead of) the other class of sites previously mentioned.

Although most drug specificity studies on GABA binding have been carried out under conditions where radioactive ligand was bound to a mixture of these two subpopulations of GABA binding sites which differ in GABA affinity (121), we have recently determined by kinetic manipulation (Lummis and Olsen, unpublished) that both sites have receptor-like specificity. Furthermore, the two subpopulations have a remarkably similar order of preference for a series of GABA analogues (121), indicating that the two sites may be related to each other. Whereas we were not able to interconvert GABA binding sites from one affinity state to another by a limited number of assay conditions varying from the standard 50 mM Tris-citrate, pH 7.1, 0 °C (12), it now appears that such interconversion may be effected in chloride ion-containing buffers by various drugs which interact with the receptor-ionophore system (30, 31) (see below).

Drugs which appear to act directly (and competitively in binding studies) at the GABA receptor sites are primarily physiological agonists (15, 21). The possible use of such agents as anticonvulsants has been discussed above. Very few examples have been found of compounds which inhibit GABA receptor binding and show GABA antagonist and/or convulsant activity.

Convulsant drugs which inhibit GABA receptor binding include bicuculline ($IC_{50} = 1$ μM), strychnine ($IC_{50} = 10$ μM); d-tubocurarine ($IC_{50} = 100$ μM) and benzyl penicillin ($IC_{50} = 50$ μM) (2, 11, 13, 22). The convulsant action of bicuculline is considered likely to be due to GABA antagonism (21), but the question of whether bicuculline actually acts at the GABA recognition site is not yet firmly established.

Strychnine is considered to inhibit glycine synapses (at the receptor-ionophore level) much more potently than GABA synapses (21), although an inhibition of GABA synapses by high concentrations of strychnine is possible. Strychnine binding to brain membranes is inhibited by glycine (141) (at least partially) and by anions (141), suggesting a possible coupling of strychnine receptors to chloride ionophores (see discussion of GABA ionophores below). Although it has not been established that glycine ionophores and GABA ionophores are distinct, they appear pharmacologically different, but perhaps with some overlap. Bicuculline ($IC_{50} = 5 \mu M$) inhibits radioactive strychnine binding (142) with a similar potency to its block of GABA binding. However, strychnine inhibits radioactive bicuculline binding ($IC_{50} = 3 \mu M$) (135) much less well than its own binding ($K_D = 3$ nM) (141). The bicuculline site in the GABA receptor-ionophore complex may thus have a low affinity for strychnine (relative to strychnine's affinity for glycine receptor-ionophores), and/or a bicuculline-strychnine binding site may be common to both GABA and glycine regulated chloride ion channels. We have recently observed (Olsen, unpublished) that 10 μM strychnine, like bicuculline, interferes with the coupling of GABA, barbiturate, and benzodiazepine receptors as described below.

d-Tubocurarine is known as a potent cholinergic antagonist and the weak effect on GABA receptor binding is not likely to be important. Benzyl penicillin, on the other hand, inhibits GABAergic synapses (45, 46, 74), probably at the level of the ion channels rather than at the GABA receptor (45, 112). The effect on GABA binding might be at the active site or via an allosteric site.

B. Picrotoxinin binding

Catalytic hydrogenation of a double bond in picrotoxinin allowed introduction of ^{3}H into the reduced product, α-dihydropicrotoxinin (DHP), which was shown to have biological activity only slightly lower than that of picrotoxinin. This radioactive ligand was demonstrated to bind specifically to synaptic membrane fragments from crayfish muscle (23) (a tissue containing picrotoxin-sensitive GABA synapses (143, 144)) and mammalian brain, but not to nonneural tissues (2, 11, 24). The binding dissociation constant was 1-2 μM, comparable to the pharmacologically active concentration of the drug (23). The number of binding sites B_{max} in rat cortex was 5-10 pmol/mg, about three times the level of GABA receptor sites. DHP binding sites appear to be distinct from GABA receptor sites by various criteria (25), while showing a similar brain regional and subcellular distribution (25, 27). The relatively low affinity binding causes technical problems in that the ratio of specifically bound ligand to background (signal:noise ratio) is unfavorable and barely acceptable for quantitative measurements (24). Nevertheless, [^{3}H]DHP is a unique and valuable ligand for labeling a class of drug receptor sites which binds many CNS depressant and excitatory agents, and so far the only successful ligand for these sites, which seem to be related to the chloride ion channels which are regulated by GABA receptors (2, 27, 29, 39).

DHP binding is inhibited by biologically active but not inactive chemical analogues of picrotoxin (2, 11, 23, 24). Several other convulsant drugs inhibit DHP binding, as shown in Table 1. These include the cage compounds such as bicyclophosphates and tetramethylene disulfotetramine, which block GABA synaptic activity (49, 50) but do not inhibit GABA receptor binding up to 0.1 mM (145). Other inhibitors of DHP binding include excitatory barbiturates (such as DMBB and CHEB (28, 29)) and an excitatory benzodiazepine analogue of diazepam, RO5-3663 (27, 29). These compounds inhibit DHP binding in submicromolar concentrations (26, 29) and inhibit GABA synaptic activity (47, 79). Pentylenetetrazole also inhibits [^{3}H] DHP binding ($\cong 10$ μM) (Leeb-Lundberg and Olsen, unpublished), and blocks GABA synapses (45, 75-78). Therefore [^{3}H] DHP labels high affinity convulsant drug receptor sites in brain membranes which are circumstantially related to GABA receptor-ionophores.

DHP binding is also inhibited by numerous CNS depressant drugs, including hypnotic barbiturates (at 1-100 μM) (2, 28), anxiolytic pyrazolopyridines like etazolate = SQ 20009 (at $\cong 1$ μM) (26, 39), and numerous anticonvulsants including benzodiazepines (at 0.1-100 μM) (27, 29), barbiturates (at 1 μM-1 mM) (24, 28, 29) and other substances, such as diphenylhydantoin (24), carbamazepine, and chlormethiazole (at 0.1-1 mM) (146). The potency of these drug effects on DHP binding correlates roughly with depressant activity (e.g., pentobarbital and secobarbital more potent than phenobarbital and metharbital (28)). Binding potency also correlates well with activity of barbiturates in enhancing the postsynaptic chloride conductance activated by GABA (60, 91), and with the effective reversal by barbiturates of the antagonism by bicuculline (55, 99) and picrotoxin (72) of GABAergic synaptic transmission. The concentrations of anesthetic/hypnotic and anticonvulsant drugs which inhibit DHP binding are rather high but still consistent with known pharmacological doses (59, 100). Further evidence for the relevance of these picrotoxin/barbiturate binding sites to pharmacological activity and to the GABA receptor-ionophore is provided by the interaction of these sites with benzodiazepine and GABA receptor binding sites *in vitro* as described below. [³H] DHP binding is also inhibited weakly by valproic acid ($\cong$ 1 mM) and ethanol ($\cong$ 30 mM) (M. K. Ticku, unpublished).

The inhibition of DHP binding by benzodiazepines (27, 29), on the other hand, does not seem to correlate with the CNS depressant activities of this class of drug, which can however, be correlated with high-affinity benzodiazepine binding (17, 18). The excitatory benzodiazepine (RO5-3663), however, inhibits DHP binding much more potently (0.1 μM) than it blocks [³H] benzodiazepine binding ($\cong$ 10 μM) (27), indicating a likely action at DHP sites. The other benzodiazepines inhibit DHP binding in a specific (e.g. nitrazepam > diazepam > chlordiazepoxide > RO5-4864) and even stereospecific (e.g., RO 11-6896 > RO 11-6893) manner, but the order of potency of a series of compounds (e.g., diazepam > clonazepam, flunitrazepam) did not agree with potency (27) in either high-affinity [³H] benzodiazepine binding (17, 18) or in anxiolytic, anticonvulsant, or muscle relaxant activity (147). The inhibition of DHP binding by benzodiazepines could still represent a direct or allosteric effect of a pharmacologically relevant subpopulation of benzodiazepine binding sites, but the [³H] DHP binding sites appear distinct from the high-affinity [³H] benzodiazepine binding sites described below.

C. Benzodiazepine binding

[³H] Diazepam binds to high affinity sites (K_D = 4 nM, $B_{max} \cong$ 1 pmol/mg membrane protein) in mammalian brain showing á chemical specificity correlating with the activity of a series of benzodiazepines as CNS depressant agents with anxiolytic, anticonvulsant, sedative-hypnotic, and muscle relaxant actions (17, 18, 148). Further evidence that these binding sites mediate the psychopharmacological effects of the benzodiazepines is provided by specific *in vivo* binding which correlates with drug action (149-150), and modification of this binding as expected by drug treatment, lesions, seizures, and mutations which modify CNS activity

(151-160) (see ref. (16) for a review of this topic). The specificity of benzodiazepine receptor binding also correlates well with potentiation of GABA *in vivo* (161).

Benzodiazepine binding sites appear to be localized in neurons (151, 162) according to a brain regional distribution similar to but not identical to that of GABA and DHP binding sites (27, 151-154, 163). The same sites can be labeled with the higher affinity (K_D = 0.5 nM) ligand [³H] flunitrazepam (164), which also has photoaffinity label activity, binding irreversibly to the receptor protein following irradiation by ultraviolet light (162). This binding protein has a molecular weight of about 50 000 as determined by polyacrylamide gel electrophoresis in sodium dodecylsulfate (162); further study by another group has indicated that multiple peptides in the 50-60 000 molecular weight range are labeled by this photoaffinity label in some brain regions (165).

[³H] Diazepam or flunitrazepam binding, as already described, is inhibited potently by pharmacologically active benzodiazepines, but by very few other drugs. One important exception is the triazolopyridazine class of anxiolytic drugs such as CL218, 872, which potently inhibit benzodiazepine binding (166). The anticonvulsant diphenylhydantoin is a weak inhibitor ($\cong$ 200 μM) of benzodiazepine binding (M. Karobath, unpublished), as is the convulsant, pentylenetetrazole (167), and the minor tranquilizer, meprobamate (R. W. Olsen, unpublished). It is not yet known whether these interactions are pharmacologically relevant.

A similarity between DHP binding sites and benzodiazepine binding sites exists, and that is the inhibition of both by purines and related endogenous brain substances. The existence of high affinity binding sites in brain for exogenous compounds like the benzodiazepines and picrotoxin-related convulsants suggests that previously unidentified endogenous ligands may exist for these receptors, in analogy to the opioid peptides found in brain which appear to be the endogenous ligands for morphine receptors (168). The search for endogenous benzodiazepine receptor ligands has revealed a weak inhibition ($\cong$ 0.1 mM) by various purines and related substances, including inosine, hypoxanthine (167, 169), related purines (170), and nicotinamide (171). DHP binding is likewise inhibited by naturally occurring purines (e.g., adenine, hypoxanthine at 0.1 mM), and their meta-bolites (e.g., allantoin, uric acid) and pyrimidines (e.g., cytosine at 0.1 mM) (29, 172). Note that these molecules are chemical analogues of the exogenous CNS active agents, the barbiturates and diphenyl-hydantoin. It is possible that one of these natural substances or a related substance may be an endogenous CNS depressant or excitatory substance. DHP binding is inhibited by crude extracts of brain (172), and other endogenous inhibitors of benzodiazepine binding have been isolated, including β-carbolines (173) (metabolites of tryptophan including the excitatory drugs, harmaline and harmane), and some peptides (138, 174). Indeed, whereas one receptor site for exogenous drugs which modulate the action of GABA receptor-ionophores might reasonably be expected, two such sites hardly seems likely, and one might therefore conclude that there is a good possibility of finding an endogenous ligand for either the benzodiazepine receptors and/or for the picrotoxinin/-barbiturate receptors.

D. Receptor interactions

Early studies on GABA receptor binding found no perturbations by drugs thought to act on the receptor-ionophore complex, neither by picrotoxinin (2, 11, 22), nor by barbiturates (2), nor by benzodiazepines (21, 22). Likewise, DHP binding was not perturbed by GABA receptor ligands (2, 24), nor significantly inhibited by chloride ions (24, 25).

An interesting study of anion effects on GABA receptors (136) revealed that although GABA agonist binding was not very sensitive to ions, the affinity of the antagonist bicuculline was dramatically enhanced by certain anions, an effect also observed with radioactive bicuculline methiodide binding (135). Examination of the anion specificity of this effect reveals a striking similarity in those anions able to enhance bicuculline binding affinity (135, 136) and those able to permeate the ion channels involved in spinal cord postsynaptic inhibitory potentials (175), now considered to be GABAergic (72). This observation strongly suggests that the bicuculline binding site (GABA receptor?) is coupled to chloride channels; anion ligands for the channels cause allosteric perturbations of bicuculline binding. This same anion

specificity now appears to govern many of the interactions between components of the GABA receptor-ionophore complex. Nevertheless, in earlier work the importance of the physiological ions (chloride) to the assays was not fully appreciated, and most GABA binding was done in the sodium-free buffer Tris-citrate (3), which also happened to lack chloride ions.

Benzodiazepine receptor binding affinity is enhanced by the same anions (19, 176), suggesting a coupling of these binding sites to the chloride ion channels involved in GABA-mediated postsynaptic inhibitory potentials. Consistent with this observation and the neurophysiological evidence for the involvement of GABA in the actions of benzodiazepines, the binding affinity of benzodiazepines is enhanced by GABA and related agonists, and reversed by bicuculline (16, 34, 164, 176–181). Benzodiazepine binding activity was also found to be protected against heat denaturation by GABA receptor ligands and certain anions (182). Although some GABA agonists did not enhance benzodiazepine binding under the usual assay conditions at 0 °C (183, 184), these 'inactive' analogues could reverse the enhancement caused by GABA and the active analogues (185); other analogues acted as 'partial agonists' in this regard, enhancing benzodiazepine binding to a lower maximal extent than GABA and thus able to partly inhibit the effect of GABA when the 'partial agonist' was present in excess over GABA (185, 186). The relative activities of GABA agonists for enhancing or blocking enhancement of benzodiazepine binding (185) agree with their potency for activating postsynaptic chloride channels (187) or for receptor binding (13—15, 185). However, the effective concentrations are all about five-fold higher than even the lower affinity GABA receptor binding sites, e.g., 1-2 μM GABA is needed for enhancement of benzodiazepine binding (177, 185), compared to 0.1-0.3 μM for the 'low affinity' K_{D2} (121, 122). The concentrations of GABA agonists needed to enhance benzodiazepine binding are lowered slightly by using more physiological conditions (37° and chloride ions (188)), but the discrepancy in apparent affinities for direct binding and the indirect effect on benzodiazepine binding is not yet explained. Perhaps the enhancement involves some nonequilibrium effect; alternatively a low affinity GABA binding site or a low affinity conformational state of the known binding sites might be coupled to benzodiazepine receptors.

GABA binding *in vitro* was enhanced by benzodiazepines in one study (189), but this effect has proved difficult to reproduce (9, 32, 124, 190). Two other preliminary reports of benzodiazepine enhancement of GABA binding suggest that the effect may be very sensitive to the conditions of assay and membrane preparation (32, 191). In particular, an endogenous protein modulator 'GABA-modulin' has been reported to mediate the GABA-benzodiazepine interaction; this modulator is apparently easily washed away or metabolically altered (190) so that the interactions are lost. The well-documented perturbation of benzodiazepine binding by GABA suggests that the opposite effect ought to be observable under appropriate conditions. The protection by GABA of benzodiazepine binding activity during heat inactivation (182) has been extended to show a similar GABA protection against inactivation of benzodiazepine binding by the protein reagent iodoacetamide (192). These effects were also observable in the reciprocal direction, with benzodiazepines protecting GABA binding activity from inactivation by the two treatments (192), showing that at least some of the benzodiazepine and GABA binding proteins are at least sometimes physically coupled in the membranes.

The same group further demonstrated that the enhancement of benzodiazepine binding by GABA was retained by detergent-solubilized preparations (192, 193), a result now confirmed by several workers (190, 194–196) (R. W. Olsen, unpublished). The soluble benzodiazepine and GABA binding activities were also observed to co-migrate on sucrose gradients (196–198) and to be co-purified on a benzodiazepine affinity column (198) showing that at least part of the two binding activities were found together in the same complex, at least under some conditions. Under other conditions, benzodiazepine binding activity free of GABA binding (199–202) and GABA binding activity free of benzodiazepine binding (122, 203) have also apparently been observed.

Benzodiazepine binding in membranes is also enhanced in affinity by another class of drugs which are not GABA receptor ligands, the anxiolytic pyrazolopyridines, e.g., etazolate, or SQ 20 009 (33, 34). This effect is dependent on chloride ions and reversed by picrotoxin (40).

This latter observation was the first report of an interaction between picrotoxin and the benzodiazepine receptor, and therefore, indirectly, with the GABA receptor, since benzodiazepine and GABA receptors are coupled, at least in part. Studies in our laboratory have shown that this interaction with benzodiazepine receptors by etazolate occurs at the picrotoxinin/barbiturate receptor site (26, 39). Etazolate and analogues competitively inhibit [^{3}H] DHP binding at concentrations similar to those effective in enhancing benzodiazepine binding (1–10 μM); picrotoxinin competitively inhibits the etazolate enhancement of benzodiazepine binding at concentrations similar to the binding affinity ($\cong$ 1 μM) for the picrotoxin receptor sites (26, 39) (Leeb-Lundberg, Snowman & Olsen, unpublished).

Interactions with benzodiazepine receptor binding were also observed for the other drugs previously described to inhibit [^{3}H] DHP sites. Convulsants such as isopropylbicyclophosphate, tetramethylene disulfotetramine, and the benzodiazepine RO5-3663 act like picrotoxin to block the enhancement by etazolate of benzodiazepine binding (26, 39). Depressants like anesthetic/hypnotic barbiturates act like etazolate to enhance benzodiazepine binding (36, 39). This effect occurs at concentrations similar to those inhibiting [^{3}H] DHP binding (e.g., 0.1 mM for pentobarbital) and is competitively inhibited by micromolar picrotoxinin (36). This *in vitro* effect appears to involve a pharmacologically relevant barbiturate receptor site, since the relative potency of a series of barbiturates ((−) DMBB > secobarbital > pentobarbital > hexobarbital > phenobarbital) to enhance benzodiazepine binding correlated highly with both anesthetic activity (204) and with potency in reversing synaptic antagonists of GABA action (55, 99). Furthermore, this enhancement is dependent on the presence of anions such as chloride, and only those anions which permeate GABA-regulated ionophores (175), as described above for bicuculline binding (135) and baseline benzodiazepine binding (19, 176). These barbiturate effects on binding assays appear relevant to the electrophysiological measurements of barbiturate enhancement of chloride conductance activated by GABA (60, 90, 91). A recent report demonstrated that ethanol (20 mM) can also enhance benzodiazepine binding in a picrotoxin-sensitive manner (205).

The action of pentobarbital on benzodiazepine

binding is not additive with the effect of etazolate, both reaching a common maximal effect, consistent with action at a common, picrotoxin binding site (39). On the other hand the action of just maximal etazolate or pentobarbital on benzodiazepine binding is additive with the effect of GABA (39), (Leeb-Lundberg *et al.* unpublished) consistent with action at two different sites. The barbiturate and etazolate effects occur in the absence of GABA and do not appear to be mediated by GABA receptors since they are not blocked by GABA analogues such as THIP, imidazole acetate, or piperidine-4-sulfonate (38, 39), (Leeb-Lundberg *et al.* unpublished), which reverse GABA enhancement of benzodiazepine binding (185, 186). Barbiturate and etazolate enhancement are, however, at least partially inhibited by submicromolar concentrations of the GABA antagonist bicuculline (Leeb-Lundberg *et al.*, unpublished) and the mechanism of this apparently allosteric interaction merits investigation.

A less than perfect correlation was obtained between IC_{50} values for barbiturate reversal of [³H] DHP binding (2, 28) and EC_{50} values for enhancement of benzodiazepine binding (36). The picrotoxin reversal of the latter shows that the barbiturate receptor site involved is a picrotoxinin binding site. Since the displacement of [³H] DHP binding by some drugs indicate a likely heterogeneity in DHP binding sites (27–29), it is likely that the population of sites involved in allosteric coupling to benzodiazepine receptors is a subpopulation of the total DHP binding sites. The nature of the other DHP binding sites is not yet known and their identification will require further studies.

Another question in the barbiturate-benzodiazepine receptor interactions involves the convulsant barbiturates, such as (+) DMBB and CHEB, already mentioned as potent inhibitors of [³H] DHP binding (2, 28). These compounds and a few other barbiturates such as (+) pentobarbital do have depressant activity at high doses and/or long times of application, but also cause 'preanesthetic excitation' and direct stimulation of neurons at lower doses and/or earlier times (72, 206). The inhibition of [³H] DHP binding (212) and the enhancement of GABA (31) and benzodiazepine (36) binding by barbiturates is stereospecific. Our current studies are aimed at determining whether qualitative or quantitative differences between bar-

biturates having different pharmacological actions can be observed with respect to interactions with the GABA receptor-ionophore complex.

Anticonvulsant barbiturates and some nonbarbiturates such as carbamazepine, diphenylhydantoin, and chlormethiazole also inhibit [³H] DHP binding but do not enhance quilibrium benzodiazepine binding (146). Some weak sedative-hypnotic barbiturates seem to enhance benzodiazepine binding but to a lower maximal effect than the more potent compounds like pentobarbital (although solubility limits in some cases prevent the measurement of full dose-response curves). These weak or inactive enhancing agents can, however, by virtue of competing for the picrotoxinin/barbiturate receptor sites, lower the enhancement of benzodiazepine binding by the more potent compounds such as pentobarbital (146) (Leeb-Lundberg & Olsen, unpublished). Thus some anticonvulsants interact with this barbiturate receptor in a qualitatively different manner from the anesthetic-hypnotic barbiturates; current studies seek to determine whether this *in vitro* effect can be related to anticonvulsant drug action in cells and *in vivo*. Further evidence for the role of this barbiturate/picrotoxinin receptor in the GABA receptor-ionophore is provided by recent observations of effects on GABA binding by ligands which bind to the barbiturate/picrotoxinin sites. As mentioned previously, barbiturates do not perturb GABA binding to well-washed membranes assayed at 0° in sodium and chloride free media (2). The first report of an interaction of GABA receptors and picrotoxinin/barbiturate receptors was the demonstration that etazolate (now shown to act via the barbiturate/picrotoxinin site (26, 39)) could potentiate the GABA enhancement of benzodiazepine binding and reciprocally, GABA could enhance the etazolate enhancement of benzodiazepine binding (38, 207). These interactions appeared to be dependent on the presence of chloride ions (38, 40). This was followed by a report that the convulsant benzodiazepine RO5-3663 (a DHP site ligand (27, 29)) reversed the enhancement by GABA of benzodiazepine binding (35), an effect also seen for picrotoxin and isopropyl bicyclophosphate at 37° in chloride containing buffer (208). Barbiturates were also observed to potentiate the GABA enhancement of benzodiazepine binding (37) (in addition to the enhancement of baseline benzodiazepine binding (36)). A more dramatic result supporting coupling between the GABA and barbiturate receptors was the observation of an increase in B_{max} for GABA receptor binding *in vitro* in the presence of etazolate and chloride ions.

Barbiturates were recently reported to enhance GABA receptor binding (32); this effect was observed only part of the time and only with membranes which had been prepared by very gentle techniques, involving no osmotic shock, no sonic disruption, no freeze-thaw steps, and no detergent (32), suggesting that the barbiturate receptor and/or its coupling to the GABA receptor was a rather fragile entity.

We have now observed reproducible enhancement by barbiturates of GABA receptor binding (31) (Olsen & Snowman, unpublished). Since the membrane preparation used by Johnston & Willow (32) may contain residual endogenous GABA, we have employed more rigorously washed membranes, either the freeze-thaw, thoroughly disrupted and washed bovine cortex membranes we routinely employ for GABA receptor binding (8, 9), or osmotically shocked and dialyzed fresh rat brain membranes. Barbiturate enhancement was observed only in chloride-containing media (31). Indeed, the anion specificity and barbiturate potency profile (31) (Olsen & Snowman, unpublished) were identical to that which we found for barbiturate enhancement of benzodiazepine binding (36), demonstrating that the same barbiturate-/picrotoxinin receptor is involved and this receptor is coupled to GABA receptors.

The effect of barbiturates on GABA receptor binding in chloride solutions involves a greater than 100% enhancement in some brain regions, but the relative enhancement varies with brain region, indicating a variation in coupling between the two types of drug receptor. Barbiturate enhancement can be observed with various ligands, [³H] GABA, [³H] muscimol, [³H] isoguvacine, or [³H] piperidine-4-sulfonic acid (Olsen & Snowman, unpublished). Scatchard plots suggest an increase in the apparent number of sites B_{max} rather than a change in affinity (31), although an increase in affinity for a class of binding sites with normally undetectably low affinity is probably involved. This hypothetical low affinity class of GABA receptors may be relevant to some of the other receptor interactions such as those of GABA-benzodiazepine described above.

Thus there are three classes of drug receptors related to GABA action on chloride ion channels – receptors for GABA, benzodiazepines, and barbiturates. By virtue of *in vitro* allosteric interactions between these three receptors they appear to be coupled in a protein complex situated in the postsynaptic membrane. Fig. 1 describes a model for the GABA receptor-ionophore complex incorporating the three classes of drug receptors (those for GABA, picrotoxinin/barbiturates, and benzodiazepines) which control the GABA-activated chloride channels.

Conclusions

Table 1 summarizes observations regarding the interactions of various convulsant and anticonvulsant drugs with the GABA system, especially the binding studies with the various components of the GABA receptor-ionophore complex. Each item has been discussed in the previous section, and references are given there as well as in the table.

The drugs are divided into two major categories: I. depressants, and II. excitants. Within each category the drugs are grouped as GABA-related (category I or II), barbiturate-related (category I), picrotoxin-related (category II) or benzodiazepine-related (category I).

In category IA are listed GABA and three agonist analogues, muscimol, THIP, and 3-aminopropane sulfonic acid (as representatives of this class). Their success as anticonvulsants appears to depend on how well they can cross the blood-brain barrier. Cetyl-GABA and Progabamide are examples of hydrophobic GABA analogues synthesized with the objective of obtaining compounds which penetrate the brain. DABA and nipecotic acid are examples of GABA uptake inhibitors, with clinical use, however, again limited by penetration of the brain. Baclofen, or lioresal, is not very active on the best characterized GABA synapses (209) and appears to have more potent actions via presynaptic inhibition involving a unique class of GABA receptors showing a pharmacology different from those GABA receptors discussed here (210). The last five compounds: amino oxyacetic acid, gabaculine, γ-vinyl GABA, γ-acetylenic GABA, and valproic acid, are reportedly inhibitors of the GABA degradative enzyme, GABA transaminase; these drugs show variable success with respect to both raising brain GABA levels and anticonvulsant activity. The action of valproic acid may also involve postsynaptic potentiation of GABA action by an unknown mechanism.

In category IB are listed the benzodiazepines and other drugs with possible benzodiazepine-like CNS depressant activity. Representative examples of benzodiazepines are diazepam, chlordiazepoxide, flunitrazepam and clonazepam. CL218, 872 is an example of a triazolopyridazine type of minor tranquilizer, which inhibits high affinity benzodiazepine receptor binding. Meprobamate may also act at this site (unpublished). The other four entries are examples of naturally-occurring substances which inhibit benzodiazepine receptor binding with nanomolar affinities (β-carboline carboxylate ethyl ester) to millimolar affinities (nicotinamide and various purines, such as hypoxanthine and adenosine). These compounds have some CNS depressant activities (171, 211), although some analogues might also possess excitatory activity (213).

Category IC contains the barbiturates and substances of related pharmacological activity, roughly speaking. Pentobarbital and related anesthetic-hypnotics inhibit DHP binding and allosterically enhance benzodiazepine and GABA receptor binding in a chloride-dependent and picrotoxin-sensitive manner. This property is shared by the pyrazolopyridine anxiolytics such as etazolate, cartazolate, and tracazolate (191). These compounds share some but not all of the pharmacological profile of benzodiazepines and barbiturates. They are not yet well characterized regarding their potential for enhancing GABA-activated chloride conductance. Another compound which seems to share the properties of pentobarbital in perturbing the GABA receptor-ionophore system, albeit rather weakly, is ethanol. It will be interesting to see how relevant these effects on the GABA system are to the complex action of this widely used drug. The anticonvulsants such as phenobarbital (and related barbiturates), chlormethiazole, and carbamazepine inhibit DHP binding but do not enhance benzodiazepine binding or GABA binding. Since the anticonvulsants bind to the same receptor site as the anesthetic-hypnotics, they can actually reverse the enhancement by pentobarbital of the other two receptors. Diphenylhydantoin may fit into this category as well, since it inhibits DHP binding (at 10^{-4} M) without enhancing the other receptors; it

also inhibits benzodiazepine binding at 3×10^{-4} M. Two other substances which are likely to act on this system in a manner resembling phenobarbital and/or diphenylhydantoin are ethosuximide and trimethadione, which have similar chemical structures and pharmacological action. These compounds have yet to be tested on the *in vitro* system. Valproic acid is a weak inhibitor of DHP binding and does not enhance the binding of benzodiazepines or GABA, so it may also affect the GABA system in a manner similar to phenobarbital. Nevertheless, it is difficult to determine the relevance to *in vivo* drug action for these rather weak *in vitro* interactions.

Finally, there are naturally occurring substances such as allantoin, hypoxanthine and related purines (adenine, uric acid) and pyrimidines (cytosine) which inhibit DHP binding. As in the case of the putative endogenous inhibitors of benzodiazepine binding, further pharmacological studies on these natural substances may shed light on their relevance to the action and regulation of GABAergic synapses.

In category IIA are listed excitatory agents related to GABA. Bicuculline is considered the classical antagonist of GABA synapses and inhibits GABA receptor binding. Its affinity is enhanced by anions able to permeate the GABA ionophore. Strychnine is considered the classical glycine antagonist but also has a weak affinity (10 μM) for the bicuculline site (compared to 10 nM for glycine-sensitive strychnine binding sites). Benzyl penicillin blocks GABA synaptic responses and inhibits both GABA binding and DHP binding with an IC_{50} of 100 μM, with the latter site possibly the most directly involved.

Also in category IIA are compounds which specifically or nonspecifically inhibit GABA synthesis at the level of L-glutamic acid decarboxylase: mercaptopropionic acid, allylglycine, and the hydrazides. Likewise included is the bacterial protein exotoxin produced by *Clostridium tetani*; tetanus toxin inhibits nonspecifically the release of neurotransmitter GABA from nerve endings.

In category IIB are compounds which block GABA stimulated chloride conductance at sites other than the GABA receptor. The classic example is picrotoxinin (a small molecular weight non-nitrogenous plant substance with convulsant activity), related naturally occurring analogues such as tutin, and the reduced analogue, α-dihydropicrotoxinin, which we have employed as a radioactive probe ($[^3H]$ DHP) of the drug receptor site mediating the action of picrotoxinin.

Other excitatory agents behaving like picrotoxinin in this system and binding potently ($\leqslant 1 \mu M$) to DHP sites include the 'convulsant' barbiturates such as DMBB and CHEB, the convulsant cage compounds such as isopropyl bicyclophosphate and tetramethylene disulfotetramine (TETS), and the 'convulsant' benzodiazepine, RO5-3663.

Pentylenetetrazole has some affinity ($\cong 10 \mu M$) for the $[^3H]$ DHP binding sites and may also act via this system, although another site of action for this convulsant with greater affinity is also a good possibility. Pentylenetetrazol also inhibits benzodiazepine binding weakly ($100 \mu M$), so these *in vitro* interactions with the GABA system may not be coincidental. Pentylenetetrazol is the only excitatory agent reported to inhibit benzodiazepine binding, although endogenous ligands such as β-carbolines, purines, and peptides might be excitatory. Another excitatory agent which has not yet been examined in this sytem is bemegride. Because of its structural similarities to barbiturates, this compound might very likely act at the picrotoxinin/barbiturate receptor sites.

The table shows that at least 50 substances with convulsant and anticonvulsant activity have been linked to the neurotransmitter GABA. Although the evidence for this link is certainly not compelling for all the compounds listed, the link is firmly established for many of them and makes the relationship of the others to GABA reasonable and certainly worth further study. The inescapable conclusion is that GABA synapses are relevant to seizure disorders. Hopefully, these clues to the disease process and treatment will provide rapid new developments regarding this important clinical problem.

Acknowledgement

The time involved in preparation of this review was supported by a Research Career Development Award (#NS 00224 from the National Institutes of Neurological, Communicative Disorders, and Stroke).

References

1. Meldrum, B., 1979. In: GABA-Neurotransmitters (Krogsgaard-Larsen, P., Scheel-Kruger, J. & Kofod, H., eds.), pp. 390–405, Munksgaard, Copenhagen.
2. Olsen, R. W., Ticku, M. K., Greenlee, D. & Van Ness, P., 1979. In: GABA-Neurotransmitters (Krogsgaard-Larsen, P., Scheel-Kruger, J. & Kofod, H., eds.), pp. 165–178, Munksgaard, Copenhagen.
3. Enna, S. J. & Snyder, S. H., 1975. Brain Res. 100: 81–97.
4. Nistri, A., Constanti, A. & Krnjević, K., 1980. In: Receptors for Neurotransmitters and Peptide Hormones (Pepeu, G., Kuhar, M. J. & Enna, S. J., eds.), Adv. Biochem. Psychopharmacol. Vol. 21, pp. 81–90, Raven Press, New York.
5. Curtis, D. R., 1979. In: GABA-Neurotransmitters (Krogsgaard-Larsen, P., Scheel-Kruger, J. & Kofod, H., eds.) pp. 17–27, Munksgaard, Copenhagen.
6. McBurney, R. N. & Barker, J. L., 1978. Nature 274: 596–597.
7. Zukin, S. R., Young, A. B. & Snyder, S. H., 1974. Proc. Natl. Acad. Sci. USA 71: 4802–4807.
8. Greenlee, D. V., Van Ness, P. C. & Olsen, R. W., 1978. Life Sci. 22: 1653–1662.
9. Napias, C., Bergman, M. O., Van Ness, P. C., Greenlee, D. V. & Olsen, R. W., 1980. Life Sci. 27: 1001–1011.
10. Coyle, J. T. & Enna, S. J., 1976. Brain Res. 111: 119–133.
11. Olsen, R. W., Greenlee, D., Van Ness, P. & Ticku, M. K., 1978. In: Amino Acids as Chemical Transmitters (Fonnum, F., ed.), pp. 467–486, Plenum Press, New York.
12. Olsen, R. W. & Mikoshiba, K., 1978. J. Neurochem. 30: 1633–1636.
13. Greenlee, D. V., Van Ness, P. C. & Olsen, R. W., 1978. J. Neurochem. 31: 933–938.
14. Enna, S. J., Ferkany, J. W. & Krogsgaard-Larsen, P., 1979. In GABA-Neurotransmitters (Krogsgaard-Larsen, P., Scheel-Kruger, J. & Kofod, H., eds.) pp. 191–200, Munksgaard, Copenhagen.
15. Krogsgaard-Larsen, P., Hjeds, H., Curtis, D. R., Lodge, D. & Johnston, G. A. R., 1979. J. Neurochem. 32: 1717–1724.
16. Tallman, J. F., Paul, S. M., Skolnick, P. & Gallager, D. W., 1980. Science 207: 274–281.
17. Squires, R. F. & Braestrup, C., 1977. Nature 266: 732–734.
18. Möhler, H. & Okada, T., 1977. Science 198, 849–851.
19. Costa, T., Rodbard, D. & Pert, C. B., 1979. Nature 277: 315–317.
20. Haefely, W., Polc, P., Schaffner, R., Keller, H. H., Pieri, L. & Möhler, H., 1979. GABA-Neurotransmitters (Krogsgaard-Larsen, P., Scheel-Kruger, J. and Kofod, H., eds.) pp. 357–375, Munksgaard, Copenhagen.
21. Johnston, G. A. R., 1978. Ann. Rev. Pharmacol. Toxicol. 18: 269–289.
22. Olsen, R. W., Ticku, M. K., Van Ness, P. C. & Greenlee, D., 1978. Brain Res. 139, 277–294.
23. Olsen, R. W., Ticku, M. K. & Miller, T., 1978. Mol. Pharmacol. 14, 381–390.
24. Ticku, M. K. Ban, M. and Olsen, R. W., 1978. Mol. Pharmacol. 14: 391–402.

25. Ticku, M. K., Van Ness, P. C. Haycock, J. W., Levy, W. B. & Olsen, R. W., 1978. Brain Res 150: 642–647.

26. Leeb-Lundberg, F. & Olsen, R. W., 1980. In: Psychopharmacology and Biochemistry of Neurotransmitter Receptors (Yamamura, H. I., Olsen, R. W. & Usdin, E., eds.) pp. 593–606, Elsevier, New York.

27. Leeb-Lundberg, F., Napias, C. & Olsen, R. W., 1981. Brain Res., in the press.

28. Ticku, M. K. & Olsen, R. W., 1978. Life Sci. 22: 1643–1651.

29. Olsen, R. W., Leeb-Lundberg, F. & Napias, C., 1980. Brain Res. Bull. 5, Suppl. 2: 217–221.

30. Placheta, P. & Karobath, M., 1980. Eur. J. Pharmacol. 62: 225–228.

31. Olsen, R. W., Snowman, A. & Leeb-Lundberg, F., 1981. Fed. Proc. Abstracts, in press.

32. Johnston, G. A. R. & Willow, M., 1981. In: GABA and Benzodiazepine Receptors (Costa, E., DiChiara, G. & Gessa, G., eds.) Adv. Biochem. Psychopharmacol. Vol. 26, pp. 191–198, Raven Press, New York.

33. Beer, B., Klepner, C. A., Lippa A. S. & Squires, R. F., 1978. Pharmacol. Biochem. Behav. 9: 849–851.

34. Williams, M. & Risley, E. A., 1979. Life Sci. 24: 833–841.

35. O'Brien, R. A. & Spirt, N. M., 1980. Life Sci. 26: 1441–1445.

36. Leeb-Lundberg, F., Snowman, A. & Olson, R. W., 1980. Proc. Natl. Acad. Sci. USA, 77: 7468–7472,

37. Skolnick, P., Paul, S. & Barker, J. L., 1980. Eur. J. Pharmacol. 65, 125–127.

38. Sieghart, W., Placheta, P., Supavilai, P. & Karobath, M., 1981. In: GABA and Benzodiazepine Receptors (Costa, E., DiChiara, G. & Gessa, G., eds.) Adv. Biochem. Psychopharmacol. Vol. 26, pp. 121–128, Raven Press, New York.

39. Olsen, R. W. & Leeb-Lundberg, F., 1981. In: GABA and Benzodiazepine Receptors (Costa, E., DiChiara, G. & Gessa, G. eds.) Adv. Biochem. Psychopharmacol. Vol. 26, pp. 93–102, Raven Press, New York.

40. Supavilai, P. & Karobath, M., 1979. Eur. J. Pharmacol. 60, 111–113.

41. Tower, D. B., 1976. In: GABA in Nervous System Function (Roberts, E., Chase, T. N. & Tower, D. B., eds.) pp. 461–478, Raven Press, New York.

42. Horton, R. W., 1980. Br. Res. Bull. 5, Suppl. 2, pp. 605–608.

43. Ribak, C. E., Harris, A. B., Vaughn, J. E. & Roberts, E., 1979. Science 205, 211–214.

44. Barker, J. L., Nicoll, R. A. & Padjen, A., 1975. J. Physiol. 245: 521–548.

45. Macdonald, R. L. & Barker, J. L., 1978. Neurology (Minneapolis) 28: 325–330.

46. Straughan, D. W., 1974. Neuropharmacol. 13: 495–508.

47. Schlosser, W. & Franco, S., 1979. J. Pharmacol. Exp. Ther. 211: 290–295.

48. Geller, H. M., 1979. Neurosci. Lett. 15: 313–318.

49. Bowery, N. G., Collins, J. F. & Hill, R. G., 1976. Nature 261: 601–603.

50. Dray, A., 1975. Neuropharmacol. 14: 703–705.

51. Simmonds, M. A., 1980. Neuropharmacol. 19: 39–45.

52. Goldstein, D. B., 1973. J. Pharmacol. Exp. Thera. 168: 1–9.

53. Cooper, B. R., Viik, K., Ferris, R., & White, H. L., 1980. Br. Res. Bull. 5, Suppl. 2, pp. 815–820.

54. Straughan, D. W., 1978. Adv. Pharmacol. Thera. 2: 19–27.

55. Dray, A. & Bowery, N. G., 1979. In: GABA-Neurotransmitters (Krogsgaard-Larsen, P., Scheel-Kruger, J. & Kofod, H., eds.) pp. 376–389, Raven Press, New York.

56. Enna, S. J. & Maggi, A., 1979. Life Sci. 24: 1727–1738.

57. Bartholini, G., 1980. Br. Res. Bull. 5, Suppl. 2, pp. 487–490.

58. Lippa, A. S., Klepner, C. A., Benson, D. I., Critchett, D. J., Sano M. C. & Beer, B., 1980. Br. Res. Bull. 5, Suppl. 2, pp. 861–866.

59. Haefely, W. E., 1980. Br. Res. Bull. 5, Suppl. 2, pp. 873–878.

60. Macdonald, R. L. & Barker, J. L., 1979. Brain Res. 167: 323–326.

61. Löscher, W. & Frey, H. H., 1979. Naunyn. Schmiedebergs Arch. Pharmacol. 296: 263–269.

62. Metcalf, B. W., 1979. Biochem. Pharmacol. 28: 1705–1712.

63. Enna, S. J., Maggi, A., Worms, P. & Lloyd, K. G., 1980. Muscimol: Br. Res. Bull. 5, Suppl. 2, pp. 461–464.

64. Krogsgaard-Larsen, P., 1980. Mol. Cell. Biochem. 31: 105–121.

65. Meldrum, B., Pedley, T., Horton, R., Anlezark, G. & Franks, A., 1980. Br. Res. Bull. 5, Suppl. 2, pp. 685–690.

66. Frey, H.-H., Popp, C. & Löscher, W., 1979. Neuropharmacology 18: 581–590.

67. Fariello R, G, & Golden G. T., 1980. Br. Res. Bull. 5, Suppl. 2, pp. 691–700.

68. Krogsgaard-Larsen, P., Johnston, G. A. R., Lodge, D. & Curtis, D. R., 1977. Nature 268, 53–54.

69. Meldrum, B. & Horton, R., 1980. Eur. J. Pharmacol 61: 231–237.

70. Frey, H.-H. & Löscher, W., 1980. Neuropharmacol. 19: 217–220.

71. Morselli, P. L., Bossi, L., Henry, J. F., Zarifian, E. & Bartholini, G., 1980. Br. Res. Bull. 5, Suppl. 2, pp. 411–424.

72. Nicoll, R. A. & Wojtowicz, J. M., 1980. Brain Res. 191: 225–237.

73. Hochner, B., Spira, M. E. & Werman, R., 1976. Brain Res. 107: 85–103.

74. Dingledine, R. & Gjerstad, L., 1979. Brain Res. 168: 205–209.

75. Macdonald, R. L. & Barker, J. L., 1977. Nature 267: 720–721.

76. Nicoll, R. A. & Padjen, A., 1976. Neuropharmacol. 15: 69–71.

77. Scholfield, C. N., 1979. Br. J. Pharmacol. 67: 443P–444P.

78. Pellmar, T. C. & Wilson, W. A., 1977. Science 197: 912–913.

79. Downes, H. & Williams, J. K., 1969. J. Pharmacol. Exp. Thera. 168: 283–289.

80. Nestoros, J. N., 1980. Science 209: 708–710.

81. Macdonald, R. L. & Bergey, G. K., 1979. Brain Res. 170: 558–562.

82. Hayashi, T. & Negishi, K., 1979. Brain. Res. 175: 271–278.

83. Geller, H. M., Abstr. Soc. Neurosci. 6: 538 (1980) #184.5.

84. Raabe, W. & Ayala, G. F., 1976. Brain Res. 105: 597–601.

85. Ayala, G. F., Lin, S. & Johnston, D., 1977. Brain Res. 121: 245–258.

86. Deisz, R. A. & Lux, H. D., 1977. Neurosci. Lett. 5, 199–203.

87. Hershkowitz, N. & Ayala, G. F., 1980. Soc. Neurosci. Abstr. 6, 183 (#64.6).

88. Naik, S. R., Naid, P. R. & Sheth, U. K., 1978. Psychopharmacol. 57: 103–107.

89. Davidoff, R. A., J. C. Hackman & V. Grayson. Br. Res. Bull, 5, Suppl. 2, pp. 665–672.

90. Barker, J. L. & McBurney, R. N., 1979. Proc. R. Soc. Lond. 206: 319–327.

91. Ransom, B. R. & Barker, J. L., 1976. Brain Res. 114: 530–535.

92. Evans, R. H., 1979. Brain Res. 171: 113–120.

93. Schlosser, W. & Franco, S., 1980. Neuropharmacol. 18: 377–381.

94. Tsuchiya, T. & Fukushima, H., 1978. Eur. J. Pharmacol 48: 421–424.

95. Brown, D. A. & Constanti, A., 1978. Br. J. Pharmacol. 63: 217–224.

96. Curtis, D. R. & Lodge, D., 1977. Nature 270: 543–544.

97. Lebeda, F. J., Brown, T. H. & Johnston, D., 1980. Soc. Neurosci. Abstr. 6, 183 (#64.8).

98. Nicoll, R. A., Eccles, J. C., Oshima, T. C. & Rubia, F., 1975. Nature 258: 625–627.

99. Bowery, N. G. & Dray, A., 1978. Br. J. Pharmacol. 63: 179–215.

100. Richards, C. D., 1972. J. Physiol. 227: 749–767.

101. Fink, B. R. (ed.), 1980. Molecular Mechanisms of Anesthesia, Progress in Anesthesiology, Vol. 2, Raven Press, New York.

102. Collins, G. G., 1980. Brain Res. 290: 517–528.

103. Potashner, S. J., Lake, N., Langlois, E. A., Plouffe, L. & Lecavalier, D., 1980. Br. Res. Bull. 5, Suppl. 2, pp. 659–665.

104. Costa, E. & Guidotti, A., 1979. Ann. Rev. Pharmacol. Toxicol. 19: 531–545.

105. Sepinwall, J. & Cook, L., 1980. Br. Res. Bull. 5, Suppl. 2, pp. 839–848.

106. Waddington, J. L., 1978. Eur. J. Pharmacol. 51: 417–422.

107. Schmidt, R. F., Vogel, M. E., Zimmermann, M., 1967. Naunyn-Schmiedebergs Archives Pharmacol. 258: 69–82.

108. Dray, A. & Straughan, D. W., 1976. J. Pharm. Pharmacol. 28: 314–315.

109. Curtis, D. R., Lodge, D., Johnston, G. A. R. & Brand, S. J., 1976. Brain Res. 118: 344–347.

110. Raabe, W. & Gumnit, R. J., 1977. Epilepsia 18: 117–120.

111. Nistri, A. & Constanti, A., 1978. Neuropharmacol. 17: 127–135.

112. Simmonds, M. A., 1980. Nature 284: 558–560.

113. Polzin, R. L. & Barness, C. D., 1979. Neuropharmacol. 18: 431–434.

114. Okamoto, K. & Sakai Y., 1979. Br. J. Pharmacol. 65: 277–285.

115. Gallager, D. W., 1978. Eur. J. Pharmacol, 49: 133–143.

116. Zakusov, V. V., Ostrovskaya, R. U., Kozhechkin, S. N., Markovich, V. V., Molodavkin, G. M. & Voronina, T. A., 1977. Arch. Int. Pharmacodyn. Ther. 229: 313–326.

117. Geller, H. M., Hoffer, B. J. & Taylor, D. A., 1980. Fed. Proc. 39: 3016–3023.

118. Montarolo, P. G., Raschi, F. & Strata, P., 1979. Brain Res. 162: 358–362.

119. Macdonald, R. & Barker, J. L., 1978. Nature 271: 563–564.

120. Choi, D. W., Farb, D. H. & Fischbach, G. D., 1979. Nature 269: 342–344.

121. Olsen, R. W., Bergman, M. O., Van Ness, P. C., Lummis, S. C., Watkins, A. E., Napias, C. & Greenlee, D. V., 1981. Mol. Pharmacol. in the press.

122. Olsen, R. W., 1981. In: Psychopharmacology and Biochemistry of Neurotransmitter Receptors (Yamamura, H. I., Olsen, R. W. & Usdin, E., eds.) pp. 537–550, Elsevier, New York.

123. Lloyd, K. G. & Dreksler, S., 1978. In: Amino Acids as Chemical Transmitters (Fonnum, F., ed.) pp. 457–466, Plenum Press, New York.

124. Olsen, R. W., Van Ness, P. C., Napias, C., Bergman, M. & Tourtellotte, W. W., 1980. In: Receptors for Neurotransmitters and Peptide Hormones (Pepeu, G., Kuhar, M. J. & Enna, S. J., eds.) Adv. Biochem. Psychopharmacol. Vol. 21, pp. 451–460, Raven Press, New York.

125. Simantov, R., Oster-Granite, M. L., Herndon, R. M. & Snyder, S. H., 1976. Brain Res. 105, 365–371.

126. Campochiaro, R., Schwarcz, R. & Coyle, J. T., 1977. Brain Res. 136, 501–511.

127. Biggio, G., Corda, M. G., De Montis, G., Stefanini, E. & Gessa, G. L., 1980. Brain Res 193: 589–593.

128. Waddington, J. L. & Cross, A. J., 1980. Br. Res. Bull. 5, Suppl. 2, 825–828.

129. Guidotti, A., Gale, K., Suria, A. & Toffano, G., 1979. Brain Res. 172: 566–571.

130. Enna, S. J., Bennett, J. P., Bylund, D. B., Snyder, S. H., Bird, E. D. & Iversen, L. L., 1976. Brain Res. 116, 531–537.

131. Olsen, R. W., Reisine, T. D. & Yamamura, H. I., 1980. Life Sci. 27, 801–808.

132. Beaumont, K., Chilton, W., Yamamura, H. I. & Enna, S. J., 1978. Brain Res. 148: 153–162.

133. Morin, A. M. & Wasterlain, C., 1980. Life Sci. 26: 1239–1245.

134. Krogsgaard-Larsen, P., Snowman, A., Lummis, S. C. & Olsen, R. W., 1981. J. Neurochem, in the press.

135. Möhler, H. & Okada, T., 1977. Nature 267: 65–67.

136. Enna, S. J. & Snyder, S. H., 1977. Mol. Pharmacol. 13: 442–453.

137. Wong, D. T., Bymaster, F. P. & Lane, P. T., 1980. Br. Res. Bull. 5, Suppl. 2, pp. 853–856.

138. Toffano, G., Guidotti, A. & Costa, E., 1978. Proc. Natl. Acad. Sci. USA 75, 4024–4028.

139. Johnston, G. A. R. & Kennedy, S. M. E., 1978. In: Amino Acids as Chemical Transmitters (Fonnum, F., ed.) pp. 507–516, Plenum Press, New York.

140. Yoneda, Y. & Kuriyama, K., 1980. Nature 285: 670–673.

141. Young, A. B. & Snyder, S. H., 1974. Proc. Nat. Acad. Sci. USA 71: 4002–4005.

142. Goldinger, A. & Müller, W. E., 1980. Neurosci. Lett 16: 91–95.

143. Takeuchi, A. & Takeuchi, N., 1969. J. Physiol. 205: 377–391.

144. Ticku, M. K. & Olsen, R. W., 1977. Biochim. Biophys. Acta 464: 519–529.

145. Ticku, M. K. & Olsen, R. W., 1979. Neuropharmacol. 18: 315–318.

146. Leeb-Lundberg, F., Snowman, A. & Olsen, R. W., 1981. Fed. Prcc. Abstracts, in the press.

147. Randall, L. O., Schallek, W., Sternbach, L. H. & Ning, R. Y., 1974. In: Psychopharmacology Agents III (Gordon, M., ed) pp. 175–281, Academic Press, New York.

148. Paul, S. M., Syapin, P. J., Paugh, B. A., Moncada, A. & Skolnick, P., 1979. Nature 281: 688–689.

149. Mazière, M., Godot, J. M., Berger, G., Baron, J. C., Comar, D., Cepeda, C., Menini, C. & Nauquet, R., 1981. In: GABA and Benzodiazepine Receptors (Costa, E., DiChiara, G. & Gessa, G., eds.) Adv. in Biochem. Psychopharmacol. Vol. 26, pp. 273–286, Raven Press, New York.

150. Duka, T., Hollt, V. & Herz, A., 1979. Brain Res. 179: 147–156.

151. Young, W. S. & Kuhar, M. J., 1979. Nature 280, 393–395.

152. Shibuya, H., Gale, K. & Pert, C. B., 1980. Eur. J. Pharmacol. 62: 243–244.

153. Chang, R. S., Tran, V. T. & Snyder, S. H., 1980. Brain Res. 190: 95–110.

154. Biggio, G., Corda, M. G., Lamberti, C. & Gessa, G. L., 1979. Eur. J. Pharmacol. 58: 215–216.

155. Möhler, H., Okada, T. & Enna, S.J., 1978. Brain Res. 156: 391–395.

156. Gallager, D. W., Thomas, J. W. & Tallman, J. F., 1978. Biochem. Pharmacol. 27: 2745–2749.

157. Gallager, D. W., Mallorga, P. & Tallman, J. F., 1980. Brain Res. 180: 209–220.

158. Speth, R. C., Bresolin, N., Mimaki, T., Deshmukh, P. P. & Yamamura, H. I., 1981. In: GABA and Benzodiazepine Receptors (Costa, E., DiChiara, G. & Gessa, G., eds.) Adv. in Biochem. Psychopharmacol. Vol. 26, pp. 27–39, Raven Press, New York.

159. Paul, S. M. & Skolnick, P., 1978. Science 202: 892–894.

160. McNamara, J. O., Peper, A. M. & Patrone, V., 1980. Proc. Natl. Acad. Sci. USA 77: 3029–3032.

161. Nestoros, J. N., 1980. Br. Res. Bull. 5, Suppl. 2, pp. 849–852.

162. Möhler, H., Battersby, M. K. & Richards, J. G., 1980. Proc. Natl. Acad. Sci. USA 77: 1666–1670.

163. Placheta, P. & Karobath, M., 1979. Brain Res. 178: 580–583.

164. Wastek, G. J., Speth, R. C., Reisine, T. D. & Yamamura, H. I., 1978. Eur. J. Pharmacol. 50: 445–447.

165. Sieghart, W. & Karobath, M., 1980. Nature 286, 285–287.

166. Squires, R. F., Benson, D. I., Braestrup, C., Coupet, J. Klepner, C. A., Myers, V. & Beer, B., 1979. Pharmacol. Biochem. Behav. 10: 825–830.

167. Marangos, P. J., Paul, S. M., Parma, A. M., Goodwin, F. K., Syapin, P. & Skolnick, P., 1979. Life Sci. 24: 851–858.

168. Snyder, S. H. & Childers, S. R., 1979. Ann. Rev. Neurosci. 2: 35–64.

169. Asano, T. & Spector, S., 1979. Proc. Natl. Acad. Sci. USA 76: 977–981.

170. Davies, L. P., Cook, A. F., Poonian, M. & Taylor, K. M., 1980. Life Sci. 26: 1089–1095.

171. Möhler, H., Polc, P., Cumin, R., Pieri, L. & Kettler, R., 1979. Nature 278: 563–565.

172. Olsen, R. W. & Leeb-Lundberg, F., 1980. Eur. J. Pharmacol. 65: 101–104.

173. Braestrup, C., Nielsen, M. & Olsen, C. E., 1980. Proc. Natl. Acad. Sci. USA 77: 2288–2292.

174. Davis, L. G. & Cohen, R. K., 1980. Biochem. Biophys. Res. Comm. 92: 141–148.

175. Araki, T., Ito, M. & Oscarsson, O., 1961. J. Physiol. 159: 410–435.

176. Martin, I. L. & Candy, J. M., 1980. Neuropharmacol. 19: 175–179.

177. Tallman, J. F., Thomas, J. W. & Gallager, D. W., 1978. Nature 274: 383–385.

178. Karobath, M. & Sperk, G., 1979. Proc. Natl. Acad. Sci. USA 76: 1004–1006.

179. Briley, M. S. & Langer, S. Z., 1978. Eur. J. Pharmacol. 52: 129–132.

180. Chiu, T. H. & Rosenberg, H. C., 1979. Eur. J. Pharmacol. 56: 337–345.

181. Dudai, Y., 1979. Brain Res. 167: 422–425.

182. Squires, R. F., 1981. In: GABA and Benzodiazepine Receptors (Costa, E., DiChiara, G. & Gessa, G., eds.) Adv. Biochem. Psychopharmacol. Vol. 26, pp. 129–138, Raven Press, New York.

183. Maurer, R., 1979. Neurosci. Lett. 12: 65–68.

184. Karobath, M., Placheta, P., Lippitsch, M. & Krogsgaard-Larsen, P., 1979. Nature 278: 748–749.

185. Braestrup, C., Nielsen, M., Krogsgaard-Larsen, P. & Falch, E., 1979. Nature 280: 331–333.

186. Karobath, M. & Lippitsch, M., 1979. Eur. J. Pharmacol. 58: 485–488.

187. Barker, J. L. & Mathers, D. A., 1980. Soc. Neurosci. Abstr. 6, 189 (#67.2).

188. Supavilai, P. & Karobath, M., 1980. Neurosci. Lett. 19: 337–341.

189. Guidotti, A., Toffano, G., Baraldi, M., Schwartz, J. P. & Costa, E., 1979. In: GABA-Neurotransmitters (Krogsgaard-Larsen, P., Scheel-Kruger, J. & Kofod, H., eds.) pp. 406–415, Munksgaard, Copenhagen.

190. Massotti, M., Guidotti, A. & Costa, E., 1981. In: GABA and Benzodiazepine Receptors (Costa, E., DiChiara, G. & Gessa, G., eds.) Adv. Biochem. Psychopharmacol. Vol. 26, pp. 19–26, Raven Press, New York.

191. Meiners, B. A. & Salama, A. I., 1980. Soc. Neurosci. Abstr. 6, 189 (#67.4).

192. Gavish, M. & Snyder, S. H., 1980. Nature 287: 651–652.

193. Gavish, M. & Snyder, S. H., 1980. Life Sci. 26: 579–582.

194. Sherman-Gold, R. & Dudai, Y., 1980. Brain Res. 198: 485–490.

195. Fong, J. & Goldstein, M., 1980. Soc. Neurosci. Abstr. 6, 255 (#94.13).

196. Asano, T. & Ogasawara, N., 1980. Life Sci. 26: 607–613.

197. Asano, T. & Ogasawara, N., 1980. Life Sci. 26: 1131–1137.

198. Gavish, M. & Snyder, S. H., 1980. Soc. Neurosci. Abstr. 6, 236 (#89.2).

199. Yousufi, M. A. K., Thomas, J. W. & Tallman, J. F., 1979. Life Sci. 25: 463–470.

200. Lang, B., Barnard, E. A., Chang, L. R. & Dolly, J. O., 1979. FEBS Lett. 104: 149–153.

201. Bymaster, F. P. & Wong, D. T., 1980. Soc. Neurosci. Abstr. 6, 252 (#94.3).

202. Chiu, T. H. & Rosenberg, H. C., 1980. Fed. Proc. 39, 1006 (Abstr. #3889).

203. Greenlee, D. V. & Olsen, R. W., 1979. Biochem. Biophys, Res. Comm. 88: 380–387.

204. Butler, T. C., 1942. J. Pharmacol. 74: 118–128.

205. Burch, T. & Ticku, M. K., 1980. Eur. J. Pharmacol. 67: 325–326.

206. Huang, L.-Y. and Barker, J. L., 1980. Science 207: 195–197.
207. Supavilai, P. & Karobath, M., 1980. Eur. J. Pharmacol. 62: 229–233.
208. Karobath, M., Drexler, G. & Supavilai, P., 1981. Life Sci. 28: 307–313.
209. Waddington, J. L. & Cross, A. J., 1980. Br. Res. Bull. 5, Suppl. 2: 503–505.
210. Bowery, N. G., Hill, D. R., Hudson, A. L., Doble, A., Middlemiss, D. N., Shaw, J. & Turnbull, M., 1980. Nature 283: 92–94.
211. Skolnick, P., Syapin, P. J., Paugh, B. A., Moncada, V., Marangos, P. J. & Paul, S. M., (1979) Proc. Natl. Acad. Sci. USA 76: 1515–1518.
212. Ticku, M. K., 1980. Brain Res. Bull. 5: 919–923.
213. Tenen, S. S. & Hirsch, J. D., 1980. Nature 288, 609–610.
214. Ticku, M. K. & Burch, T., 1980. Biochem. Pharmacol. 29: 1217–1220.

Received December 23, 1980.

The stimulation of ion fluxes in brain slices by glutamate and other excitatory amino acids

Vivian I. Teichberg, Ora Goldberg* and Alberto Luini
Depts. of Neurobiology and Organic Chemistry, The Weizmann Institute of Science, Rehovot, Israel

Summary

The stimulation of ion movements by excitatory amino acids in brain slices allows the study of various events related to the process of excitatory neurotransmission. Presynaptic mechanisms of uptake of putative neurotransmitters can be followed by the influx of Na^+ ions. Postsynaptic depolarizations due to the activation of action potentials or of ionophores associated with specific receptors can be monitored by measurements of the rate of efflux of radioactive tracer ions. Thus, the pharmacological properties of the excitatory amino acid receptors can be investigated as well as those of their putative endogenous effectors.

Introduction

The ability of glutamate to increase ion movements in brain was first noticed in 1950 by Terner *et al.* (1) who reported that the addition of L-glutamate to sliced brain tissue increases the K^+ content. These investigators were, however, unable to provide an explanation to this phenomenon. Four years later, it was observed by Hayashi (2) that injection of the brain metabolites L-glutamate and L-aspartate into various regions of the brain caused convulsions. On the basis of this observation Hayashi proposed that glutamate might have, in addition to its role in cerebral metabolism, a modulating role in brain excitability. Unaware of these results, Curtis *et al.* (3) found in 1960 that L-glutamate, iontophoretically applied on cortical neurones, produced an excitatory effect, manifested by a depolarization of the neuronal membrane (4). The decrease in membrane potential, following glutamate application to neurones, was interpreted as due to alterations in membrane permeability to the ions K^+, Na^+ and Cl^-, or to some of them (5). From measurements of Na^+ and K^+ levels in cortical slices exposed to glutamate, Bradford &

McIlwain (6), calculated that glutamate brings about a fivefold increase in the permeability of the tissue to Na^+, relative to K^+ (6). Following these pioneering studies, the effects of glutamate on brain tissue were extensively investigated, mainly by electrophysiological techniques. Several aspects of the glutamate problem were thus clarified, yet the precise role of this amino acid in brain function remains to be elucidated.

The purpose of this article is to review the contributions of studies of glutamate-stimulated ion movements in brain slices to the understanding of the neuronal excitatory actions of glutamate and other acidic amino acids.

I. Na^+ dependent uptake of glutamate

The assignment to glutamate of a putative role in excitatory neurotransmission requires the fulfilment of a series of criteria for its identification as a genuine neurotransmitter. Among these, the existence of mechanisms of degradation or uptake of glutamate needs to be established, in order to account for the inactivation of the neurotransmitter

Molecular and Cellular Biochemistry 39, 281–295 (1981). 0300-8177/81/0391-0281/$03.00.

released in the synaptic cleft. Bennet *et al.* (7) investigated this question using synaptosomal preparations of cerebral cortex and spinal cord. They incubated synaptosomes in the presence of 10^{-5} M and 10^{-3} M glutamate and studied the accumulation of this amino acid with respect to ionic requirements, metabolic inhibitors, structural analogues and ontogeny. An uptake of glutamate was shown to take place via two systems operating at different glutamate concentrations. The low affinity uptake has a large capacity and transports 200 mmole of glutamate per gram tissue per minute at 37 °C with a K_m of 1.2×10^{-3} M. The high affinity uptake has a relatively small capacity and transports only 50 mmole of glutamate per gram tissue per minute with a K_m of 3.3×10^{-5} M. A third uptake system of a very high affinity for glutamate ($K_m = 2 \mu$M) has recently been identified (8). The low and the high affinity systems were found to differ in their requirements for external Na^+ ions. Whereas the rate of low affinity uptake is decreased by two fold in the absence of Na^+, the rate of high affinity uptake decreases by more than twenty fold. The high affinity system was found to transport glutamate against a concentration gradient (estimates of the intracellular glutamate concentration vary in the range of 5–10 mM depending on the CNS region (9)), only in the presence of a favourable gradient of Na^+ ions. In the absence of external Na^+ ions or in the presence of ouabain, which, by blocking the Na^+/K^+ ATPase, causes a dissipation of the transmembrane ion gradients, only a small accumulation of glutamate was found to take place most probably via the low affinity uptake system. It is clear, thus, that the high affinity transport of glutamate functions by coupling the uptake of glutamate with the uptake of Na^+ ions and that the electrochemical Na^+ gradient which is maintained by the Na^+/K^+ ATPase provides the driving force for this cotransport. The stoechiometry of the glutamate Na^+ coupling was established by Stallcup *et al.* (10) who measured simultaneously the rate of uptake of $^{22}Na^+$ and [^{3}H]-glutamate into the cerebellar nerve cell line ϵ'. Two Na^+ ions were found to be transported for every glutamate molecule. Considering the various values of the rate of glutamate uptake in brain slices reported in the literature (7, 11, 12), one can deduce

that the uptake of glutamate contributes to the entry of 15–60 μ equiv of Na^+/g tissue/h. The existence of a high affinity glutamate uptake system is often taken as an argument in favour of a neurotransmitter role for glutamate. The glutamate uptake systems are present not only in nerve terminals but are also in glia (13). This finding suggests a role of the high affinity glutamate transport systems not in the inactivation of the released neurotransmitter but rather in the maintenance of a steady concentration of glutamate in the cerebrospinal fluid (CSF). Glutamate is present in brain at the concentration of 5–10 mM and in the CSF at the concentration of 30 μM (9). Accordingly, following its electrochemical gradient, glutamate should leak constantly from its intracellular pools. In the absence of high affinity uptake systems, the CSF concentration of glutamate could easily reach the threshold required for neuronal excitation which is estimated to be around 0.1 mM (5). Considering the CSF concentrations of glutamate and its threshold concentration for neuronal excitation, one expects that if indeed glutamate is a neurotransmitter it should be released in the synaptic cleft at mM concentrations (14). Of the various glutamate uptake systems, the low affinity transport system with an affinity for glutamate in the mM range, is more likely to play a role in the inactivation of the neurotransmitter.

II. Na^+ movements associated with glutamate induced depolarization: Na^+ uptake studies

Curtis *et al.* (4) found that the application of glutamate on a toad spinal cord, produces a potent excitatory effect characterized by an acceleration of spike potentials and a decrease in the membrane potential. This depolarization, which is accompanied by an increase in membrane conductance (15), has been attributed to an influx of Na^+ ions (16). A strong argument in favour of this hypothesis was presented by Hösli & Hösli (17) who prevented a glutamate-induced depolarization of spinal cord neurones maintained in tissue culture by the removal of Na^+ ions from the bathing medium.

The question of the ionic mechanisms underlying the excitatory actions of glutamate and other acidic amino acids prompted Bradford & McIlwain (6) to investigate the levels of Na$^+$ and K$^+$ ions in glutamate treated cerebral tissues. Within one minute of addition, L-glutamate as well as other acidic amino acids such as L-aspartate, DL-homocysteate and L-α-aminodipate, produced a significant change in the tissue content of Na$^+$ ions while not affecting the potassium content. The average change was 590 μ equiv Na/g tissue/h, whereas the normal turnover of Na$^+$ ions in unstimulated tissue was 175–275 μ equiv Na/g tissue/h. On the basis of the tissue levels of Na$^+$ and K$^+$ and the membrane potential after short exposures to glutamate, Bradford & McIlwain calculated the relative permeabilities of cerebral cells to Na$^+$ and K$^+$, using a modified Goldman equation. Not taking into account the contribution of glia to the tissue levels of Na$^+$, they found that glutamate increases by five fold the tissue permeability to sodium relative to that to potassium. However, since the measured increase in tissue permeability to Na$^+$ ions originates in the activation of glutamate receptor-linked ionophores as well as of action potential Na$^+$ channels, the calculated increase in Na$^+$ permeability relative to that of K$^+$ could not reasonably account for the primary action of L-glutamate. A puzzling finding of Bradford & McIlwain was that although glutamate increased the frequency of action potentials it did not affect, under their experimental conditions, the tissue levels of K$^+$. In a later paper, Harvey & McIlwain (18) found that glutamate does indeed cause a loss of tissue K$^+$ ions. During the first minute of incubation with glutamate, the rate of K$^+$ loss was 660 μ equiv/g tissue/h. The K$^+$ lost after the addition of glutamate was regained later due to the activation of the Na$^+$/K$^+$ ATPase. This finding provides the most likely explanation for the observation of Terner et al. (1) that glutamate increases the K$^+$ content of brain slices. In order to assess the contribution of glutamate activated action potential Na$^+$ channels to the glutamate-induced Na$^+$ movements in brain slices, McIlwain et al. (19) studied the effects of tetrodotoxin (TTX), a neurotoxin known to block the action potential Na$^+$ channels. It was found that while TTX markedly limited the changes of tissue levels of Na$^+$ caused by glutamate, it did not affect the K$^+$ levels. A closer analysis of the effects of TTX on glutamate-induced Na$^+$ movements led Pull et al. (20) to suggest that tetrodotoxin and

glutamate might not compete for a common site. This was the first suggestion that glutamate-induced Na$^+$ movements measured in the presence of tetrodotoxin could possibly shed some light on the specific ion channels (ionophores) associated with glutamate receptors. Aware of this possibility, Biziere & Coyle (21) initiated a study of the effects of kainic acid, a conformationally restricted analogue of glutamate, on the Na$^+$ and K$^+$ levels of rat striatal slices incubated in vitro. Kainic acid was found to cause an increase in striatal sodium levels comparable to that observed with glutamate. Kainic acid was however about a thousand fold more potent than glutamate as its effects were observed already at a concentration of 0.1 μM. This cyclic amino acid further differed from glutamate in that it did not increase the intracellular K$^+$ levels. Since kainate and glutamate did not exhibit additive effects on Na$^+$ uptake, Biziere & Coyle suggested that these two compounds may activate the same Na$^+$ channel, while producing sometimes separate effects. It should be pointed out that the Na$^+$ and K$^+$ levels of striatal slices incubated with kainate or glutamate were measured after 60 min of incubation and therefore could not be easily related to the primary permeability changes produced by these excitants.

The studies reviewed above suggest that glutamate and other acidic amino acids cause in brain slices Na$^+$ movements which result not only from their interactions with receptors controlling the membrane permeability but also from the activation of action potential Na$^+$ channels, Na$^+$/K$^+$ ATPase, and Na$^+$ dependent uptake systems. The limitations of these studies are due mainly to the fact that ion uptake methods which require extreme care give rise to results with very poor signal to noise ratio and a relatively large margin of error. Therefore their use in routine pharmacological studies of the excitatory action of acidic amino acids has been limited.

III. Na$^+$ movements resulting from the interactions of excitatory amino acids with receptors: ^{22}Na$^+$ efflux studies

Biochemical methods based on measurements of ion movements that result from neurotransmitter-receptor interactions have been of great assistance

284

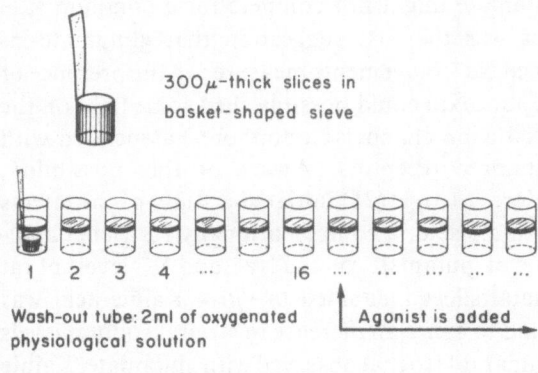

300μ-thick slices in
basket-shaped sieve

Wash-out tube: 2ml of oxygenated
physiological solution | Agonist is added

① INCUBATE 30'-60' IN PHYSIOLOGICAL SOLUTION CONTAINING THE
RADIOACTIVE TRACER ION.

② WASH-OUT OF RADIOACTIVITY-ONE TRANSFER/MIN.

③ COUNT THE RADIOACTIVITY IN EACH WASH-OUT TUBE.

④ CALCULATE THE CONTENT OF RADIOACTIVITY IN THE SLICES AS
A FUNCTION OF TIME: C_t

⑤ CALCULATE SPECIFIC EFFLUX RATE R_t

$$R_t = \frac{C_{(t-\Delta t)} - C_t}{C_{(t-\Delta t)}\Delta t}$$

Fig. 1. A scheme of the tracer ion efflux assay. C_t is the tracer ion content of the slices at time t, and $C_{(t-\Delta t)}$ is the content at $(t-\Delta t)$.

in the study of the receptors of acetylcholine (22, 23), γ-aminobutyric acid (24) and noradrenaline (25). Ion flux methods have also been used to study the properties of the action potential Na^+ channels (26–29) and of voltage dependent Ca^{++} channels (30). In brain slices, ion movements induced by L-glutamate and other excitatory amino acids have been observed, as described above. However, due to methodological difficulties such measurements have not been used in pharmacological studies of amino acid receptors.

Since excitatory amino acids depolarize the neuronal membrane by increasing its permeability to Na^+ ions, one expects an increased traffic of Na^+ ions to take place in both directions across the membrane. The increased efflux of Na^+ ions taking place upon exposure to an excitatory amino acid can therefore be used for monitoring its interaction with a membrane receptor. The principle of the method that we have developed to investigate the pharmacological properties of the excitatory amino acid receptors in the rat brain is outlined in Fig. 1. Rat striatal slices are first loaded with a radioactive tracer ion (i.e. $^{22}Na^+$, $^{42}K^+$, $^{86}Rb^+$, $^{36}Cl^-$, $^{51}Cr^{+++}$)

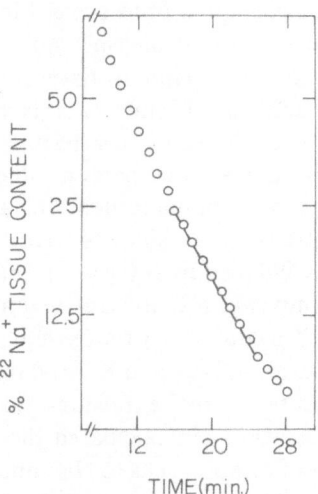

Fig. 2. Evolution of the $^{22}Na^+$ tissue content, expressed as percent of the amount of the ion remaining in the slices 5 min after the start of the wash-out. Every point represents a mean value from at least three determinations. The standard deviation never exceeded 20% of the respective means.

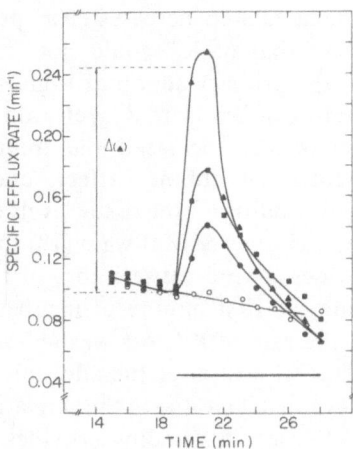

Fig. 3. Effect of L-glutamate on the specific $^{22}Na^+$ efflux rate from striatal slices. The black horizontal bar indicates the time of exposure to L-glutamate at the following concentrations: 0.3 mM (●), 1 mM (■), 3 mM (▲). Basal $^{22}Na^+$ efflux rate (O). The stimulatory effect, Δ, of 3 mM glutamate is shown. Every point represents a mean value from at least three determinations. The standard deviation never exceeded 20% of the respective means.

and the radioactivity is then washed-out by repetitive transfers of the slices into wash-out vessels containing a non-radioactive physiological solution. At one point in this series of transfers, when the bulk of the radioactivity present in the extracellular space has been removed, the slices are exposed to an effector which is tested for its ability to increase the membrane ionic permeability. At the end of the wash-out, the radioactivity present in each wash-out vessel and that left in the slices is measured. The results of the wash-out are expressed in terms of a specific $^{22}Na^+$ efflux rate, R_t (for definition see Fig. 1). This procedure allows a standardization of the results as they become independent of the amount of slices used or the actual amount of radioactivity released.

In Fig. 2, we show a semi-log plot of the evolution of the $^{22}Na^+$ tissue content as a function of time (1 transfer/min). As seen, the Na^+ content decreases in an almost linear manner from 14 min onwards, indicating that the rate of $^{22}Na^+$ efflux is constant for most of that period. The same data can be expressed in terms of a specific efflux rate (Fig. 3). The basal rate of $^{22}Na^+$ efflux is stabilized around a value of 0.1 min^{-1} for the time period between 16 and 25 min. If the striatal slices are transferred into vessels containing L-glutamate or any other excitatory amino acid, one observes a bell-shaped evolution of the specific $^{22}Na^+$ efflux rate, the maximal levels being dependent on the effector concentration. The stimulatory effect of an effector on the specific efflux rate is expressed in terms of Δ, a parameter equal to the difference between the average values of the specific efflux rates measured during the two minutes before and the two minutes after the exposure to the effector (Fig. 3).

1. Origin of the excitatory amino acid induced increase in $^{22}Na^+$ efflux rate

Theoretically, several mechanisms can account for the glutamate-induced increase in the specific $^{22}Na^+$ efflux rate described in Fig. 3.

a. Glutamate is known to depolarize neurones and to induce spike discharges (3, 4, 5). The large increase in the permeability of the neuronal membrane to Na^+ accompanying the rising phase of action potentials could contribute to the glutamate-induced acceleration of $^{22}Na^+$ efflux.

b. The activation of the Na^+/K^+ ATPase, following the glutamate-induced depolarization, may lead to an increased removal of intracellular Na^+ ions.

c. Glutamate may activate polysynaptic pathways causing the release of various neurotrans-

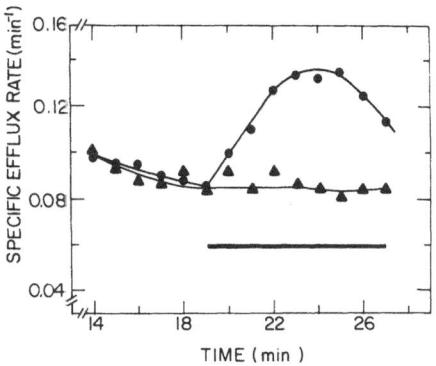

Fig. 4. Effect of 10^{-4} M veratridine on the specific $^{22}Na^+$ efflux rate in the presence (▲) or absence of 10^{-7} tetrodotoxin (●). The black horizontal bar indicates the time of exposure to veratridine. Every point represents a mean value from three determinations. The standard deviation never exceeded 20% of the respective means.

mitters which affect the permeability of the postsynaptic membrane to Na^+ ions.

d. Glutamate may cause a specific opening of Na^+ channels (ionophores) linked to glutamate receptors.

The following series of experiments were carried out in order to evaluate the involvement of each of the above mentioned mechanisms to the glutamate-induced increase in $^{22}Na^+$ efflux rate.

a. Action potentials

The effect on the $^{22}Na^+$ efflux rate of veratridine, a neurotoxin known to maintain the Na^+ action potential channel in an open state, was studied. Figure 4 shows that veratridine at 10^{-4} M causes an increased $^{22}Na^+$ efflux from rat striatal slices. The concentration of 10^{-4} M was chosen since it corresponds to the K_m of veratridine in various systems (27–30). In order to prove that the observed veratridine-induced increased efflux is a measure of the steady state activity of the action potential Na^+ channel, we tested whether the increase in $^{22}Na^+$ efflux could be blocked by tetrodotoxin (TTX), a specific inhibitor of the action potential Na^+ channel. The veratridine dependent $^{22}Na^+$ efflux was found to be completely blocked by 10^{-7} M TTX (Fig. 4). On the other hand, the rate of the glutamate-stimulated $^{22}Na^+$ efflux from rat striatal slices was not affected by 10^{-7} M TTX. We therefore conclude that the glutamate-induced increase in $^{22}Na^+$ efflux rate is not due to spike discharges.

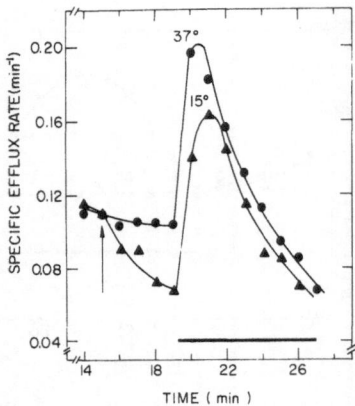

Fig. 5. Effect of temperature on the basal and glutamate-stimulated specific ^{22}Na$^+$ efflux rate. At the arrow, the temperature was shifted from 37° (●) to 15° (▲). The black horizontal bar indicates the time of exposure to 2 mM L-glutamate. Every point represents a mean value from at least three determinations. The standard deviation never exceeded 20% of the respective means.

b. Na$^+$/K$^+$ ATPase

The Na$^+$/K$^+$ activated ATPase is an enzyme known to be highly sensitive to temperature, the Q_{10} of which varies from 3 to 4 depending on the enzyme origin (31). The effects of temperature on the basal and glutamate stimulated ^{22}Na$^+$ efflux rates are shown in Fig. 5. The wash-out was performed by transferring the rat striatal slices for the first 15 min through vessels containing a physiological solution at 37 °C and then into vessels maintained at 15 °C. A control wash-out curve was carried out at a constant temperature of 37 °C. The decrease in temperature had an immediate effect on the basal ^{22}Na$^+$ efflux rate reducing it within 4 min from a value of 0.11 min^{-1} to a value of 0.07 min^{-1}. However, temperature had no effect on the gluta-mate stimulated ^{22}Na$^+$ efflux. Analysis of the results in terms of Δ values gives Δ = 0.073 min^{-1} at 37 °C and Δ = 0.072 min^{-1} at 15 °C. The increased efflux of ^{22}Na$^+$ caused by glutamate is therefore not due to the activation of a Na$^+$/K$^+$ ATPase.

c. Polysynaptic pathways

The release of neurotransmitters is known to be abolished in physiological solutions containing low Ca^{++} and high Mg^{++} concentrations. We have therefore studied the effect of glutamate on ^{22}Na$^+$ efflux rates in the presence of 0.02 mM Ca^{++} and 10 mM Mg^{++} concentrations. These conditions were found not to affect either the basal or the glutamate-stimulated ^{22}Na$^+$ efflux rate.

d. Receptor mediated increase in membrane permeability

In the absence of active processes, the efflux of ^{22}Na$^+$ depends on the membrane permeability, the intracellular ^{22}Na$^+$ concentration and the membrane potential (electric field factor) (32). The contribution of the electric field factor to the stimulated ^{22}Na$^+$ efflux can be assessed by conducting the experiments under conditions preventing the glutamate-induced depolarization, for instance, in a physiological medium in which Na$^+$ has been replaced by a non-permeating cation like choline. In such a case, the stimulated ^{22}Na$^+$ efflux should decrease by a factor which is a function of the difference between the potential of a depolarized and a resting membrane. Indeed, in the absence of extracellular Na$^+$, glutamate was found to increase the ^{22}Na$^+$ specific efflux to a rate which was two thirds of that observed in the Na$^+$ containing medium (33). Thus, the existence of an increased ^{22}Na$^+$ efflux in the absence of depolarization supports the proposition that the effects of gluta-mate are due to its interactions with receptors controlling the membrane permeability.

To determine whether the glutamate-stimulated increase in membrane permeability might involve other ions besides Na$^+$, we have tested the effects of glutamate on rat striatal slices preloaded with either ^{42}K$^+$, ^{86}Rb$^+$, ^{36}Cl$^-$, ^{51}Cr^{+++} or [^{14}C]glutamate. L-glutamate was found to increase the ^{42}K$^+$ and ^{86}Rb$^+$ efflux rate during the first two minutes of exposure, from basal efflux rates of about 0.05 min^{-1} to 0.08 min^{-1}. As in the case of ^{22}Na$^+$, the specific efflux rate of ^{42}K$^+$ or ^{86}Rb$^+$ first increased and then decreased even through glutamate was still present. The efflux rate of ^{51}Cr^{+++}, ^{36}Cl$^-$ or [^{14}C]glutamate was not affected by glutamate. The finding that L-glutamate increases the efflux of both ^{22}Na$^+$ and ^{42}K$^+$ does not necessarily indicate that these effluxes take place through the same mixed channels. As glutamate is known to exert on cerebellar neurones an inhibitory action which is not mediated by Cl$^-$ ions (34), it is possible that the glutamate-induced increase in ^{42}K$^+$ efflux is mediated by a glutamate receptor responsible for a hyperpolarizing inhibitory action. The heterogeneity of receptors for glutamate and other excitatory amino acids is discussed below.

2. Origin of the effector-induced decrease in ion efflux rates

At least two mechanisms can account for the decrease in the specific efflux rates subsequent to the glutamate-induced increase in these rates:

a. Prolonged exposures to glutamate induce receptor desensitization which makes the system unresponsive to further additions of glutamate.

b. The increase in membrane permeability leads to the exhaustion of the intracellular pools of radioactive tracer ion.

Fig. 6 illustrates the results of experiments in which striatal slices, incubated with $^{22}Na^+$, were treated with 1 mM and 2 mM L-glutamate. Fig. 6A is a control curve showing the variation in the specific $^{22}Na^+$ efflux rate upon transfer of the slices at t = 29 min into solutions containing 1 mM glutamate. Fig. 6B shows the results of transferring the slices into tubes containing 1 mM L-glutamate solutions from t = 13 min to t = 29 min, followed by transfers into 2 mM L-glutamate solutions from t = 29 min to t = 37 min. There is a marked increase in the specific efflux rate upon exposure to the first dose of glutamate but the rate goes back to its basal level within 7–8 min and is not affected by exposure to a higher concentration of L-glutamate. Fig. 6C shows that when the slices are first exposed for 7 min to 1 mM L-glutamate, then washed during 9 min and exposed again to a dose of 1 mM L-glutamate, the second exposure does not cause an increase in the specific efflux rate. In Fig. 7, the same types of experiments are repeated using striatal slices preincubated in a physiological solution containing $^{86}Rb^+$. Since the effects of L-glutamate on the $^{86}Rb^+$ or $^{42}K^+$ specific efflux rate are not as marked as those on the $^{22}Na^+$ efflux rate, relatively high concentrations of L-glutamate were used in these experiments. Fig. 7A shows that 5.5 mM L-glutamate increases the specific $^{86}Rb^+$ efflux rate from 0.038 min^{-1} to 0.055 min^{-1}. Exposure of the slices first to 0.5 mM L-glutamate during 9 min and then to 5.5 mM L-glutamate produces an increase of the specific efflux rate from a value of 0.043 min^{-1} at the end of the first addition to a value of 0.051 min^{-1} at the end of the second (Fig. 7B). If a washing period of 5 min is introduced between the two exposures to L-glutamate, the second addition of 5.5 mM L-glutamate causes an increase of the specific efflux rate from 0.038 min^{-1} to 0.057^{-1} (Fig.

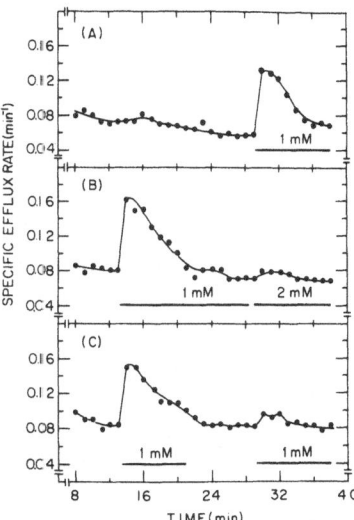

Fig. 6. Effect of successive exposures to L-glutamate on the specific $^{22}Na^+$ efflux rate from striatum slices. A. Exposure to 1 mM L-glutamate; B. Conditioning exposure to 1 mM L-glutamate followed by a test exposure to 2 mM L-glutamate; C. Conditioning exposure to 1 mM L-glutamate followed by a wash-out period and exposure to 1 mM L-glutamate.

Every point represents a mean value from at least three determinations. The standard deviation never exceeded 20% of the respective means.

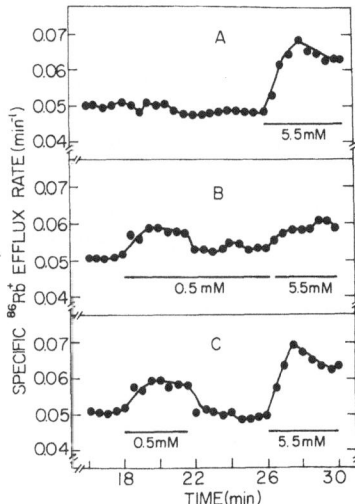

Fig. 7. Effect of successive exposures to L-glutamate on the specific $^{86}Rb^+$ efflux rate from striatum slices. A. Exposure to 5.5 mM L-glutamate; B. Exposure to 0.5 mM L-glutamate followed by 5.5 mM L-glutamate. C. Exposure to 0.5 mM L-glutamate followed by a wash-out period and exposure to 5.5 mM L-glutamate.

Every point represents the mean value from at least three determinations. The standard deviation never exceeded 20% of the respective means.

7C). A qualitative difference exists, thus, between the repetitive effects of glutamate on the specific $^{22}Na^+$ efflux rate and on the $^{86}Rb^+$ efflux rate. It may appear that glutamate causes a reversible desensitization of the glutamate receptor – K^+ ionophore complex and an irreversible desensitization of the glutamate receptor – Na^+ ionophore complex. However, it has been reported that the glutamate depolarization does not cause desensitization (3, 17, 35, 36). Therefore, one ought to consider the alternative explanation for the bell shaped time dependence of the specific efflux rate, namely, that the glutamate-induced increase in membrane permeability brings about an exhaustion of the intracellular pools of radioactive tracer ion. Using the compartmental analysis of Daniel (37), we have shown (33) that a depletion process alone could fully account for the decrease in efflux rates of both $^{22}Na^+$ and $^{86}Rb^+$. The differential effect of repetitive additions of glutamate on the $^{22}Na^+$ and the $^{86}Rb^+$ efflux rates is tentatively suggested to be due to the larger depletion of $^{22}Na^+$ relative to $^{86}Rb^+$ ions taking place during the excitation of dendritic synapses (38). As the change in the permeability to Rb^+ is much smaller than that to Na^+, only a transient depletion of the Rb^+ localized in the dendritic branches would take place and these ions could be replenished by diffusion from the cell body once the glutamate stimulus is removed. To summarize, the bell shaped evolution of efflux rates in the presence of glutamate, other excitatory amino acids and veratridine (Fig. 4) can be explained by the following processes: a) The effector causes an enhancement in the membrane permeability to ions and increases the tracer ion efflux rate; b) In the absence of desensitization, a depletion of the tracer ion pools takes place causing a decrease in the efflux rate.

3. Pharmacological properties of excitatory amino acids receptors

a. Agonists

Glutamate increases the specific $^{22}Na^+$ efflux rate in a dose dependent manner (Fig. 3). In Fig. 8, the values of Δ are plotted as a function of the logarithm of the bath concentrations of three excitatory effectors: L-glutamate, kainate and N-methyl-D-aspartate. At high concentrations of these effectors, Δ reaches a maximal value of 0.18

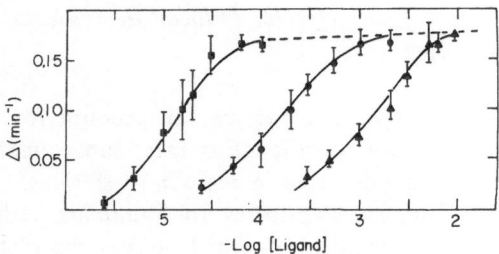

Fig. 8. Dose-response curves for N-methyl-D-aspartate (■), kainate (●) and L-glutamate (▲). Each point represents the mean value (±S.D.) of 6 experiments. The parameter Δ is defined in the text.

min^{-1}. The same maximal Δ value is reached with all the other ligands tested. Since large receptor occupancy may lead to an exhaustion of $^{22}Na^+$ ions in the effector-sensitive pools before receptor saturation is reached, it is most probable that the maximal rate observed in all cases is not the rate corresponding to true receptor saturation. Therefore apparent effector-receptor affinities cannot be deduced. As seen in Fig. 8, the threshold of increased $^{22}Na^+$ efflux rates is observed at very different concentrations of effectors. Comparing the concentrations of N-methyl-D-aspartate, kainate and L-glutamate giving rise to identical Δ values, one can nevertheless establish the order of efficacy of these effectors. Thus, N-methyl-D-aspartate and kainate are respectively 50 and 8 times more potent than L-glutamate in increasing $^{22}Na^+$ specific efflux rates. In Table 1, we have listed, according to the order of their potency, the various effectors tested. This list includes several new agonists that were synthesized in our laboratory (39). Their structures are presented in Fig. 9. Table 1 lists also various compounds that were found to be devoid of agonist properties. They include antagonists of amino acid excitation such as γ-glutamylglycine, 2-amino-5-phosphonovalerate, DL-2-aminosuberate, diethyl glutamate, and neurotransmitters such as noradrenaline, Substance P and γ-aminobutyric acid (GABA). The latter, while ineffective in increasing the $^{22}Na^+$ specific efflux rate, increased significantly the $^{36}Cl^-$ efflux from striatal slices (Fig. 10). This effect of GABA could be blocked to the extent of 75% by 50 μM picrotoxinin, an established GABA antagonist. Table 1 includes also the results of experiments carried out in order to determine whether cyclic nucleotides may be involved in the membrane

Table 1. Relative potency of excitatory amino acids in inducing a $^{22}Na^+$ efflux from preloaded rat striatum slices.

N-Methyl-D-aspartate	50.0	L-Glutamate	1.0
DL-Homocysteate	11.0	D-Aspartate	0.6
Kainate*	8.0	L-Aspartate	0.6
Quisqualate	6.4	Dihydrokainate*	0.6
Kainate methyl ketone*	5.2	Cephalosporin C	0.5
Allokainate methyl ketone*	4.6	L-Glutamate-γ-monohydroxamate	0.2
Carboxy-kainate*	2.5	L-Proline	0.2
Carboxy-allokainate*	2.3	Hydroxykainate*	0.2
Piperidinedicarboxylic acid	1.2	Dihydroxykainate*	0.1
D-Glutamate	1.2	Phenylthio-hydroxykainate*	0.1

* For the structure of this compound see Fig. 9.

All amino acids were tested at least at two concentrations, 0.1 mM and 1 mM. N-Methyl-D-aspartate and DL-homocysteate were tested at 30 μM. The following compounds tested at 3 mM, were found to be devoid of agonist properties: DL-α-aminopimelate, LL-α-ε-diaminopimelic acid, L-α-aminosuberate, diethyl glutamate, DL-α-methylglutamate, N-acetylkainate, GABA, γ-D-glutamylglycine, 2-amino-5-phosphonovalerate, carbamylcholine, glutarate, norepinephrine. The following compounds tested at 1 mM, were found to be devoid of agonist properties: N-acetyl-L-aspartate, N-acetyl-DL-aspartate, L-glutamate-γ-hydrazine. The following compounds were found not to affect the response to 0.5 mM L-glutamate: 10 mM dithiothreitol, 10^{-5} M Substance P, 1 mM theophylline, 10 mM Na F.

permeability changes induced by excitatory amino acids. It is known that the action of certain neurotransmitters on receptors is associated with changes in the levels of cyclic nucleotides (40) that may control, by so far unknown mechanisms, the neurotransmitter-induced permeability changes (41). When added to brain slices, glutamate and other acidic amino acids have been found to increase the formation of cyclic AMP (42) and cyclic GMP (43–45). Theophylline was shown to block the glutamate-induced formation of cyclic AMP (42). However, when tested in the $^{22}Na^+$ efflux assay in the presence of glutamate, theophylline was found to be devoid of activity. The glutamate-induced increase in $^{22}Na^+$ efflux was also unaffected by the presence in the medium of NaF, a stimulator of adenylate cyclase. It is therefore reasonable to assume that the effects of glutamate on the $^{22}Na^+$ specific efflux rate and on the formation of cyclic nucleotides are not inter-related.

The affinities of the excitatory amino acids to their receptors could provide significant information on the relationships between the structures of the effectors and the potency of their excitatory action. The order of efficacy of the various amino acids tested, as presented in Table 1, cannot, however, be taken as an indication of the order of their receptor affinities. This limitation is due to the fact that amino acid uptake and degradation processes as well as the existence of diffusion barriers may influence the effector concentration near the membrane. Therefore, the bath concentration of the amino acid may not reflect its actual concentration in the vicinity of the receptor. It can be shown, however, that the contribution of diffusion delays to this problem may be neglected. The diffusion of a substance from the bulk phase into a slice is analogous to the problem of diffusion in a plane sheet described by Crank (46), where the tortuosity of the slice (47) has to be taken into account. With a diffusion coefficient for L-glutamate of 1.1×10^{-5} cm^2/s and a tortuosity factor of 1.6, (47), one can calculate that after 60 s, in the absence of uptake or degradation processes, the concentration of L-glutamate in the middle of a 300 μ thick slice will be 95% of that present in the bulk phase. The validity of these calculations for brain slices has been established experimentally by Bradford & McIlwain (6).

The question of glutamate concentration at the receptor level is of importance for the understanding of the results concerning the minimal concentrations of this amino acid necessary for eliciting an excitatory response. Electrophysiological studies (5) and $^{22}Na^+$ efflux measurements (see Fig. 8) have

290

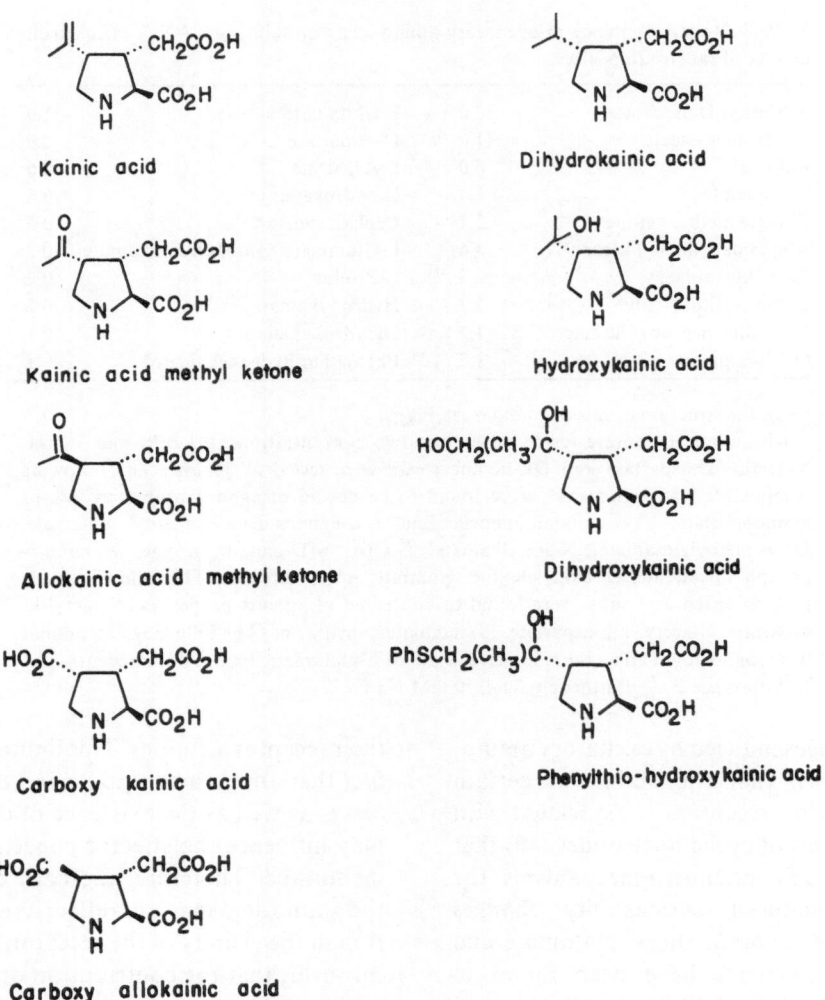

Fig. 9. Structures of kainic acid analogues.

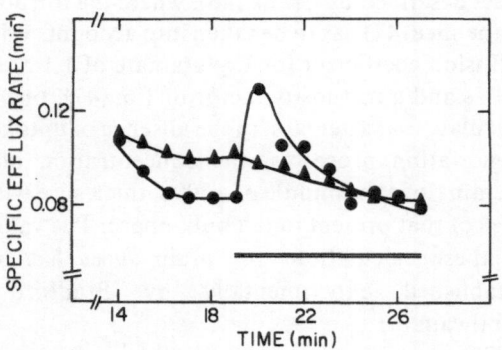

Fig. 10. Effect of 3 mM GABA on the specific ^{36}Cl (●) and $^{22}Na^+$ (▲) efflux rates from preloaded rat striatal slices. The black horizontal bar indicates the time of exposure to GABA. Every point represents a mean value from at least three determinations. The standard deviation never exceeded 20% of the respective means.

shown that the activity of glutamate is observed at a concentration of about 0.1 mM. This concentration is most probably lower than that needed for the occupancy of 50% of the glutamate receptor population. There is, however, a discrepancy between these data and the results obtained from measurements of the binding of [^{3}H]glutamate to brain membranes, which indicate the presence of high affinity binding sites with K_D's of 11 nM, 80 nM (48) and 700 nM (49, 50). In view of the high concentration of glutamate in the cerebrospinal fluid (30 μM (9)), one can assume that these glutamate binding sites will be saturated *in vivo*. Therefore, these sites are not likely to be involved in the excitatory action of glutamate and their physiological role remains to be elucidated. On the other hand, the concentration of glutamate needed to

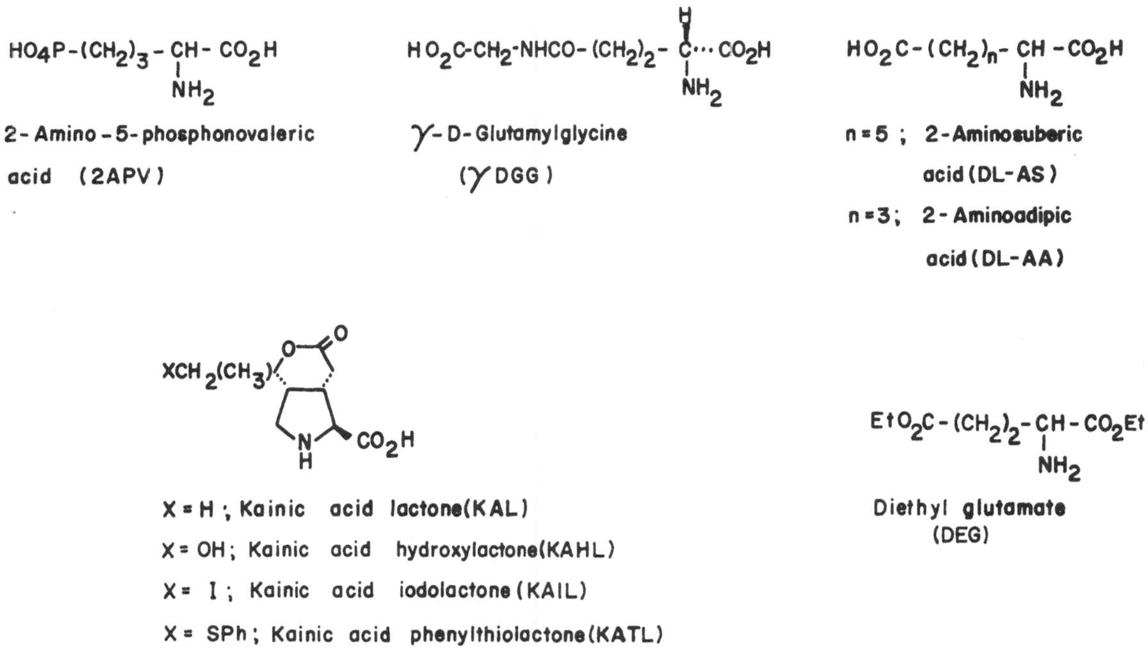

HO$_4$P-(CH$_2$)$_3$-CH-CO$_2$H
$\quad\quad\quad\quad\quad$|
$\quad\quad\quad\quad\quad$NH$_2$

2-Amino-5-phosphonovaleric
acid (2APV)

HO$_2$C-CH$_2$-NHCO-(CH$_2$)$_2$-C$\cdots$CO$_2$H
$\quad\quad\quad\quad\quad\quad\quad\quad\quad\quad$|
$\quad\quad\quad\quad\quad\quad\quad\quad\quad\quad$NH$_2$

γ-D-Glutamylglycine
(γDGG)

HO$_2$C-(CH$_2$)$_n$-CH-CO$_2$H
$\quad\quad\quad\quad\quad\quad\quad$|
$\quad\quad\quad\quad\quad\quad\quad$NH$_2$

n=5 ; 2-Aminosuberic
$\quad\quad\quad$acid (DL-AS)

n=3 ; 2-Aminoadipic
$\quad\quad\quad$acid (DL-AA)

XCH$_2$(CH$_3$)

X = H ; Kainic acid lactone (KAL)

X = OH; Kainic acid hydroxylactone (KAHL)

X = I ; Kainic acid iodolactone (KAIL)

X = SPh; Kainic acid phenylthiolactone (KATL)

EtO$_2$C-(CH$_2$)$_2$-CH-CO$_2$Et
$\quad\quad\quad\quad\quad\quad\quad$|
$\quad\quad\quad\quad\quad\quad\quad$NH$_2$

Diethyl glutamate
(DEG)

Fig. 11. Structures of antagonists of excitatory amino acids.

elicit an increase in the specific ^{22}Na$^+$ efflux seems to be within a reasonable physiological range. It may be a reflection of the rather weak affinity of glutamate for its receptors. Such a weak affinity may fulfil a physiological role by preventing fluctuations in the concentration of glutamate in the cerebrospinal fluid from giving rise to neuronal excitation.

b. Antagonists

In order to investigate in more detail the pharmacological properties of the excitatory amino acid receptors, we have tested several antagonists of amino acid induced excitation (51–54) as well as various kainic acid analogues that were synthesized in our laboratory (55). The structures of the tested compounds are shown in Fig. 11. None of these compounds caused an increase in the specific ^{22}Na$^+$ efflux rate. However, when added, together with specific agonists, all of them displayed an antagonist activity. An example of the antagonism of the effect of kainic acid by kainic acid hydroxylactone is illustrated in Fig. 12. The extent of inhibition is determined by comparing the values of Δ obtained for the agonist in the absence and in the presence of the antagonist. Using this method we have carried out a systematic study of the antagonism of the

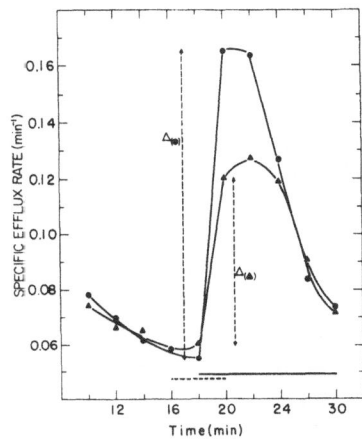

Fig. 12. Effect of kainic acid (100 μM) on the specific ^{22}Na$^+$ efflux rate in the absence (●) or presence of 3 mM kainic acid hydroxylactone (▲). The full and the broken horizontal bars indicate the times of exposure to kainic acid and to kainic acid hydroxylactone, respectively. In these experiments the transfer of the slices from one wash-out tube to the other was done once in two minutes. Every point represents a mean value from at least three determinations. The standard deviation never exceeded 20% of the respective means.

response to four excitatory amino acids: N-methyl-D-aspartate, quisqualate (QA), L-glutamate, and kainate (KA) (Fig. 13). The very different profiles of antagonism that are observed can be accounted

292

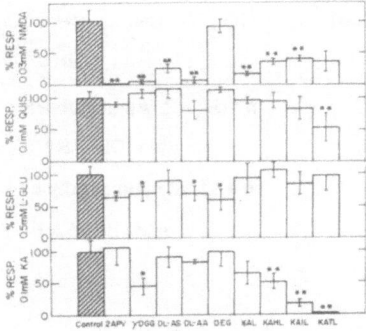

Fig. 13. Antagonism of the increase in specific $^{22}Na^+$ efflux rate produced by excitatory amino acids on $^{22}Na^+$-preloaded rat striatal slices. The agonists were used at the following concentrations. N-methyl-D-aspartate, 30 μM; quisqualate, 100 μM; L-glutamate, 1 mM; kainate, 100 μM; The antagonists were used at the following concentrations: 2-amino-5-phosphonovalerate (2-APV), 30 mM; γ-D-glutamylglycine (γ-DGG), 1 mM; DL-α-aminosuberate (DL-AS), 1 mM; DL-α-aminoadipate (DL-AA), 3 mM; diethyl glutamate (DEG), 10 mM, kainic acid lactone (KAL), 2 mM; kainic acid hydroxylactone (KAHL), 3 mM; kainic acid iodolactone (KAIL), 2 mM; kainic acid phenyl-thiolactone (KATL), 1 mM. The bars indicate means $\pm$S.D., based on at least 3 determinations.

*: p < 0.05 and **: p < 0.01 respectively, by the Student t test.

for by assuming the existence of heterogenous populations of excitatory amino acids receptors. Four types of receptors are so far pharmacologically distinguishable in the rat striatum: The 'NMDA' receptor, the 'quisqualate' receptor, the 'glutamate' receptor and the 'kainate' receptor. Excitatory amino acids such as DL-homocysteate and D-glutamate, which are antagonized by the same compounds antagonizing NMDA would act on the 'NMDA' receptor, whereas L-aspartate would act at the 'L-glutamate' receptor. The existence of heterogenous populations of receptors and in particular that of distinct receptors for L-glutamate and kainate, has been suggested previously (51–54, 56). However, in the cat spinal cord, the presence of only three types of receptors has been proposed and no specific receptors have been assigned to L-glutamate and L-aspartate.

The presence of distinct receptors for glutamate and kainate can be deduced not only from pharmacological considerations but also from experiments in which the ability of glutamate to increase $^{86}Rb^+$ efflux rates is compared to that of kainate. Table 2 shows that glutamate and kainate, tested at concentrations equipotent in increasing $^{22}Na^+$

Table 2. Comparison of the effects of glutamate and kainate on the specific efflux rates of $^{86}Rb^+$.

Effector	% Increase in specific efflux rate	
	$^{22}Na^+$	$^{86}Rb^+$
Glutamate 3 mM	160 ± 10	34 ± 10
Kainate 0.6 mM	150 ± 10	10 ± 1

efflux rates, differ markedly in their ability to increase the outward movement of $^{86}Rb^+$ ions. These results indicate that glutamate and kainate do not induce the same permeability changes (56). Glutamate may increase the membrane permeability to both Na^+ and K^+ ions (via a single or separate ionophores) whereas kainate appears to modify the membrane permeability mainly to Na^+ ions.

The antagonists presented in Fig. 11 may be divided into two classes, according to their structures. The first consists of acidic α-amino carboxylic acids in which the second acidic function (CO_2H or PO_4H) is removed from the α-carbon by a chain of three or five atoms. The compounds of this type antagonize mainly the response to NMDA (Fig. 13). The second class of antagonists includes bicyclic amino acid lactones, all of which derive chemically from kainic acid. These compounds which can be considered as conformationally restricted glutamate or kainate analogues possess only one acidic (carboxyl) group. The other carboxyl initially present in kainic acid is incorporated into a lactone function. As seen in Fig. 13 the lactones antagonize the responses to both NMDA and kainate. KAL and KAHL (Fig. 11) are more specific for NMDA while those bearing more bulky substituents, KAIL and KATL, block the response to kainate more efficiently than that to NMDA. The available data do not allow, however, a clear-cut differentiation between the structural requirements for the antagonism of the responses to NMDA and kainate. Of the other agonists tested, the effects of quisqualate are inhibited to a moderate extent by KATL while no antagonist blocks effectively the responses to glutamate and aspartate. The discovery of such antagonists, either by drug screening or by synthesis is of utmost importance for the further pharmacological characterization of amino acid receptors.

Some mention should be given to the properties of diethyl glutamate (DEG). This compound, at 10 mM, was found to be a weak antagonist of glutamate and aspartate (Fig. 13) and not of NMDA, kainate or quisqualate. These findings are in contrast with the reported effects of diethyl glutamate as an antagonist of both glutamate and quisqualate on Renshaw cells (57), or of the effects of glutamate on hippocampal neurones (58, 59). However, in agreement with our results it has also been shown that diethyl glutamate is an extremely variable antagonist of glutamate being unreliable, poorly selective and of low potency (60).

c. Endogenous excitatory neurotransmitters

The possible existence of multiple classes of receptors for excitatory amino acids raises the question of the identity of the natural ligands for these receptors. In the striatum, several observations have led to the suggestion that glutamate is the neurotransmitter of the cortico-striatal pathway: L-glutamate is taken up by cortico-striatal nerve terminals (61) from where it can also be released upon K^+ depolarization (62, 63). Furthermore, diethyl glutamate was found to block the excitation of striatal neurones produced by cortical stimulation (64). However, in view of the poor specificity and potency of diethyl glutamate as a glutamate antagonist, the assignment to glutamate of a transmitter role in the striatum is not yet warranted. A detailed comparison of the excitatory action of glutamate with that of the natural neurotransmitter is still missing.

If glutamate were a genuine neurotransmitter in the striatum, one would expect its depolarizing action to be blocked by the same antagonists as those blocking the postsynaptic effects of the natural excitatory neurotransmitter released by stimulation of the presynaptic nerve terminals. We have examined this possibility by studying the effects of amino acid antagonists on K^+-induced $^{22}Na^+$ effluxes from striatal slices. Exposure of the slices to a depolarizing dose of K^+ (40 mM) caused an increase in the $^{22}Na^+$ specific efflux rate with a $\Delta = 0.11 \, min^{-1}$. Since this effect is abolished in the absence of Ca^{++} ions, it can be assumed that the K^+-induced $^{22}Na^+$ efflux is due to a K^+-evoked depolarization of nerve terminals causing the release of endogenous excitatory neurotransmitters that act on subsynaptic receptors controlling the membrane permeability to Na^+ ions. Selected antagonists were tested for their ability to block the Ca^{++} dependent K^+-induced $^{22}Na^+$ efflux. Fig. 14

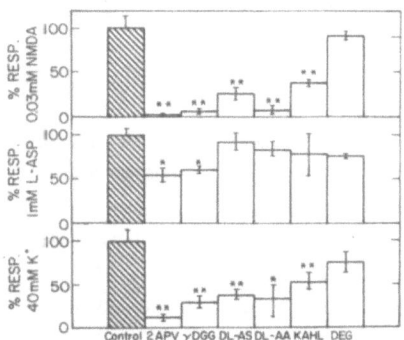

Fig. 14. Antagonism of the increase in specific $^{22}Na^+$ efflux rate produced by 30 μM N-methyl-D-aspartate, 1 mM L-aspartate and 40 mM K^+ on $^{22}Na^+$-preloaded rat striatal slices. The slices were depolarized by 40 mM K^+ (substituted for Na^+) in the presence of 2 mM Ca^{++} and 1.2 mM Mg^{++}. The antagonists were used at the same concentrations as in figure 13. The bars indicate means ±S.D., based on at least three determinations.
*: $p < 0.05$, and **: $p < 0.01$, by the student t-test.

shows that this effect can indeed be blocked by antagonists of excitatory amino acids. However, the profile of antagonism of the endogenous neurotransmitter differs markedly from that obtained with exogenously applied glutamate or aspartate (Fig. 13). On the other hand it is quite similar to the observed effects of the antagonists on the response to NMDA. These results suggest therefore the release of an 'NMDA-like' substance with pharmacological properties different from those of glutamate or aspartate. The fact that the various antagonists do not inhibit the K^+- and the NMDA-depolarization to the same extent as well as the finding that diethyl glutamate exerts some antagonist effect (Fig. 14), suggest that a release of glutamate does also take place concomitantly with that of an 'NMDA-like' substance. However, the contribution of released glutamate to the K^+-evoked $^{22}Na^+$ efflux is not as important as that of the 'NMDA-like' substance. The suggestion of the release of an 'NMDA-like' substance with neurotransmitter properties is supported by a growing number of reports showing that in other brain areas, NMDA antagonists depress both the synaptic and NMDA-evoked excitation (51, 53, 65, 66). Since the response of Renshaw cells to L-aspartate is blocked by 2-amino-5-phosphono-valerate and by γ-D-glutamylglycine as effectively as that of the natural neurotransmitter released upon stimulation of the dorsal roots, it has been proposed that L-aspartate might be the natural

294

ligand of the NMDA receptor (54). In the striatum, however, the response to L-aspartate is not blocked effectively by 2-amino-5-phosphonovalerate or by γ-D-glutamylglycine (Fig. 14). One can therefore rule out the possibility that in striatal slices L-aspartate is responsible for the K$^+$ evoked increase in ^{22}Na$^+$ efflux rate.

Although no evidence can be provided to implicate glutamate and aspartate in the major interneuronal transactions of the striatum, the possibility that these amino acids are still genuine neurotransmitters in other brain areas cannot be ruled out. The suggestion that the excitatory amino acids naturally occurring in brain are unlikely transmitter candidates in the striatum raises now the question of the chemical identity of the 'NMDA-like' substance. Since this compound acts as transmitter of a subsynaptic NMDA-receptor, answers will have to be provided as to the localisation and functions of the other receptors and to the nature of their endogenous effector(s).

Acknowledgements

The authors thank N. Tal and R. Kuperman for excellent technical assistance. This research was supported by grants from the Délégation Générale à la Recherche Scientifique et Technique, the Israel Commission for Basic Research and the US-Israel Binational Science Foundation. A.L. is on leave from the Istituto Mario Negri, Milan and is a recepient of an EMBO-postdoctoral fellowship. V.I.T. is an incumbent of the Mark Stanley Shriro Career Development Chair.

References

1. Terner, C., Eggleston, L. V. & Krebs, H. A., 1950. Biochem. J. 47: 139–149.
2. Hayashi, T., 1954. Keio J. Med. 3: 183–192.
3. Curtis, D. R., Phillis, J. W. & Watkins, J. C., 1959. Nature 183: 611–612.
4. Curtis, D. R., Phillis, J. W. & Watkins, J. C., 1960. J. Physiol. 150: 656–682.
5. Curtis, D. R. & Watkins, J. C., 1965. Pharmacol. Rev. 17: 347–391.
6. Bradford, H. F. & McIlwain, H., 1966. J. Neurochem. 13: 1163–1177.
7. Bennett, J. P. Jr., Logan, W. J. & Snyder, S. H., 1973. J. Neurochem. 21: 1533–1550.
8. Campbell, G. Lem. & Shank, R. P., 1978. Brain Res. 153: 618–622.
9. Curtis, D. R. & Johnston, G. A. R., 1974. Ergebn. der. Physiol. 69: 97–188.
10. Stallcup, W. B., Bulloch, K. & Baetge, E. E., 1979. J. Neurochem. 32: 57–65.
11. Balcar, V. J. & Johnston, G. A. R., 1972. J. Neurobiol. 3: 295–301.
12. Johnston, G. A. R., Kennedy, S. M. & Twitchin, B., 1979. J. Neurochem. 32: 121–127.
13. Roberts, P. J. & Watkins, J. C., 1975. Brain Res. 85: 120–125.
14. Shank, R. P. & Aprison, M. H., 1979. Glutamic Acid: Advances in Biochemistry and Physiology (Filer, L. J. Jr., Garattini, S., Kare, M. R., Reynolds, W. A. & Wurtman, R. J., eds.), pp. 139–150. Raven Press, New York.
15. Krnjevic, K. & Schwartz, S., 1967. Exp. Brain Res. 3: 306–319.
16. Zieglgänsberger, W. & Puil, E. A., 1973. Exp. Brain Res. 17: 35–49.
17. Hösli, L. & Hösli, E., 1978. Rev. Physiol. Biochem. Pharmacol. 81: 136–188.
18. Harvey, J. A. & McIlwain, H., 1968. Biochem. J. 108: 269–274.
19. McIlwain, H., Harvey, J. A. & Rodriguez, G., 1969. J. Neurochem. 16, 363–370.
20. Pull, I., McIlwain, H. & Ramsey, R. L., 1970. Biochem. J. 116: 181–187.
21. Biziere, K. & Coyle, J. T., 1978. J. Neurochem. 31: 513–520.
22. Kasai, M. & Changeux, J. P., 1971. J. Memb. Biol. 6: 1–23.
23. Catterall, W. A., 1975. J. Biol. Chem. 250: 1776–1781.
24. Ticku, M. K. & Olsen, R. W., 1977. Biochim. biophys. Acta 464: 519–529.
25. Mauger, J. P., Moura, A. M. & Worcel, M., 1978. Br. J. Pharmacol. 64: 29–36.
26. Catterall, W. A. & Nirenberg, M., 1973. Proc. Nat. Acad. Sci. USA 70: 3759–3763.
27. Catterall, W. A., 1975. Proc. Nat. Acad. Sci. USA 72: 1782–1786.
28. Stallcup, W. B., 1977. Brain Res. 135: 37–53.
29. Palfrey, C. & Littauer, U. Z., 1976. Biochem. Biophys. Res. Commun. 72: 209–215.
30. Stallcup, W. B., 1979. J. Physiol. 286: 525–540.
31. Charnock, J. S., Cook, D. A. & Casey, R., 1971. Arch. Biochem. Biophys. 147: 323–329.
32. Katz, B., 1966. 'Nerve Muscle and Synapse', McGraw Hill, New York.
33. Teichberg, V. I., Goldberg, O., Tal, N. & Luini, A., 1980. Neurotransmitters and their Receptors (Littauer, U. Z., Dudai, Y., Silman, I., Teichberg, V. I. & Vogel, Z., ed.), pp. 349–368, John Wiley, N. Y.
34. Yamamoto, C., Yamashita, H. & Chujo, T., 1976. Nature 262: 786–787.
35. Krnjevic, K. & Phillis, J. W., 1963. J. Physiol. 165: 274–304.
36. Ransom, B. R., Bullock, P. N. & Nelson, P. G., 1977. J. Neurophysiol. 40: 1163–1177.
37. Daniel, E. E., 1975. Methods in Pharmacology 3: 699–721.
38. Curtis, D. R., Duggan, A. W., Felix, D., Johnston, G. A. R., Tebecis, A. K. & Watkins, J. C., 1972. Brain Res. 41: 283–301.

39. Goldberg, O., Luini, A. & Teichberg, V. I., 1980. Tetrahedron Lett. 21: 2355–2358.

40. Nathanson, J. A., 1977. Physiol. Rev. 57, 157–256.

41. Greengard, P., 1976. Nature, 260: 101–108.

42. Shimizu, H., Ichishita, H. & Odagiri, H., 1974. J. Biol. Chem. 249: 5955–5962.

43. Ferrendelli, J. A., Chang, M. M. & Kinscherf, D. A., 1974. J. Neurochem. 22, 535–540.

44. Mao, C. C., Guidotti, A. & Costa, A., 1974. Brain Res. 79: 510–514.

45. Garthwaite, J. & Balazs, R., 1978. Nature 275, 328–329.

46. Crank, J., 1956. The Mathematics of Diffusion, Oxford at the Clerendon Press.

47. Nicholson, C., Phillips, J. M. & Gardner-Medwin, A. R., 1979. Brain Res. 169: 580–584.

48. Biziere, K., Thompson, H. & Coyle, J. T., 1980. Brain Res. 183: 421–423.

49. Baudry, M. & Lynch, G., 1980. Proc. Nat. Acad. Sci. USA 77, 2298–2302.

50. Foster, A. C. & Roberts, P. J., 1978. J. Neurochem. 31: 1467–1777.

51. Davies, J. & Watkins, J. C., 1979. J. Physiol. 297: 621–635.

52. McLennan, H. & Lodge, D., 1979. Brain Res. 169: 83–90.

53. Watkins, J. C., 1980. Trends in Neurosciences 3: 61–64.

54. Davies, J., Evans, R. H., Francis, A. A., Jones, A. W. & Watkins, J. C., 1980. Neurotransmitters and their Receptors (Littauer, U. Z., Dudai, Y., Silman, I., Teichberg, V. I. & Vogel, Z. ed.), pp. 333–348, John Wiley, N.Y.

55. Goldberg, O., Luini, A. & Teichberg, V. I., 1981. Neuroscience Lett. (in press).

56. Hall, J. G., Hicks, T. P. & McLennan, H., 1978. Neuroscience Lett. 8, 171–175.

57. McLennan, H. & Lodge, D., 1979. Brain Res. 169: 83–90.

58. Segal, M., 1976. Br. J. Pharmac. 58: 341–345.

59. Spencer, H. J., Gribkoff, V. K., Cotman, C. W. & Lynch, G., 1976. Brain Res. 105: 471–481.

60. Clarke, G. & Straughan, D. W., 1977. Neuropharmacology 16: 391–398.

61. McGeer, P. L., McGeer, E. G., Scherer, U. & Singh, K., 1977. Brain Res. 128: 369–373.

62. Reubi, J. C. & Cuenod, M., 1979. Brain Res. 176: 185–188.

63. Rowlands, G. J. & Roberts, P. J., 1980. Exp. Brain Res. 39: 239–240.

64. Spencer, H. J., 1976. Brain Res. 102: 91–101.

65. Evans, R. H., Francis, A. A., Hunt, K., Oakes, D. J. & Watkins, J. C., 1979. Br. J. Pharmacol. 67: 591–603.

66. Biscoe, T. J., Davies, J., Dray, A., Evans, R. H., Francis, A. A., Martin, M. R. & Watkins, J. C., 1977. Europ. J. Pharmacol. 54: 315–316.

Received December 30, 1980.

Alterations of central GABAergic activity in neurologic and psychiatric disorders: evaluation through measurements of GABA and GAD activity in cerebrospinal fluid

Theodore A. Hare

Dept. of Pharmacology, Thomas Jefferson University, 1020 Locust Street, Philadelphia, PA 19107, U.S.A.

Introduction

Glutamic acid decarboxylase (GAD) is generally thought to be the primary catalyst mediating the formation of γ-aminobutyric acid (GABA), which in turn is thought to be the main inhibitory neurotransmitter in the central nervous system (CNS) (1). For this reason GAD activity in CNS tissue has been widely investigated because of the possibilities that it may serve a role in the regulation of central GABAergic activity or that it may provide a reflection of CNS GABAergic alterations associated with certain neurologic or psychiatric disorders. Efforts to elucidate the involvement of GAD alterations in the pathology of CNS disorders have benefitted from studies of animal models and human autopsy tissue (e.g., 2–8). However, in many instances it has not been possible to develop entirely suitable animal models. The diseased human would be the only perfect model for these disorders except, of course, human brain tissue can seldom be studied except at autopsy. Thus, especially in clinical studies, variables are difficult to control and great care must be exercised in extrapolating data to the living human condition.

Cerebrospinal fluid (CSF) bathes the CNS and tends to reflect individual variations in the state of activity of adjacent nervous tissue (9, 10). CSF is readily available from patients; however, in the past procedures for studying neurotransmitters in CSF have not been available. Recent advances of technique have provided reliable methods so that now neurotransmitters can be accurately measured in CSF. Numerous studies have demonstrated that for many of the CNS neurotransmitters, CSF levels or that of metabolites are correlated with CNS activities (reviewed in 17, 18).

A general hypothesis underlying studies of neurotransmitters in CSF is that alterations of the central activities of neurotransmitter substances are associated (either as a cause or consequence) with CNS disorders. Since the brain functions as an integrated network of many neurotransmitters systems it is probable that pathologic processes result when imbalances exist between two or more of these systems. Recent studies of GABA in CSF have demonstrated the utility of neurotransmitter measurements in CSF for studying neurologic and psychiatric disorders – providing the realization that deficiency of GABA function is an underlying defect for many of the degenerative-type disorders (19–28).

Evidence has been presented which supports the contention that GABA levels in lumbar CSF provide a reflection of alterations in central GABAergic activity. For example, the concentration of GABA in cisternal CSF correlates with its relative level in brain (29) and significant correlations between ventricular or cisternal CSF GABA levels and brain GABA concentrations have been demonstrated following the administration of drugs known to alter brain GABA levels in animals (29, 30). CSF is not contaminated by peripheral GABA in the presence of an intact blood-brain barrier and there is little correlation between peripheral and central GABA concentrations (29–31). The existence of rostrocaudal concentration gradients have been demonstrated in sequential aliquots of human lumbar CSF suggesting that the GABA in CSF obtained at the lumbar level also

Molecular and Cellular Biochemistry 39, 297–304 (1981). 0300-8177/81/0391-0297/$01.60.

reflects brain GABAergic activity (11, 14, 17, 19, 32, 33). Initial clinical investigations further support this concept documenting low GABA levels (12, 24, 34–42) in lumbar CSF from patients with disorders known to be associated with CNS GABA deficiencies (3, 7, 43–46).

Based on this rationale quantification of the GABA content in lumbar CSF has become a widely-used method of studying pathologic and drug-induced alterations in central nervous system GABAergic metabolism (9, 12, 22, 27, 29, 33–40, 47–52). Alterations in central nervous system GABAergic activity as reflected by changes in CSF GABA levels have been reported to occur in numerous neurologic and psychiatric disorders (9, 22, 24, 26, 33–37, 40, 47–53). Thus quantification of GABA content in CSF offers a method of studying GABAergic activity in living patients which does not require brain biopsy with its associated morbidity and avoids the vagaries of extrapolation from animal models or post mortem tissue. Recent studies (54, 55) have demonstrated that similar procedures can be utilized to measure GAD activity in CSF offering further refinement of data concerning central GABAergic activity as reflected in CSF.

In view of the exciting possibility that coordinated and careful study of the balances between the various neurotransmitters in CSF would significantly aid in the elucidation of specific underlying pathologic mechanisms of CNS disorders, it is important that the initial studies with each of the neurotransmitters be critically evaluated so that valid conclusions will be reached leading eventually to appropriate comparisons among the neurotransmitters.

Critical Evaluation of Studies of GABA in CSF

The early literature on GABA in CSF contains several key discrepencies which evidently resulted from differences among assay procedures as well as from inadequate regard for both in vivo and in vitro variations influencing GABA content.

GABA assay procedures

Human CSF GABA has been measured by ion-exchange/fluorometric (I-E/F) (11, 56, 57), radio-receptor (RR) (14), gas chromatography/mass spectrometric (GC/MS) (15, 16, 34) and enzymatic methods (58, 59). The I-E/F, RR and GC/MS procedures have been compared (34, 60) and provided generally consistent data, whereas the enzymatic procedure has been criticized (12, 56), evidently lacking specificity and sensitivity and providing data inconsistent with that of the other three methods. Of the three available procedures for reliably measuring GABA in CSF, the I-E/F and RR methods have been most widely used for clinical investigations and of these two the I-E/F method evidently is the more precise. For example, calculation of data reported using the RR assay (34, 47–49) reveals mean standard deviations to be ±49% of the mean GABA values, whereas similar calculation of data reported (22, 26, 33, 40) from corresponding patient groups when the I-E/F method was used reveals mean standard deviations to be 27% of the mean GABA values. This difference of precision could be highly significant in view of the numerous reports suggesting differences which are not statiscally significant between controls and patients. Thus the I-E/F GABA method is currently the prefered assay for clinical investigations of GABA in CSF.

In vivo variations

In several of the initial studies of GABA in human CSF, control groups were comprised of patients with miscellaneous neurologic disorders other than the subject disorder (15, 34, 35, 47–49). As discussed above subsequent studies have demonstrated that GABAergic deficiency is a characteristic of a variety of neurologic and psychiatric disorders leading to the conclusion that well-controlled reference populations are essential for clinical CSF GABA studies. Recent extensive studies (26, 32, 33, 40, 61) of CSF GABA from normal individuals have confirmed the significant influence of the rostrocaudal gradient for GABA especially in females and further demonstrated the significant influence of age and sex on CSF GABA content. Fig. 1 presents a summary of the data from these studies. These results illustrate that alterations of GABA content are associated even with the normal pathology of aging and point out the requirement that control and experimental populations be separated on the basis of sex and grouped in specific matching age ranges.

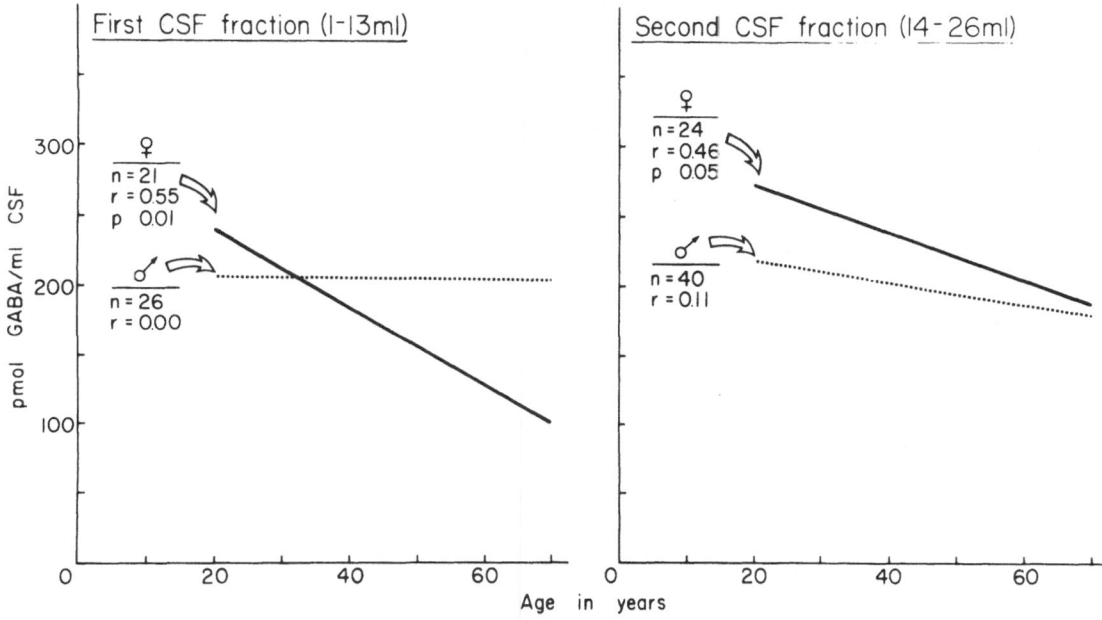

Fig. 1. *In vivo* variations of GABA in human CSF based on age and sex. Lines show results of linear regression analyses of data from CSF of normal human volunteers. Figure redrawn from data presented in ref. 32.

Many neurologic and psychiatric disorders affect age- and/or sex-specific populations and therefore invalid conclusions would be drawn if comparisons were made with control individuals unmatched with respect to age and sex distribution. The data summarized in Fig. 1 shows that unmatched control populations heavily weighted with elderly females would have lower mean CSF GABA levels than would be appropriate for comparison with experimental groups, containing more males of younger age. This difficulty can be illustrated by considering conflicting conclusions which have recently been published based upon evaluations of GABA in CSF from psychiatric patient groups (25, 26, 33, 47–49, 62). In some of these studies (47–49) the results are biased by major disparities existing among patient and/or control groups with respect to age and sex distribution.

In a study by Post et al. (26) GABA levels in the second 13 ml CSF fraction from both male and female depressed patients had been shown to be lower but not significantly different from those of corresponding normal volunteers of similar age range. In a similar study also utilizing CSF from normal volunteers of matching age range Gerner and Hare (33) found the GABA levels in the first 13 ml CSF fraction to be significantly reduced in both

male and female depressed patients and, as in the previous study found the levels in the second CSF fraction to be lower than but not significantly different from that of the normals.

In another study, Gold et al. (47) reported a seemingly more dramatic reduction of GABA in CSF from depressed patients in comparison to that of patients with various neurological disorders. In the latter study however, it seems appropriate to question whether the GABA differences were biased by differences in the age and sex distributions between the two groups since only one of the seventeen depressed patients (mean age 45) and four of the neurologic patients (mean age 52) were male. Thus in view of the propensity of older females to have low CSF GABA it is possible, depending on the precise age distribution (not specified), that the age and sex descrepencies could have produced an exaggeration of the GABA differences.

In the same report (47) and a subsequent expanded report (48) it was concluded that GABA in CSF from a group of psychotic patients was not significantly different from that of either depressed or the neurologic control group. For these comparisons the age and sex distributions were especially inappropriate however because the

300

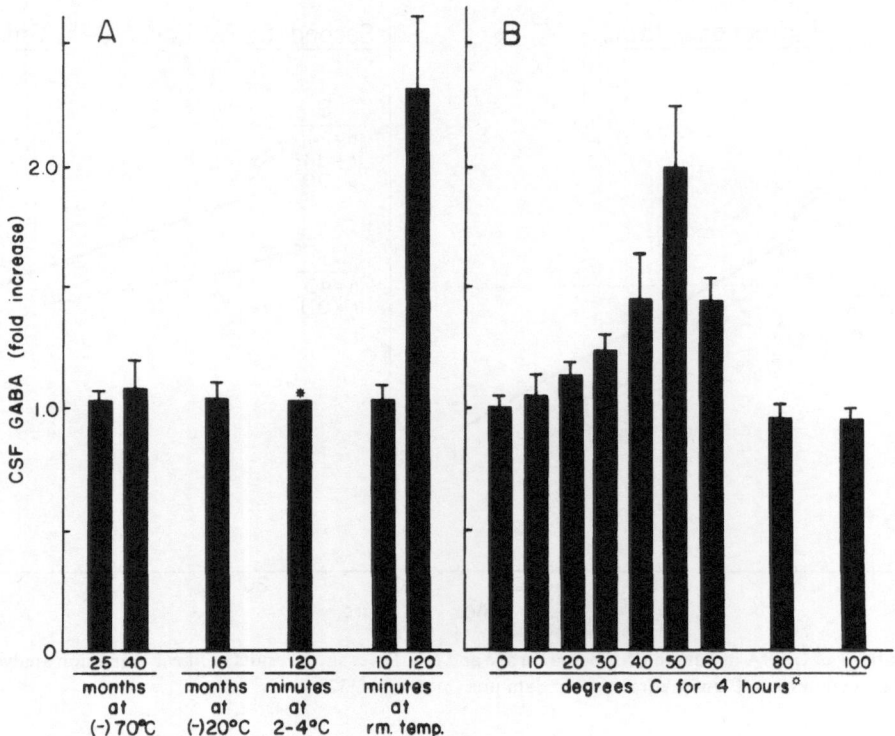

Fig. 2. In vitro alterations of GABA in untreated (i.e. not deproteinized) human CSF as the result of storage under various conditions. Bars show mean (+SE) fold increase of GABA relative to that of the same CSF prior to storage. A. Redrawn from data presented in ref. 21 and 65. *Pool of CSF from 10 individuals. B. Redrawn from data presented in ref. 54. ° Duplicate analyses of duplicate incubations of two pools of CSF from 3 and 6 individuals.

psychotic group consisted of nine men and five women (subsequently 11 men and eight women) of considerably younger age (mean 25 years). Similar desparities of age and sex distribution exist between psychiatric and non-psychiatric control groups in a report by McCarthy et al. (49) which concluded that GABA in CSF of chronic schizophrenic is elevated relative to that of non-psychiatric. On the other hand, Van Kammen et al. (22) found GABA in CSF from schizophrenic patients to be significantly reduced in comparison to that of normal volunteers. Subsequent evaluation of the data (62) following division into male and female groups of matching age ranges, revealed that the significant reduction was limited to the female schizophrenic patients. This result is compatable with data of Gerner and Hare (33) who also compared GABA levels in CSF from schizophrenic patients and normal volunteers. In this study the values from male patients were lower but not significantly different from age matched normals; whereas, the values from female patients were substantially

lower (173 ± 25 pmol/ml vs 224 ± 20 pmol/ml) than age matched normals although the low number (N = 3) of female patients precluded statistical comparison.

Thus a critical review of the literature to date suggests that GABAergic activity as reflected in CSF, may be reduced in both depressed and psychotic patients and that this reduction is more prominent in women. In order to evaluate GABA alterations it is evident that great care must be exercized in drawing comparisons with reference populations because influences based on age and sex even in normal individuals are of similar magnitude to that resulting from the disorder.

In vitro GABA alterations during CSF procurement, storage and analysis

Other discrepancies in the literature evidently resulted as a consequence of inadequate regard for in vitro GABA alterations. For example, various values were reported for normal or control individuals ranging from undetectable to 913 pmol/ml (15, 32–37, 56, 58, 59, 61–64). Similar discrepancies exist for values reported from various neurologic and psychiatric patient groups (22, 26, 28, 34, 40, 47–49, 58, 59, 63). Fig. 2 illustrates the results of recent studies which have demonstrated that to a substantial degree, these discrepancies resulted from previous inadequate regard for in vitro GABA alterations which can occur in CSF during sample procurement, storage and analysis (12, 21, 54, 56, 64, 65).

As summarized in Fig. 2a Grossman et al. (64) showed that GABA levels are unstable in untreated CSF at room temperature producing a two-fold increase during two hours. Bohlen et al. (56) also reported that GABA levels increase about ten-fold in untreated CSF during 50 hours at room temperature. Subsequently, (21, 65) the GABA increase was found to be linear with respect to time reaching significant levels after only about 10 min at room temperature. The GABA level was found to be stable for two hours in chilled (2–4 °C) CSF and to be stable to long term storage in frozen CSF. As shown in Fig. 2b., it has been demonstrated (54) that these GABA increases (i.e. in untreated CSF) are entirely secondary to enzyme action, because study of the differential influence of temperature (0–100 °C) revealed a progressive increase of GABA content reaching a maximum at 50 °C but no increase in CSF incubated at 80 °C or 100 °C.

At least part of the increase of GABA in untreated CSF evidently results from GAD activity as shown by a study in which 'live' and 'boiled' CSF was incubated in the presence and absence of glutamate (5 mM) and B₆ (0.025 mM) (55). In that study the GABA level remained unchanged in the tubes which contained 'boiled' CSF. In the tubes which contained the 'live' CSF the GABA levels increased as shown in the table below.

| Exogenous | GABA increase (pmol/ml) | | |
Glu & B₆	30 min	60 min	100 min
–	97	131	171
+	129	203	326

The above results evidently demonstrate the presence of GAD activity in CSF and further suggest that the in vitro increases in the untreated CSF may result from conversion of endogenous glutamic acid to GABA. In addition it can be presumed that GABA is continuously being formed

in the CSF in vivo and that the level observed in lumbar specimens represents some combination of GABA secreted into CSF and that formed in situ via GAD action. Thus the GABA level observed in lumbar CSF reflects combined GABA plus GAD activity and it should be possible to distinguish the two contributions through measurement of GAD activity as well as GABA. GAD activity itself may reflect GABAergic function but measurement of both parameters in patient and control CSF could provide a substantially refined reflection of central GABAergic activity.

Grossman et al. (65) utilized acid deproteinization to terminate enzyme activity and found that the increase of CSF GABA was reduced but not entirely eliminated (Fig. 3). The remaining instability was attributed to hydrolysis of GABA containing peptides because homocarnosine, a dipeptide of GABA and histidine, was found to be hydrolyzed to its constituent amino acids when stored in dilute acid under conditions which produce increases of GABA content in CSF.

Thus, there are two mechanisms which produce in vitro alterations of CSF GABA levels: (a) at

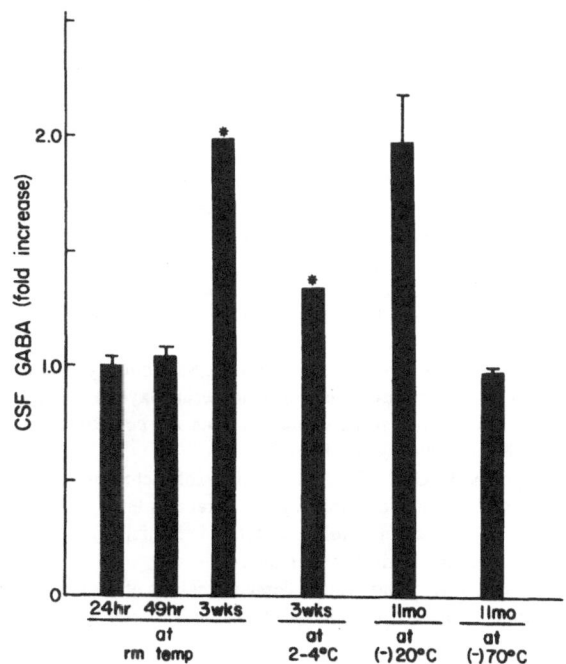

Fig. 3. In vitro alterations of GABA in acid deproteinized human CSF as the result of storage under various conditions. Bars show mean (+SE) fold increases of GABA relative to that of the same CSF prior to storage. Redrawn from data presented in ref. 65. *pool of CSF from 10 individuals.

302

physiological pH, the increase is entirely secondary to GAD and perhaps other enzyme activity (54); and (b) at acid pH the increase is evidently secondary to chemical hydrolysis (65). It has been pointed out (9, 12, 21, 54, 65, 66) that these in vitro alterations appear to explain much of the conflicting data in the literature. It is clear therefore that future clinical studies should utilize only standardized protocols which have been demonstrated to yield no artefactual alterations, that precise assay procedures should be selected to avoid exposure of the sample to acid conditions and/or elevated temperature and that values be compared with data from properly matched control populations.

References

1. Roberts, E., Chase, T. N. & Tower, D. B. (eds.), 1976. GABA in Nervous System Function, New York, Raven Press.
2. Bird, E. D., MacKay, A. V. P., Rayner, C. N. & Iversen, L. L., 1973. Reduced glutamic acid decarboxylase activity of postmortem brain in Huntington's chorea. Lancet 1: 1090–1092.
3. Bird, E. D., Iversen, L. L., 1974. Huntington's chorea: Postmortem measurement of glutamic acid decarboxylase, choline acetylase and dopamine in basal ganglia. Brain 97: 457–472.
4. McGeer, P. L., McGeer, E. G., Fibiger, H. C., 1973. Choline acetylase and glutamic acid decarboxylase in Huntington's chorea. Neurology 23: 912–917.
5. McGeer, P. L., McGeer, E. G., 1976. The GABA system and function of the basal ganglia: Huntington's disease, In: GABA in Nervous System Function, Roberts, E., Chase, T. N., Tower, D. B., eds.) New York, Raven Press, pp. 487–496.
6. Stahl, W. L., Swanson, P. D., 1974. Biochemical abnormalities in Huntington's chorea brains. Neurology 24: 913–819.
7. Urquhart, N., Perry, T. L., Hansen, S., Kennedy, J., 1975. GABA content and glutamic acid decarboxylase activity in brain of Huntington's chorea patients and control subjects. J. Neurochem. 24: 1071–1075.
8. Spokes, E. G. S., 1979. An analysis of factors influencing measurements of dopamine, noradrenaline, glutamate decarboxylase and choline acetylase in human post-mortem brain tissue. Brain 102: 333–346.
9. Wood, J. H., 1980. Neurochemical analysis of cerebrospinal fluid. Neurology (Minneap) 30: 645–651.
10. Wood, J. H., 1980. Physiology, pharmacology and dynamics of cerebrospinal fluid. In: Neurobiology of Cerebrospinal Fluid I (Wood, J. H. ed.) New York, Plenum Publishing Corp., pp. 1–16.
11. Hare, T. A., Manyam, N. V. B., 1980. Rapid and sensitive ion-exchange/fluorometric method for measuring GABA in physiological fluids. Anal. Biochem. 101: 349–355.
12. Hare, T. A., Manyam, N. V. B., Glaeser, B. S., 1980. Evaluation of cerebrospinal fluid γ-aminobutyric acid content in neurological and psychiatric disorders. In: Neurobiology of Cerebrospinal Fluid I (Wood, J. H. ed.) New York, Plenum Publishing Corp., pp. 171–187.
13. Ziegler, M. G., Lake, C. R., Wood, J. H., Ebert, M. H., 1980. Norepinephrine in cerebrospinal fluid: Basic studies, effects of drugs and disease. In: Neurobiology of Cerebrospinal Fluid I (Wood, J. H. ed.) New York, Plenum Publishing Corp., pp. 141–152.
14. Enna, S. J., Wood, J. H., Snyder, S. H., 1977. γ-aminobutyric acid (GABA) in human cerebrospinal fluid: radioreceptor assay. J. Neurochem. 28: 1121–1124.
15. Huizinga, J. D., Teelken, A. W., Muskiet, F. A. J., et al., 1978. Gamma-aminobutyric acid determination in human cerebrospinal fluid by mass-fragmentography. J. Neurochem. 30: 911–913.
16. Faull, K. P., DoAmaral, J. R., Berger, P. A., et al., 1978. Mass spectrometric identification and selected ion monitoring quantitation of gamma-aminobutyric acid (GABA) in human lumbar cerebrospinal fluid. J. Neurochem. 31: 1119–1122.
17. Wood, J. H., 1980. Sites of origin and CSF concentration gradients: Neurotransmitters, their precursors and metabolites and cyclic nucleotides. In: Neurobiology of Cerebrospinal Fluid I (Wood, J. H. ed.) New York, Plenum Publishing Corp., pp. 53–62.
18. Chase, T. N., 1980. Neurochemical alterations in Parkinson's disease. In: Neurobiology of Cerebrospinal Fluid I (Wood, J. H. ed.) New York, Plenum Publishing Corp., pp. 207–218.
19. Wood, J. H., Hare, T. A., Enna, S. J., Manyam, N. V. B., 1980. Sites of origin and rostrocaudal concentration gradients of GABA in cerebrospinal fluid. Brain Res. Bull. 5 (suppl 2) 111–114.
20. Hare, T. A., Wood, J. H., Manyam, N. V. B., et al., 1980. Selection of control populations for clinical cerebrospinal fluid GABA investigations based on comparison with normal volunteers. Brain Res. Bull. 5 (Suppl 2): 721–724.
21. Hare, T. A., Grossman, M. H., Wood, J. H., et al., 1980. Factors influencing concentrations of GABA in cerebrospinal fluid. Brain Research Bull. 5 (Suppl 2): 725–730.
22. Van Kammen, D. P., Sternberg, D. E., Hare, T. A., et al., 1980. Schizophrenia: Low spinal fluid GABA levels? Brain Res. Bull. 5 (Suppl 2): 731–636.
23. Prasad, A. L. N., Fahn, S., 1980. GABA levels in CSF of neurological patients by high performance liquid chromatography. Brain Res. Bull. 5 (Suppl 2): 737–740.
24. Manyam, N. V. B., Hare, T. A., Katz, L., 1980. Cerebrospinal fluid GABA levels in involuntary movement disorders. Brain Res. Bull. 5 (Suppl 2): 741–746.
25. Wood, J. H., Hare, T. A., Glaeser, B. S., Brooks, B. R., Ballenger, J. C., Post, R. M., 1980. Cerebrospinal fluid GABA variations with seizure type and cerebellar stimulation in man. Brain Res. Bull. (Suppl 2): 747–754.
26. Post, R. M., Ballenger, J. C., Hare, T. A., et al., 1980. Cerebrospinal fluid GABA in normals and patients with affective disorders. Brain Res. Bull. 5 (Suppl 2): 755–760.
27. Brooks, B. R., Ziegler, M. G., Lake, C. R., Wood, J. H., Enna, S. J., Engel, W. K., 1980. Cerebrospinal fluid

norepinephrine and free γ-aminobutyric acid in amyotrophic lateral sclerosis. Brain Res. Bull. 5 (Suppl 2): 765–768.

28. Teychenne, P. F., Zeigler, M. G., Lake, C. R., Enna, S. J., 1980. Effects of dopaminergic drugs in cerbrospinal fluid GABA concentration in Parkinson's disease. Brain Res. Bull. 5 (Suppl 2): 769–772.

29. Bohlen, P., Huot, S., Paltreyman, M. G., 1979. The relationship between GABA concentrations in brain and cerebrospinal fluid. Brain Res. 167: 267–305.

30. Loscher, N., 1979. GABA in plasma and cerebrospinal fluid of different species. Effects of γ-acetylenic GABA, γ-vinyl GABA, and sodium vaporoate. J. Neurochem. 32: 1587–1591.

31. Kuriyama, K., Sze, P. Y., 1971. Blood-brain barrier to ³H-γ-aminobutyric acid in normal and aminooxyacetic acid-treated animals. Neuropharmacology 10: 103–108.

32. Hare, T. A., Wood, J. H., Manyam, B, V., Gerner, R. H., Ballenger, J. C., Post, R. M. Central nervous system γ-aminobutyric acid activity in man related to age and sex as reflected in cerebrospinal fluid. Arch. Neurol., in press.

33. Gerner, R. H., Hare, T. A. CSF GABA in normals, depression, schizophrenia, mania and anorexia nervosa, Am. J. Psychiatry, in press.

34. Enna, S. J., Stern, L. Z., Wastek, G. J., et al., 1977. Cerebrospinal fluid gamma-aminobutyric acid and variations in neurological disorders. Arch. Neurol. 34: 683–685.

35. Glaeser, B. S., Vogel, W. H., Oleweiler, D. B., et al., 1975. GABA levels in cerebrospinal fluid of patients with Huntington's chorea. Biochem. Med. 12: 380–385.

36. Manyam, N. V. B., Hare, T. A., Katz, L., et al., 1978. Huntington's disease: Cerebrospinal fluid GABA levels in at-risk individuals. Arch. NEUROL. (Chic) 35: 728–730.

37. Manyam, N. V. B., Hare, T. A., Katz, L., 1979. Cerebrospinal fluid GABA levels in Huntington's disease, 'at risk' for Huntington's disease and normal controls. In: Advances in Neurology (Chase, T. N., Wexler, N. S. & Barbeau, A., ed.) New York, Raven Press, Vol. 23, pp. 547–556.

38. Manyam, N. V. B., Hare, T. A., Katz, L., 1980. Effect of isoniazid on cerebrospinal fluid and plasma GABA levels in Huntington's disease. Life Sci. 26: 1303–1308.

39. Manyam, B. V., Katz, L., Hare, T. A., Kaniefski, K., Tremblay, R. D. Isoniazid induced elevation of CSF GABA levels and effects on chorea in Huntington's disease. Ann. Neurol., in press.

40. Manyam, N. V. B., Katz, L., Hare, T. A., et al., 1980. Cerebrospinal fluid GABA levels in various neurologic disorders. Arch. Neurol. (Chic) 37: 352–355.

41. Wood, J. H., Hare, T. A., Glaeser, B. S., Ballenger, J. C., Post, R. M., 1979. Cerebrospinal fluid GABA reductions in seizure patients, Neurology 29: 1203–1208.

42. Enna, S. J., Ziegler, M. G., Lake, C. R., Wood, J. H., Brooks, B. R., Butler, I. J., 1980. CSF GABA: Correlation with CSF and blood constituents and alterations in neurological disorders, In: Neurobiology of Cerebrospinal Fluid I (Wood, J. H., ed.) New York, Plenum Publishing Corp., pp. 189–196.

43. Perry, T. L., Hansen, S., Kloster, M., 1973. Huntington's chorea: Deficiency of gamma-aminobutyric acid in brain, N. Eng. J. Med. 288: 337–342.

44. Van Gelder, N. M., Sherwin, A. L., Rasmussen, T., 1972. Amino acid content of epileptogenic human brain: Focal versus surrounding regions, Brain Res. 40: 385–389.

45. Ribak, C. E., Harris, A. B., Vaughn, J. E., Roberts, E., 1979. Inhibitory GABAergic nerve terminals decrease at sites of focal epilepsy. Science 205: 211–214.

46. Spokes, E. G. S., 1980. Neurochemical alterations in Huntington's chorea. A study of post mortem brain tissue, Brain 103: 179–210.

47. Gold, B. I, Bowers, M. B., Roth, R. H., Sweeney, D. W., 1980. GABA levels in CSF of patients with psychiatric disorders. Am J Psychiatry 137: 362–364.

48. Bowers, M. B., Jr., Gold, B. I., Roth, R. H., 1980. CSF GABA in psychotic disorders. Psychopharmacology 70: 279–282.

49. McCarthy, B. W., Gomes, U. R., Neethling, A. C., Shanley, B. C., Toljaard, J. J. F., Polgieter, L., Roux, J. T., 1981. γ-Aminobutyric acid concentration in cerebrospinal fluid in schizophrenia. J. Neurochem. 36: 1406–1408.

50. Post, R. M., Ballenger, J. C., Hare, T. A., Bunney, W. E., Jr., 1980. Lack of effect of carbamazepine on gamma-aminobutyric acid levels in cerebrospinal fluid. Neurology (minneap) 30: 1008–1011.

51. Wood, J. H., Glaeser, B. S., Hare, T. A., Sode, J., Brooks, B. R., Van Beuren, J. M., 1977. Cerebrospinal fluid GABA reductions in seizure patients evoked by cerebellar surface stimulation. J. Neurosurg. 47: 582–589.

52. Grove, J., Schecter, P. J., Tell, G., Koch-Weser, J., Sjoerdsma, A., Warter, J.-M., Marescaux, C., Rumbach, 1981. Increased gamma-aminobutyric acid (GABA), homocarnosine and β-alanine in cerebrospinal fluid of patients treated with γ-vinyl GABA (4-amino-hex-5-enoic acid). Life Sci. 28: 2431–2439.

53. Ziegler, M. G., Brooks, B. R., Lake, C. R., Wood, J. H., Enna, S. J., 1980. Norepinephrine and γ-aminobutyric acid in amyotrophic lateral sclerosis. Neurology (Minneap) 30: 99–106.

54. Hare, T. A., Wood, J. H., Manyam, B. V. Clinical implications of enzyme-mediated alterations of γ-aminobutyric acid in human cerebrospinal fluid, Arch. Neurol., in press.

55. Hare, T. A., Manyam, B. V., Tremblay, R. D. Quantification of GAD activity in human cerebrospinal fluid, submitted.

56. Bohlen, P., Schechter, P. J., van Damme, W., Coquillat, G., Dosch, J.-C. & Koch-Weser, J., 1978. Automatic assay of gamma-aminobutyric acid in human cerebrospinal fluid, Clin. Chem. 24: 256–260.

57. Glaeser, B. S., Hare, T. A., 1975. Measurement of GABA in human cerebrospinal fluid, Biochem. Med. 12: 274–282.

58. Achar, V. S., Welch, K. M. A., Chabi, E., Bartosh, K., Meyer, J. S., 1976. Cerebrospinal fluid gamma-aminobutyric acid in neurologic disease, Neurology 26: 777–780.

59. Lichtshtein, D., Dobkin, J., Ebstein, R. P., Biederman, J., Rimon, R., Balmaker, R. H., 1978. Gamma-aminobutyric acid (GABA) in the CSF of schizophrenic patients before and after neuroleptic treatment, Brit. J. Psychiat. 132: 145–148.

60. Wood, J. H., Glaeser, B. S., Enna, S. J. Hare, T. A., 1978. Verification and quantification of GABA in human cerebrospinal fluid. J. Neurochem. 30: 291–293.

61. Hare, T. A., Wood, J. H., Ballenger, J. C., Post, R. M., 1979.

304

γ-Aminobutyric acid in human cerebrospinal fluid: normal values, Lancet ii: 574–535.

62. Van Kammen, D. P., Sternberg, D. E., Hare, T. A., Ballenger, J. C., Marder, S. R., Post, R. M., Bunney, W. E., Jr., Spinal fluid GABA levels in schizophrenia. Life Sci., in press.
63. Chase, T. N., Tamminga, C. A., 1979. GABA system participation in human motor cognitive and endocrine function, in Krogsgaard-Larsen, P., Scheel-Kruger, J., Kofod, H. (eds.). GABA-Neurotransmitters: Pharmacochemical, Biochemical and Pharmacological Aspects, New York, Academic Press, pp. 283–294.
64. Grossman, M. H., Hare, T. A., Tourtellotte, W. W., Alderman, J. L., Katz, L., Manyam, N. V. B., 1977. GABA measurement in human cerebrospinal fluid. Basic consideration, Soc. Neurosci. Abstr. 3: 407.
65. Grossman, M. H., Hare, T. A., Manyam, N. V. B., et al., 1980. Stability of GABA levels in CSF under various conditions of storage. Brain Research 182: 99–106.
66. Wood, J. H., 1980. Technical aspects of clinical and experimental cerebrospinal fluid investigations. In: Neurobiology of Cerebrospinal Fluid I (Wood, J. H. ed.) New York, Plenum Publishing Corp., pp. 71–96.

Received June 23, 1981.

Cellular compartments of GABA in brain and their relationship to anticonvulsant activity

Michael J. Iadarola* and Karen Gale
*Dept. of Pharmacology, Georgetown University Schools of Medicine and Dentistry, Washington, D.C., USA. *Present address: Duke VA Neurology Research Laboratory, VA Hospital, Durham, N.C., USA.*

Summary

The effects of GABA-elevating agents were examined with respect to the cellular compartments in which GABA increases occurred and the brain region(s) that mediate the anticonvulsant activity of these compounds. Changes in GABA occurring in the presence and absence of GABAergic nerve terminals were estimated in vivo using rats in which the GABA projection to the substantia nigra (SN) was destroyed on one side of the brain. One week post-operatively, the GABA concentration in the denervated SN was 10–20% of control. The net increase in GABA content of the denervated SN was compared to that of the intact SN after intraperitoneal injection of amino-oxacetic acid (AOAA), di-n-propylacetate (DPA) and γ-vinyl GABA (GVG). In the intact SN, all drugs produced significant increases in GABA. In the denervated SN, both AOAA and GVG produced marked increases in GABA (nearly equivalent to those obtained in the intact SN) whereas DPA was without effect. It therefore appears that the DPA-induced elevation of GABA depends upon the presence of GABAergic nerve terminals whereas AOAA and GVG primarily elevate GABA in non-nerve terminal compartments. An increase in GABA associated with nerve terminals was obtained with GVG only after a latency of more than 12 h following a single injection. The time course of elevation of nerve terminal-associated GABA coincided with the time course of anticonvulsant action of GVG; both effects were maximal at 60 h after a single injection. Taken together, our results indicate that the ability of DPA, AOAA and GVG to protect against chemically- and electrically-induced seizures is directly correlated with increases in nerve terminal GABA and not related to increases in other GABA compartments.

Localization of the anatomical site that mediates anticonvulsant activity was examined using intracerebral injections of GVG into fore-, mid- and hindbrain areas. Blockade of tonic hindlimb extension in the maximal electroshock test and blockade of tonic and clonic seizures produced by pentylenetetrazol and bicuculline was obtained by microinjection of GVG (10 μg) into the ventral tegmental area of the midbrain. Injections of GVG (10–40 μg) into forebrain areas (striatum, thalamus) or into hindbrain (pontine tegmentum) were without anticonvulsant activity. Anticonvulsant effects of midbrain GVG were correlated with GABA elevation (3–4 fold) within a 1.5 mm radius of the injection site; these effects were obtained within 6 h and lasted three to four days after a single treatment. After four days seizure activity returned to control. No changes in spontaneous motor activity or reflexes accompanied the GVG injections. Similar but shorter lasting anticonvulsant effects were obtained with the direct GABA receptor agonist muscimol (50 ng) injected into the midbrain site. On the other hand, doses of muscimol up to 500 ng placed in the rostral pontine tegmentum were without anticonvulsant effect, despite the appearance of marked sedation.

The time to peak anticonvulsant activity after midbrain microinjection of GVG (6 h) was considerably more rapid than that after intraperitoneal injection (60 h). Compartmental analysis revealed that nerve terminal associated GABA was elevated by 6 h after GVG when the direct microinjection route was used. These results suggest that GABAergic synapses in the midbrain may be critically involved in the control of seizure propagation.

Molecular and Cellular Biochemistry 39, 305–330 (1981). 0300-8177/81/0039-0305/$05.20.

306

Introduction

Investigation of the physiology, biochemistry, pharmacology and anatomy of GABA and GABA-containing neural systems, continues to reveal the rich complexities associated with this neuroactive amino acid (see recent symposia 1, 2, 3). Advances in the pharmacology of GABA-mimetic agents have resulted in the development of compounds that can selectively activate GABA receptors (4, 5, 6, 7), inhibit the synthetic and degradative enzymes for GABA (8, 9) or affect the neuronal and glial uptake processes for GABA (10, 11). This has already had a significant impact on our understanding of the role of GABA in convulsions and a range of other CNS functions including feeding (12), cardiovascular control (13), motor activity (14) and release of pituitary hormones (15). Before this impact can be fully realized however, we need to gain an understanding of the way in which the drugs interact with GABA metabolism and utilization in vivo. While we have some knowledge of biochemical actions of these drugs in vitro, the complexities of GABA transmission in vivo (see Section 3) do not permit a simple extrapolation to be made between the homogenate and the intact organism. For example, the synthesis, degradation and uptake of GABA appear to take place in a variety of cellular compartments, both neuronal and non-neuronal (16, 17); thus, compounds that inhibit the enzymatic degradation of GABA may cause an increase in GABA at multiple cellular sites. The most likely site for an increase in GABA to exert a functional impact on GABAergic synaptic transmission would be in GABAergic nerve terminals. On the other hand, an increase in GABA associated with GABAergic neuronal perikarya or glial cells might be less likely to directly affect GABAergic synaptic transmission. Hence, the functional consequences of a drug-induced increase in GABA levels may be critically dependent upon the site or cellular compartment in which the increase takes place.

The present article discusses a number of investigations we have made with drugs that elevate brain GABA. Our approach has focused on the relationship between drug-induced elevation of GABA and anticonvulsant effects. The experiments address the problem of localization of drug action in terms of (1) the cellular compartment in which the GABA increase takes place and (2) the area of the brain that may mediate the anticonvulsant activity. Three compounds that increase brain GABA by distinct mechanisms were used in these studies: di-n-propylacetate (DPA, sodium valproate, Depakene[(R)]), amino-oxyacetic acid (AOAA) and γ-vinyl GABA (GVG).

In the next sections, the metabolism of GABA and a brief historical account of the relationship between GABA and anticonvulsant activity are outlined followed by a discussion of the biochemical and pharmacological effects of the three drugs. In particular, the literature pertaining to the suppression of seizures and the correlation between anticonvulsant action and increases in brain GABA will be examined.

1.1 GABA metabolism

The pathways of GABA metabolism in the CNS have been extensively characterized and are briefly presented here in order to illustrate the steps at which DPA, AOAA and GVG and other compounds interact with GABA metabolism (Fig. 1).

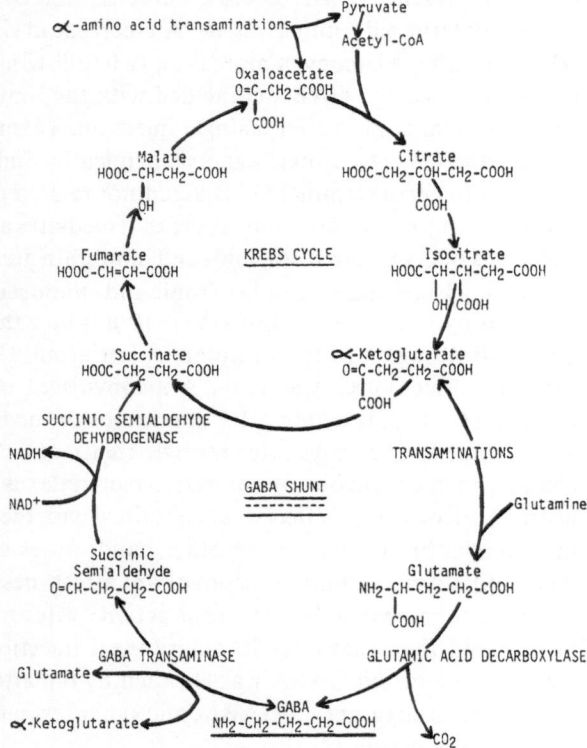

Fig. 1. The GABA shunt and its relationship to intermediary metabolism.

GABA is synthesized from glutamic acid in an irreversible decarboxylation reaction catalyzed by the enzyme glutamic acid decarboxylase (GAD, L-glutamate-l-carboxylyase, EC 4.1.1.15) which requires pyridoxal phosphate as the cofactor (36). The catabolism of GABA proceeds via two sequential reactions. The first step is a reversible transamination reaction catalyzed by the enzyme GABA-transaminase (GABA-T, γ-aminobutyric acid-α-oxoglutaric acid aminotransferase EC 2.6.1.19) which also requires pyridoxal phosphate as cofactor. Alpha-ketoglutaric acid serves as the amino-acceptor and the reaction products are succinic-semialdehyde (from GABA) and glutamic acid (from alpha-ketoglutarate). Succinic semialdehyde is further oxidized in an NAD^+ linked reaction by succinic semialdehyde dehydrogenase (SSADH, SSA-NAD$^+$-oxidoreductase, EC 1.2.1.16) to yield succinic acid, which then may enter the tricarboxylic acid cycle. For this reason the GABA metabolic pathway is referred to as the 'GABA shunt' and represents an alternate pathway that bypasses the portion of the Krebs cycle which converts alpha-ketoglutarate to succinate. More details on the enzymology, additional metabolites of GABA and intercellular relationships can be found in references 16, 36, 37 and 38.

1.2 GABA and its relationship to anticonvulsant activity: some historical highlights

GABA was initially isolated from brain by two groups working independently in 1950 (18, 19). A specific physiological action of GABA was not described until nearly seven years later when Bazemore, Elliott and Florey (20, 21) demonstrated that GABA could block discharges from the crayfish stretch receptor. Furthermore, it was known that an inhibitory substance (Factor 'I') was present in mammalian brain extracts that also blocked crayfish stretch receptor discharges. GABA was identified as the principle active substance in Factor I preparations which suggested that GABA might have an inhibitory role in brain function as well (21). About this same time it was shown that intracarotid or intraventricular injection of GABA or its β-hydroxy derivative into cats could suppress chemically-induced seizures (22). Topical administration of GABA to cerebral or cerebellar cortex of cats was demonstrated to reverse or block the

surface negative wave evoked by superficial electrical stimulation (23). GABA applied topically to cerebral cortex was also able to block the convulsive effects of electrical stimulation (24). All of these physiological findings were consistant with the hypothesis that GABA acted as an inhibitory neuroactive substance. Clinically, oral doses of GABA were shown to be effective in controlling epileptic seizures in a small number of patients (25). The usefulness of this treatment was limited by the difficulty of increasing cerebral GABA content after systemic administration of GABA (26).

Seizures induced by certain hydrazides such as thiosemicarbazide and semicarbazide were found to be associated with a decrease in brain GABA levels resulting from an inhibition of GAD activity (27). The requirement for pyridoxal phosphate as a cofactor for GAD led to renewed interest in infantile convulsions resulting from dietary deficiency of vitamin B_6 (28, 29) as well as photic induction of seizures after administration of hydrazides and B_6 antimetabolites (30). More recently, seizures produced by the convulsant agents picrotoxin and bicuculline have been correlated with the ability of these agents to block the synaptic GABA receptor-ionophore complex (31, 32).

The possibility of suppressing seizures by the pharmacological manipulation of brain GABA was first explored by Baxter and Roberts (33) with the compound hydroxylamine. In vitro hydroxylamine had been demonstrated to inhibit both GAD and GABA-T through an action on the enzymes' pyridoxal phosphate cofactor. However the strength of attachment of cofactor to apoenzyme was found to be greater for GABA-T than for GAD; addition of excess cofactor could reverse hydroxylamine inhibition of GAD but not GABA-T. These findings suggested that administration of hydroxylamine in vivo would preferentially inhibit GABA-T and result in a net elevation of brain GABA. As predicted from the in vitro studies, hydroxylamine elevated brain GABA upon systemic administration in a variety of species (24, 33, 34). Concurrently, Roberts and his co-workers investigated the effects of hydroxylamine on electrically induced seizure-after discharge in cat cerebral cortex. Hydroxylamine reduced both the duration of the after discharge as well as its ability to propagate to additional cortical recording sites. This reduction in seizure activity was paralleled by greater than twofold increases in cortical GABA levels (24). Although hydroxylamine was effective in enhancing GABAergic activity, the numerous toxic effects of this agent, including methemoglobinemia, limited its usefulness. The discovery of hydroxylamine was a milestone in the pharmacology of GABA and inaugurated an area of research which is currently being pursued. It also formed the basis from which many other drugs with similar actions were developed and investigated (9, 35) three of which (DPA, AOAA and GVG) are the subject of this article.

2. Biochemistry of GABA elevation

2.1 Biochemistry of GABA-T inhibitors

One of the most extensively studied GABA elevating agents has been amino-oxyacetic acid (AOAA) a structural analogue of hydroxylamine, first introduced by Wallach in 1961 (39). Like hydroxylamine, AOAA is a potent inhibitor of GABA-T in vivo and in vitro and is thought to work by interacting with the carbonyl group of the pyridoxal phosphate cofactor of GABA-T. The synthetic enzyme for GABA, glutamic acid decarboxylase (GAD) also utilizes pyridoxal phosphate; thus AOAA is also capable of inhibiting GABA synthesis. However, based on in vitro studies, the attachment of the pyridoxal cofactor to the apoenzyme appears to be stronger for GABA-T than for GAD; therefore, the inhibition of GAD but not GABA-T can be reversed by addition of excess pyridoxal phosphate (34, 35). This may explain why in vivo, AOAA preferentially inhibits GABA-T with a relatively weak action on GAD (40). The inhibition of GABA-T after systemic administration is long lasting (more than 12 h) and associated with marked (2–5 fold) increases in brain GABA concentration (39, 41, 42). In high doses, AOAA is capable of causing inhibition of GAD activity accompanied by seizures (40, 43).

More recently a new class of GABA-T inhibitors has been developed known as catalytic or 'suicide' inhibitors (9, 44). These analogs of the naturally occurring substrate have a latent reactive group incorporated into their structure. They bind at the enzyme's active site and, during catalytic turnover, generate a reactive intermediate which can form a covalent bond with an active site amino acid. Since the activity of such a compound requires both recognition and catalytic activation by the target enzyme, the resulting interactions are usually highly specific as well as irreversible. Ethanolamine-0-sulfate (EOS) was the first catalytic inhibitor described for GABA-T. Although EOS acted with specificity and elevated brain GABA, it did not readily penetrate the blood brain barrier (45). Soon after the introduction of EOS, Jung and Metcalf (46) developed gamma-acetylenic GABA, and Rando and Bangerter (47) characterized gabaculine, isolated from the bacteria *Streptomyces toyocaenis* (48). Both compounds caused irreversible inactivation of GABA-T and marked elevation of brain GABA after systemic administration (49, 50).

Further studies by Jung and colleagues revealed that gamma-acetylenic GABA significantly inhibited GAD activity although other pyridoxal-dependent enzymes such as aspartate transaminase and alanine transaminase were not affected (50). The lack of specificity of the acetylenic derivative led to the development of gamma-vinyl GABA (GVG) which is relatively devoid of GAD inhibitory activity (51). GVG, administered peripherally, inhibits brain GABA-T and produces pronounced (up to fivefold) and prolonged (several days) elevation of brain GABA (52). Given intraperitoneally, GVG is approximately one-tenth as potent as gamma-acetylenic GABA. However, very little difference in potency exists between the acetylenic and vinyl derivatives when assayed for GABA-T inhibitory activity in vitro (the $IC_{50} = 1.5$ and 3.5×10^{-4} M for acetylenic and vinyl GABA, respectively) (53). The different potencies after systemic administration appear to be due to poorer penetration of the vinyl derivative into the CNS.

The GABA-T inhibitors thus far discussed, cause several fold increases in brain GABA levels. In contrast, di-n-propylacetate (DPA) causes an elevation of brain GABA which is considerably less dramatic. Godin and colleagues first described the GABA elevating properties of this drug and attributed it to the ability of DPA to inhibit GABA-T (54). The inhibition of GABA-T by DPA was competitive, with Ki of 1.4×10^{-3} M with respect to GABA (55). Subsequently, Fowler et al. (56) suggested that the inhibitory action of DPA could not be characterized as clearly competitive and reported a Ki of 4.2×10^{-2} M for the aldimine form of GABA-

T; a value considerably higher than reported by Simler et al. (55). The high Ki observed suggested that GABA-T inhibition might not be the mechanism by which DPA elevated brain GABA. This notion was further reinforced when DPA was shown to inhibit succinic semialdehyde dehydrogenase (SSADH) with a Ki (1.5×10^{-3} M) similar to that reported by Simler et al. (55) for inhibition of GABA-T (57). More recently DPA has been reported to be a potent inhibitor of the enzyme aldehyde reductase (Ki = 8.5×10^{-5} M) (58). Aldehyde reductase can catalyze the reduction of succinic semialdehyde to γ-hydroxybutyrate. This pathway may be an alternative route for GABA degradation, although its importance in vivo is not known. The enzyme may be identical to that which reduces the aldehyde metabolites of biogenic amines (however, it may be a distinct entity, see 59). Although the inhibition constants for GABA-T and SSADH seem rather high, plasma and brain levels in the near millimolar range are achieved with anticonvulsant doses of DPA (60, 61, 62). This suggests that the DPA induced increase in brain GABA may be related to an inhibition of GABA-T and/or SSADH in vivo. It is also possible that additional mechanisms such as an effect of GABA synthesis, precursor availability, intracellular pH etc. may participate in the action of DPA on GABA. To date the characterization of the mechanism on action of DPA is considerably less complete than that of AOAA and GVG.

Changes in free brain amino acid profiles have also been examined for DPA, AOAA and GVG. Of 35 amino compounds measured in whole rat brain only two were found to change after DPA (400 mg/kg ip): GABA (increased by 30–40%) and aspartate (decreased by 32–45%) (63, 64, 65). The changes in the two amino acids followed a remarkably similar time course (63). AOAA and GVG produced increases in GABA, homocarnosine, hypotaurine and β-alanine (64, 66, 67, 68). The latter three compounds occur in concentration 1/20th to 1/40th that of GABA and the physiological significance of drug-induced alteration in their concentrations in unknown. GVG also caused small decreases in threonine and glutamine; no effect was seen on the levels of approximately thirty other brain amino compounds (68).

The prolonged increase in brain GABA levels produced by GVG appears to interact with brain polyamine metabolism. A delayed elevation (at about 16 h) of brain putrescine concentration occurs following a single dose of GVG. Since in vivo administration of GVG has little direct effect on activity of enzymes involved in putrescine metabolism the alterations in putrescine have been suggested to be an indirect consequence of GABA elevation (69, 70).

2.2 Pharmacology of GABA-T inhibitors

To evaluate the functional effects of GABAergic drugs in intact unanesthetized animals, anticonvulsant seizure models have often been employed. Despite the fact that anticonvulsant effects of AOAA and GVG and DPA have been studied in several experimental models, it has been difficult to formulate a coherent relationship between their anticonvulsant activity and their effects on brain GABA. Three main issues appear to be involved in attempting to evaluate whether an increase in GABA is responsible for the functional effects of AOAA, GVG and DPA: 1) temporal relationship between changes in GABA and anticonvulsant activity 2) degree of GABA elevation required for a given amount of seizure protection 3) relationship between GABA levels and seizure protection when GABA synthesis inhibitors are combined with inhibitors of GABA degradation. The literature relevant to each of these issues will be discussed briefly below.

2.2.1 Temporal relationship between changes in GABA and anticonvulsant activity

In a detailed investigation of AOAA's time-course of action, Kuriyama et al., (71) found that the peak activity against maximal electroshock seizures occurred between one and two hours after AOAA, whereas, after six hours no protection was observed. In addition, seizure protection from the convulsant agent pentylenetetrazol followed a similar time-course with greater protection at two hours than at six hours. The elevation in brain GABA did not parallel the seizure protection: a greater accumulation of GABA had occurred by six hours than by two hours. The temporal dissociation between antiseizure activity and increased GABA levels resulted in considerable speculation as to whether the two effects were related (71). Subsequent studies, also using the mouse, were unable to confirm these observations. AOAA was found to be as effective at six hours as at two hours against seizures induced by allylglycine, hydrazine, picrotoxin, pentylentetrazol and hyperbaric oxygen (72). Loscher and Frey (41) demonstrated that a close correlation existed between AOAA-induced increases in brain GABA content, GABA-T inhibition and elevations in the thresholds for maximal electroshock and tonic- and clonic-pentylene-tetrazol-induced seizures. The duration of maximal anticonvulsant activity in the three tests extended from two to eight h following injection; the elevation in GABA followed a similar pattern.

In contrast to the controversy surrounding AOAA's time course of activity, a very close correlation has been observed between the time course of brain GABA increases and seizure protection after DPA in all experiments that have examined the two variables (55, 63, 73, 74). Unlike AOAA, DPA has a rapid onset (within 15 min) and short duration of action (less than 2 h) with respect to GABA increases and anticonvulsant effects. The tests in which the anticonvulsant efficacy of DPA has been demonstrated include audiogenic seizures in mice (55, 60, 63, 74), amygdala kindled seizures (62), ethanol-withdrawal seizures (75), photosensitive epilepsy in baboons (76), seizures induced by picrotoxin, pentylenetetrazol, bicuculline, 3-mercaptopropionic acid (77), maximal electroshock seizures (73), and hyperbaric oxygen (78). The activity of DPA in electroshock seizure models is included in an extensive review by Simon and Penry (79).

The effect of catalytic inhibitors of GABA-T in various seizures models has been studied mainly by Schechter and colleagues, in mice (52, 80, 81, 82). Using the audiogenic model, these authors found that the time-course of whole-brain GABA elevation paralleled seizure protection after treatment with GVG. There was also a dose-related correlation between elevated brain GABA content and audiogenic seizure suppression. However, GVG failed to block seizures induced by bicuculline, picrotoxin or pentylenetrazol, given 4 h following GVG treatment (81, 82). This observation is somewhat paradoxical, because 4 h after GVG whole brain GABA levels are maximally elevated. The lack of effect against seizures induced by GABA-receptor antagonists (e.g. bicuculline) suggests that the increase in GABA (4 h after GVG) is not substantially affecting the amount of GABA at receptor sites. Based on the similarity of the doses of GVG and GABA ($>$1 g/kg) needed to exert anticonvulsant effects after peripheral administration, it has recently been suggested that the *acute* anticonvulsant activity of GVG may involve a direct activation of GABA receptors (83); although the IC_{50} value (4.1×10^{-3} M) in the GABA receptor binding assay is rather high (53).

2.2.2 Degree of GABA elevation required for seizure protection

A striking difference between GVG, AOAA and DPA is the degree of increase in brain GABA that occurs in association with anticonvulsant effects. Briefly, the antiseizure activity of DPA is seen with whole brain GABA increases in the range of 30–60% over control, whereas antiseizure actions of AOAA and GVG occur only with GABA increases between 200–400% over control (41, 69, 71). Obviously, if the change in GABA content is the common mechanism by which these compounds exert their anticonvulsant activity, then the precise nature of their interactions with the GABA system must differ in some important respect.

In a previous report (84) we examined the possibility that DPA or AOAA may selectively affect the GABA content of different brain regions. With doses of AOAA and DPA (20 and 400 mg/kg, respectively) that produced nearly equivalent effects on whole rat brain GABA an examination of six discrete brain areas revealed that the profile of GABA increases across areas generated by DPA was distinct from that obtained with AOAA. In superior colliculus and cerebellum DPA (400 mg/kg) produced a significantly greater elevation of GABA than did AOAA (20 mg/kg). On the other hand AOAA had a significantly greater effect on GABA in frontal cerebral cortex than did DPA. The 400 mg/kg dose of DPA blocked maximal electroshock seizures much more effectively than did 20 mg/kg AOAA; this raised the possibility that those brain areas which respond better to DPA might contain GABAergic synapses which play a role in seizure protection.

It might be expected, then, that a higher dose of AOAA, which produced increases in GABA equivalent to that of DPA in all areas, would result in an equivalent degree of seizure protection.

However, when we administered AOAA in a dose (40 mg/kg) that elevated GABA in all brain areas examined to an extent at least as great as that seen after DPA (400 mg/kg), only a partial reduction (50% decrease in the mean duration of tonic hindlimb extension in the MES test) in seizure response was obtained. In contrast, the 400 mg/kg dose of DPA completely abolished tonic hindlimb extension. Furthermore, with GVG, we found it possible to elevate GABA in all brain areas several-fold higher than can be obtained with DPA without obtaining protection against MES seizures (e.g. when rats are tested 12 h after GVG) (85). Thus, there remain apparent discrepancies between the degree of seizure protection and the degree of GABA elevation associated with DPA, AOAA and GVG which cannot be resolved simply on the basis of different regional responses.

This problem prompted us to question whether these drugs exert their effects on the same compartments of GABA. It seemed possible for example, that a relatively small increase in GABA in GABAergic nerve-terminals could have a greater functional impact (with respect to synaptic transmission) than a large GABA increase occurring in neuronal cell bodies or glial cells (see section 5).

2.2.3 Interactions between GABA synthesis inhibitors and GABA elevating agents

Most studies in which inhibitors of GABA degradation have been combined with GABA synthesis inhibitors were conducted in the early 1960s before many of the complexities of the GABA system such as the subcellular location of GAD and GABA-T were known. The drug combinations (elevating agent followed by synthesis inhibitor) were: hydroxylamine plus thiosemicarbazide (86), AOAA plus thiosemicarbazide (87, 88, 89), and hydrazine plus semicarbazide (90). After these treatments, seizures occurred despite elevated concentrations of total brain GABA. These results led to the conclusion that the increase in brain GABA was not related to the anticonvulsant activity of the GABA elevating agents. A more conservative interpretation of the data is that there is no simple relationship between the concentration of *total brain* GABA and protection from convulsions. In fact, recent subcellular fractionation studies of brain after convulsant doses of GABA elevating agents have revealed that decreases in nerve-

terminal (synaptosomal) GABA occurred with hydrazine or AOAA despite increases in total brain GABA (91, 92).

Thus, the only conclusion which can be drawn from the data in the literature is that there is not a straightforward correspondence between total brain GABA levels and seizure susceptibility (93). However, at the same time there is no evidence to support the conclusion that the anticonvulsant activity of GABA-elevating agents is not mediated by a GABAergic system. In all likelihood, GABAergic systems may be subject to a variety of manipulations which have varying degrees of functional impact depending upon features which are considerably more subtle and complex than steady-state levels of whole brain GABA. Some of these features will be discussed in the next section.

3. Complexities of studying GABAergic transmission in the CNS

Several characteristics of the GABA system complicate our understanding of the neurotransmitter role of this amino acid. These include the regional distribution in brain, the types of circuits in which GABA-containing neurons are found and the cellular localization of the synthetic and degradative pathways for GABA. Each of these features will be discussed below in the context of the difficulties which each poses for the interpretation of pharmacological and neurochemical studies of GABAergic function.

3.1 Regional distribution of GABA in brain

A distinct regional profile with respect to GABA levels in brain has been observed in several species. The highest concentration of GABA is found in the substantia nigra (SN), an area rich in GABA-containing nerve terminals. On the other hand, the cerebellar cortex contains a relatively low concentration of GABA, nearly eight times lower than that in SN (94, 95). Unlike the monamines and acetylcholine, which are frequently restricted to specific brain nuclei, GABA or GAD activity can be measured in almost every brain nucleus (94–100). It therefore appears to be rather ubiquitously, albeit unevenly, distributed in the CNS. Similarly, receptor binding sites for GABA, and electrophysiological responses to iontophoretically applied GABA, have been measured in almost every brain nucleus examined (31, 101–103). GABA-containing neurons are often of the type which project over short distances, generally intrinsic to a nucleus (Golgi type II interneurons) and less frequently of the type which participate in long distance pathways between brain regions. An additional feature of GABAergic neurons, and one which perhaps follows from their ubiquitous distribution, is that they may be found synapsing upon each other, connected in series. In the basal ganglia, for example, it is likely that GABAergic neurons intrinsic to striatum form synapses with GABAergic neurons projecting to SN; the GABAergic terminals in SN may in turn synapse upon GABAergic nigral cells, some of which project to thalamus (104, 105) and superior colliculus (106). Such circuitry makes it difficult to predict the specific functional impact of a pharmacological manipulation of GABAergic transmission, since an augmentation of GABAergic transmission in one brain nucleus may indirectly cause inhibition of GABAergic activity in an adjacent area.

In view of the variations in GABA content of different brain nuclei, and the fact that GABAergic neurons in different nuclei may play mutually counterposing roles, it is evident that measurement of whole brain GABA cannot provide functionally interpretable information. In fact, measurement of whole-brain GABA content would be highly insensitive to those changes in GABA taking place only in a few selected nuclei, changes which may be sufficient to markedly influence specific behavioral and physiological functions.

3.2 Compartmentation

The synthesis of GABA in the CNS takes place primarily, but probably not exclusively, in GABAergic neurons (107). In particular, axon terminals of GABAergic neurons possess a marked capacity for synthesizing GABA, which is then likely to be available for release into the synapse (108). Once released, GABA can then be taken back up into the GABAergic nerve endings (and presumably reutilized), or into glial cells or the cell bodies of GABAergic neurons (107, 109–111). Uptake of GABA into neuronal cell bodies and glial cells is thought to play a major role in the inactivation of

synaptically released GABA, although this has not been conclusively established (107, 110, 112–114).

Neuronal perikarya and glia comprise the cellular compartments which contain the most significant activity of GABA-T (115–118); it is probably these compartments in which the bulk of GABA degradation occurs. Under normal conditions, therefore, steady-state GABA levels are likely to be proportional to the density of GABAergic nerve-endings in a given brain region. However, in conditions where the degradation of GABA is blocked, GABA may be expected to accumulate in compartments other than (or, in addition to) the nerve terminal compartment. Likewise, when exogenous GABA is applied to brain tissue (often this is done in large concentrations or in the presence of a GABA-T inhibitor), it may be taken up into cellular compartments other than GABAergic nerve endings.

A further consideration is that significant concentrations of GABA can be measured in brain tissues in which the GABAergic neurons have been completely destroyed (119). Similarly, pure glial or glioma cell cultures contain measurable amounts of GABA, indicating that these cells probably have the capacity to synthesize, as well as to take up and degrade GABA (120, 121). As a result, manipulations of GABA metabolism need not exert an exclusive effect on nerve-terminal related GABA, and conversely, changes in GABA content need not necessarily reflect alterations relevant to synaptic transmission.

The following sections will review some of the experiments we have performed examining 1) GABA elevation in various cellular compartments 2) the relationship of compartmental GABA increases to anticonvulsant and 3) localization of the brain site at which GABA-agonist drugs exert their anticonvulsant action.

4. Assessment of anticonvulsant activity

The rationale for using anticonvulsant activity as a functional endpoint in our studies was twofold. First, interactions between drugs that affect the brain GABA system and convulsions have been well documented. Secondly drugs that augment the activity of GABA neural function may be of potential clinical importance (e.g. DPA, which is used clinically for epilepsy) and one of our goals is to discriminate aspects of drug action that are relevant to, or predictive of, anticonvulsant activity.

The primary seizure model employed was the maximal electroshock seizure (MES) test. The MES test is a widely employed seizure model and consists of delivering, via electrodes placed on the cornea, an electric stimulus that is supra-maximal for eliciting a seizure; for the rat the stimulus parameters are: 150 mA, 60 Hz, 200 ms (122, 123). The resultant seizure is of a stereotyped pattern composed of an initial tonic flexion followed by tonic extension of the limbs. The customary end-point for assessing anticonvulsant activity is blockade of the tonic extension of the hindlimbs. Since low doses of the GABA elevating agents were observed to shorten the duration of tonic hindlimb extension without producing outright blockade, the *duration* of this phase was timed in order to increase the sensitivity of the test. In addition to the MES test, we employed the chemoconvulsants pentylenetetrazol (PTZ, administered subcutaneously, 90 mg/kg or intravenously, 40 mg/kg) and bicuculline (administered intravenously, 0.25 mg/kg). The latter agent has been demonstrated to be a GABA receptor antagonist (31). PTZ like MES is widely used in anticonvulsant drug screening programs (124).

Intravenous injection of bicuculline or PTZ produced a tonic seizure within 1–3 s. The behavioral manifestations were similar for both drugs and the maximal response observed was tonic *forelimb* extension. Animals were observed for the presence or absence of seizures and the following scale was used to rate the severity of the seizures:

0   = No seizure
0.5 = Mild clonic seizure (forepaw clonus)
1   = Moderate clonic seizure (with twisting of the body)
2   = Severe clonic seizure (explosive motor activity)
3   = Tonic forelimb extension (the maximal response seen with the doses of both convulsants used).

In some experiments PTZ was adminstered subcutaneously in order to determine the effect of varying the route of administration had on anticonvulsant activity. The resulting seizures were of a stereotyped nature, consisting of one or more clonic seizures followed by tonic forelimb extension. The onset of symptoms was more gradual than with intravenous administration and the scale used to rate the severity of these seizures reflects this fact:

0 = No seizure
1 = Mild clonic seizure (forepaw clonus)
2 = Severe clonic seizure (explosive motor activity)
3 = Severe clonic seizure within the first 10 min
4 = Severe recurrent clonic seizures without a tonic seizure
5 = Steady clonic seizure activity with animal lying on its side
6 = Same as in 5 but within the first 10 min
7 = Tonic forelimb extension (TFE)
8 = TFE within 20 min
9 = TFE within 10 min
10 = TFE within 3 min

5. Elevation of GABA and cellular compartmentation

We were interested in testing the hypothesis that a major portion of the GABA increase produced by AOAA and GVG might be sequestered in compartments that do not directly participate in GABA-mediated synaptic transmission. To do this, we needed an in vivo preparation that was relatively devoid of GABAergic nerve terminals in which we could assess the effect of AOAA, GVG and DPA. For this purpose, we exploited certain unique features of the GABAergic system in the substantia nigra (SN).

The reason for selecting the SN as a model system was twofold: a) this nucleus has the highest GABA content of all brain nuclei and b) at least 80% of the GABA content of the SN is associated with GABAergic nerve-terminals, most of which arise from cell bodies which are located several millimeters away (in the forebrain). This anatomical arrangement makes it possible to sever the GABA-containing projections to the SN without causing direct injury to the nucleus itself (see Fig. 2). The normal intact SN is therefore representative of a GABA nerve-terminal *rich* area, while the denervated SN is representative of a GABA nerve-terminal *poor* area (comprised of glial cells, GABAergic cell bodies and possibly a small popu-

314

Table 1. Cellular elements constituting the GABA-containing compartments in the intact and lesioned tissues of the in vivo preparations.

	Afferent nerve terminals	Cell bodies of efferents	Glia	Interneurons
Intact S. Nigra	*	*	*	?
Denervated S. Nigra	0	*̲	*	?
Intact striatum	?	*	*	*̲
Kainic acid lesioned striatum	?	0	*̲	0

The stars indicate the presence of a particular compartment; underlined stars denote the elements that contribute the majority of the GABA. The zeros indicate those pools deleted by the lesion. GABAergic interneurons, although not directly demonstrated in the nigra, may also contribute to the GABA pool of the intact and denervated SN, hence the question mark. Similarly, GABA containing afferent terminals from a GABAergic projection to the striatum have not been demonstrated but may exist. (The kainic acid lesioned striatum is discussed in section 7.)

lation of their local collaterals). We will refer to the pool of GABA remaining in the denervated SN as the 'cellular-metabolic' or 'non-nerve terminal' pool. (Table 1).

5.1 Characterization of the GABA-denervated SN

A number of investigations have demonstrated that unilateral hemitransections anterior to the SN cause a loss of nigral GABA (128–131). In characterizing such lesions the extent of loss of nigral GABA was found to be dependent upon the rostrocaudal level of the transection (129, 130). Because we intended to study drug effects in the GABA denervated SN we required a technique that would reliably ensure a complete loss of nigral GABA-containing afferents. Our modifications of the technique are described in Fig. 2. The transecting probe was angled in order to eliminate GABA containing afferents arising from the tail of the caudate nucleus and yet not cause any direct damage to the SN (132).

In an initial series of 44 operated rats the nigral GABA content was reduced to less than 25% in the majority of the animals (88%). Further application of the hemitransection procedure has shown that complete lesions leave 10 to 15% GABA remaining in the SN of the lesioned hemisphere. The degeneration of the GABA terminals is also reflected by a

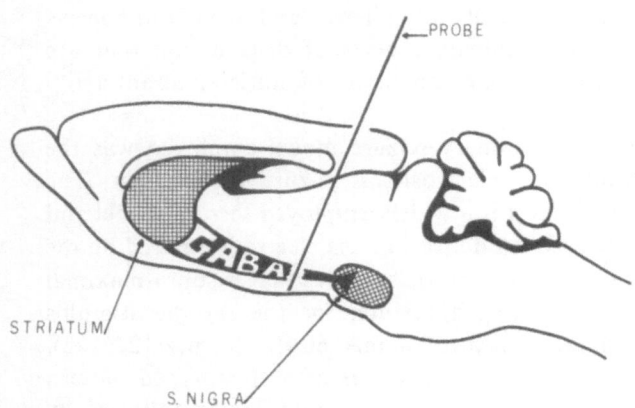

Fig. 2. Hemitransection technique illustrated schematically in a parasagittal section of rat brain. Cerebral hemitransection was performed using a stereotaxic apparatus (David Kopf) with the incisor bar 5 mm above the interaural line. A stainless steel loop, mounted in an electrode carrier, was inclined in the anteroposterior plane at an angle of 6.3° from vertical with the lower tip directed rostrally. The probe entered the cortex at AP +3.0 and was lowered to intercept the base of the brain 1–2 mm anterior to the SN. The probe was moved 5 mm laterally from the midline by manipulating the electrode carrier. The lateral movement was repeated 3–4 times, adjusting the vertical depth as necessary in order to follow the contours of the base of the skull. Transections posterior to the SN were made with the probe in a vertical position; the probe entered the cortex at AP +0.2 and was moved medio-laterally as was done for the anterior transections. Use of a blunt tipped probe allowed us to reliably sever nerver fibers at the base of the brain with only a minimum of bleeding. Seven to ten days were allowed postoperatively for degeneration to occur before drugs were administered (132).

loss of GAD activity; after complete lesions, the percent GAD activity remaining is 10–15% of that in the SN from the intact hemisphere (Fig. 3). Unilateral hemitransections were also placed posterior to the SN to determine whether neurons from caudal brain areas sent GABA-containing terminals to the SN. No significant change in GABA content was observed in the SN from the lesioned or intact hemispheres (N = 5).

In order to evaluate the functional state of the denervated SN, we monitored turning behavior in response to drugs directly microinjected into the SN (Tables 2 and 3). Unilateral injection of GABA agonists into the SN causes a rat to turn in circles in a direction contralateral to the injection site and produces a contralateral postural asymmetry. On the other hand, GABA antagonists produce the opposite effects: ipsilateral turning and postural asymmetry (133). In the intact SN microinjection of

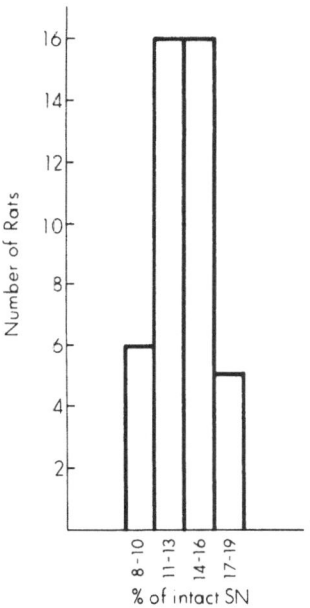

Fig. 3. Frequency histogram: range of GAD activity remaining in SN after hemitransection. Lesioned animals were grouped according to per cent GAD remaining in comparison to the contralateral intact SN. Number of rats per group is plotted on the ordinate. The total number of animals represented is 43. The mean per cent remaining was 13.6%. (Data were kindly provided by Dr. M. Casu).

isoniazid, a drug that blocks GABA synthesis (27), caused ipsilateral circling behavior indicating that functionally the drug acts as an antagonist. Microinjection of isoniazid into the denervated SN revealed that the ability of INH to induce turning behavior was dependent upon the presence of forebrain GABAergic nerve terminals. In animals with 20% or less GABA remaining in the SN, isoniazid injection into the denervated SN failed to induce either turning behavior or postural asymmetry (Table 2). Partially lesioned animals which had 25–30% GABA remaining in SN still showed ipsilateral circling in response to intranigral isoniazid, although the response was significantly attenuated compared to unlesioned controls.

A similar situation was encountered with microinjections of AOAA into the intact and denervated SN (Table 3). Unilateral microinjection of AOAA into the intact SN produced dose-related contralateral circling behavior similar to what is observed with GABA agonists (14). As was seen with isoniazid, complete GABAergic denervation of the SN (10–20% GABA remaining) abolished AOAA-induced turning. Sub-total denervation resulted in

an attenuated but, nonetheless, significant amount of turning behavior and indicates that the AOAA induced turning is also dependent upon the presence of forebrain GABAergic nerve terminals.

Parenthetically, it may be of interest to note that the rapid onset (within minutes) and short duration (40–60 min) of the AOAA-induced turning suggest that this effect may not be due to an increase in GABA. Rather the circumscribed time course suggests that the effects of *locally* applied AOAA may be mediated by a transient release of GABA from presynaptic endings or, possibly, by inhibition of release of an excitatory transmitter. Since AOAA seems to have little direct effect on GABA receptors (134–135), stimulation of turning through activation of GABA receptors does not appear to be a likely mechanism.

In contrast to AOAA and isoniazid, microinjection of the direct GABA receptor agonist muscimol (50 mg) into the SN produced vigorous contralateral turning regardless of whether the forebrain GABAergic input was present (Table 2). The presence of this behavior in response to muscimol after complete GABAergic denervation suggests that the cell bodies of nigral efferents remain functionally intact. Biochemical and behavioral observations of the development of GABA-receptor supersensitivity in nigral neurons following surgical hemitransection or lesions of the striatum also support this conclusion (136, 137). Taken together, the results obtained with isoniazid, AOAA and muscimol demonstrate that, from a functional

Table 2. Turning behavior after intranigral injection of muscimol or ioniazid in hemitransected rats (total turns in 3 min).

GABA remaining	Treatment					
(% of Intact SN)	Saline		Isoniazid		Muscimol	
	ipsi	contra	ipsi	contra	ipsi	contra
100% (intact)	2.0	3.0	29.0	1.0	0	53.0
25–30%	3.5	2.0	14.5	0.5	0	55.0
10–20%	4.0	1.0	5.0	2.0	0	50.0

Injections were made stereotaxically into the denervated SN 7–10 days after the hemitransection procedure. Muscimol (0.4 nmol) was infused in a volume of 0.5 μl over 3 min. Isoniazid (1.0 μmol) was infused in a volume of 1 μl over 5 min. Values represent the mean number of complete turns (total over a 3 min period) for a group of 4–6 rats. GABA content of the intact and denervated SN was measured three days after the injection in order to allow drug effects to wear off. (Adapted from 132).

standpoint, forebrain derived GABA nerve terminals in the SN can be completely eliminated following the denervation procedure without directly damaging the perikarya of nigral efferent neurons. Based on these results, the denervated SN appeared to be a suitable preparation in which to study compartmental increases in GABA after treatment with DPA, AOAA and GVG.

5.2 Drug-induced elevation of GABA in the intact and denervated SN

Fig. 4 summarizes the results obtained after intraperitoneal injection of DPA (300 mg/kg),

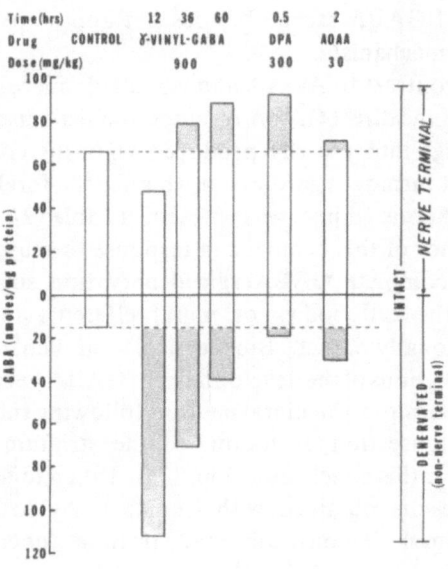

Fig. 4. The effect of GVG, DPA, and AOAA on GABA content of the intact and GABA-denervated SN. In this figure the *total* length of a bar represents the GABA content of the intact SN. The portion of the bar that extends below the horizontal axis represents the GABA content of the GABA-denervated SN. The GABA content of the denervated SN was subtracted from that of the intact SN to obtain the nerve terminal associated GABA level. The control level of GABA in the nerve terminal and non-nerve terminal compartments is shown in the first bar and demarcated by the dotted lines. The net increase due to drug treatment, in both compartments, is indicated by the shaded portion of each bar. Each bar represents the mean GABA value from at least six animals. Animals were sacrificed by focussed microwave irradiation of the head for 4 s. All drug-induced increases in GABA in the intact and denervated SN were significantly different from the respective controls except for DPA in the denervated SN. Criterion for significance was p < 0.05. Comparisons were made by analysis of variance and Duncan's new multiple range test. (Reproduced with permission from 145).

Table 3. Effect of AOAA on rotational behavior after injection into the intact or denervated SN.

Treatment	AOAA dose (μg)	N	Turns/min	
Intact Rats			ipsi	contra
	0.5	(3)	0.2 ± 0.2	0.4 ± 0.3
	1.0	(5)	0	5.3 ± 0.5*
	2.0	(4)	0	12.1 ± 3.5*
	4.0	(5)	0	26.0 ± 8.8*
Hemitransected rats	4.0			
Subtotal denervation (25–30% GABA remaining)		(3)	0	6.7 ± 2.3*
Complete denervation (10–20% GABA remaining)		(12)	0	0

The number of animals in each group is indicated in parentheses. The values represent the mean ± SEM of the average number of turns counted over a three minute period for each animal. Turning was measured at 20 min after the end of the infusion. In order to assess the completeness of the lesion three days were allowed to elapse between the AOAA infusion and sacrifice of the rats.

* Denotes responses significantly different (p < 0.05) from 0.5 μg. Comparisons were made by ANOVA and Duncan's new multiple range test.

AOAA (30 mg/kg) and GVG (900 mg/kg) to rats that had undergone the GABA-denervation procedure 7–10 days previously. In this figure we have tried to represent the compartmental nature of the drug-induced changes in GABA. The *total* length of each bar represents the GABA level measured in the intact SN. The portion of the bar that extends below the horizontal midline represents the GABA level measured in the denervated SN. The GABA content of the intact SN was 81 ± 2.7 nmoles/mg protein, that of the denervated SN was 15 ± 2.0 nmoles/mg protein. Subtracting the GABA content of the denervated SN from that of the intact SN yields an estimate of the GABA content of the nerve terminal compartment (the portion of the bar extending above the horizontal midline). Three groups of rats were sacrificed at 12, 36 and 60 h after a single injection of GVG. The GABA level of the intact SN was greatly elevated at 12 h and the elevation was sustained through 36 h (160 and 150 ± 8 nmoles/mg protein respectively) but began to decrease by 60 h (127 ± 5.3). At 12 hours GVG produced a large increase in GABA in the denervated SN (112 ± 7.3). However the GABA content was significantly diminished by 36 h (71 ± 3.8) and was still lower by 60 h (39 ± 3.1). The net increases in GABA due to the drug treatments are depicted by the shaded areas in Fig. 4. At 12 h the net increase in GABA in the denervated SN (97 nmoles/mg protein) was actually greater than that in the intact SN (79 nmoles/mg protein). Since the increase in GABA on the denervated side can account for all of the GABA increase on the intact side, we may conclude that the increase in nigral GABA occurring within 12 h after GVG treatment does not depend upon the presence of nigral GABAergic terminals. At 36 h after GVG the situation began to change; a greater net increase was observed in the SN on the intact side than on the denervated side (Fig. 4). The separation between the GABA concentrations of the intact and denervated tissues became more apparent at 60 hours; at this time nearly half of the increase in GABA in the intact SN was associated with the presence of nerve terminals (85).

The GABA-denervated SN was also used to evaluate compartmental increases in GABA after treatment with DPA and AOAA (last two bars of Fig. 4). In the SN of the intact hemisphere DPA (300 mg/kg) and AOAA (30 mg/kg) produced significant elevations of GABA which were of similar magnitude (net increase = 32 and 22 nmoles/mg protein respectively). In the denervated SN, AOAA caused a significant increase in GABA; the net increase (18 nmoles/mg protein) could account for more than 80% of the net increase seen in the intact SN. Consequently only a small part of the GABA increase in the intact SN can be attributed to the nerve terminal-dependent compartment. In contrast, DPA failed to significantly elevate the GABA content of the denervated SN; more than 90% of the increase in GABA after DPA was found to be dependent upon the presence of GABA nerve terminals. Thus, in the relative absence of GABA nerve terminals, the GABA elevating effect of DPA appears to be lost whereas the GABA elevating effect of AOAA is retained (138).

These data suggest that, in fact, a large portion of the GABA elevation seen with AOAA and GVG is associated with compartments other than GABA-ergic nerve terminals. This is perhaps because these compartments contain a large amount of GABA-T. Our observations are consistent with studies that have demonstrated marked effects of GABA-T inhibition in non-neuronal cells and neural tissues that are not known to contain GABA terminals (139, 140) as well as with subcellular fractionation studies (141, 142). Since these compounds probably influence nerve-terminal GABA only after other compartments of GABA have been elevated severalfold, it is understandable that relatively large increases in total GABA are required to elicit GABA-related physiological effects with these drugs (143, 144).

On the other hand, the results obtained with DPA demonstrate that increases in nerve-terminal GABA can be obtained in the absence of large effects on other GABA compartments. This observation is supported by the subcellular fractionation studies of Sarhan and Seiler (142) which demonstrated a selective effect of DPA on synaptosomal GABA. Thus, although the total GABA increase after DPA is modest (compared to AOAA and GVG), it appears to be almost exclusively nerve-terminal associated.

5.3 Correlation of anticonvulsant activity with increases in GABA in the nerve terminal compartment

To determine whether the changes in GABA content of a particular compartment were correlated with functional effects we tested DPA, AOAA and GVG for anticonvulsant activity against maximal electroshock seizures.

The time course of GVG activity was examined after a single injection of 900 mg/kg. There was no reduction in THE duration at 12 h, a 28% reduction at 36 h and a 45% reduction at 60 h. This same time course of anticonvulsant activity was seen using doses of 600 and 1600 mg/kg. In all cases maximal effects were obtained at 60 h. At this time THE was completely blocked with the 1600 mg/kg dose (85). It is evident that the onset and peak of anticonvulsant activity in the MES test directly parallels the time course of the increase in nerve terminal GABA. Since peak activity after GVG occurred at 60 h we determined the dose dependency of anti-MES activity at that time (Fig. 5). The dose that was effective in reducing THE duration by 50% (ED$_{50}$) was 933 mg/kg. AOAA and DPA were also active in the MES test. AOAA was the most potent of the three drugs with an ED$_{50}$ of 42 mg/kg. The toxicity of AOAA at or above 60 mg/kg (about a

318

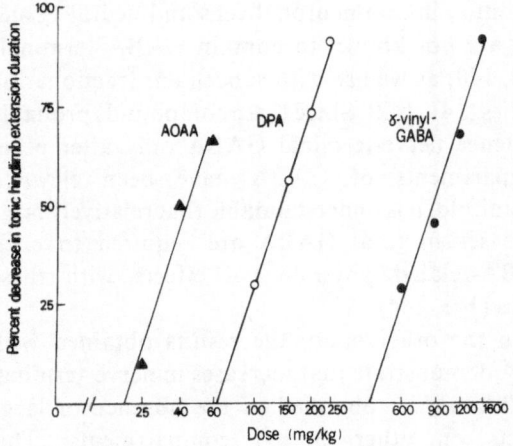

Fig. 5. Suppression of tonic hindlimb extension (THE) as a function of dose of AOAA, DPA and GVG. The mean duration of THE for each drug-treated group was subtracted from that of vehicle-injected controls and expressed as a percentage of the control mean (8 s). Data obtained with GVG were from rats tested only once, 60 h after drug administration. The values obtained from animals treated with 600 and 1600 mg/kg in this experiment were comparable to those obtained in the time course experiments discussed in the text. The dose-effect relationships obtained for DPA and AOAA were from separate groups of rats tested 30 min and 2 h after injection, respectively. N = 10–12 animals per dose for each drug.

15% mortality occurred at this dose) precluded the use of higher doses (Fig. 5). The dose of AOAA used in our biochemical studies (30 mg/kg) reduced the duration of THE by 18%. DPA was of intermediate potency with an ED_{50} of 140 mg/kg; a 90% reduction in THE duration was observed with a dose of 300 mg/kg.

To explore the correlation between changes in nerve-terminal GABA and anticonvulsant activity in the MES test, the data from rats with transections were used to estimate the proportional

changes in GABA in the two compartments. As discussed above, the difference in GABA content between the denervated and intact SN represents the nigral GABA associated with nerve terminals. These values are presented in Table 4, along with the percent reduction in THE duration associated with each treatment. The values reveal that the percent increase in the nerve-terminal pool is positively correlated (r = +0.93) with anticonvulsant activity in the MES test. This relationship is presented graphically in Fig. 6. On the other hand, GABA increases in the nigra as a whole (intact SN) and in the non-nerve terminal compartment, do not

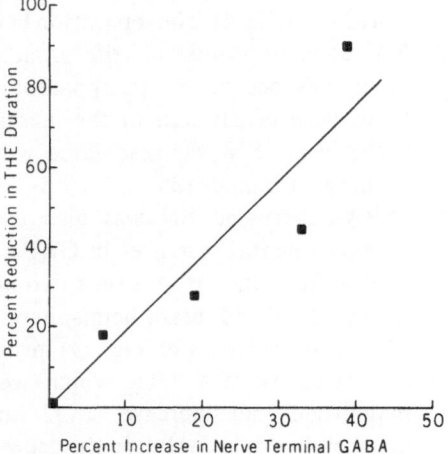

Fig. 6. Relationship between per cent reduction in THE duration in the MES test and per cent increase in nerve terminal associated GABA. The graph was derived from the data of Table 4. Three drug treatments are represented: GVG 900 mg/kg at 12 h (origin), 36 h (2nd point), 60 h (3rd point); AOAA 30 mg/kg at 2 h (1st point); and DPA 300 mg/kg at 0.5 h (4th point). The correlation coefficient between the two variables was 0.93. The best fitting line was calculated by the method of least squares. (Reproduced with permission from 145).

Table 4. Relationship between suppression of THE in the MES test and compartmental increases in GABA.

Treatment	Suppression of THE	Increase in GABA (% over control)		
		Total	Non-nerve terminal	Nerve terminal
GVG (12 hrs)	0%	98%	646%	0%
GVG (36 hrs)	28%	85%	373%	19%
GVG (60 hrs)	45%	57%	160%	33%
DPA (0.5 hrs)	90%	36%	28%	39%
AOAA (2 hrs)	18%	25%	100%	7%

The percent changes in the various compartments were calculated from the data in Fig. 4. Total refers to the per cent increase observed in the intact SN.
Adapted from 145 and 85.

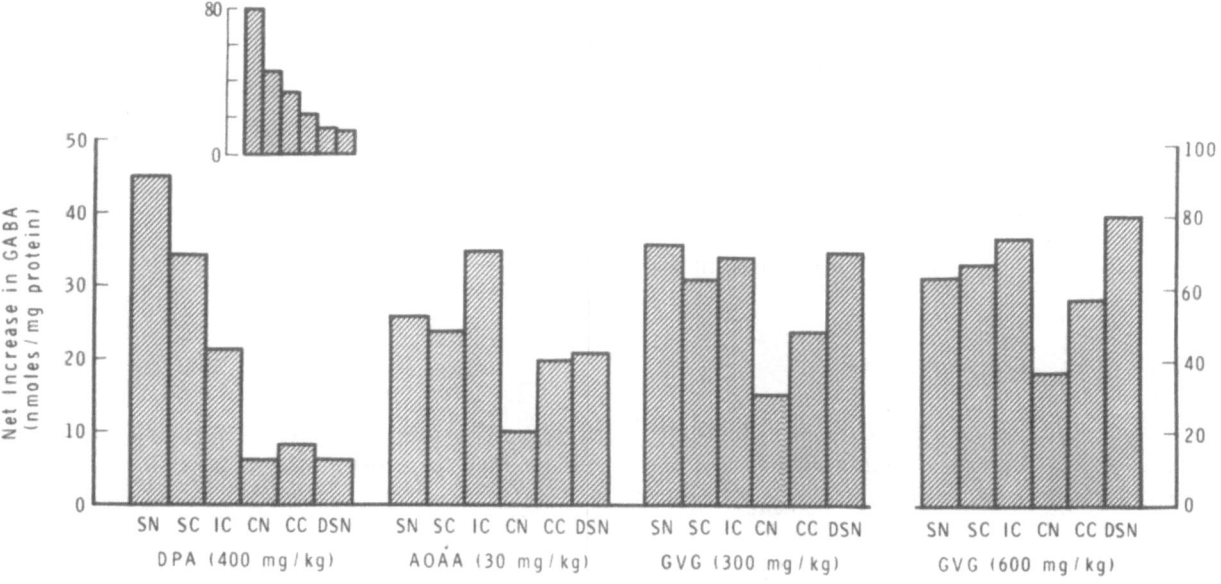

Fig. 7. Net increase in GABA after DPA, AOAA, and GVG in five areas of rat brain. The last bar for each drug treatment represents the net increase in the GABA-denervated SN (DSN). The areas are rank ordered from highest to lowest according to the control GAD activity. GAD activity was found to be directly proportional to the control GABA levels across the different areas. The control GABA levels of the different areas are shown in the small insert at the top of the graph. Drug-induced increases in GABA in all areas were significantly different from control ($p < 0.05$) except for DPA in the denervated SN. Comparisons were made by ANOVA and Duncan's new multiple range test. Net increases in GABA with DPA were directly correlated ($r = 0.96$) with the GAD activity in the different areas. The scale on the left pertains to DPA, AOAA and GVG 300 mg/kg; the scale on the right pertains to GVG 600 mg/kg. The scale on the inset denotes the GABA content of the different areas in nmoles/mg protein. N = 4–5 rats per group. (Reproduced with permission, from 145).

positively correlate with seizure protection. These data demonstrate that changes in GABA which occur in the non-nerve terminal pools may actually conceal the degree of change in GABA in the functionally relevant (nerve terminal) compartment. Moreover, the relatively undramatic effect of DPA on GABA levels takes on a different meaning when we realize that this is simply due to its lack of effect on the non-nerve terminal compartment. While we cannot exclude the possibility that DPA may have anticonvulsant effects mediated by mechanisms other than GABA, our data suggest that the DPA-induced increase in nerve terminal GABA is sufficient to predict marked anticonvulsant activity in the electroshock seizure model.

5.4 Elevation of GABA in various brain regions as a function of the density of GABAergic innervation

The relationship between the DPA-induced increases in GABA and the presence of GABAergic nerve terminals is further supported by the effect of this drug on GABA in different brain areas. Since it is well known that the regional variation exists in brain with respect to the density of GABAergic nerve terminals, it might be expected that alterations in the profile of regional GABA concentrations may reflect the compartment most affected by drug treatment. The increase in GABA after DPA, AOAA and GVG was measured in the SN as well as four other brain areas, each with different amounts of GABA and GAD activity. DPA was found to increase GABA in direct proportion to the GAD activity and GABA level of each area (Fig. 7).

In contrast to DPA, both AOAA and GVG produced net increases in GABA which varied relatively little variations across brain areas, and the magnitude of the change was independent of the normal steady-state GABA content (Fig. 7). Furthermore, the net increase in most areas was similar to the increase in GABA in the denervated SN (included in Fig. 7 for comparison). This

320

analysis supports the interpretation that AOAA and GVG exert their predominant effect on a pool of GABA that is independent of GABAergic nerve terminals (145).

6. Elevation of brain GABA: localization of anticonvulsant action using intracerebral microinjection of GVG

6.1 Effects on seizures and GABA levels

The irreversible nature of GABA-T inhibition produced by GVG was a major advantage for localizing its site of anticonvulsant action in the brain. Preliminary studies indicated that after GVG microinjection, GABA levels remained markedly elevated for a period of days, offering the possibility of testing anticonvulsant action several hours or days after a single application of drug. Furthermore, the drug appeared to spread quite readily through brain tissue (146) allowing us to increase GABA over large areas, thus simplifying the initial process of surveying the brain for sites of anticonvulsant activity.

Microinjections were made stereotaxically into ether anesthetized rats (150–200 g). The five brain areas injected (illustrated schematically in Fig. 8) were: 1) both striata (20 μg GVG into the head of the caudate-putamen of each hemisphere). 2)

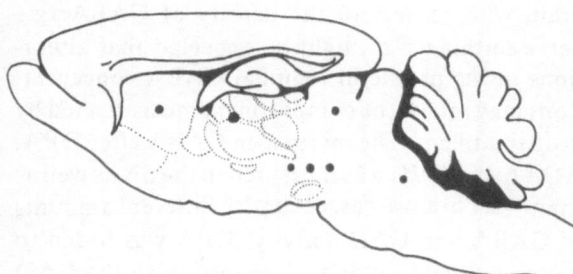

Fig. 8. Schematic parasagittal section through rat brain illustrating sites of GVG injection. The brain regions injected are indicated by the black circles. Each circle represents a separate group of rats. GVG was dissolved in normal saline and the volume of fluid injected was 1–1.5 μl. The rate of injection, controlled by an infusion pump, was 0.2 μl/min. The cannula was left in place for one minute following the end of the injection. Control animals were injected with saline alone. Infusions into the striatum and superior colliculus were bilateral.

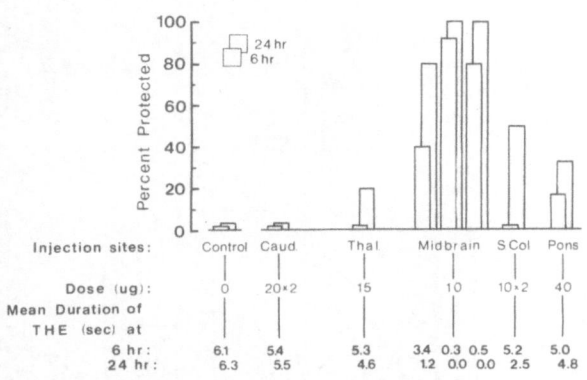

Fig. 9. Effect of intracerebral GVG on maximal electroshock seizures. The graph portion of the figure depicts the per cent of animals protected from THE 6 and 24 h after microinjection of GVG into the brain sites indicated below the bars and in Fig. 8. The mean duration of THE for each of the groups is shown at the bottom of the graph. There were 5–6 rats in each group. Abbreviations: Caud., Caudate nucleus; Thal., thalamus; S. Col., superior colliculus.

Thalamus, (15 μg GVG into the region of ventral anterior/ventral medial nuclei). 3) Both superior colliculi (10 μg GVG into each hemisphere). 4) Ventral midbrain reticular formation, (10 μg GVG into the region ventral to the central gray, 1.0–1.5 mm lateral to the midline in the left hemisphere). 5) Pontine reticular formation, (40 μg GVG just caudal and ventral to the left dorsal tegmental nucleus). Following the injection 6 h recovery time was allowed before animals were challenged in the MES test; each group was tested again at 24 h.

The results, presented in Fig. 9, demonstrate that, at 6 h after GVG, the only placements effective in blocking THE were the ventral midbrain sites. The anticonvulsant effect of GVG in the ventral midbrain appeared to require spread of the drug across the midline because animals in which the midbrain injection was placed more than 1.5 mm lateral to midline, did not show maximal seizure protection until the 24 h test time. Groups receiving injections into the thalamus, superior colliculus and pontine reticular formation showed partial protection only after 24 h. This may have been due to diffusion of GVG into the midbrain region (see biochemical results below).

The volume of tissue affected by GVG was

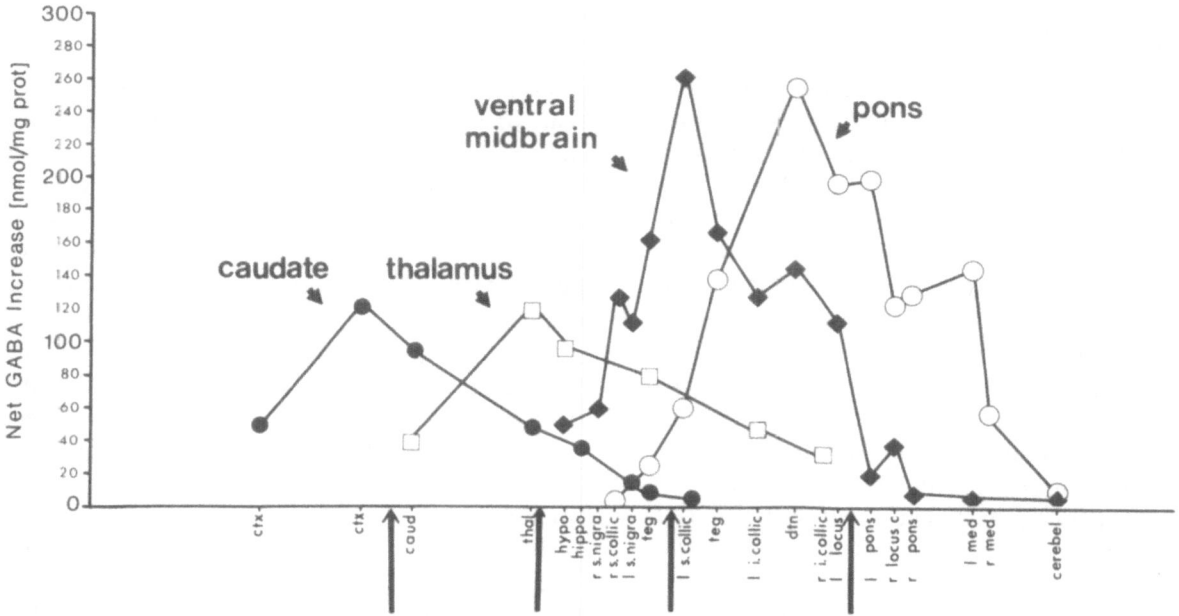

Fig. 10. Regional GABA elevation after microinjection of GVG. The volume of tissue affected by GVG at 6 h was ascertained by measuring the GABA increases in different regions along the neuraxis. The areas are plotted along the abscissa in terms of distance from the injection sites. Injection sites were 3–4 mm apart. The relative location of the injections is indicated by the arrows. Some areas were assayed bilaterally and are indicated by right (r) and left (l). The ordinate is scaled in terms of the net increase in GABA produced by GVG, (over and above control values). The doses of GVG and the injection sites correspond to those illustrated in Fig. 8 and 9. Abbreviations from left to right are: Ctx, cerebral cortex; caud, caudate nucleus; thal, thalamus; hypo, hypothalamus; hippo, hippocampus; s. nigra, substantia nigra; s. collic, superior colliculus; teg, midbrain tegmentum; i collic, inferior colliculus; dtn, dorsal tegmental nucleus; locus, locus ceruleus; med, medulla; cerebel, cerebellum.

assessed by measuring the GABA levels in a number of different areas from rats in each of the micro-injection groups (Fig. 10). All injections produced pronounced (3–4 fold) increases in GABA in the vicinity of the injection site. At 6 h after GVG, maximal elevation of GABA was observed to extend over an area within a 1.5 mm radius of the injection site. By 24 h all tissues within a radius of 3 mm showed maximal GABA elevations. At 6 h after the ventral midbrain injection of GVG, the midbrain tegmentum, substantia nigra, superior and inferior colliculi and dorsal tegmental nucleus contained 2.5–4-fold more GABA than controls. On the other hand the GABA content of the medulla, cerebellum and spinal cord was not significantly elevated 6 h after midbrain GVG injection and we can therefore conclude that GABA increases in these areas are not required for the anticonvulsant effect of GVG as measured in the MES test. Conversely, severalfold elevation of GABA in the striatum, hippocampus, thalamus

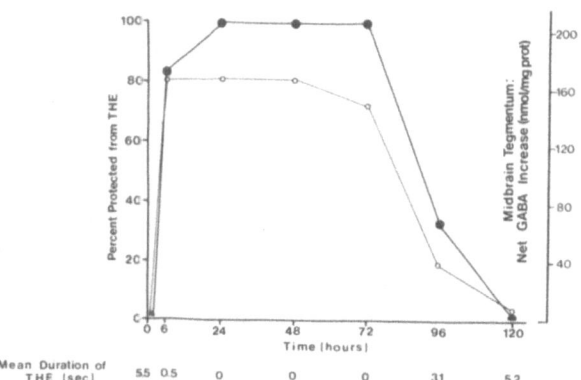

Fig. 11. Time course of seizure protection and GABA elevation after unilateral midbrain microinjection of GVG. The filled circles show the per cent protected from THE in the MES test (n = 6). The open circles show the net increase in GABA measured in the midbrain tegmentum in the vicinity of the injection site. The mean duration of THE at each time point is shown below the graph.

and hypothalamus (after forebrain GVG), or in the pons and medulla (after hindbrain GVG), was evidently not sufficient to confer protection in the MES test (147).

The duration of seizure protection after a single ventral midbrain injection of GVG was determined in another group of rats (Fig. 11). Complete blockade of THE was observed for 72 h. Partial recovery of THE was observed on the fourth day and return to normal duration of THE in all rats took place by the fifth day after injection. The increase in GABA (measured in the midbrain tegmentum) paralleled the timecourse of anticonvulsant activity: a maximal elevation was achieved by 6 h and maintained through 72 h. On the fourth day after midbrain injection the net increase in GABA was approximately 25% of that measured at the earlier time points. Thus, recovery of normal seizure activity appears to correlate with the decline in GABA levels.

Throughout the course of these studies the rats receiving GVG microinjections exhibited no overt alterations in motor function. All animals were alert and active; rats receiving midbrain injection of GVG appeared to be somewhat more active (with respect to spontaneous motor activity), while rats receiving striatal or pontine injections were slightly less active than controls.

Further experimentation revealed that midbrain injection of GVG produced a broad spectrum of anticonvulsant activity. In these studies we used bilateral injections of lower doses of GVG into the ventral midbrain tegmentum; control rats received equivalent volumes of saline microinjected into the same sites. Four different seizure models were tested: MES, intravenous pentylenetetrazol (PTZ), sub-cutaneous PTZ and intravenous bicuculline. GVG (at 6 h) provided complete protection against MES seizures and bicuculline-induced convulsions and significantly attenuated convulsions induced by intravenous PTZ (Table 5). Partial protection was also observed against subcutaneously administered PTZ.

These data demonstrate that the irreversible inhibition of GABA degradation in the ventral midbrain tegmentum can suppress or eliminate the motor manifestations of generalized convulsions. This protection is associated with marked and long-lasting increases in GABA, comparable to the GABA increases observed in the midbrain when

Table 5. Seizure protection following bilateral injections of GVG and Muscimol into ventral mesencephalic tegmentum.

| Microinjection | Time | Dose | Seizure Model | | | |
| | | | MES | PTZ | | Bicuculline |
				40 mg/kg iv	90 mg/kg sc	0.25 mg/kg iv
Control (No injection)			6.6 ± 0.6	2.9 ± 0.2	8.8 ± 0.3	2.6 ± 0.2
Saline	2.5 h		4.8 ± 0.2	2.3 ± 0.2		
	5.0		6.5 ± 0.7	2.5 ± 0.3		
	6.0		6.3 ± 0.4	2.6 ± 0.2	8.7 ± 0.4	2.1 ± 0.3
	8.0		6.1 ± 0.5	2.8 ± 0.3		
GVG	6.0 h	5 µg	0.6 ± 0.6*	1.2 ± 0.4*	4.2 ± 0.4*	0.5 ± 0.2*
Muscimol	2.5 h	25 ng	1.8 ± 0.6*	1.0 ± 0.2*		
		50 ng	0.0 ± 0*			
	5.0 h	25 ng	4.8 ± 2.1	1.3 ± 0.9		
		50 ng	3.8 ± 1.5*			
		75 ng	0.7 ± 0.7*			
	8.0 h	50 ng	6.0 ± 0.7	2.6 ± 0.4		

N = 4–6 per group
* Significantly different from saline microinjected rats $p < 0.05$, Student's t test.
The values for MES represent the mean duration of tonic hindlimb extension. The values for PTZ and Bicuculline are derived from the scale used to rate the severity of the seizures (see section 4).

GVG was administered systemically in anticonvulsant doses (85). Since elevation of GABA in the hindbrain or forebrain was not associated with protection from MES seizures our data raise the possibility that GABAergic synapses in the midbrain may be critically involved in the physiological and pharmacological control of seizure propagation.

6.2 Role of GABA receptors in seizure protection

To verify the importance of midbrain GABA receptors for the control of seizure expression we examined the ability of the directly acting GABA receptor agonist, muscimol, to confer seizure protection after microinjection into the ventral midbrain tegmentum. Bilateral injection of muscimol (25–75 ng/injection) into the vicinity of the substantia nigra was found to reduce the duration of THE in a dose-dependent fashion (Table 5). The midbrain injection of muscimol also significantly reduced the severity of seizures induced by intravenous PTZ. In contrast to the effects of GVG, the effects of the muscimol injections were relatively short-lasting; by 8 hours the seizure response to MES as well as to intravenous PTZ had returned to normal.

Our observation that the direct activation of midbrain GABA receptors provides protection against electrically- and chemically-induced seizures, further supports the proposal that GABAergic synapses in the ventral midbrain are involved in the control of the spread of generalized seizure activity. The specificity of this anatomical location is further underscored by our observation that doses of muscimol as high as 500 ng, microinjected into the pontine reticular formation failed to protect against MES seizures (data not shown). Furthermore, injections of microgram amounts of muscimol into the cisterna magna failed to protect against either chemically or electrically induced seizures (J. Seppinwall, personal communication).

The ventral midbrain injections (Table 5) were just superior to the SN and suggest that anticonvulsant activity may involve activation of GABAergic synapses in this nucleus. Evidence for the involvement of the SN in seizure mechanisms is somewhat limited. However, metabolic activity and presumably synaptic activity, as measured with the 2-deoxyglucose technique, has been demonstrated

to increase during the active motor phase of seizures induced by intravenous injection of the excitatory agent kainic acid (148). In addition, the SN has also been implicated in the propagation of seizure activity generated from cerebral cortex (see discussion in 149).

While these observations are suggestive of nigral participation, it must be realized that regions adjacent to the injection site (red nucleus, subthalamic nucleus midbrain reticular formation etc.) are also potential neural substrates for the anticonvulsant effects of the GABA agonists. We are presently attempting to identify with greater anatomical precision, the structures which are critical for the GABA-receptor mediated anticonvulsant activity. This necessitates the use of chronic intracerebral cannulas, which will allow us to assess the actions of GABA receptor agonists (e.g. muscimol) within several minutes of microinjection, thus minimizing the intracerebral spread of the drug.

6.3 Compartmental increases in GABA after direct microinjection of GVG

One of the striking differences between systemic administration of GVG and the direct microinjection of GVG into the midbrain was the latency to onset of anticonvulsant activity. After midbrain injection of GVG peak anticonvulsant action was achieved within hours whereas days were required after systemic treatment. Since we have previously established a correlation between the time course of seizure protection and elevation of nerve-terminal GABA after systemic injection of GVG, we were interested in determining whether the more rapid onset of anticonvulsant effects after intracerebral applicaiton of GVG was also accompanied by a short latency increase in nerve-terminal GABA. To answer this question, Dr. Casu working in our laboratory, has examined the effect of intranigral microinjection of GVG in the GABA-denervated SN (150). Seven to ten days after unilateral hemitransections rats were anesthetized with ether and GVG (5 μg) was infused into the denervated SN and into the contralateral intact SN. The animals were sacrificed at 1.5, 2, 3 and 6 h after the GVG infusion and the GABA content of the denervated and intact SN was determined (Fig. 12). At each time point a significantly greater net increase in GABA was obtained in the intact SN than in the denervated SN.

324

The difference between the net increase in the intact SN and the net increase in the denervated SN reflects the increase that has taken place in the nerve terminal compartment. The maximal GABA elevation in the nerve terminal compartment was obtained at 6 h and was maintained for at least 24 h after microinjection (not shown).

7. Glial contribution to the cellular-metabolic compartment

Many of the efferents from the SN zona reticulata appear to be GABAergic, including projections to superior colliculus (106) and thalamus (104, 105). GABAergic cell bodies in SN could, therefore, contribute to the accumulation of GABA after drug treatment in the denervated SN. Thus the GABA-denervated SN provides an in vivo model of the glial and neural perikarya compartments, but does not allow the respective contribution of *each* to be evaluated. In order to examine a mainly *glial* compartment, we again took advantage of the well-defined neurochemical anatomy of the basal ganglia. The striatum (caudate-putamen) in the rat contains GABAergic neurons which give off terminals within the nucleus (i.e. intrinsic) as well as GABAergic neurons which send their projections out to other nuclei (such as SN). Virtually all of these neurons can be destroyed by microinjecting

the neurotoxin, kainic acid (KA) directly into the striatum, while fibers of passage and terminals afferent to the region are largely spared (125, 126). Since there are no known GABAergic projections to the caudate-putamen, KA treatment would be expected to destroy all neuronally-related GABA compartments, leaving primarily a glial compartment. Consistent with this expectation is the observation that KA lesions result in more than a 65% loss of GABA in the caudate-putamen (127).

Kainic acid (total of 2 μg) was injected unilaterally at two sites in the striatum located about 2 mm apart in order to ensure a complete destruction of intrinsic neuronal perikarya. After 5–6 weeks GVG was microinjected bilaterally into the intact and kainic acid-lesioned striatum and the rats were sacrificed at 1.5, 3, 6 and 24 h following the GVG injection (Fig. 13). The microinjection route was used to minimize any contribution of GABA from surrounding tissues.

In the intact striatum GVG caused a progressive increase in GABA content between 1.5 and 6 h. The net increase at 6 h was 90 nmoles/mg protein which represents above a fivefold increase compared to control GABA levels. No further increase was observed at 24 h indicating that the GABA level had reached a plateau by 6 h.

The KA-lesioned striatum was able to accumulate significant amounts of GABA although the net increase was significantly less than that of the intact

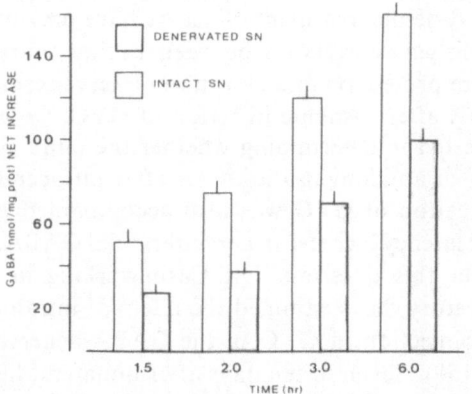

Fig. 12. Net increase in GABA in the intact and denervated SN after direct intranigral injection of GVG. Seven to ten days after unilateral hemitransection rats were given bilateral intranigral injections of GVG (5 μg) and sacrificed at 1.5, 2, 3 and 6 h after the injection, GVG caused significant increases at all times in both the intact and denervated SN. The difference between the two bars (significant at all time points, p < 0.05) represents the net increase in the nerve terminal compartment. Each set of bars is the mean + SEM of values obtained from six rats (153).

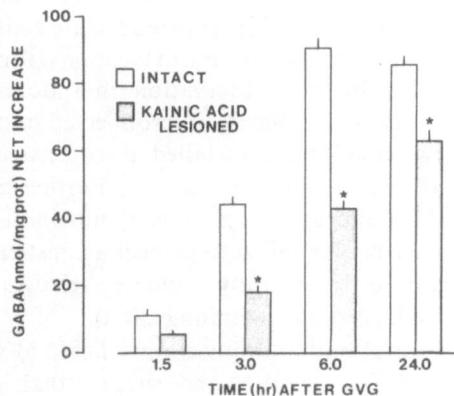

Fig. 13. Net increase in GABA in the intact and kainic acid lesioned striatum following intrastriatal injection of GVG (bilateral, 20 mg/injection). The mean (±SEM) control GABA content of the intact and kainic acid lesioned striatum was 24 ± 0.5 and 9 ± 1.5 n moles/mg protein respectively. There were 5–6 animals/time point. * significant at p < 0.05.

striatum. It is interesting to note that, unlike the intact striatum the KA-lesioned striatum does not reach a plateau at 6 h but continues to slowly accumulate GABA between the 6 and 24 h time points. The mechanism of this slow phase of accumulation is presently not clear, but may reflect a difference in the regulation of synthesis or accumulation of GABA in the KA-lesioned tissue.

These data indicate that a measurable amount of GABA synthesis occurs in the relative absence of GABAergic nerve terminals and cell bodies in the KA lesioned striatum. These results must be interpreted however, with some caution. It is possible that the metabolism of the cells which survive the trauma of a KA lesion may not be completely normal. Neuronal activity may also influence glial metabolism in intact tissue and, thus, their removal after KA lesion may in turn affect glial GABA metabolism. In addition, it is not possible to unequivocally determine whether all neuronally related GAD activity is eliminated by the lesion although studies of amino acid precursor-product relationships in the KA lesioned striatum suggest that this tissue represents a single compartment system (151).

Another limitation of the KA-lesioned striatum is that, unlike denervation of the SN, the KA lesion results in a significant loss of tissue and tissue protein, as a result it may be misleading to compare the intact to KA-lesioned tissue on a per mg protein basis. However if we compare them on a *per nucleus* basis, the following relationship emerges: the initial rate of GABA accumulation in the intact striatum is 1.0 nmole/min/nucleus and in the KA-lesioned striatum is 0.15 nmole/min/nucleus. Viewed from this perspective the contribution of the 'glial' compartment to the overall GABA accumulation appears to be relatively minor. Thus, the cell body compartment may be postulated to be an important synthetic source of GABA. For example, in our comparison of the intact and denervated SN, we have observed that the rate of accumulation in the denervated SN is 50% of the intact SN (despite the fact that the in vitro GAD activity is less than 20% of the intact SN; ref. 150). These considerations suggest that, while GABAergic cell bodies contain a relatively small amount of GAD, this compartment may be highly active and therefore, can contribute disproportionately to GABA accumulation in vivo. The relative contribution of

GABAergic nerve terminals vs GABAergic perikarya to the overall rate of accumulation in a given nucleus will, of course, depend on the respective densities (or activities) of GABAergic afferents vs GABAergic efferents in that structure.

8. Conclusions

It is apparent that the problem of correlating drug-induced increases in GABA with functional effects has been complicated by the multi-compartmental nature of the GABA elevation. The various lesion preparations we employed distinguish, either directly or indirectly, three cellular compartments: a nerve terminal dependent compartment and two nerve terminal independent compartments, one associated mainly with GABAergic neuronal perikarya and the other associated with glial cells (referred to together as the non-nerve terminal or cellular-metabolic compartment).

AOAA and GVG, two well defined GABA-T inhibitors appear to be capable of elevating GABA in all three compartments. The preponderant effect of these two drugs appears to be associated with the non-nerve terminal compartments. The GABA increase in the nerve terminal compartment is relatively small and tends to be overshadowed by the larger (several-fold) increases in the non-nerve terminal compartments.

Unlike AOAA and GVG, the GABA increase induced by DPA appears to be predominantly related to the nerve terminal compartment; an increase occurs only when this compartment is present in the tissue. A unique relationship between DPA and nerve terminal GABA is also evident in Fig. 7 which shows that the net increase in GABA produced by DPA in different brain areas directly correlates with the density of GABAergic innervation in each area.

Our observations on compartmentalization of GABA increases may help to explain some of the paradoxical results obtained when drugs that elevate brain GABA are examined for functional effects. One such paradox concerns the magnitude of GABA elevation produced by AOAA and GVG compared to DPA and protection from experimental seizures. The antiseizure effects of the former two drugs is associated with much larger increases in GABA than those seen with anticonvulsant doses of DPA. However, our data suggest that DPA interacts with a pool of GABA that seems to be closely linked to synaptic transmission; the effect of DPA on this pool is at least as great as the effect of AOAA or GVG. Another paradox involves the time course of anticonvulsant effects and GABA increases after GVG. At early time periods after GVG, no effect on MES seizures was observed despite a maximal elevation of brain GABA. Conversely, at a time when the total GABA was declining, seizure protection became evident. However, analysis of compartmentalized changes in GABA after GVG revealed that nerve terminal related GABA increased in parallel with the development of anticonvulsant activity. In addition a close temporal correlation between increases in nerve terminal GABA and seizure protection was also observed after intracerebral microinjection of GVG. Thus, increases in nerve terminal GABA appear to reliably predict functional effects such as seizure protection.

Suppression of seizures is only one functional correlate of enhanced GABAergic activity; recently our laboratory has examined the effects of AOAA, GVG and DPA using another system involving GABAergic control of nigro-striatal dopamine neurons (see Gale and Casu, this volume). Systemic administration of the dopamine receptor antagonist haloperidol provokes a compensatory increase in dopamine neuronal activity. One manifestation to this excess activity is an increased affinity of the enzyme tyrosine hydroxylase (TH) for its pteridine cofactor. The haloperidol-induced activation of dopamine neurons (and TH) is, in part, regulated by the striato-nigral GABA projection. Thus, augmentation of GABAergic transmission in this pathway would be reflected by a reversal of the haloperidol-induced activation of striatal TH. DPA was found to be completely effective in reversing the haloperidol effect on TH. The action of DPA was dose-dependent and occurred in conjunction with increases in nigral GABA in the range of 15–45% over control. In addition the action of DPA could be blocked by bicuculline indicating that it was mediated by GABA receptors. AOAA produced a partial reversal of the haloperidol effect on TH, but this occurred only in conjunction with a large increase in nigral GABA (100% over control) (152). Moreover, a striking parallelism between the time course for reversal of the haloperidol effect and the time course of anticonvulsant activity was

seen with GVG. For both functional endpoints, peak action occurred at 60 h after systemic administration and at 6 h after direct intranigral injection of GVG (153). Thus, the predictive value of increases in nerve terminal GABA holds not only across drugs and routes of administration, but across experimental measurements.

It is noteworthy that the route of administration markedly influences the time course of action of GVG. This may be related to the fact that GVG penetrates the blood-brain barrier poorly. As a result, higher local intracerebral concentrations of drug are achieved by the microinjection route than are obtained following systemic administration. A high local concentration of GVG may favor uptake of GVG into GABA nerve terminals where it can inhibit GABA-T and increase GABA. Conversely, after systemic administration GVG may be preferentially taken up into GABAergic cell bodies and glia with relatively little drug entering the nerve terminal compartment. It is possible that GVG may enter the terminals quite readily but intra-terminal conditions may not favor catalytic inhibition of GABA-T unless a relatively high intra-terminal GVG concentration is achieved. In any case, direct intracerebral injection produces a rapid increase in nerve terminal GABA which in turn appears to result in a functional augmentation of GABAergic synaptic transmission.

It is somewhat puzzling however, that in the case of systemic administration we obtain increases in the nerve terminal compartment of GABA at a time well beyond that required for the primary effects of the drug on GABA-T (52). Perhaps GABA itself or GVG-inactivated GABA-T molecules, which accumulate in the GABAergic perikarya are subsequently sent to the nerve terminals via axoplasmic transport, resulting in a net increase in nerve terminal GABA.

Lastly, a broad spectrum anticonvulsant action has been obtained with direct microinjection of GVG as well as the GABA receptor agonist muscimol into the ventral midbrain area. In contrast, GABA elevations in the forebrain and hindbrain were without anticonvulsant effects. The elevation of GABA in the ventral midbrain paralleled the time course of anticonvulsant activity. Furthermore the initial development of anticonvulsant activity was accompanied by an increase in nerve terminal associated GABA. Further studies are in progress to determine the exact site in the midbrain region that mediates the anticonvulsant effects.

In conclusion, it is likely that the physiological and behavioral effects of GABA elevating agents, in particular the anticonvulsant actions, are a function both of their ability to elevate GABA in nerve terminals and their ability to exert this effect in specific brain regions.

References

1. DeFeudis, F. V. & Mandel, P., 1981. Amino Acid Neurotransmitters; Adv. in Biochem. Psychopharmacol. Vol. 29, Raven Press, New York.

2. Costa, E., DiChiara, G. & Gessa, G. L., 1981. GABA and Benzodiazepine Receptors, Adv. in Biochem. Psychopharmacol. Vol. 26, Raven Press, New York.

3. Lal, H., 1980. GABA Neurotransmission, Brain Res. Bull. 5: Suppl 2.

4. Bartholini, G., Scatton, B., Zivkovic, B. & Lloyd, K. G., 1979. GABA-Neurotransmitters (Krogsgaard-Larsen, P., Scheel-Kruger, J. & Kofod, H., eds) Academic Press, New York, pp. 326–334.

5. Johnston, G. A. R., Allan, R. D., Kennedy, S. M. E. & Twitchin, B., 1979. (Krogsgaard-Larsen, P., Scheel-Kruger, J. & Kofod, H., eds) Academic Press, New York, pp. 149–168.

6. Krogsgaard-Larsen, P. & Johnston, G. A. R., 1978. J. Neurochem. 30: 1377–1382.

7. Enna, S. J. & Maggi, A., 1979. Life Sci. 24: 1727–1738.

8. Chrystal, E., Bey, P. & Rando, R. R., 1979. J. Neurochem. 32: 1501–1507.

9. Metcalf, B. W., 1979. Biochem. Pharmacol. 28: 1705–1712.

10. Schousboe, A., Thorbek, P., Hertz, L. & Krogsgaard-Larsen, P., 1979. J. Neurochem. 33: 181–189.

11. Brehm, L., Krogsgaard-Larsen, P. & Jacobsen, P., 1979. GABA-Neurotransmitters (Krogsgaard-Larsen, P., Scheel-Kruger, J. & Kofod, H., eds) Academic Press, New York, pp. 247–262.

12. Grandison, L. & Guidotti, A., 1977. Neuropharmacol. 16: 533–536.

13. DiMicco, J. A., Gale, K., Hamilton, B. & Gillis, R. A., 1979. Science 204: 1106–1109.

14. Scheel-Kruger, J., Arnt, J. & Magelund, G., 1977. Neurosci. Lett. 4: 351–354.

15. Grandison, L. & Guidotti, A., 1979. Endocrinology 105: 754–759.

16. Baxter, C. F., 1976. GABA in Nervous System Function. (Roberts, E., Chase, T. N. & Tower, D. B., eds) Raven Press, New York, pp. 61–87.

17. Iversen, L. L., 1978. Psychopharmacology: A Generation of Progress (Lipton, M. A., DiMascio, A. & Killam, K. F., eds) Raven press, New York, pp. 25–38.

18. Awapara, J., Landua, A. J., Fuerst, R. & Seale, B., 1950. J. Biol. Chem. 187: 35–39.

19. Roberts, E. & Frankel, S., 1950. J. Biol. Chem. 187: 55–63.

20. Bazemore, A. W., Elliott, K. A. C. & Florey, E., 1956. Nature 178: 1052–1053.

21. Bazemore, A. W., Elliott, K. A. C. & Florey, E., 1957. J. Neurochem. 1: 334–339.

22. Hayashi, T., 1959. J. Physiol. 145: 570–578.

23. Purpura, D. P., Girado, M., Smith, T. G., Callan, D. A. & Grundfest, H., 1959. J. Neurochem. 3: 238–268.

24. Eidelberg, E., Baxter, C. F., Roberts, E. & Saldias, C. A., 1960. Inhibition in the Nervous System and γ-Aminobutyric Acid (Roberts, E., Baxter, C. F., Van Harreveld, A., Wiersma, C. A. G., Adey, R. & Killam, K. F., eds) Pergamon Press, New York, pp. 365–370.

25. Tower, D. B., 1960. Inhibition in the Nervous System and γ-Aminobutyric Acid (Roberts, E., Baxter, C. F., Van Harreveld, A., Wiersma, C. A. G., Adey, R. & Killam, K. F. eds) Pergamon Press, New York, pp. 562–578.

26. Van Gelder, N. M. & Elliott, K. A. C., 1958. J. Neurochem. 3: 139–143.

27. Killam, K. F. & Bain, J. A., 1957. J. Pharmacol. Exp. Ther. 119: 255–262.

28. Coursin, D. B., 1960. Inhibition in the Nervous System and γ-Aminobutyric Acid (Roberts, E., Baxter, C. F., Van Harreveld, A., Wiersma, C. A. G., Adey, W. R. & Killam, K. F. eds) Pergamon Press, New York, pp. 294–301.

29. Tower, D. B., 1958. Nutrition Rev. 16: 161–164.

30. Reilly, R. H., Killam, K. F., Jenney, E. H., Marshall, W. H., Tausig, T., Apter, N. S. & Pfeiffer, C. C., 1953. J. Am. Med. Assoc. 152: 1317–1321.

31. Kelly, J. S. & Beart, P. M., 1975. Handbook of Psychopharmacol. (Iversen, L. L., Iversen, S. D. & Snyder, S. H., eds.) Vol. 4, Plenum Press, New York, pp. 129–209.

32. Ryall, R. W., 1975. Handbook of Psychopharmacol. (Iversen, L. L., Iversen, S. D. & Snyder, S. H., eds.) Vol. 4, plenum Press, New York, pp. 83–128.

33. Baxter, C. F. & Roberts, E., 1959. Proc. Soc. Exp. Biol. and Med. 101: 811–815.

34. Baxter, C. F. & Roberts, E., 1961. J. Biol. Chem. 236: 3287–3294.

35. Tapia, R., 1975. Handbook of Psychopharmacol. (Iversen, L. L. Iversen, S. D. & Snyder, S. H., eds.), Vol. 4, Plenum Press, New York, pp. 1–58.

36. Roberts, E. & Eidelberg, E., 1960. Internatl. Rev. Neurobiol. 2: 279–331.

37. Roberts, E., Wein, J. & Simonsen, D. G., 1964. Vitamins and Hormones 22: 503–559.

38. Cooper, J. R., Bloom, F. E. & Roth, R. H., 1978. The Biochemical Basis of neuropharmacology, Oxford Univ. Press, new York, pp. 223–258.

39. Wallach, D. P., 1961. Biochem. Pharmacol. 5: 323–331.

40. Tapia, R , Pasantes, H., Perez de la Mora, M., Ortega, B. G. & Massieu, G. H., 1967.

41. Loscher, W. & Frey, H. H., 1978. Biochem. Pharmacol. 27: 103–108.

42. Kuriyama, K., Roberts, E. & Rubenstein, M. K., 1966. Biochem. Pharmacol. 15: 221–236.

43. Wood, J. D. & Peesker, S. J., 1973. J. Neurochem. 20: 379–387.

328

44. Rando, R. R., 1974. Science 185: 320–324.
45. Fowler, L. J. & John, R. A., 1972. Biochem. J. 130: 569–573.
46. Jung, M. J. & Metcalf, B. W., 1975. Biochem. Biophys. Res. Comm.
47. Rando, R. R. & Bangerter, F. W., 1976. J. Am. Chem. Soc. 98: 6762–6764.
48. Kobayashi, K., Miyazawa, S. & Terahara, A., 1976. Tetrahedron Lett. 7: 537–540.
49. Matsui, Y. & Deguchi, T., 1977. Life Sci. 20: 1291–1296.
50. Jung, M. J., Lippert, B., Metcalf, B. W., Schechter, P. J., Bohlen, P. & Sjoerdsma, A., 1977. J. Neurochem. 28: 717–723.
51. Lippert, B., Metcalf, B. W., Jung, M. J. & Casara, P., 1977. Eur. J. Biochem. 74: 441–445.
52. Schechter, P. J., Trainer, Y., Jung, M. J. & Bohlen, P., 1977. Eur. J. Pharmacol. 45: 319–328.
53. Loscher, W., 1980. J. Neurochem. 34: 1603–1608.
54. Godin, Y., Heiner, L., Mark, J. & Mandel, P., 1969. J. Neurochem. 16: 869–873.
55. Simler, S., Ciesielski, L., Maitre, M., Randrianarisoa, H. & Mandel, P., 1973. Biochem. Pharmacol. 22: 1701–1708.
56. Fowler, L. J., Beckford, J. & John, R. A., 1975. Biochem. Pharmacol. 24: 1267–1270.
57. Harvey, P. K. P., Bradford, H. F. & Davison, A. N., 1975. FEBS Lett. 52: 251–254.
58. Whittle, S. R. & Turner, A. J., 1978. J. Neurochem. 31: 1453–1459.
59. Kaufman, E. E., Nelson, T., Goochee, C. & Sokoloff, L., 1979. J. Neurochem. 32: 699–712.
60. Ciesielski, L., Maitre, M., Cash, C. & Mandel, P., 1975. Biochem. Pharmacol. 24: 1055–1058.
61. Dickinson, R. G., Harland, R. C., Ilias, A. M., Rodgers, R. M., Kaufman, S. N., Lynn, R. K. & Gerber, N., 1979. J. Pharmacol. Exp. Ther. 211: 583–595.
62. Albertson, T. E., Peterson, S. L., Stark, L. G. & Baselt, R. C., 1981. Neuropharmacol. 20: 95–97.
63. Schechter, P. J., Trainer, Y. & Grove, J., 1978. J. Neurochem. 31: 1325–1327.
64. Perry, T. L. & Hansen, S., 1978. J. Neurochem. 30: 679–684.
65. Kukino, K. & Deguchi, T., 1977. Chem. Pharm. Bull. 25: 2257–2261.
66. Perry, T. L. & Hansen, S., 1973. J. Neurochem. 21: 1167–1175.
67. Perry, T. L., Urquhart, N., Hansen, S. & Kennedy, J., 1974. J. Neurochem. 23: 443–445.
68. Perry, T. L., Kish, S. J. & Hansen, S., 1979. J. Neurochem. 32: 1641–1645.
69. Seiler, N., Bink, G. & Grove, J., 1979. Neurochem. Res. 4: 425–435.
70. Seiler, N., Bink, G. & Grove, J., 1980. Neuropharmacol. 19: 251–258.
71. Kuriyama, K., Roberts, E. & Rubinstein, M. K., 1966. Biochem. Pharmacol. 15: 221–236.
72. Wood, J. D. & Peesker, S. J., 1975. J. Neurochem. 25: 277–282.
73. Lust, W. D., kupferberg, H. J., Yonekawa, W. D., Penry, J. K., passoneau, J. V. & Wheaton, A. B., 1978. Molec. Pharmacol. 14: 347–356.

74. Horton, R. W., Anlezark, G. M., Sawaya, M. C. B. & Meldrum, B. S., 1977.
75. Goldstein, D. B., 1979. J. Pharmacol. Exp. Ther. 208: 223–227.
76. Meldrum, B. S., Anlezark, G. M., Ashton, C. G., Horton, R. W. & Sawaya, M. C. B., 1977. Post-traumatic Epilepsy, Pharmacological Prophylaxis of Epilepsy (Majkowski, J., ed.) pp. 139–153.
77. Stone, W. E., 1977. Epilepsia 18: 507–514.
78. Wood, J. D., Durham, J. S. & Peesker, S. J., 1977. Neurochem. Res. 2: 707–715.
79. Simon, D. & Penry, J. K., 1975. Epilepsia 16: 549–573.
80. Schechter, P. J., Tranier, Y., Jung, M. J., Sjoerdsma, A., 1977. J. Pharmacol. Exp. Ther. 201: 606–612.
81. Schechter, P. J. & Trainer, Y., 1977. Psychopharmacol. 54: 145–148.
82. Schechter, P. J. & Trainer, Y., 1978. Enzyme-Activated Irreversible Inhibitors (Seiler, N., Jung, M. J. & Koch-Weser, J., eds.) Elsevier, Amsterdam, pp. 149–162.
83. Loscher, W., 1980. N.S. Arch. Pharmacol. 315: 119–128.
84. Iadarola, M. J., Raines, A. R. & Gale, K., 1979. J. Neurochem. 33: 1119–1123.
85. Gale, K. & Iadarola, M. J., 1980. Science 208: 288–291.
86. Baxter, C. F. & Roberts, E., 1960. Proc. Soc. Exp. Biol. Med. 104: 426–427.
87. DaVanzo, J. P., Greig, M. E. & Cronin, M. A., 1961. Am. J. Physiol. 201: 833–837.
88. Roa, D. P., Tews, J. K. & Stone, W. E., 1964. Biochem. Pharmacol. 13: 477–487.
89. Murakami, Y., Abe, M. & Murakami, K., 1976. J. Neurochem. 26: 655–656.
90. Maynert, E. W. & Kaji, H. K., 1962. J. Pharmacol. Exp. Ther. 137: 114121.
91. Abe, M. & Matsuda, M., 1977. J. Biochem. 82: 195–200.
92. Wood, J. D., Russell, M. P., Kurylo, E. & Newstead, J. D., 1979. J. Neurochem. 33: 61–68.
93. Wood, J. D., 1975. Prog. in Neurobiol. 5: 77–95.
94. Okada, YU., Nitsch-Hassler, C., Kim, J. S., Bak, I. J. & Hassler, R., 1971. Exp. Brain Res. 14: 514–518.
95. Fahn, S. & Cote, L. J., 1968. J. Neurochem. 15: 209–213.
96. Tappaz, M. L., Brownstein, M. J. & Palkovits, M., 1976. Brain Res. 108: 371–379.
97. Massari, V. J., Gottesfeld, Z. & Jacobowitz, D. M., 1976. Brain Res. 118: 147–151.
98. Tappaz, M. L., Brownstein, M. J. & Kopin, I. J., 1977. Brain Res. 125: 109–121.
99. van der Heyden, J. A. M. & Korf, J., 1979. J. Neurochem. 33: 857–861.
100. Albers, R. W. & Brady, R. O., 1959. J. Biol. Chem. 234: 926–928.
101. Enna, S. J., Kuhar, M. J. & Snyder, S. H., 1975. Brain Res. 43: 168–174.
102. Placheta, P. & Karobath, M., 1979. Brain Res. 178: 580–583.
103. DeFeudis, F. V., 1977. Prog. in Neurobiol. 9: 123–145.
104. Kilpatrick, I. C., Starr, M. S., Fletcher, A., James, T. A. & MacLeod, N. K., 1980. Exp. Brain Res. 40: 45–54.
105. MacLeod, N. K., James, T. A., Kilpatrick, I. C. & Starr, M. S., 1980. Exp. Brain Res. 40: 55–61.

106. Vincent, S. R., Hattori, T. & McGeer, E. G., 1978. Brain Res. 151: 159–164.

107. Hertz, L., 1979. Prog. in Neurobiol. 13: 277–323.

108. Fonnum, F. & Walberg, F., 1973. Brain Res. 54: 115–127.

109. Schon, F. & Kelly, J. S., 1974. Brain Res. 66: 275–288.

110. Iversen, L. L., Dick, F., Kelly, J. S. & Schon, F., 1975. Metabolic Compartmentation and Neurotransmission (Berl, S., Clarke, D. D. & Schneider, D., eds) Plenum Press, new York, pp.65–89.

111. Hutchinson, H. T., Werrbach, K., Vance, C. & Haber, B., 1974. Brain Res. 66: 265–274.

112. Lodge, D., Curtis, D. R. & Johnston, G. A. R., 1978. J. Neurochem. 31: 1525–1528.

113. Yarbrough, G. G., 1978. Can. J. Physiol. Pharmacol. 56: 443–446.

114. Frey, H. H., Popp, C. & Loscher, W., 1979. Neuropharmacol. 18: 581–590.

115. Kuriyama, K., 1976. GABA in Nervous System Function (Roberts, E., Chase, T. N. & Tower, D. B., eds) Raven Press, New York, pp. 187–196.

116. Barber, R. & Saito, K., 1976. GABA in Nervous System Function (Roberts, E., Chase, T. N. & Tower, D. B., eds) Raven Press, New York, pp. 113–132.

117. Van Gelder, N. M., 1965. J. Neurochem. 12: 231–237.

118. Hyde, J. C. & Robinson, N., 1974. J. Neurochem. 23: 365–367.

119. Schwarcz, R., Bennett, J. P. & Coyle, J. T., 1977. Ann. Neurol. 2: 299–303.

120. Wu, P. H., Durden, D. A. & Hertz, L., 1979. J. Neurochem. 32: 379–390.

121. Kohl, R. L., Quay, W. B. & Perez-Polo, J. R., 1980. J. Neurochem. 34: 1792–1795.

122. Toman, J. E P., Swinyard, E. A. & Goodman, L. S., 1946. J. Neurophysiol. 9: 231–239.

123. Woodbury, L. A. & Davenport, V. D., 1952. Arch. Int. Pharmacodyn. 92: 97–107.

124. Krall, R. L., Penry, J. K., White, B. G., Kupferberg, H. J. & Swinyard, E. A., 1978. Epilepsia 19: 409–428.

125. Coyle, J. T., Molliver, M. E. & Kuhar, M. J., 1978. J. Comp. Neurol. 180: 301–324.

126. Zaczek, R., Schwarcz, R. & Coyle, J. T., 1978. Brain Res. 152: 626–632.

127. Schwarcz, R. & Coyle, J. T., 1977. Brain Res. 127: 235–249.

128. Kim, J. S., Bak, I. J., Hassler, R. & Okada, Y., 1971. Exp. Bain Res. 14: 95–104.

129. Hattori, T., McGeer, P. L., Fibiger, H. C. & McGeer, E. G., 1973. Brain Res. 54: 103–114.

130. Fonnum, F., Gottesfeld, Z. & Grofova, I., 1978. Brain Res. 143: 125–138.

131. Ribak, C. E., Vaughn, J. E. & Roberts, E., 1980. Brain Res. 192: 413–420.

132. Gale, K. & Iadarola, M. J., 1980. Brain Res. 183: 217–223.

133. Pycock, C. J., 1980. Neurosci. 5: 461–514.

134. Buu, N. T. & Van Gelder, N. M., 1974. Br. J. Pharmacol. 52: 401–406.

135. Knjevic, K. & Schwartz, S., 1968. Structure and Function of Inhibitory Neural Mechanisms (Von Euler, S., Skoglund, S. & Soderberg, U., eds.) Pergamon Press, New York, pp. 419–427.

136. Guidotti, A., Gale, K., Suria, A. & Toffano, G., 1979. Brain Res. 172: 566–571.

137. Waddington, J. L. & Cross, A. J., 1978. Nature 276: 618–620.

138. Iadarola, M. J. & Gale, K., 1979. Eur. J. Pharmacol. 59: 125–129.

139. Beart, P. M., Kelly, J. S. & Schon, F., 1974. Biochem. Soc. Transac. 2: 266–268.

140. Waniewski, R. A. & Suria, A., 1977. Life Sci. 21: 1129–1142.

141. Wood, J. D., Kurylo, E. & Newstead, J. D., 1978. Can. J. Biochem. 56: 667–672.

142. Sarhan, S. & Seiler, N., 1979. J. Neurosci. Res. 4: 398–421.

143. Bell, J. A. & Anderson, E. G., 1974. Neuropharmacol. 13: 885–894.

144. Gottesfeld, Z., Kelly, J. S. & Renaud, L. P., 1972. Brain Res. 11: 319–335.

145. Iadarola, M. J. & Gale, K., 1980. Brain Res. Bull. 5: Suppl. 2, pp. 13–19.

146. Palfreyman, M. G., Huot, S., Lippert, B. & Schechter, P. J., 1979. GABA-Neurotransmitters (Krogsgaard-Larsen, P., Scheel-Kruger, J. & Kofod, H., eds.) Academic Press, New York, pp. 432–446.

147. Gale, K. & Iadarola, M. J., 1980. Eur. J. Pharmacol. 68: 233–235.

148. Collins, R. C., McLean, M. & Olney, J., 1980. Life Sci. 27: 855–862.

149. Faeth, W. H., Walker, A. E. & Andy, O. J., 1954. Epilepsia, 3rd Series, 3: 37–48.

150. Casu, M. & Gale, K., 1981. Life Sci., 29: 681–688.

151. Nicklas, W. J., Nunez, R., Berl, S. & Duvoisin, R., 1979. J. Neurochem. 33: 839–844.

152. Casu, M. & Gale, K., 1981. J. Pharmacol. Exp. Ther. 217: 177–180.

153. Casu, M. & Gale, K., 1981. Fed. Proc., 40: 290.

Received May 18, 1981.
Revision received September 15, 1981.

Pteroylpolyglutamates

Roy L. Kisliuk

Dept. of Biochemistry and Pharmacology, Tufts University, Boston, MA 02111 U.S.A.

Summary

Reduced derivatives of the vitamin pteroylglutamic acid (folic acid) are essential coenzymes for the biosynthesis of purine nucleotides, methionine, thymidylate and for many other enzyme catalyzed reactions involving the transfer, oxidation and reduction of single carbon units. Pteroylglutamic acid is found in tissues in the form of poly-γ-glutamyl derivatives of varying chain length. The present review covers the detection, distribution, synthesis, degradation, coenzyme function and inhibitory activities of pteroyl-γ-glutamates. The biosynthesis and inhibitory activities of poly-γ-glutamyl derivatives of methotrexate, an analog of pteroylglutamic acid having antitumor activity, are also considered. An hypothesis on the coenzymatic role of pteroylpoly-γ-glutamates in the coordination of sequential enzymatic steps in the metabolism of single carbon units is presented.

Introduction

Pteroylpolyglutamates, the tissue forms of folate (PteGlu) coenzymes (Fig. 1), are receiving increasing attention not only because of their role in the metabolism of thymidylate, methionine, purines and many other compounds (1, 2, 3), but because methotrexate (4), a folate analog having antitumor activity (5), is also converted to polyglutamate forms (3) which may be important in considering the selectivity of methotrexate toxicity toward tumor cells. The present review will emphasize recent literature on the biological activities of these compounds.

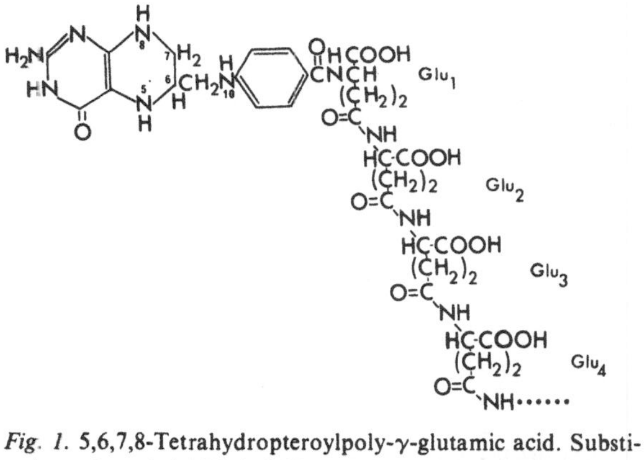

Abbreviations used

PteGlu, pteroylglutamic acid, folic acid; H_2PteGlu, 7,8-dihydrofolic acid; H_4PteGlu, 5,6,7,8-tetrahydrofolic acid. Forms with additional γ-glutamyl groups are numbered with a subscript indicating the total number of Glu residues (6). MTX, methotrexate; MTX (+ Glu_1), methotrexate having one additional γ-Glu residue. pAB, paraaminobenzoic acid.

Fig. 1. 5,6,7,8-Tetrahydropteroylpoly-γ-glutamic acid. Substitutions: 5-methyl (CH_3), 5,10-methylene (CH_2), 5,10-methenyl (CH), 5-formyl (CHO), 10-formyl (CHO) and 5-formimino (CH=NH).

Molecular and Cellular Biochemistry 39, 331–345 (1981). 0300-8177/81/0391-0331/$03.00.
© 1981, Martinus Nijhoff/Dr W. Junk Publishers, The Hague.

Preparation

In addition to the isolation of $PteGlu_7$ from yeast (7) and $10\text{-}CHO\text{-}H_4PteGlu_3$ from *Clostridium* (8), polyPteGlu derivatives have been synthesized chemically (9, 10, 11, 12). The procedure used most commonly is that of Krumdieck and Baugh (10, 13, 14) which employs a modification of the Merrifield solid phase peptide synthetic method. This procedure leads to $PteGlu_n$ which may then be converted to reduced metabolites (Fig. 1) such as $H_2PteGlu_n$ (13, 15, 16), $H_4PteGlu_n$ (13, 17, 18), $5\text{-}CHO\text{-}H_4PteGlu_n$ (19), $10\text{-}CHO\text{-}H_4PteGlu_n$ (17, 20), and $5\text{-}CH_3\text{-}H_4PteGlu_n$ (21, 22) by procedures analogous to those used for the corresponding $PteGlu_1$ derivatives. $H_4PteGlu_n$ derivatives containing the natural (13, 17, 19, 20, 21, 22, 23) and unnatural (13, 21) configurations at C-6 have been prepared.

Determination of $PteGlu_n$ in tissues

The difficulties in determining the length of γ-Glu chains in tissues have been stressed repeatedly (24, 25, 26, 27, 28, 29). In addition to low tissue concentrations and variable numbers of Glu residues, the chemical properties of individual compounds vary with the state of oxidation of the pteridine ring and with the different single carbon constituents. In addition, hydrolases are present in many tissues which catalyze the cleavage of γ-Glu bonds (Table 9). Maruyama et al. (24) state '. . . there is at present no chemical method that allows the simultaneous determination of chain length and nature of the one-carbon substituent'. In order to simplify the problem, chemical methods were sought which produced $pABGlu_n$ from total tissue $PteGlu_n$ derivatives. Although both oxidative and reductive methods appeared to suffice, more recently it has been observed that $5\text{-}CH_3\text{-}H_4PteGlu$, often the major tissue folate, is not cleaved by either procedure (Table 1) and new

Table 1. Products of degradative treatment of PteGlu derivatives[a]

	Treatment		
PteGlu derivative	$KMnO_4$ (Ref. 25) (1)	Zn-HCl (Ref. 26) (2)	Modified sequential procedure[b] (Refs. 28, 29) (3)
$PteGlu_1$	$pABGlu_1$	$pABGlu_1$	$pABGlu_1$
$PteGlu_7$	$pABGlu_7$	$pABGlu_7$	$pABGlu_7$
$10\text{-}CHO\text{-}PteGlu_1$	$N\text{-}CHO\text{-}pABGlu_1$	$N\text{-}CHO\text{-}pABGlu_1{}^c$	$pABGlu_1$
$10\text{-}CHO\text{-}PteGlu_7$	$N\text{-}CHO\text{-}pABGlu_7$	–	$pABGlu_7$
$10\text{-}CH_3\text{-}PteGlu_1$	$N\text{-}CHO\text{-}pABGlu_1$	$N\text{-}CH_3\text{-}pABGlu_1$	$pABGlu_1$
$7,8\text{-}H_2\text{-}PteGlu_1$	$pABGlu_1$	$pABGlu_1$	$pABGlu_1$
$5,6,7,8\text{-}H_4\text{-}PteGlu_1$	$pABGlu_1$	$pABGlu_1$	$pABGlu_1$
$5\text{-}CH_3\text{-}H_2\text{-}PteGlu_1$	$5\text{-}CH_3\text{-}H_2\text{-}PteGlu_1$	$5\text{-}CH_3\text{-}H_4\text{-}PteGlu_1$	$pABGlu_1$
$5\text{-}CH_3\text{-}H_4\text{-}PteGlu_1$	$5\text{-}CH_3\text{-}H_2\text{-}PteGlu_1$	$5\text{-}CH_3\text{-}H_4\text{-}PteGlu_1$	$pABGlu_1$
$5,10\text{-}CH_2\text{-}H_4\text{-}PteGlu_1$	$N\text{-}CHO\text{-}PteGlu_1$	–	$pABGlu_1$
$5,10{=}CH\text{-}H_4\text{-}PteGlu_1$	$N\text{-}CHO\text{-}PteGlu_1$	$N\text{-}CH_3\text{-}pAbGlu_1$	$pABGlu_1$
$5\text{-}CHO\text{-}H_4\text{-}PteGlu_1$	$pABGlu_1$	$N\text{-}CH_3\text{-}pABGlu_1$	$pABGlu_1$
$10\text{-}CHO\text{-}H_4\text{-}PteGlu_1$	$N\text{-}CHO\text{-}PteGlu_1$	$N\text{-}CH_3\text{-}pABGlu_1$	$pABGlu_1$
$5\text{-}CHNH\text{-}H_4\text{-}PteGlu_1$	–	–	$pABGlu_1$
$pABGlu_1$	$pABGlu_1$	$pABGlu_1$	$pABGlu_1$
$N\text{-}CH_3\text{-}pABGlu_1$	$pABGlu_1$	$N\text{-}CH_3\text{-}pABGlu_1$	$pABGlu_1$
$N\text{-}CHO\text{-}pABGlu_1$	$N\text{-}CHO\text{-}pABGlu_1$	$N\text{-}CHO\text{-}pABGlu_1{}^c$	$pABGlu_1$
Aminopterin	$pABGlu_1$	$pABGlu_1$	–
Methotrexate	$N\text{-}CHO\text{-}pABGlu_1$	$N\text{-}CH_3\text{-}pABGlu_1$	–

[a] The pteridine cleavage product from $PteGlu_n$, $H_2PteGlu_n$ and $H_4PteGlu_n$ under condition (1) is largely pteridine-6-carboxylic acid (28). The pteridines formed under conditions (2) and (3) or from 1 carbon substituted PteGlu derivatives are not yet defined.

[b] HCl, $NaBH_4$, H_2O_2-$KMnO_4$ pH 9.

[c] Some reduction to $N\text{-}CH_3\text{-}pABGlu$ occurs.

procedures have been developed which yield unsubstituted $pABGlu_n$ from the known $PteGlu_n$ derivatives. These new procedures involve acid treatment, which converts all CHO and CHNH derivatives to the =CH- form, followed by reduction with $NaBH_4$ to $5-CH_3-H_4PteGlu$ derivatives. These are then oxidized to $5-CH_3-H_2PteGlu$ derivatives and then cleaved in acid. $CH_2-H_4PteGlu_n$, $H_2PteGlu_n$ and $H_4PteGlu_n$ are also cleaved to unsubstituted $pABGlu_n$ in this procedure. Using sequential acidification, oxidation and reduction, Eto and Krumdieck (28) distinguished three pools of PteGlu derivatives: 1) $5,10-CH_2-H_4$, H_4 and H_2, 2) $5-CH_3-H_4$ and 3) $5,10=CH-H_4$, $10-CHO-H_4$, $5-CHO-H_4$ and $5-CHNH-H_4$. It is not known whether the length of the polyGlu chains differs in one or another of these pools as compared with that determined for total $PteGlu_n$ derivatives.

$pABGlu_n$ can be separated according to the number of Glu residues by high-performance liquid chromatography (30, 31) or by chromatography of azo dyes formed in the Bratton-Marshall test (32). They may be quantitated by the Bratton-Marshall test or by working with pAB having a radioactive marker (28). Since the Bratton-Marshall test is relatively insensitive (standard curve made with 0.01–0.1 umoles), new methods

are contemplated utilizing radioactively labeled N-1-naphthylethylenediamine for diazotization. The Bratton-Marshall test has the important advantage that it avoids the necessity of equilibrating tissues with radioactive precursors (28).

Direct amino acid analysis has been employed to determine polyGlu chain length (7, 8, 33). More often a combination of diethylaminoethyl-cellulose chromatography, microbiological assay and treatment with γ-Glu hydrolases are used (34, 35, 36, 37). Generally in a given series of polyGlu derivatives, the longer the chain, the greater the affinity for diethylaminoethyl-cellulose (10, 13). However, the elution from diethylaminoethyl-cellulose is also altered by the state of oxidation of the pteridine (13) and by the various substitutions (33). After isolation, the $PteGlu_n$ derivatives can be assayed microbiologically before and after treatment with γ-Glu hydrolases which catalyze the formation of $PteGlu_1$ or $PteGlu_2$ derivatives (Table 9). *Streptococcus faecium* shows greatly diminished growth on PteGlu forms having more than two Glu residues, whereas with *Lactobacillus casei* diminished growth occurs with derivatives having more than three Glu residues (Table 2). An increase in microbial growth activity after hydrolase treatment therefore indicates the presence of long chain polyGlu deriva-

Table 2. Growth factor activity of some PteGlu derivatives for microorganisms (32, 42, 43, 44, 45, 46).

Compound	*Pediococcus cerevisiae* (ATCC 8081)	*Streptococcus faecium* (ATCC 8043)	*Lactobacillus casei* (ATCC 7469)
Pte	–	+	–
$PteGlu_1$	–	+	+
$PteGlu_2$	–	+	+
$PteGlu_3$	–	–	+
$PteGlu_4$	–	–	$\pm^a$
$PteGlu_5$	–	–	–
$PteGlu_6$	–	–	–
$PteGlu_7$	–	–	–
$H_2PteGlu_1$	–	+	+
$H_4PteGlu_1$	+	+	+
$5-CHO-H_4PteGlu_1$	+	+	+
$5-CHO-H_4PteGlu_2$	+	+	+
$5-CHO-H_4PteGlu_3$	$+^b$	–	+
$5-CH_3-H_4PteGlu_1$	–	–	+

[a] $PteGlu_4$, $PteGlu_5$, $PteGlu_6$ and $PteGlu_7$ are 66%, 20%, 4% and 3% as active, respectively, as $PteGlu_1$ for *L. casei* (44, 45).

[b] Two studies report $5-CHO-H_4PteGlu_3$ as active in supporting the growth of *P. cerevisiae* (42, 43) and one study reports it to be inactive (33).

tives. Microorganisms can also distinguish different types of PteGlu$_1$ compounds (Table 2) as can high-performance liquid chromatography (31), thin-layer chromatography (38), Sephadex-G-10 chromatography (39) and ultraviolet spectral analysis (40).

A method has recently been reported to determine the Glu chain length of CH$_2$-H$_4$PteGlu$_n$ by attaching them to *Lactobacillus casei* thymidylate synthase by reaction with FdUMP. The electrophoretic mobility of the resulting complexes is a linear function of Glu chain length (41).

PteGlu and 5-CHO-H$_4$PteGlu are not known to occur in vivo and are most likely artefacts of extraction and isolation. For example, 5-CHO-H$_4$PteGlu is formed from 10-CHO-H$_4$PteGlu on heat treatment of tissue extracts (35).

Distribution

In spite of the pitfalls encountered in determining polyGlu chain lengths discussed above, there are consistent differences in length found in different organisms and in different metabolic states of the same organism (Table 3). Perhaps the best understood situation is that of Coliphage T4D which contains H$_2$PteGlu$_6$ as a baseplate structural component (47, 48, 49). Neither H$_2$PteGlu$_5$ nor H$_2$PteGlu$_7$ will serve in its place. Most of the PteGlu chains found in the *E. coli* host are shorter (Table 3). However, T4D infection causes the formation of very long chains which are cleaved to H$_2$PteGlu$_6$ by T4D induced hydrolase activity. T4D mutant 28$^-$ lacks this hydrolase activity.

Most of the bacteria examined have PteGlu$_3$ or PteGlu$_4$ as the predominant form (Table 3). Yeast and *Neurospora* have longer chains (PteGlu$_6$ and PteGlu$_7$ predominate), whereas animal livers are

Table 3. Percent distribution of PteGlu chain lengths in various cell types.

Cell type	Glu residues								
	(1)	(2)	(3)	(4)	(5)	(6)	(7)	(8)	(9)
Procaryotes:									
Bacillus subtilis (43, 60)		6	88	3	1				
Clostridium acidi-urici (8)			100						
Corynebacterium (29)				100					
Escherichia coli B (48)	11		48	16	12	8	4	1	
Escherichia T4D infected (48)	6		48	16	15	11	4	2	
Escherichia T4D 28$^-$ infected (48)	7		30	16	17	13	6	3	7[a]
Coliphage T4D						100			
Lactobacillus casei-									
1) high PteGlu medium (61)	3		9	59	23	5			
2) low PteGlu medium (62)						8	14	42	19
Streptococcus faecium (61)	16	4	20	55					
Eucaryotes:									
Guinea pig liver (62)				5	85	10			
Hamster liver (62)				30	51	13	2		
Human lymphocytes (63)	4	1	11	24	21	22	13	4	
Monkey liver (64)				24	46	15			
Rat liver (62, 65)				9	66	25			
Quail liver- (66)									
1) regular diet				12	56	26	6		
2) high casein diet				6	47	38	8		
Neurospora crassa- (67)									
1) regular medium					14	80		6[b]	
2) high glycine medium						56	24	20[b]	
Saccharomyces cerevisiae (62)						12	71	13	

[a] High molecular weight PteGlu derivatives eluted with HCl

[b] Eight or more Glu residues

intermediate between the two (PteGlu$_5$ predominates). PteGlu$_5$ also predominates in Chinese hamster ovary cells (50). There is a shift to longer Glu chain lengths in *Neurospora* grown on a high glycine medium, in *L. casei* grown on a low PteGlu medium and in quail liver from animals fed a high casein diet. The reason for these changes observed in *L. casei*, *Neurospora* and quail under varying nutritional regimens is not determined but all three altered situations might benefit from increased efficiency of PteGlu coenzyme activity brought about by longer Glu chain lengths.

Other biological materials found to contain PteGlu derivatives with three or more Glu residues include: *Physalia physalis* (Portugese Man-of-War) (35), *Candida utilis* (33), *Diplococcus pneumoniae* (51), soybean (52), wheat, pea, spinach, radish and corn plants (53, 54), *Euglena gracilis* (55), plant mitochondria and chloroplasts (53, 56), chicken liver (57), human liver (58) and human red blood cells (42). The major form in human plasma is 5-CH$_3$-H$_4$PteGlu$_1$ (59).

Coenzyme function

Table 4 lists the K$_m$ values for a number of PteGlu requiring enzymes as a function of polyGlu chain length. As the sources, purity and conditions of assay vary greatly, these results should be taken only to indicate general trends. In only two instances out of 58 trials were the K$_m$ values higher for any polyGlu form than for the corresponding Glu$_1$ derivative. These two instances are found with the H$_2$PteGlu reductases obtained from human acute myelogenous leukemia and human lymphocytic leukemia respectively. Even with these two enzymes, the lowest K$_m$ values are found with H$_2$PteGlu$_7$. It would be of interest to extend these studies to include the H$_2$PteGlu$_2$, H$_2$PteGlu$_4$ and H$_2$PteGlu$_6$ derivatives to determine the maximum K$_m$. With the L1210 H$_2$PteGlu reductase, little or no change in K$_m$ was found on increasing the Glu chain length. (PteGlu polyGlu synthetase (vide infra) appears to differ from the enzymes listed in Table 4 in that the K$_m$ values increase with increasing Glu chain length. With the *Corynebacterium* PteGlu synthetase, for example, CH$_2$-H$_4$PteGlu$_2$ has a greater than 20 fold higher K$_m$ than that for H$_4$PteGlu$_1$ (68).)

A particularly striking effect is seen (Table 4) with AICAR transformylase from chicken liver in which the K$_m$ value decreases 350 fold when the Glu$_4$ substrate replaces the Glu$_1$ substrate. Pig liver CH$_2$-H$_4$PteGlu reductase shows a stepwise decrease in K$_m$ through Glu$_6$.

The only enzyme so far discovered which has an absolute requirement for a polyGlu substrate is the vitamin B$_{12}$-independent 5-CH$_3$-H$_4$PteGlu-homocysteine transmethylase (Table 4). The enzymes from *N. crassa* and *S. cerevisiae* will utilize 5-CH$_3$-H$_4$PteGlu$_2$ as substrate, whereas the *E. coli* enzyme requires 5-CH$_3$-H$_4$PteGlu$_3$. The high K$_m$ values for the *N. crassa* and *S. cerevisiae* enzymes as compared with the *E. coli* enzyme, may relate to the fact that the polyGlu chains found in *N. crassa* and *S. cerevisiae* are much longer than those found in *E. coli* (Table 3). The transmethylase from the former sources may therefore prefer substrates with longer Glu chains.

In those instances where a mixture of diastereoisomers at C-6 of H$_4$PteGlu are employed as substrates (Table 4), the possibility of inhibition caused by the polyGlu derivative of the unnatural diastereoisomer must be considered. In the cases so far studied, *L. casei* thymidylate synthase is so inhibited whereas the vitamin B$_{12}$ dependent 5-CH$_3$-H$_4$PteGlu-homocysteine transmethylase and CH$_2$H$_4$PteGlu reductase of rat liver are not.

Calf thymus thymidylate synthase differs from the other thymidylate synthases listed in that increasing the Glu chain length did not lower the K$_m$ value.

Alterations in V$_{max}$ with polyGlu substrates are usually ±100% of those obtained with the corresponding Glu$_1$ substrate and are often lower with the polyGlu forms (15, 17, 20, 23).

Other enzymes which have been studied with polyGlu substrates include ribothymidyl synthase from *Streptococcus faecalis* (69), which shows a rate six times faster with CH$_2$-H$_4$PteGlu$_5$ as substrate than with CH$_2$-H$_4$PteGlu$_1$ and serine hydroxymethyltransferase from *Clostridium cylindrosporum* with which incompletely characterized PteGlu$_n$ derivatives were much more effective cofactors than H$_4$PteGlu$_1$ (70).

The kinetic mechanism of pig liver CH$_2$-H$_4$PteGlu reductase (15) differs depending on whether short or long chain polyGlu substrates are employed. With CH$_2$-H$_4$PteGlu$_{1-3}$ ping-pong bi-bi kinetics in

336

Table 4. The effect of polyglutamyl chain length on K_m values of PteGlu requiring enzymes.

Enzyme	Source	K_m (uM) Glu residues						
		(1)	(2)	(3)	(4)	(5)	(6)	(7)
1. H_2PteGlu Reductase	L1210 (16)	1.4	ND	1.2	ND	0.8	ND	1.3
2. H_2PteGlu Reductase	Human (16) Erythrocytes	6	ND	4.2	ND	1.3	ND	1.3
3. H_2PteGlu Reductase	Human Acute (16) Myelogenous Leukemia	4	ND	10	ND	1.5	ND	0.6
4. H_2PteGlu Reductase	Human Acute (16) Lymphocytic Leukemia	3.5	ND	1.8	ND	9.3	ND	0.8
5. Thymidylate Synthase	Lactobacillus (23) casei	24	15	2	2.1	1	1.2	1.8
6. Thymidylate Synthase	Escherichia[a] coli	11	4.4	3.7	c	c	c	4.2
7. Thymidylate Synthase	Coliphage T2[a]	9.2	4.6	2	7	c	6	3
8. Thymidylate Synthase	Calf Thymus[b]	16	ND	13	ND	ND	ND	15
9. Thymidylate Synthase	Human Acute (72) Myelogenous Leukemia	31[d]	ND	ND	ND	2.2[d]	ND	ND
10. 5-CH_3H_4PteGlu-homocysteine transmethylase (B_{12}-dependent)	Bovine Brain (22)	73	ND	24	ND	28	ND	22
11. 5-CH_3H_4PteGlu-homocysteine transmethylase (B_{12}-dependent)	Rat Liver (21)	12.6	ND	ND	ND	7.4	ND	ND
12. CH_2-H_4PteGlu Reductase	Pig Liver (15)	7.1	5.2	1.7	0.6	0.3	0.1	0.5
13. CH_2-H_4PteGlu Reductase	Rat Liver (21)	17	ND	ND	ND	2	ND	ND
14. 10-CHO-H_4PteGlu Synthetase	Pig Liver (17)	89	ND	2	ND	ND	ND	ND
15. 10-CHO-H_4PteGlu Synthetase	Clostridium cylindrosporum (8)	290	ND	25	ND	ND	ND	ND
16. CH_2-H_4PteGlu Dehydrogenase	Pig Liver (17)	25	ND	7	ND	3	ND	3
17. CHNHGlu-H_4PteGlu Forminotransferase	Pig Liver (17)	48	ND	31	ND	4	ND	5
18. AICAR Transformylase	Chicken Liver (20)	353	ND	6	1	2	2	3

Table 4. (Cont.)

Enzyme	Source	K_m (uM) Glu residues						
		(1)	(2)	(3)	(4)	(5)	(6)	(7)
19. Ketopantoate Hydroxymethyl Transferase	*Escherichia* (73) *coli*	330[d]	250[d]	180[c]	100[d]	100[d]	170[d]	290[d]
20. 5-CH$_3$-H$_4$PteGlu homocysteine transmethylase (B$_{12}$-independent)	*neurospora* (74) *crassa*	–	960[d]	820[c]	ND	ND	ND	ND
21. 5-CH$_3$-H$_4$PteGlu homocysteine transmethylase (B$_{12}$-independent)	*Saccharomyces* (74) *cerevisiae*	–	430[d]	380[c]	ND	ND	ND	ND
22. 5-CH$_3$-H$_4$PteGlu homocysteine transmethylase (B$_{12}$-independent)	*Escherichia* (75) *coli*	–	–	4.7[d]	ND	ND	ND	ND

ND = not determined

– = no activity

[a] Kisliuk, R. L., Gaumont, Y., Maley, G., Maley, F. & Galivan, J., unpublished work

[b] Dwivedi, C. M. & Kisliuk, R. L., unpublished work

[c] do not follow Michaelis-Menten kinetics

[d] mixture of diastereoisomers at C-6

which the enzyme bound flavin is alternately reduced by NADPH and reoxidized by CH$_2$Pte-Glu$_{1-3}$ are observed. With CH$_2$-H$_4$PteGlu$_{4-7}$ as substrates it appears that the reduction of CH$_2$-H$_4$-PteGlu$_{4-7}$ is no longer fully rate limiting and that either product release or flavin reduction by NADPH partially controls the rate of the reaction.

Both L1210 H$_2$PteGlu reductase and *E. coli* thymidylate synthase show a remarkable lack of specificity when tested with Pte analogs containing polyLys side chains in place of polyGlu (71). For example, H$_2$-Nα-Pte-Nϵ-(di-α-lysyl)Lys was 1.2 times as active as H$_2$PteGlu$_1$ as a substrate for L1210 H$_2$PteGlu reductase and the corresponding H$_4$-Nα-Pte-Nϵ-(di-α-lysyl)Lys derivative was 0.67 times as active as H$_4$PteGlu$_1$ as a substrate for *E. coli* thymidylate synthase. Thus changing the polarity from the negative Glu residues to the positive polyLys did not result in large differences in cofactor activity with either enzyme.

Enzyme inhibition by polyPteGlu derivatives

The effect of polyGlu chain length on enzyme inhibition is shown in Table 5. With all 14 enzymes listed the polyGlu derivatives are more inhibitory than the corresponding Glu$_1$ forms, often by as much as 100 to 200 fold. The situation differs with the H$_2$PteGlu reductase from L1210 cells. MTX (+ Glu$_1$) was no more inhibitory than MTX (76, 77, 78). Displacement studies showed further that MTX (+ Glu$_1$), MTX (+ Glu$_2$) and MTX (+ Glu$_6$) have similar affinities for the H$_2$PteGlu reductases from L1210 and guinea pig liver (77).

In the case of pig liver CH$_2$-H$_4$PteGlu reductase (Table 5), the strong inhibition by H$_2$PteGlu$_n$ could be of physiological significance in that a decrease in the CH$_2$-H$_4$PteGlu$_n$/H$_2$PteGlu$_n$ ratio would result in decreased CH$_2$-H$_4$PteGlu$_n$ reduction, sparing CH$_2$H$_4$PteGlu$_n$ for purine and pyrimidine biosynthesis (15). Similarly, H$_2$PteGlu$_n$ resulting from the action of thymidylate synthase could result in thymidylate synthase inhibition, sparing H$_4$PteGlu$_n$ for other reactions (13).

Table 5. Enzyme inhibition by PteGlu$_n$ derivatives.

| Enzyme | Source & ref. | Inhibitor | Concentration (uM) for 50% inhibition Total # of Glu residues | | | | | | |
			(1)	(2)	(3)	(4)	(5)	(6)	(7)
1. Formimino H$_4$PteGlu Formiminotransferase	Pig Liver (17)	PteGlu	70	ND	13	ND	1	ND	2
2. Methenyl H$_4$PteGlu Cyclohydrolase	Pig Liver (17)	PteGlu	195	ND	60	ND	18	ND	18
3. Methylene H$_4$PteGlu Reductase	Pig Liver (15)	H$_2$PteGlu[b]	11	3	3	2	0.8	0.6	0.7
4. Thymidylate Synthase	*Lactobacillus casei* (13)	PteGlu	150	30	0.8	0.4	0.4	0.6	0.7
5. Thymidylate Synthase	*Lactobacillus casei* (13)	H$_2$PteGlu	300	20	3	ND	ND	3	ND
6. Thymidylate Synthase	*Lactobacillus casei* (13)	H$_4$PteGlu[c]	>100[d]	ND	30	ND	ND	ND	2
7. Thymidylate Synthase	*Lactobacillus casei* (84)	Methotrexate	44	ND	0.2	ND	ND	ND	0.2
8. Thymidylate Synthase	*Escherichia coli* (84)	PteGlu	180	11	5	4	4	5	4
9. Thymidylate Synthase	*Escherichia coli* (19)	CHO-H$_4$PteGlu	200	20	3	3	2	1	ND
10. Thymidylate Synthase	*Escherichia coli* (84)	Methotrexate	100	ND	1	ND	ND	ND	1
11. Thymidylate Synthase	Coliphage T2 (84)	PteGlu	70	8	8	8	8	9	10
12. Thymidylate Synthase	Coliphage T2 (84)	Methotrexate	20	ND	2	ND	ND	ND	2
13. Thymidylate Synthase	Calf thymus[a]	PteGlu	80	15	10	8	ND	3	3
14. Thymidylate Synthase	Calf thymus[a]	Methotrexate	20	ND	2	ND	ND	ND	1

[a] Dwivedi, C. M. and Kisliuk, R. L., unpublished work
[b] using the corresponding H$_4$PteGlu$_n$ substrate in each instance;
[c] unnatural configuration at C-6
[d] K_i = 50 uM, ND = not determined

H$_2$PteGlu$_5$ forms a tight complex with FdUMP and L1210 thymidylate synthase (79). This might explain why pretreatment with MTX enhances fluorouracil toxicity over that obtained when the two drugs are given simultaneously, that is, the H$_2$PteGlu$_n$ which would be expected to accumulate after MTX treatment, would combine with FdUMP to form an inactive complex. Similarly, CH$_2$-H$_4$PteGlu$_3$ enhances the inhibitory activity of the phosphonate derivative of FdUMP (23). Therefore tests of the inhibitory activity of pyrimidine analogs for thymidylate synthase which employ H$_4$PteGlu$_1$ as substrate (80), may underestimate their inhibitory potency.

CH$_3$-H$_4$PteGlu plays a role in regulating the activity of cystathionine-γ-synthase from *Neurospora crassa* (81). This enzyme catalyzes the formation of cystathionine from O-acetylhomoserine and cysteine and has an absolute and specific requirement for CH$_3$-H$_4$PteGlu for activity, CH$_3$-H$_4$PteGlu$_7$ being much more active than CH$_3$-H$_4$-PteGlu$_2$. The function of cystathionine-γ-synthase is to provide homocysteine for methionine formation. It is inhibited by S-adenosylmethionine. Thus CH$_3$-H$_4$PteGlu and S-adenosylmethionine reciprocally control the synthesis of the methyl group acceptor homocysteine.

It may be that serine hydroxymethyltransferase is regulated by CH$_3$-H$_4$PteGlu as well. Weak inhibition of this enzyme from rabbit liver by CH$_3$-H$_4$PteGlu$_1$ (K_i = 9 × 10^{-5}) (82) would be expected to be enhanced by elongation of the polyGlu chain. This inhibition would lead to a decrease in the amount of serine used to supply single carbon units for purine, pyrimidine and methionine formation and an increase in the serine used for gluconeogenesis (83).

In vitro enzymatic synthesis of polyGlu derivatives

The mutant Chinese hamster ovary cell line AUXB1 lacks PtepolyGlu synthetase and will grow only if glycine, adenosine and thymidine or high concentrations of 5-CHO-H_4PteGlu are supplied in the medium (50, 85). The inability to convert PteGlu derivatives to their polyGlu forms leads to leakage of the monoGlu forms from the cells. Another mutant, AUXB3, which requires only glycine and adenosine for growth, lacks the ability to add Glu residues to H_4PteGlu$_3$ (86). In this instance the shorter PteGlu derivatives apparently suffice for thymidylate synthesis but not for purines and glycine. A single enzyme appears to be responsible for PtepolyGlu synthesis. In humans, the gene coding for this enzyme is found on chromosome 9 (87). In the hope of designing an inhibitor of PtepolyGlu synthetase which might lead to selective inhibition of cell growth, many workers are studying the properties of the enzyme.

Some of the enzyme systems examined are listed in Table 6. The *Corynebacterium* enzyme is highly purified, the *E. coli* and rat liver enzymes partially purified and the Chinese hamster ovary cell and sheep liver enzymes are in crude extracts. All of the enzymes require Mg^{++} and K^+ for activity. The pH optimum is high, in three instances being above pH 9. ATP is required with dATP having equal or greater activity. Complete specificity for Glu incorporation has been observed so far, neither aspartate, glycine, methionine nor a wide variety of potential Glu replacements were active (68, 88). The aspartate analog of MTX was also inactive (88).

The activity of a number of substrates relative to H_4PteGlu$_1$ are listed in Table 7. A Pte moiety is required for activity and many congeners of PteGlu including aminopterin, MTX, homofolate derivatives and the unnatural diastereoisomer of H_4PteGlu are active. The synthesis of polyGlu derivatives of these analogs must be considered in evaluating the cytotoxicity of these substances in view of the inhibitory potency of polyGlu analogs for many enzymes (Table 5).

The relative activities of various substrates differ greatly with the source of the enzyme. The most active substrate for the *E. coli* enzyme was 10-CHO-H_4PteGlu$_1$, being seven times as active as H_4PteGlu$_1$. With the *Corynebacterium* and rat liver enzymes, H_4PteGlu$_1$ was substantially more active than 10-CHO-H_4PteGlu$_1$. Preliminary results with a mouse liver system show H_2PteGlu$_1$ as more active than H_4PteGlu$_1$ (91).

Both the *E. coli* and *Corynebacterium* enzymes catalyze the formation of H_2PteGlu$_1$ from H_2Pte (dihydrofolate synthetase activity) as well as the addition of a second Glu residue (68, 92). With the *E. coli* enzyme it has been observed that separate active sites on the same protein are involved in adding Glu$_1$ to H_2Pte and in adding Glu$_1$ to H_2PteGlu$_1$ (92). This system does not add any more Glu residues beyond the formation of H_2PteGlu$_2$ (89, 92) and therefore does not account for the longer Glu chains found in *E. coli* (Table 3).

The *Corynebacterium*, Chinese hamster ovary cell, rat liver and sheep liver systems can synthesize derivatives with longer Glu chains. The synthesis of longer chains is favored by low H_4PteGlu$_1$ concentration, H_4PteGlu$_2$ and H_4PteGlu$_3$ derivatives being

Table 6. Properties of PtepolyGlu synthetases from various sources.

Properties	Source				
	Escherichia coli (89)	*Corynebacterium* (68)	Chinese hamster (85) ovary cells	Sheep liver (90)	Rat liver (88)
Molecular weight	43 000	53 000	ND	ND	69 000
pH optimum	9.4	10	9.5	8.4	8.4
Mg^{++} requirement	+	+	+	+	+
K^+ requirement	+	+	+	+	+

Table 7. Substrate specificity of PteGlu PolyGlu synthetase.

Substrate	Activity relative to $H_4PteGlu_1$ (%).			
	E. coli (89, 92)	*Corynebacterium* (68)	Chinese hamster (85) ovary	Rat liver (88)
1. (dl)-$H_4PteGlu_1$	100	100	100	100
2. (dl)-$H_4PteGlu_2$	ND	0.6	a	ND
3. (dl)-$H_4PteGlu_3$	ND	0.1	a	ND
4. (dl)-5,10-CH_2-$H_4PteGlu_1$	162	101	ND	64
5. (dl)-5,10-CH_2-$H_4PteGlu_2$	ND	3	ND	ND
6. (dl)-5,10-CH_2-$H_4PteGlu_3$	ND	0.2	ND	ND
7. (dl)-10-CHO-$H_4PteGlu_1$	707	26	ND	54
8. (dl)-10-CHO-$H_4PteGlu_2$	ND	3	ND	ND
9. (dl)-10-CHO-$H_4PteGlu_3$	ND	0.2	ND	ND
10. (dl)-5-CHO-$PteGlu_1$	0	37	71	27
11. (dl)-5-CH_3-$PteGlu_1$	0	8	17	48
12. $PteGlu_1$	16	0.2	3	47
13. Pte (D) Glu_1	ND	ND	ND	0
14. $H_2PteGlu_1$	0	10	ND	84
15. (dl) H_4Pte	ND	15	ND	ND
16. H_2Pte	a	14	ND	ND
17. Aminopterin	a	1	ND	100
18. (dl)-10-CHO-H_4 Aminopterin	346	ND	ND	ND
19. Methotrexate	ND	0.2	ND	100
20. Asp analog of Methotrexate	ND	ND	ND	0
24. (dl)-H_4-Homofolate	ND	ND	56	ND
25. (dl)-11-CHO-H_4-Homofolate	388	ND	ND	ND
26. (dl)-5-CH_3-H_4-Homofolate	ND	ND	ND	15
27. pAB	0	ND	ND	ND
28. $pABGlu_1$	ND	0	ND	ND

ND = not determined.
a   active but quantitative data not comparable to that given due to different conditions.

much poorer substrates for the enzyme than $H_4PteGlu_1$ derivatives (Table 7). The rat liver system synthesizes $H_4PteGlu_5$ which is a poor substrate and a powerful inhibitor of the enzyme (88). Therefore this system is capable of terminating polyGlu synthesis at Glu_5 which could account for the preponderance of Glu_5 derivatives in liver (Table 3).

Biosynthesis of methotrexate polyGlu derivatives

A wide variety of animal tissues can readily incorporate MTX into polyGlu forms (Table 8) (3). MTX ($+ Glu_1$) and MTX ($+ Glu_2$) are most commonly found in the tissue with MTX ($+ Glu_3$) formed on more prolonged exposure. In Chinese hamster ovary cells the same enzyme that acts on PteGlu derivatives acts on MTX derivatives (105).

Table 8. Conversion of methotrexate to PolyGlu forms by various tissues.

Tissue	
In vivo	
1. Human red blood cells (93)	+
2. Human bone marrow cells (94)	+
3. Human liver (95)	+
4. Rat liver (96, 97)	+
5. Rat thymus (97)	−
6. Rat small intestine (97)	−
7. Mouse small intestine (100)	±
8. Mouse L1210 cells (77, 100)	+
In vitro	
1. Cultured human breast cancer cells (98)	+
2. Human diploid fibroblasts (99)	+
3. Mouse L1210 cells (78)	+
4. Ehrlich ascites tumor cells (rat) (101)	+
5. Reuber H35 Rat hepatoma (102, 103)	+
6. Rat hepatocytes (104)	+
7. Chinese hamster ovary cells (105)	+
8. Chinese hamster ovary cells deficient (105) in polyGlu synthetase	−
9. Baby hamster kidney cells (105)	+
10. Baby hamster kidney cells resistant to MTX (105)	+

Once formed, the MTX ($+ Glu_n$) derivatives can exchange with MTX bound to $H_2PteGlu$ reductase. MTX ($+ Glu_1$), MTX ($+ Glu_2$) and MTX ($+ Glu_6$) have the same affinity for L1210 $H_2PteGlu$ reductase as does MTX (77). Synthesis of MTX ($+ Glu_n$) commences after the $H_2PteGlu$ reductase in the cells is saturated. This is particularly noticeable in cells containing a high level of this enzyme (77, 105).

Intestine and thymus form MTX ($+ Glu_n$) derivatives poorly (Table 8). This suggests that conversion to polyGlu forms is not a prerequisite for MTX toxicity since intestinal cells are sensitive to MTX intoxication. A role for MTX ($+ Glu_n$) in MTX toxicity has not been conclusively demonstrated.

The incorporation of H_2-aminopterin to polyGlu forms in *Pediococcus cerevisiae* has been reported (106).

PolyGlu hydrolases

Enzymes capable of hydrolysing γ-Glu amide bonds are widely distributed in nature and are commonly referred to as conjugases because they are capable of liberating $PteGlu_1$ and $PteGlu_2$ from conjugated ($PteGlu_n$) forms. Those which have been highly purified are listed in Table 9 along with some of their properties. Enzymes from different sources cleave the γ-Glu chain at different points but require a free carboxy terminal residue for activity. Those having a pH optimum near 4.5 are considered to be of lysosomal origin. The beef liver enzyme is a glycoprotein which contains Zn^{++}. It is not clear how or if these presumed lysosomal

Table 9. Properties of some Poly-γ-Glu hydrolases.

Source	Action	Molecular weight	pH optimum
Beef liver (107)	Endopeptidase $PteGlu_n \rightarrow PteGlu_1 + Glu_{n-1}$ $Glu_{n-1} \rightarrow n\text{-}1(Glu_1)$	108 000	4.5
Chicken intestine (108)	Endopeptidase $PteGlu_n \rightarrow PteGlu_2 + Glu_{n-2}$	80 000	7.5
Chicken liver (109)	Exopeptidase (Carboxypeptidase) $PteGlu_n \rightarrow PteGlu_1 + n\text{-}1(Glu_1)$	60 000	4.1, 5.2
Chicken pancreas (110)	Exopeptidase (Carboxypeptidase) $PteGlu_n \rightarrow PteGlu_2 + n\text{-}2(Glu_1)$	130 000	7.8

342

activities are related to PteGlu$_n$ metabolism in vivo. The pancreatic and intestinal enzymes with higher pH optima are most likely involved in the conversion of PteGlu$_n$ derivatives to PteGlu$_1$ and PteGlu$_2$ derivatives to facilitate intestinal absorption since long chain PteGlu derivatives are not absorbed in the intestine. Some doubt that conjugases are involved in the digestion of PteGlu$_n$ in humans has been expressed (111). The PteGlu$_n$ hydrolase of human pancreatic juice has a pH optimum below 5, a value practically never found in the lumen of the proximal human intestine. It is therefore proposed that monoGlu forms are more significant than polyGlu forms in human nutrition.

A biological role for a PtepolyGlu hydrolase is clearly indicated in the case of the enzyme coded by gene 28 of Coliphage T4D discussed above in the Distribution section (48, 49). H$_2$PteGlu$_6$ is a specific structural component in the tail plate of this phage and is formed by hydrolase action from compounds with longer Glu chains. Conjugase from hog kidney can reversibly inactivate Coliphage T4D by binding to H$_2$PteGlu$_6$ in situ under conditions where hydrolysis of the γ-Glu bonds does not take place (112).

Animal hydrolases are not able to cleave the α-amide bond between Pte and Glu. Bacterial enzymes have been identified which do catalyze this reaction (113, 114).

A convenient radioactive assay for PteGlu$_n$ hydrolases was developed by Krumdieck and Baugh (115, 116, 117). Microbiological methods have also been developed (118).

An hypothesis on the role of PtepolyGlu derivatives as coenzymes

Many PteGlu requiring enzymes occur in groups with the apparent purpose of channeling metabolites (17, 119, 120, 121, 122, 123, 124, 125). The likely function of the polyGlu chain would be to coordinate the activities of a given group of enzymes. The carboxy terminal Glu would be attached to an anchor protein (as suggested by Mackenzie and Baugh (17)) by a salt link while the Pte portion of the molecule proceeds sequentially from enzyme to enzyme. Examples of such metabolic sequences would be:
1) serine hydroxymethyltransferase $\rightarrow$ thymidylate synthase $\rightarrow$ H$_2$PteGlu reductase

2) serine hydroxymethyltransferase $\rightarrow$ CH$_2$-H$_4$PteGlu reductase $\rightarrow$ CH$_3$-H$_4$PteGlu, homocysteine transmethylase
3) serine hydroxymethyltransferase $\rightarrow$ CH$_2$-H$_4$PteGlu dehydrogenase $\rightarrow$ AICAR transformylase (or GAR transformylase)
4) CHNH-H$_4$PteGlu formiminotransferase $\rightarrow$ CHNH-H$_4$PteGlu cyclodeaminase

Serine hydroxymethyltransferase would be a central distribution point because serine is the main source of single carbon units. Serine hydroxymethyltransferase from rabbit liver is a tetramer (126) and it could be that individual monomers connect with pathways 1), 2) and 3).

The Pte head would move from one enzyme to the next influenced by the substituent at the 5, 10 positions and the state of oxidation of the ring. That is, the Pte configuration would alter its relationship with its polyGlu tail at each successive metabolic step. At pH 7.4 poly-γ-Glu is rod shaped due to the repulsion of the negatively charged COO$^-$ groups (127). These charges could be neutralized at specific points along the chain by divalent metal ions or basic groups on the protein, allowing the chain to bend as it moves from one protein to the next. (Mg^{++} exerts a powerful influence on the interaction of Coliphage T2 and E. coli thymidylate synthases with PteGlu$_6$ (128).) Under conditions of dietary stress (Table 3) where the action of degradative enzymes such as the glycine cleavage enzyme (129) and formiminoGlu-PteGlu formiminotransferase (130) would be required, the increase in the length of the Glu chains would enable the coenzymes to gain access to these enzymes which under normal circumstances are out of reach.

Acknowledgement

Work from the authors' laboratory was supported by Grant CA 10914 from the National Cancer Institute.

Publication of papers delivered at a workshop on folyl and antifolyl polyglutamates, organized by I. D. Goldman, B. Chabner and J. Bertino, held May 21–23, 1981, and sponsored by the National Cancer Institute, is anticipated during 1981.

References

1. Blakley, R. L., 1969. The Biochemistry of Folic Acid and Related Pteridines, North-Holland Publishing Co. Amsterdam.
2. Baugh, C. M. & Krumdieck, C., 1971. Ann. N.Y. Acad. Sci. 186: 7–28.
3. Covey, J. M., 1980. Life Sciences 26: 665–678.
4. Seeger, D. R., Cosulich, D. B., Smith, J. M. Jr. & Hultquist, M. E., 1949. J. Am. Chem. Soc. 71: 1753–1758.
5. Ensminger, W. D., Grindley, G. B. & Hoagland, J. A., 1979. Adv. Cancer Chemotherapy 1: 62–93. (A. Rosowsky, Ed. M. Dekker).
6. IUPAC-IUB-Tentative Rules, 1966. J. Biol. Chem. 241: 2991–2992.
7. Pfiffner, J. J., Calkins, D. G., Bloom, E. S. & O'Dell, B. L., 1946. J. Am. Chem. Soc. 68: 1392–1397.
8. Curthoys, N. P. & Rabinowitz, J. C., 1972. J. Biol. Chem. 247: 1965–1971.
9. Boothe, J. H., Mowatt, J. H., Hutchings, B. L., Angier, R. B., Waller, C. W., Stokstad, E. L. R., Semb, J., Gazzola, A. L. & Subbarow, Y., 1948. J. Am. Chem. Soc. 70: 1099–1151.
10. Krumdieck, C. L. & Baugh, C. M., 1969. Biochemistry 8: 1568–1572.
11. Godwin, H. A., Rosenberg, I. H., Ferenz, C. R., Jacobs, P. M. & Meienhofer, J., 1972. J. Biol. Chem. 247: 2266–2271.
12. Sengupta, P. K., Bieri, J. H. & Viscontini, M., 1975. Helvitca Chemica Acta 1374–1379.
13. Kisliuk, R. L., Gaumont, Y. & Baugh, C. M., 1974. J. Biol. Chem. 249: 4100–4103.
14. Krumdieck, C. L. & Baugh, C. M., 1980. Methods Enzymol. 66: 523–529.
15. Matthews, R. G. & Baugh, C. M., 1980. Biochemistry 19: 2040–2045.
16. Coward, J. K., Parameswaran, K. N., Cashmore, A. R. & Bertino, J. R., 1974. Biochemistry 13: 3889–3903.
17. MacKenzie, R. E. & Baugh, C. M., 1980. Biochim. Biophys. Acta 611: 187–195.
18. Salem, M. E., Lewis, G. P. & Rowe, P. B., 1979. Anal. Biochem. 97: 48–50.
19. Friedkin, M., Plante, L. T., Crawford, E. J. & Crumm, M., 1975. J. Biol. Chem. 250: 5614–5621.
20. Baggott, J. E. & Krumdieck, C., 1979. Biochemistry 18: 1036–1041.
21. Cheng, F. W., Shane, B. & Stokstad, E. L. R., 1975. Can. J. Biochem. 53: 1020–1027.
22. Coward, J. K., Chello, P., Cashmore, A., Parameswaran, K. N., DeAngelis, L. M. & Bertino, J. R., 1975. Biochemistry 14: 1548–1551.
23. Kisliuk, R. L., Gaumont, Y., Lafer, E., Baugh, C. M. & Montgomery, J. A., 1981. Biochemistry 20: 929–934.
24. Maruyama, T., Shiota, T. & Krumdieck, C. L., 1978. Anal. Biochem. 84: 234–240.
25. Reed, B. & Scott, J. M., 1980. Methods Enzymol. 66: 501–507.
26. Lewis, G. P. & Rowe, P. B., 1979. Anal. Biochem. 93: 91–97.
27. Baugh, C. M., Braverman, E. B., Nair, M. G., Horne, D. W., Briggs, W. T. & Wagner, C., 1979. Anal. Biochem. 92: 366–369.
28. Eto, I. & Krumdieck, C. L., 1980. Anal. Biochem. 109: 167–184.
29. Foo, S. K., Cichowicz, D. J. & Shane, B., 1980. Anal. Biochem. 107: 109–115.
30. Cashmore, A. R., Dreyer, R. N., Horvath, C., Knipe, J. O., Coward, J. K. & Bertino, J. R., 1980. Methods Enzymol. 66: 459–468.
31. Archer, M. C. & Reed, L. S., 1980. Methods Enzymol. 66: 452–459.
32. Brody, T., Shane, B. & Stokstad, E. L. R., 1979. Anal. Biochem. 92: 501–509.
33. Rao, K. N. & Noronha, J. M., 1978. Anal. Biochem. 88: 128–137.
34. Bird, O. D., McGlohon, V. M. & Vaitkus, J. W., 1965. Anal. Biochem. 12: 18–35.
35. Wittenberg, J. B., Noronha, J. M. & Silverman, M., 1962. Biochem. J. 85: 9–15.
36. Osborne-White, W. S. & Smith, R. M., 1973. Biochem. J. 136: 265–278.
37. Moran, R. G., Werkheiser, W. C. & Zakrzewski, S. F., 1976. J. Biol. Chem. 251: 3569–3575.
38. Scott, J. M., 1980. Methods Enzymol. 66: 437–443.
39. Kas, J. & Cerna, J., 1980. Methods Enzymol. 66: 443–452.
40. Rabinowitz, J. C., 1960. The Enzymes, P. D. Boyer, H. Lardy & K. Myrback, Eds., Academic Press, N.Y. Vol. 2, pp. 185–252.
41. Priest, D. G., Happel, K. K. & Doig, M. T., 1980. J. Biochem. Biophys. Methods. 3: 201–206.
42. Usdin, E., 1959. J. Biol. Chem. 234: 2373–2376.
43. Hakala, M. T. & Welch, A. D., 1957. J. Bacteriol. 73: 35–40.
44. Tamura, T., Shin, Y. S., Williams, M. A. & Stokstad, E. L. R., 1972. Anal. Biochem. 49: 517–521.
45. Shane, B. & Stokstad, E. L. R., 1976. J. Biol. Chem. 251: 3405–3410.
46. Bakerman, H. A., 1961. Anal. Biochem. 2: 558–565.
47. Kozloff, L. M. & Lute, M., 1965. J. Mol. Biol. 12: 780–792.
48. Kozloff, L. M., Crosby, L. K. & Baugh, C. M., 1979. J. Virol. 32: 497–506.
49. Kozloff, L. M., Lute, M. & Crosby, L. K., 1979. Chemistry and Biology of Pteridines, R. L. Kisliuk & G. M. Brown, Eds., Elsevier/North-Holland, pp. 309–314.
50. McBurney, M. W. & Whitmore, G. F., 1974. Cell 2: 173–182.
51. Sirotnak, F. M., Donati, G. J. & Hutchison, D. G., 1963. J. Bacteriol. 85: 658–665.
52. Iwai, K. & Nakagawa, S., 1958. Mem. Res. Inst. Food Sci. (Kyoto) 15: 49–60.
53. Clandinin, M. T. & Cossins, E. A., 1972. Biochem. J. 128: 29–40.
54. Spronk, A. M. & Cossins, E. A., 1972. Phytochem. 11: 3157–3165.
55. Lor, K. L. & Cossins, E. A., 1973. Phytochem. 12: 9–14.
56. Cossins, E. A. & Shah, S. P. J., 1972. Phytochem. 11: 587–593.
57. Noronha, J. M. & Silverman, M., 1962. J. Biol. Chem. 237: 3299–3302.

58. Whitehead, V. M., 1973. Lancet 743–745.

59. Herbert, V. & Zalusky, R., 1962. J. Clin. Invest. 41: 1263–1269.

60. Hintze, D. N. & Farmer, J. L., 1975. J. Bact. 124: 1236–1239.

61. Baugh, C. M., Braverman, E. & Nair, M. G., 1974. Biochemistry 13: 4952–4957.

62. Scott, J. M., 1976. Biochem. Soc. Trans. 4: 845–850.

63. Hoffbrand, A. V., Tripp, E. & Lavoie, A., 1977. Folic Acid Nat. Acad. Sci. (U.S.A.) pp. 110–121.

64. Brown, J. P., Davidson, G. E. & Scott, J. M., 1974. Biochim. Biophys. Acta 343: 78–88.

65. Tyerman, M. J., Watson, J. E., Shane, B., Schutz, D. E. & Stokstad, E. L. R., 1977. Biochim. Biophys. Acta 497: 234–240.

66. Thompson, R. W., Leichter, J., Cornwell, P. E. & Krumdieck, C. L., 1977. Am. J. Clin. Nutr. 30: 1583–1590.

67. Chan, P. Y. & Cossins, E. A., 1980. Arch. Biochem. Biophys. 200: 346–351.

68. Shane, B., 1980. J. Biol. Chem. 255: 5655–5662.

69. Delk, A. S., Nagle, D. P., Jr. & Rabinowitz, J. C., 1980. J. Biol. Chem. 255: 4387–4390.

70. Wright, B. E., 1956. J. Biol. Chem. 219: 873–883.

71. Plante, L. T., Crawford, E. J. & Friedkin, M., 1976. J. Med. Chem. 19: 1295–1299.

72. Dolnick, B. J. & Cheng, Y.-C., 1978. J. Biol. Chem. 253: 3563–3567.

73. Powers, S. G. & Snell, E. E., 1976. J. Biol. Chem. 251: 3786–3793.

74. Burton, E., Selhub, J. & Sakami, W., 1969. Biochem. J. 111: 793–795.

75. Whitfield, C. D., Steers, E. J., Jr. & Weissbach, H., 1970. J. Biol. Chem. 245: 390–401.

76. Jacobs, S. A., Adamson, R. H., Chabner, B. A., Derr, C. J. & Johns, D. G., 1975. Biochem. Biophys. Res. Commun. 63: 692–698.

77. Whitehead, V. M., 1977. Cancer Res. 37: 408–412.

78. Sirotnak, F. M., Chello, P. L., Piper, J. R. & Montgomery, J. A., 1978. Biochem. Pharm. 27: 1821–1825.

79. Fernandes, D. J. & Bertino, J. R., 1980. Proc. Natl. Acad. Sci. USA 77: 5663–5667.

80. DeClerq, E., Balzarini, J., Descamps, J., Bigge, C. F., Chang, C. T.-C., Kalaritis, P. & Mertes, M. P., 1981. Biochem. Pharm. 30: 495–502.

81. Selhub, J., Savin, M. A., Sakami, W. & Flavin, M., 1971. Proc. Natl. Acad. Sci. USA 68: 312–314.

82. Schirch, L. & Ropp, M., 1967. Biochemistry 6: 253–260.

83. Krebs, H. A., Hems, R. & Tyler, B., 1976. Biochem. J. 158: 341–353.

84. Kisliuk, R. L., Gaumont, Y., Baugh, C. M., Galivan, J. H., Maley, G. F. & Maley, F., 1979. Chemistry and Biology of Pteridines Kisliuk, R. L. & Brown, G. M. Eds., Elsevier/North-Holland, pp. 431–435.

85. Taylor, R. T. & Hanna, M. L., 1977. Arch. Biochem. Biophys. 181: 331–334.

86. Taylor, R. T. & Hanna, M. L., 1979. Arch. Biochem. Biophys. 197: 36–43.

87. Jones, C., Kao, F.-T. & Taylor, R. T., 1980. Cytogenet. Cell. Genet. 28: 181–194.

88. McGuire, J. J., Hsieh, P., Coward, J. K. & Bertino, J. R., 1980. J. Biol. Chem. 255: 5776–5778.

89. Masurekar, M. & Brown, G. M., 1975. Biochemistry 14: 2424–2430.

90. Gawthorne, J. M. & Smith, R. M., 1973. Biochem. J. 136: 295–301.

91. Moran, R. G. & Colman, P. D., 1980. Proc. Soc. Am. Soc. Cancer Res. 21: 25.

92. Ferone, R. & Warskow, A., 1981. Fed. Proc. 40: 1748.

93. Baugh, C. M., Krumdieck, C. L. & Nair, M. G., 1973. Biochem. Biophys. Res. Commun. 52: 27–34.

94. Witte, A., Whitehead, V. M., Rosenblatt, D. S. & Vuchich, M. J., 1980. Devel. Pharm. Therap. 1: 40–46.

95. Jacobs, S. A., Derr, J. D. & Johns, D. C., 1977. Biochem. Pharm. 26: 2310–2313.

96. Nair, M. G. & Baugh, C. M., 1973. Biochemistry 12: 3923–3927.

97. Whitehead, V. M., Perrault, M. M. & Stelcner, S., 1975. Cancer Res. 35: 2985–2990.

98. Schilsky, R. L., Bailey, B. D. & Chabner, B. A., 1980. Proc. Natl. Acad. Sci. USA 77: 2919–2922.

99. Rosenblatt, D. S., Whitehead, V. M., Vuchich, M. J., Pottier, A., Matiaszuk, N. V. & Beaulieu, D., 1981. Mol. Pharm. 19: 87–97.

100. Poser, R. G., Sirotnak, F. M. & Chello, P. L., 1980. Biochem. Pharm. 29: 2701–2704.

101. Fry, D. W., Yalowich, J. C., Hess, M. L. & Goldman, I. D., 1981. Fed. Proc. 40: 1748.

102. Galivan, J. H., 1979. Cancer Res. 39: 735–743.

103. Galivan, J. H., 1980. Mol. Pharm. 17: 105–110.

104. Gewirtz, D. A., White, J. C., Randolph, J. K. & Goldman, I. D., 1979. Cancer Res. 39: 2914–2918.

105. Whitehead, V. M. & Rosenblatt, D. S., 1979. Chemistry and Biology of Pteridines, R. L. Kisliuk & G. M. Brown, Eds., Elsevier/North-Holland, pp. 689–694.

106. Buehring, K. U. & Folsch, E., 1976. Biochim. Biophys. Acta 421: 22–32.

107. Silink, M., Reddel, R., Bethel, M. & Rowe, P., 1975. J. Biol. Chem. 250: 5982–5994.

108. Rosenberg, I. H. & Neumann, H., 1974. J. Biol. Chem. 249: 5126–5130.

109. Rao, K. N. & Noronha, J. M., 1977. Biochim. Biophys. Acta 481: 594–607.

110. Kaferstein, H. & Jaenicke, L., 1972. Hoppe-Seyler's Z. Physiol. Chem. 353: 1153–1158.

111. Elsborg, L., 1980. Danish Med. Bull. 27: 205–206.

112. Dawes, J. & Goldberg, E. B., 1973. Virology 55: 380–390.

113. Levy, C. C. & Goldman, P., 1968. J. Biol. Chem. 243: 3507–3511.

114. Albrecht, A. M., Boldizsar, E. & Hutchison, D. J., 1978. J. Bacteriol. 134: 506–513.

115. Baugh, C. M., Stevens, J. C. & Krumdieck, C. L., 1970. Biochim. Biophys. Acta 212: 116–124.

116. Krumdieck, C. L. & Baugh, C. M., 1970. Anal. Biochem. 35: 123–128.

117. Krumdieck, C. L. & Baugh, C. M., 1980. Methods Enzymol. 66: 660–662.

118. Elsenhans, B., Selhub, J. & Rosenberg, I. H., 1980. Methods Enzymol. 66: 663–667.

119. Tan, L. U. L., Drury, E. J. & MacKenzie, R. E., 1977. J. Biol. Chem. 252: 1117–1122.
120. Paukert, J. L., D'Ari-Strauss, L. & Rabinowitz, J. C., 1976. J. Biol. Chem. 251: 5104–5111.
121. Caperelli, C. A., Benkovic, P. A., Chettur, G. & Benkovic, S. J., 1980. J. Biol. Chem. 255: 1885–1890.
122. Smith, G. K., Mueller, W. T., Wasserman, G. F., Taylor, W. D. & Benkovic, S., 1980. Biochemistry 19: 4313–4321.
123. Ferone, R. & Roland, S., 1980. Proc. Natl. Acad. Sci. USA 77: 5802–5806.
124. Reddy, G. P. V. & Mathews, C. K., 1978. J. Biol. Chem. 253: 3641–3647.
125. Reddy, G. P. V. & Pardee, A. B., 1980. Proc. Natl. Acad. Sci. USA 77: 3312–3316.
126. Schirch, L. & Peterson, D., 1980. J. Biol. Chem. 255: 7801–7806.
127. Kovacs, J., Kapoor, U. R. G., Mayers, G. L., Giannasio, V. R., Giannotti, R., Senyk, G., Nitecki, E. & Goodman, J. W., 1972. Biochemistry 11: 1953–1958.
128. Maley, G. F., Maley, F. & Baugh, C. M., 1979. J. Biol. Chem. 254: 7485–7487.
129. Hiraga, K. & Kikuchi, G., 1980. J. Biol. Chem. 255: 11671–11676.
130. Tabor, H. & Wyngarden, L., 1959. J. Biol. Chem. 234: 1830–1840.

Received May 8, 1981.

Glutamate receptor binding in insects and mammals

P. A. Briley, M. T. Filbin, G. G. Lunt & P. D. Turner
Dept. of Biochemistry, Bath University, Bath, BA2 7AY, U.K.

Summary

High affinity stereospecific binding sites for L-glutamate have been reported in several regions of mammalian brain. The binding sites in the hippocampus and cerebellum have been studied more extensively than binding in other brain regions. The hippocampal and cerebellar binding sites show similar properties with respect to their pharmacology and their independence of Na^+. There is evidence, particularly good in the case of hippocampus, of mechanisms that may regulate the availability of the binding sites in both brain areas. Some progress has been made with the isolation of the hippocampal binding site but the protein has not been extensively characterised.

In the case of insect muscle, high-affinity stereospecific binding of L-glutamate to whole membrane preparations, to detergent-solubilised membranes and to isolated proteolipids has been reported. Much greater variability in the binding characteristics is seen than is the case with the mammalian brain preparations. Preliminary experiments suggest that at least four distinct binding sites may be present on insect muscle.

The complete characterisation of glutamate binding sites is at present precluded by a lack of potent agonists and antagonists. However, recent advances in the pharmacological classification of receptor sites for the excitatory amino acids in mammalian brain could provide sufficient information to permit the identification of the binding sites as synaptic receptors. Invertebrate toxins whose site of action is the insect neuromuscular junction may well prove to be useful tools with which to isolate and characterise the synaptic receptor proteins.

Introduction

The powerful excitatory effects of glutamate on mammalian brain neurones were first noted by Hayashi (1) in 1953 who postulated a neuromodulatory role for the amino acid. In 1963 Krnjevic and Phillis (2) suggested that glutamate was indeed a natural excitatory neurotransmitter in the brain and this view has been subsequently substantiated by a steady stream of reports from many laboratories (3, 4). Thus it is now generally agreed that glutamate is a major neurotransmitter in the mammalian brain and may have particular importance in the corticostriatal pathway (5, 6) and in the cerebellum (7) and hippocampus (8).

Glutamate's role as an excitatory transmitter at the insect neuromuscular junction first received attention in the mid 1960's (9, 10). Since then a wealth of evidence has accumulated that supports this suggestion (11, 12, 13, 14, 15). The bulk of this evidence however derives from electrophysiological experiments and biochemical evidence to support the proposed neurotransmitter function is not so readily available (16, 17).

The biochemical identification of a post-synaptic receptor for glutamate has proved difficult, partic-

Molecular and Cellular Biochemistry 39, 347–356 (1981).   0300-8177/81/0391-0347/$02.00.

ularly in the case of insect muscle. The successful isolation and almost complete characterisation of the nicotinic acetylcholine receptor from vertebrate muscle and from the electric organs of various species of electric fish has been made possible only by the ready availability of natural toxins that bind almost irreversibly and with very high specificity to the receptor (18, 19). The isolation of other neurotransmitter receptors has progressed more slowly but there is currently much interest in assaying synaptic receptors in their membrane-bound form as a prelude to possible isolation of the receptor protein (20).

The methods for assaying receptor sites tend to follow a common general pattern. Tissue fractions are incubated with radiolabelled ligand until the binding reaches equilibrium, after which bound ligand is separated from free ligand by rapid filtration or by centrifugation. This apparently simple procedure presents in practice, many serious problems. Firstly there is a requirement for a ligand of sufficiently high specific radioactivity to permit detection of what may be a very small number of binding sites in the tissue preparation. Secondly, the ligand should have a very high affinity for the binding site, or more precisely, the off-rate for the bound ligand should be very slow to minimise dissociation during the separation of bound from free ligand. Finally the ligand should show great specificity for the site under investigation so that binding of ligand to a small number of specific sites is not lost in an overwhelming background of nonspecific binding. It is perhaps in this last area that most of the problems of measuring glutamate binding are found, and it is worth examining this aspect of the binding experiments in some detail.

Most workers have attempted to study glutamate receptor sites by looking at the binding of glutamate itself (these studies are dealt with in detail below). The use of the natural ligand does however pose problems in that the off-rate is likely to be quite high and more importantly the assessment of the specificity of binding may be difficult. In the case of glutamate binding the specific binding component of the total binding to the tissue in question is invariably determined by the 'unlabelled ligand excess' method. In this method specific binding is eliminated by incubating in the presence of a high concentration of unlabelled ligand and specific binding is then defined as total binding

minus non-specific binding. One suspects that although this procedure is widely used, the rationale for its use is often not clearly understood, and accordingly the limitations of the method are not fully appreciated.

The method is based on the assumption that if the specific radioactivity of the radiolabelled ligand is reduced by addition of a large excess of unlabelled ligand then specific binding will become insignificant whereas non-specific binding will be essentially unchanged. This assumption may be rationalised algebraically if one considers a homogeneous population of receptor sites, R, that bind ligand, L:

$$R + L \rightleftharpoons RL$$

At equilibrium the dissociation constant K_D for the interaction is defined as:

$$K_D = \frac{[R][L]}{[RL]} \tag{1}$$

The total concentration of binding sites, B_{max} is defined as:

$$B_{max} = [RL] + [R] \tag{2}$$

therefore

$$B_{max} = [RL] + \frac{K_D[RL]}{[L]}$$

or

$$[RL] = \frac{B_{max}[L]}{K_D + [L]} \tag{3}$$

Under nearly all experimental conditions $[L] \gg [RL]$ and therefore $[L]$ may be assumed to equal $[L_T]$, where $[L_T]$ is the total ligand, i.e. bound + free and equation (3) can be written:

$$[RL] = \frac{B_{max}[L_T]}{K_D + [L_T]} \tag{4}$$

Examination of the conditions used in glutamate binding assays reveals that K_D for so-called specific-binding is comparable to or less than $[L_T]$ (usually in the micromolar range). Non-specific binding, on the other hand, is that binding in which $K_D \gg [L_T]$. In the latter case, therefore, equation (4) may be reduced to:

$$[RL] = \frac{B_{max}}{K_D}[L_T] \tag{5}$$

To examine the effects of varying concentrations of

labelled and unlabelled ligand, L can be considered to comprise L*-labelled ligand and L'-unlabelled ligand and equation 4 expands to:

$$[RL^*] + [RL'] = \frac{B_{max}\,([L^*_T] + [L'_T])}{K_D + ([L^*_T] + [L'_T])} \quad (6)$$

Making the reasonable assumption that there is no preferential binding of labelled ligand, the bound radioactivity as measured in the binding assay is [RL*] where:

[RL*] = (total bound ligand) × specific activity

$$= \frac{([RL^*] + [RL'])\,[L^*_T]}{[L^*_T] + [L'_T]} \quad (7)$$

Substituting into (7) from (6):

$$[RL^*] = \frac{B_{max}\,[L^*_T]}{K_D + [L^*_T] + [L'_T]}$$

When $K_D \ll [L'_T] \gg [L^*_T]$, that is, when a large excess of unlabelled ligand is added, then [RL*] becomes insignificant. This will be the case with specific binding; for the non-specific binding component however, equation (5) applies and this may be expanded to account for L* and L' as before:

$$[RL^*] + [RL'] = \frac{B_{max}}{K_D}\,([L^*_T] + [L'_T]) \quad (8)$$

Substituting into (7) from (8):

$$[RL^*] = \frac{B_{max}}{K_D} \cdot [L^*_T]$$

and therefore bound radioactivity is independent of $[L'_T]$.

This method defines a specific binding site as one whose K_D is lower than or comparable to the concentration of ligand present; it is clear therefore that assay of glutamate binding over a series of concentration ranges may well reveal a series of specific binding sites. That is, the specific binding sites are specific only within the context of the assay and no conclusions about their physiological relevance can be drawn without further analysis. One of the best examples of this particular pitfall is the binding of insulin to talc with a K_D in the nanomolar range (21), such binding sites behave as specific sites in this assay system. To some extent the problem can be overcome by assays in which the specific binding of the radiolabelled ligand is assessed by displacement with an excess of an unlabelled, chemically distinct ligand, i.e. an agonist or antagonist. In this case the probability of competition between labelled and unlabelled ligand for any common non-physiological high-affinity site is much less and in general the use of well-characterised structurally-distinct unlabelled ligands is to be preferred for the displacement of specific binding (22). In the case of glutamate receptor binding the lack of well-characterised potent agonists and antagonists has so far precluded the adoption of the preferred procedure.

Receptor-binding in mammalian brain

The first reports of glutamate binding to putative receptors in brain were made independently by Roberts (23) and by Michaelis et al. (24) in 1974. Both groups used ^{14}C labelled glutamate and the relatively low specific radioactivity severely limited the concentration range that was examined. Roberts (23) used the unlabelled ligand excess method to obtain the specific binding component whereas Michaelis et al. (24) used a graphical analysis of total binding data (25).

Roberts (23) reported a single binding site on cerebral cortex membranes with $K_D = 8\,\mu M$ and $B_{max} = 0.03$ nmol/mg protein. Michaelis et al. (24), who worked with membrane fractions from whole brain, saw two distinct sites, one with $K_D = 0.2\,\mu M$ and B_{max} 1.8 nmol/mg protein and a second site with $K_D = 4.4\,\mu M$ and $B_{max} = 8.8$ nmol/mg protein.

In these early binding studies the sites were not well characterised pharmacologically and it is likely that the observed binding represented a composite of postsynaptic receptors, extra-synaptic receptors and neuronal and/or glial uptake sites. Roberts (23) attempted to differentiate between synaptic receptors and uptake sites on the basis of their Na$^+$ dependence. It had been shown previously (26, 27) that glutamate uptake in brain is Na$^+$ dependent and Roberts (23) was able to demonstrate a marked difference in glutamate binding in the presence and in the absence of Na$^+$. However, it is worth bearing in mind that there are reports of substantial levels of sodium-independent specific binding of glutamate in such tissues as striated muscle (28) and in lung, liver and kidney (29). Such findings emphasize the need for extensive pharmacological characterisation of specific-binding sites before they can be unequivocally described as glutamate receptors.

More recent studies have, on the whole revealed sites of higher affinity than those mentioned above. A single population of sites with $K_D = 744$ nM and $B_{max} = 73$ pmol/mg protein was found on synaptic membranes from rat cerebellum (28). In this study the effects of a wide range of compounds on the displacement of specifically bound glutamate were in keeping with the characteristics expected for a postsynaptic glutamate receptor. However, a reappraisal by the authors of their method of preparation of the synaptic membranes has led to a reduction in the K_D to a value of about 300 nM accompanied by an increase in B_{max} to a value of 117 pmol/mg protein (30). The reasons for the increased affinity are not clear; the main differences in the membrane preparation procedure are an increased period of ultrasonication and more extensive washing of the fractions (28, 30). The authors present some preliminary data (30, 31) that support the suggestion that an endogenous inhibitor of glutamate binding may be involved. Michaelis (32) tentatively identified gangliosides as possible candidates for such an endogenous inhibitor and showed that brain gangliosides act as competitive inhibitors of glutamate binding. This effect has been interpreted as a reflection of the possible functional importance of glycosyl residues on the glutamate receptor (31), a suggestion that receives some support from other observations (33, 34) that Con A inhibits glutamate binding.

A putative glutamate receptor site has been reported in rat hippocampal membranes (35, 36) that has similar properties to the cerebellar site described by Roberts (28, 30, 31) and discussed above. Thus a sodium independent binding of glutamate is seen with a K_D of 750 nM and B_{max} of 6.5 pmol/mg protein. The pharmacological characteristics of the binding site are similar to those of the cerebellar site and the authors suggest that it represents a hippocampal postsynaptic glutamate receptor (36).

The regulation of the hippocampal binding site has been the subject of a series of studies from Baudry and Lynch. Exposure of hippocampal membranes to low concentrations of Ca^{++} results in an increased number of sites but there is no change in their K_D (36). The authors suggest that this behaviour results from activation of a Ca^{++}-regulated thiol-protease that regulates the number of glutamate receptor sites in hippocampal synaptic membranes (36). The effects are not seen in cerebellar preparations and it is suggested that they may be related to synaptic development and to the well documented long-term potentiation of transmission that can occur in the hippocampus (36). Supporting this latter involvement is the finding that repetitive electrical stimulation of hippocampal slices results in an increase in the number of glutamate binding sites but the affinity of the sites is unchanged. Evidence for an involvement of cations in the regulatory process has also been presented (38). Monovalent cations such as Li^+, Cs^+, Ru^+, K^+ and Na^+ in the low mM range all show significant inhibition of Na^+-dependent binding in hippocampal synaptic membrane preparations, whereas low μM concentrations of Ca^{++}, Mg^{++} and Mn^{++} effectively enhance the binding (37). As in the other studies the number of sites rather than their affinity is changed. As yet the precise relationship between the putative Ca^{++} activated protease and the glutamate binding site is not clear. At this stage we can however conclude that certainly in the hippocampus there appear to be endogenous mechanisms that can regulate the availability of potential synaptic receptors. Evidence that is considerably more circumstantial suggests that such mechanisms may operate in the cerebellum also since Sharif and Roberts (30) have shown that lyophillisation of membranes exposes additional binding sites but is without effect on their affinity.

Sites of much higher affinity than those discussed above have been described by Biziere et al. (39). These workers described two sites on membrane fractions from whole rat brain, having K_D values of 11 nM and of 80 nM. Roberts (31) has suggested that some of the characteristics of these sites may derive from the fact that the tissue was frozen prior to fractionation and Roberts and co-workers (30) have reported that freezing can have marked affects on glutamate binding. Roberts (31) however also reports preliminary experiments on rat striatal synaptic membranes that show the presence of a binding site of $K_D = 16.6$ nM and at least two other sites with K_D's in the high nanomolar range and suggests that the site with $K_D = 16.6$ nM may be the same as the site of higher affinity described by Biziere et al. (39). However, Roberts (31) points out that no pharmacological data for the site are available. It is perhaps worth noting that because of the concentration range of glutamate examined in most studies the 11 nM site described by Biziere et al. (37) would probably not have been detected and indeed Vincent and McGeer (40) reported that they could not detect Na^+ independent binding in rat striatum. Having regard for the characteristics of the 'unlabelled ligand excess' method it may well be that closer examination of lower concentration ranges of glutamate will reveal yet more 'specific' binding sites, but as Roberts (31) has pointed out, the physiological relevance of such high affinity sites may be far from clear.

There are few detailed reports of studies on glutamate binding to areas of the brain apart from the cerebellum and hippocampus. Head et al. (41) looked at Na^+-independent binding activity in a number of regions of the cat brain and found that binding activity was highest in the amygdaloid > hippocampus > hypothalamus = visual cortex = thalamus = caudate nucleus > olfactory lobe = tectum = cerebellum > dorsal pons = medulla > spinal cord. Unfortunately, the only region in which the binding was examined in detail was the cerebellum where two sites were identified with K_D values of 330 nM and 1.8 μM and B_{max} values of 15 pmol/mg protein and 65 pmol/mg protein respectively (41), values comparable with those discussed above. Binding to rat cortical membranes was measured by Sanderson and Murphy (42). They had particular interest in the development of glutamate receptor activity and identified a Na^+-independent site with K_D = 210 nM and B_{max} 3.01 pmol/mg protein that reached a peak of activity at about 20 days after birth. A developmental study in rat cerebellum revealed a very similar site with K_D = 220 nM and B_{max} = 10.1 pmol/mg protein that also peaked at about 20 days (43).

There have been some attempts to proceed beyond the stage of measuring the binding of glutamate to membrane-bound receptor sites and to solubilise and purify the binding component. In 1975 Michaelis (44) reported the partial purification of a glutamate binding glycoprotein by affinity chromatography on ConA-Sepharose of a Triton X-100 extract of a rat brain membrane preparation. In subsequent reports it has been claimed that this glutamate binding-glycoprotein is in fact a metallo-protein having an Fe_2S_2 grouping at the ligand binding site although no suggestions are made as to the possible function of such a grouping. The cerebellar glutamate binding site has been solubilised by treatment with Triton X-100 with little apparent change in either its affinity for glutamate or its pharmacological profile (30) there are however no reports of purification of the solubilised protein.

The ultimate goal of receptor research is to identify precisely the molecular nature of the receptor and to fully reconstitute its functional activity in a defined lipid membrane. In the case of the nicotinic acetylcholine receptor such an achievement is rapidly approaching (45, 46), but for the glutamate receptor the goal is still very distant. A very preliminary report has been made of the incorporation of the metallo-glycoprotein of Michaelis into a variety of membrane preparations and some binding activity was retained (47). Kuznetsov and colleagues have adopted several approaches to reconstitution of a functional glutamate receptor. They solubilised the hippocampal binding site with Triton X-100 and obtained a further purification of the binding protein by chromatography on Sepharose 4B. Both the Triton X-100 extract and the protein were incorporated into lipid films prepared from whole-brain phospholipids. Such films showed glutamate-induced permeability changes although with aged preparations of the binding protein spontaneous permeability changes of equal magnitude were seen in the absence of glutamate (48). More recently these workers have used what they describe as 'Triton X-100 solubilised membrane fragments' in lipid bilayer studies (49, 50). The fragments, from hippocampal synaptic membranes, are incorporated into planar lipid bilayers and as in the earlier studies glutamate-induced permeability changes are seen. Interestingly the changes are not observed unless the fragments are inserted into both sides of the membrane (50) implying that some sort of interaction between components in the two halves of the bilayer is necessary for the formation of functional channels. The authors conclude that the characteristics of the permeability changes, particularly those relating to Na^+ movements, are consistent with those of the synaptic glutamate receptor (49, 50). However, considerably more pharmacological and electrophysiological characterisation is required before this interesting system can be described as a reconstituted synaptic glutamate receptor.

The group of De Robertis has adopted an approach to the characterisation of synaptic receptors that is quite different from any of those described above. De Robertis reasoned that a synaptic receptor must be a trans-membrane protein and would therefore be expected to have a very hydrophobic exterior and that this property may be reflected in the protein's solubility characteristics (51). The group isolated hydrophobic proteins or proteolipids from a variety of sources and the isolated proteolipids showed many of the properties expected for neurotransmitter receptors. There has been much controversy in the literature over the identification of the proteolipid receptors; in some cases the criticisms (52) were ill-founded and a careful study by Donnellan et al. (53) refuted many of the arguments against the proteolipids. More recently a systematic study of the cholinergic proteolipid by Taylor (54) reconfirmed the validity of much of the work of the De Robertis group. It is perhaps worth bearing in mind that the analysis of the binding activity of proteolipids is technically difficult and the proteins do not readily lend themselves to study by the conventional techniques of protein chemistry. It is probably for these reasons that relatively few groups have pursued this approach to receptor characterisation.

Application of the proteolipid techniques to the question of the glutamate receptor resulted in the identification of three binding sites associated with proteolipids from rat cerebral cortex (55). The sites showed widely differing K_D values of 300 nM, 5 μM and 55 μM with B_{max} values of 530 pmol/mg protein, 320 nmol/mg protein and 16.6 nmol/mg protein respectively. The high affinity site showed an absolute stereospecificity for L-glutamate and in this respect resembles all the binding sites discussed above. The medium and low affinity sites did not show such discrimination. The pharmacological profile of the high affinity site was consistent with that of a synaptic glutamate receptor. The authors did not investigate the Na^+-dependence of the site and it is accordingly difficult to assess the relationship of the sites to receptor and uptake/transport mechanisms. Certainly the high affinity site shows similarities to the putative receptor sites described by others and discussed above. However, so far none of .these binding sites are sufficiently well-characterised to permit their unequivocal designation as synaptic glutamate receptors.

Glutamate receptor binding in insects

In our early studies of glutamate binding sites in insects we employed the procedures of De Robertis and his group (51). Proteolipids were extracted from the total intrathoracic musculature of the locust (Schistocerca gregaria) and two of the proteolipids showed specific binding of glutamate (56). In subsequent studies these two proteolipids were found to bind glutamate with different affinities, the values for K_D being 8 μM and 50 μM (57). The higher affinity site showed some pharmacological properties characteristic of a glutamate receptor site (57). A similar glutamate-binding proteolipid was also isolated from fly (Musca domestica) muscle (58, 69). It is worth noting that a proteolipid having very similar properties has also been isolated from shrimp muscle (60, 61) and it may be that a systematic examination of other arthropod muscles would reveal similar binding proteins. As stated above however the analysis of the glutamate binding proteolipids presents many problems and we have turned our attention to the measurement of glutamate binding to intact membrane fragments prepared from insect muscle.

Preliminary studies on a deoxycholate-solubilised preparation of whole locust muscle revealed a single class of glutamate binding sites with a $K_D = 0.5$ μM (56); the Na^+ dependence of this binding was not examined. These studies were made, as were the early measurements of the brain sites (23, 24), with ^{14}C labelled glutamate of relatively low specific radioactivity and as such suffered from a lack of sensitivity. Later studies (62) were made using membranous sub-fractions of locust muscle and an ultrafiltration technique (53) to separate bound ligand from free ligand. In these experiments (62) two binding sites specific for L-glutamate were seen which differed in their dependence on Na^+. In the absence of Na^+ a single site of $K_D = 0.53$ μM and $B_{max} = 25$ pmol/mg protein was seen, reminiscent of the site observed in the earlier studies (56). Addition of Na^+ (160 mM) to the membrane fraction revealed a second site with $K_D = 21.6$ μM and $B_{max} = 175$ pmol/mg protein. The sensitivity of the sites to a range of putative agonists and antagonists of glutamate was investigated and the results were suggestive of a receptor-like function for the higher affinity Na^+-independent site whereas the Na^+-dependent site showed some characteristics of an uptake system.

It has unfortunately proved very difficult to carry out these binding experiments in a consistently reproducible manner and we have more recently adopted a rapid filter assay based on the unlabelled ligand excess procedure (64). Under these conditions a single class of glutamate-specific binding sites is seen but the affinity is lower than in the earlier studies having a value for $K_D = 30 \, \mu M$ and $B_{max} = 52 \, pmol/mg$ protein. We have noticed that the glutamate binding characteristics of the membrane fractions change on storage and after four days at $-20 \, ^\circ C$, B_{max} is reduced by about 50%. The factors responsible for this loss of binding sites have not been identified but it is worth recalling the findings of Roberts and co-workers who find that the cerebellar binding site is also sensitive to freezing (30). Using a similar assay procedure Cleworth et al. (64) have reported the presence of two glutamate binding sites on membranous fractions from the femoral muscle of the locust (Schistocerca gregaria). No data were given that would allow an assessment of either K_D or B_{max} but the Na^+ dependency of the sites was examined. One site was rapidly saturable (with respect to glutamate binding) in the absence of Na^+ whereas in the presence of Na^+ glutamate binding increased linearly for up to 1 hour. The authors suggest that the saturable, Na^+-independent binding reflects the presence of synaptic receptors and that the Na^+-dependent component indicates uptake of glutamate into the vesiculated membrane fraction.

In our laboratory the filter assay, although an improvement on the method used in earlier studies (62) still gives very variable results and we do not consider it suitable for a detailed examination of the pharmacology of the glutamate binding sites.

In an attempt to circumvent the shortcomings of the filter assay we have recently investigated the use of rapid ultracentrifugation as a means of separating free from bound ligand (17). We found that the conditions employed for measuring binding to mammalian brain membranes (30) are not suitable for insect muscle membranes as the g force is insufficient to pellet the membrane fractions. We have therefore used an air-turbine micro centrifuge, the Beckman Airfuge. With this instrument the membrane fractions from locust muscle can be centrifuged to a tightly packed pellet in about 1 min.

Preliminary experiments with this system suggest the presence of four possible binding sites. Two of the sites show some properties expected for an uptake process with K_D values of $25 \, \mu M$ and $1 \, mM$. The other sites are of higher affinity and have some receptor-like properties, one has a $K_D = 1.3 \, \mu M$ and $B_{max} = 10.9 \, pmol/mg$ protein and may correspond to the higher affinity site ($K_D = 0.53 \, \mu M$; $B_{max} = 25 \, pmol/mg$ protein) seen in our earlier studies (62). The second high affinity site has a $K_D = 12.5 \, nM$ and $B_{max} = 0.57 \, pmol/mg$ protein, this site shows a much higher affinity than any binding site that we have previously observed in insect muscle preparations. It is emphasised that these are preliminary studies and that the binding sites have not yet been extensively characterised. It is interesting to note however that there is very good electrophysiological evidence for the presence of at least two classes of glutamate receptors on locust muscle (65, 66, 67) one might anticipate therefore that as the sensitivity of the binding assays improves two separate binding sites would be seen.

Conclusions

It is clear that there are specific high affinity binding sites for glutamate on membranes from mammalian brain and from insect muscle. It is not however possible to unequivocally identify any of the sites as a physiological synaptic receptor. Certainly in the case of the brain binding sites their behaviour is consistent with such an identity but for the insect muscle sites the evidence is still rather tenuous. Confirmation of the receptor status of the binding sites can only come from extensive study of their pharmacological characteristics. Thus the binding affinities of agonists and antagonists must correlate with the potency of those compounds in a physiological assay system in which overall receptor function is measured. It is in this area that the major problems occur because our knowledge of the pharmacology of the glutamate system is meagre compared with that of many other neurotransmitter systems. Our understanding of glutamate pharmacology is however progressing rapidly and a number of compounds are now available that are sufficiently potent for them to be useful tools in the binding studies.

Krogsgaard-Larsen and co-workers have described a new class of glutamate agonists that are

354

structurally related to ibotenic acid (68, 69, 70). The compounds are potent excitants of cat spinal neurones when administered iontophoretically (68). The rank order of potency is however not paralleled when the compounds are used as competitors in the assay of glutamate binding to rat cerebellar membranes (70). The authors provide evidence to discount the possibility that the differences reflect different receptors in the rat and the cat. We must therefore conclude that these compounds discriminate between excitatory receptors in vivo and glutamate binding sites in vitro, clearly further detailed studies may clarify the status of the cerebellar binding sites. No examination of the effects of the compounds on the insect binding sites have been reported.

The phosphonic acid analogues are a group of compounds that is also proving useful in defining more precisely the nature of glutamate binding sites. In a combined electrophysiological and binding study the compound 2-amino-4-phosphonobutyric acid (2-APB) was shown to be an antagonist of glutamate at the locust neuromuscular junction (71). Further work showed that 2-APB was not an effective inhibitor of glutamate binding to the Na^+-dependent site on locust muscle membranes (62) suggesting that the compound may discriminate between receptor and uptake sites. In mammalian brain some equivocal findings have been reported. Bioulac et al. (72) reported experiments on cerebral and cerebellar neurones in the rat in which 2-APB elicited a response equivalent to that seen with glutamate. Watkins et al. (73) however reported that iontophoretic application of 2-APB to cat spinal neurones failed to reduce excitation by glutamate. Foster and Roberts (28) reported that 2-APB inhibited the Na^+-independent binding of glutamate to the rat cerebellar site whereas earlier studies from Balcar and Johnston (27) showed that the compound was without effect on high-affinity uptake of glutamate into rat brain slices. Thus as in the insect muscle system the phosphonate appears to discriminate between putative receptor sites and uptake systems. However, it should be noted that Vincent and McGeer (40) have reported that 2-APB inhibits glutamate uptake in rat striatal synaptosomes.

The next higher homologue to 2-APB, 2 amino 4-phosphono valeric acid (2-APV) holds promise as an additional discriminatory ligand for glutamate binding sites. In what is a predominantly electrophysiological approach, Watkins and collaborators have been able to classify excitatory amino acid receptors in amphibian and mammalian central nervous system on the basis of their reponses to particular agonists (74). Thus a group of receptors has been classified as NMDA receptors on the basis of their response to N-Methyl-D-aspartate (NMDA); a separate receptor class is activated by quisqualic acid, the action of which is antagonised by glutamic acid diethyl ester (GDEE). The natural transmitter that acts at NMDE receptors is not yet known but aspartate is a strong candidate whereas glutamate is the likely transmitter at the quisqualate-sensitive receptor sites. The NMDA receptor is particularly sensitive to 2-APV whereas GDEE is almost without effect on this site. It seems likely that in binding studies both NMDE receptors and quisqualate-sensitive receptors may bind glutamate (75). Preliminary binding studies with rat cerebellar membranes revealed high affinity NMDA binding sites (76) but their relationship to glutamate binding sites known to be present also on such membranes is not clear. Binding studies using 2-APV may well help to resolve these questions. So far there are no reports of the actions of 2-APV on the insect muscle binding sites.

One can anticipate rapid developments in our understanding of relationships between the synaptic glutamate receptors and the glutamate binding sites in both mammalian brain and in insect muscle as a result of the impetus given by these new pharmacological agents. However, useful as the ibotenate analogues and the phosphonates are in characterising putative glutamate receptor sites they have limited application in the isolation and purification of the receptor protein. The successful isolation and complete purification of the nicotinic acetylcholine receptor has been critically dependent on the use of natural toxins which show highly specific, almost irreversible, binding to the acetylcholine binding site of the receptor protein (18, 19). One of these toxins, α bungarotoxin shows such specificity for this site that it has become the major diagnostic ligand for nicotinic cholinergic receptor sites in a variety of tissues. Unfortunately we have not yet discovered any natural toxin that provides such a tool with which to explore the glutamate receptor. It is well established however that there are venoms, particularly those of the braconid and sphecid wasps that contain toxins whose site of action is the insect neuromuscular junction (77, 78, 79). Further examination of such venoms may well provide the necessary tools with which to isolate and fully characterise glutamate receptors from both vertebrates and invertebrates.

References

1. Hayashi, T., 1953. Keio J. Med. 3: 183–192.
2. Krnjevic, K. & Phillis, J. W., 1963. J. Physiol. (London) 165: 274–304.
3. Curtis, D. R., 1979. Glutamic acid: Advances in Biochemistry and Physiology (Filer, L. J., Garatini, S., Kare, M. R., Reynolds, W. A. & Wurtman, R. J., eds.) pp. 163–175, Raven Press, New York.
4. Usherwood, P. N. R., 1978. Adv. Comp. Physiol. Biochem. 7: 227–309.
5. Divac, I., Fonnum, F. & Storm-Mathisen, J., 1977. Nature, 266: 377–378.
6. McGeer, E. G. & McGeer, P. L., 1976. Nature, 263: 517–519.
7. Hudson, D. B., Valcana, T., Bean, G. & Timiras, P. S., 1976. Neurochem. Res. 1: 83–92.
8. Storm-Mathisen, J., 1977. Prog. Neurobiol. 8: 119–181.
9. Kerkut, G. A., Shapira, A. & Walker, R. J., 1965. Comp. Biochem. Physiol. 16: 37–48.
10. Usherwood, P. N. R. & Machili, P., 1966. Nature 210: 633–636.
11. Usherwood, P. N. R. & Machili, P., 1968. J. Exp. Biol. 49: 341–361.
12. Beranek, R. & Miller, P. L., 1968. J. Exp. Biol. 49: 83–93.
13. Anwyl, R. & Usherwood, P. N. R., 1976. J. Physiol. (London) 254: 46–47.
14. Anderson, C. R., Cull-Candy, S. G. & Miledi, R., 1976. Nature, 261: 151–153.
15. Usherwood, P. N. R. (ed.), 1975. Insect Muscle, Academic Press, London.
16. Lunt, G. G., 1975. Insect Biochemistry and Function (Candy, D. J. & Kilby, B. A. eds.) pp. 285–306, Chapman and Hall, London.
17. Filbin, M., Lunt, G. G. & Donnellan, J. F., 1980. Receptors for Neurotransmitters Hormones and Pheromones in Insects (Sattelle, D. B., Hall, L. M. & Hildebrand, J. G., eds.) pp. 153–160, Elsevier/North Holland, Amsterdam.
18. Heidmann, T., & Changeux, J.-P., 1978. Annu. Rev. Biochem. 47: 317–357.
19. Barnard, E. A., Dolly, J. O., Lang, B., Lo, M. & Shorr, R. G., 1979. Adv. Cytopharmacol. 3: 409–435.
20. Yamamura, H. I., Enna, S. J. & Kuhar, M. J. (eds.), 1978. Neurotransmitter Receptor Binding, Raven Press, New York.
21. Cuatrecasas, P. & Hollenburg, M. D., 1975. Biochem. Biophys. Res. Commun. 62: 31–41.
22. Bennett, J. P., 1978. Neurotransmitter Receptor Binding (Yamamura, H. L., Enna, S. J. & Kuhar, M. J., eds.) pp. 57–90, Raven Press, New York.
23. Roberts, P. J., 1974. Nature, 252: 399–401.
24. Michaelis, E. K., Michaelis, M. L. & Boyarsky, L. L., 1974. Biochim. Biophys. Acta, 367: 338–348.
25. Bogdanski, D. F., Tassari, A. H. & Brodie, B. B., 1970. Biochim. Biophys. Acta, 219: 189–199.
26. Logan, W. J. & Snyder, S. H., 1971. Nature, 234: 297–299.
27. Balcar, V. J. & Johnson, G. A. R., 1972. J. Neurochem. 19: 2657–2666.
28. Foster, A. C. & Roberts, P. J., 1978. J. Neurochem. 31: 1467–1477.
29. Simon, J. R., Contrera, J. F. & Kuhar, M. J., 1976. J. Neurochem. 26: 141–147.
30. Sharif, N. A. & Roberts, P. J., 1980. J. Neurochem. 34: 779–784.
31. Roberts, P. J., 1981. Glutamate: Transmitter in the central Nervous System (Roberts, P. J., Storm-Mathisen, J. & Johnston, G. A. R., eds.) pp. 35–54. John Wiley and Sons, London.
32. Michaelis, E. K., Grubbs, R. D., Belieu, R. M. & Michaelis, M. L., 1981. Proc. Nat. Acad. Sci. U.S.A.
33. Sharif, N. A. & Roberts, P. J., 1980. Brain Res. 194: 594–597.
34. Baudry, M. & Lynch, G., 1979. Eur. J. Pharmacol. 57: 283–285.
35. Baudry, M. & Lynch, G., 1981. J. Neurochem. 26: 811–820.
36. Baudry, M. & Lynch, G., 1980. Proc. Natl. Acad. Sci. USA 77: 2298–2304.
37. Baudry, M., Oliver, M., Creager, R., Weirasko, A. & Lynch, G., 1980. Life Sci. 27: 325–330.
38. Baudry, M. & Lynch, G., 1979. Nature, 232: 748–750.
39. Biziere, K., Thompson, H. & Coyle, J. T., 1980. Brain Res. 183: 421–433.
40. Vincent, S. R. & McGeer, E. G., 1980. Brain Res. 184: 99–108.
41. Head, R. A., Tunnicliff, G., Matheson, G. K., 1980. Can. J. Biochem. 58: 534–538.
42. Sanderson, C. & Murphy, S., 1980. Dev. Neurosci, 9: 233–234.
43. De Barry, J., Vincendon, G. & Gombos, G., 1980. FEBS Letts. 109: 175–179.
44. Michaelis, E. K., 1975. Biochem. Biophys. Res. Comm. 65: 1004–1012.
45. Lindstrom, J., Anholt, R., Einarson, B., Engel, A., Osame, M. & Montal, M., 1980. J. Biol. Chem. 255: 8340–8350.
40. Wu, W. C. S. & Raftery, M. A., 1981. Biochemistry, 20: 694–701.
47. Grubbs, R. D. & Michaelis, E. K., 1979. Soc. Neurosci. Abst. 5: 304.
48. Kuznetsov, V. I. & Mogilyanskii, D. N., 1975. Stud. Biophys. 49: 61–66.
49. Kolomytkin, O. V., Kuznetsov, V. I. & Ermishkin, L. N., 1979. Deposited Doc. VINITI 1672–1679.
50. Kolomytkin, O. V., Kuznetsov, V. I. & Akoev, I. G., 1979. Zh. Biol. Khim. 1979 Abstr. 5F 46.
51. De Robertis, E., 1975. Synaptic Receptors, Marcel Dekker, New York.
52. Levinson, S. R. & Keynes, R. D., 1972. Biochim. Biophys. Acta. 288: 241–247.
53. Donnellan, J. F., Jewess, P. J. & Cattell, K. J., 1975. J. Neurochem. 25: 623–629.
54. Taylor, R. F., 1978. J. Neurochem, 31: 1183–1198.

55. De Robertis, E. & Fiszer de Plazas, S., 1976. J. Neurochem. 26: 1237–1243.
56. Lunt, G. G., 1973. Comp. Gen. Pharmacol. 4: 75–79.
57. James, R. W., Lunt, G. G. & Donnellan, J. F., 1977. Insect Biochem. 7: 247–255.
58. James, R. W., Lunt, G. G. & Donnellan, J. F., 1974. Abst. Commun. 9th Mtg. Fed. Europ. Biochem. Soc. Hungary. p. 258.
59. Fiszer de Plazas, S., De Robertis, E. & Lunt, G. G., 1977. .Gen. Pharmac. 8: 133–137.
60. Fiszer de Plazas, S. & De Robertis, E., 1973. FEBS Letts. 33: 45–48.
61. Fiszer de Plazas, S. & De Robertis, E., 1974. J. Neurochem. 23: 1115–1120.
62. James, R. W., Lunt, G. G. & Donnellan, J. F., 1977. Biochem. Soc. Trans. 5: 170–172.
63. Briley, P. A., Filbin, M. T., Lunt, G. G. & Donnellan, J. F., 1980. In Insect Neurobiology and Pesticide Action, pp. 177–184, Soc. Chem. Industry, London.
64. Cleworth, J. F., Robinson, N. L. & Usherwood, P. N. R., 1980. In Insect Neurobiology and Pesticide Action pp. 280–281, Soc. Chem. Industry, London.
65. Cull-Candy, S. G. & Usherwood, P. N. R., 1973. Nature, 246: 62–64.
66. Cull-Candy, S. G. & Usherwood, P. N. R., 1976. J. Physiol. (London) 255: 449–464.
67. Cull-Candy, S. G. & Usherwood, P. N. R., 1974. Neuropharmacol 13: 455–461.
68. Krogsgaard-Larsen, P., Honore, T., Hansen, J. J., Curtis, D. R. & Lodge, D., 1980. Nature, 284: 64–66.
69. Krogsgaard-Larsen, P., Honore, T., Hansen, J. J., Curtis, D. R. & Lodge, D., 1981. In Glutamate as a Neurotransmitter (Di Chiara, G. & Gessa, G. L., eds.) pp. 285–294, Raven Press, New York.
70. Honore, T., Lauridsen, J. & Krogsgaard-Larsen, P., 1981. J. Neurochem. 36: 1302–1304.
71. Cull-Candy, S. G., Donnellan, J. F., James, R. W. & Lunt, G. G., 1976. 262: 408–409.
72. Bioulac, B., De Tinguy-Moreaud, E., Vincent, J.-D. & Neuzil, E., 1979. Gen. Pharmacol. 10: 121–125.
73. Watkins, J. C., Curtis, D. R. & Brand, S. S., 1977. J. Pharm. Pharmacol. 29: 324.
74. Davies, J., Evans, R. H., Francis, A. A., Jones, A. W. & Watkins, J. C., 1980. In Neurotransmitters and their Receptors (Littauer, U. Z., Dudai, Y., Silman, I., Teichberg, V. I. & Vogel, Z., eds.) pp. 333–347, John Wiley and Sons Ltd., London.
75. Johnston, G. A. R., 1979. In Glutamic Acid: Advances in Biochemistry and Physiology (Filer, L. J., et al., eds.) pp. 177–185, Raven Press, New York.
76. Snodgrass, S. R., 1979. Soc. Neurosci. Abst. 5: 572.
77. Walther, C., 1980. In Insect Neurobiology and Pesticide Action, pp. 153–160, Soc. Chem. Industry, London.
78. May, T. E. & Piek, T., 1979. J. Insect. Physiol. 25: 685–691.
79. Peik, T., Mantel, P. & Jas, 1980. J. Insect Physiol. 26: 345–349.

Received June 4, 1981.

γ-Glutamyl transpeptidase: catalytic, structural and functional aspects

Suresh S. Tate and Alton Meister

Dept. of Biochemistry Cornell University Medical College, 1300 York Avenue, New York, NY 10021 U.S.A.

Summary

γ-Glutamyl transpeptidase catalyzes transfer of the γ-glutamyl moiety of glutathione to amino acids, dipeptides, and to glutathione itself; the enzyme also catalyzes the hydrolysis of glutathione to glutamate and cysteinyl-glycine. This review deals with the tissue distribution and localization of the enzyme in mammals, the catalytic properties of the enzyme (including its inhibition by reversible and irreversible inhibitors), structural studies on the enzyme, and new findings about its physiological function.

Introduction

γ-Glutamyl transpeptidase catalyzes the initial step in the utilization of glutathione in which the γ-glutamyl moiety of this tripeptide is transferred to an acceptor, which may be an amino acid, dipeptide, or glutathione itself. If the nucleophile is water, hydrolysis occurs. These three general types of reactions are illustrated in reactions [1] – [3].

Transpeptidation:

Glutathione + L-amino acid ⇌ L-γ-glu-L-amino acid + L-Cys-Gly [1]

Autotranspeptidation:

2 Glutathione ⇌ L-γ-glu-glutathione + L-Cys-Gly [2]

Hydrolysis:

Glutathione + H_2O → L-glutamate + L-Cys-Gly [3]

The reaction catalyzed by γ-glutamyltranspeptidase is of major importance in the γ-glutamyl cycle, a metabolic pathway that accounts for the enzymatic synthesis and degradation of glutathione (1, 2). The evidence that the reactions of the γ-glutamyl cycle take place in vivo and related investigations on the metabolism and function of glutathione have been reviewed (1–3). The activity of γ-glutamyl transpeptidase was first observed about 70 years ago (3, 4), and the enzyme has subsequently been studied by many investigators. The development of this area of research has been reviewed (3, 5–7). Recent work has led to the isolation of highly purified preparations of the enzyme, especially from mammalian kidney, and to elucidation of various aspects of the structure, mechanism of action, and function of this interesting enzyme. This chapter deals principally with relatively recent findings on mammalian γ-glutamyl transpeptidases; the most extensively studied enzyme is that isolated from rat kidney.

Tissue distribution and localization

When homogenates of animal tissues are assayed for γ-glutamyl transpeptidase activity, a wide range of values is found. The finding that homogenates of certain tissues exhibit low transpeptidase activity may be misleading since studies on the localization of the enzyme indicate that there are specific regions of intense enzyme activity in many tissues (see below). In most mammals, the kidney exhibits by far the highest activity. The relative activities

Molecular and Cellular Biochemistry 39, 357–368 (1981).   0300-8177/81/0391-0357/$02.40.

found in rat tissues is as follows: kidney, 100; pancreas, 20; epididymis (caput), 27; epididymis (cauda), 4; seminal vesicle, 4; jejunal crypt cells, 0.8; jejunal villus tip cells, 3.3; liver, 0.2; spleen cells, 0.2 (6). The enzyme activity has also been demonstrated in bile, seminal fluid, blood serum, and urine. It is important to note that there are significant species differences; thus, little if any γ-glutamyl transpeptidase activity is found in the blood serum of rats and mice, but the enzyme is detectable in human serum, where its elevation may be of clinical importance in the detection of liver disease (8, 9).

A gradient of transpeptidase activity has been found in the jejunum, with relatively low activity in the crypt cells and much higher activity in the differentiated villus tip cells (10). Microdissection studies of rat nephron indicate that the proximal straight tubule exhibits about twice as much transpeptidase activity than does the proximal convoluted tubule (11). The activity found in both of these regions of the nephron is nevertheless significantly higher than found in other rat tissues. Both spleen cells and peripheral blood lymphocytes have been shown to exhibit transpeptidase activity which increases several fold in response to certain mitogenic agents (12).

After introduction of histochemical methods for the localization of transpeptidase activity in tissue slices (13, 14), much effort has been directed towards localization of this enzyme in a variety of tissues and cells. Precise localization of transpeptidase is of interest in view of its proposed roles in transport and detoxification processes as well as its usefulness as an oncofetal marker. Histochemical studies indicate that, in general, high enzyme activity is seen in cells which exhibit prolific secretory or absorptive functions; these include the epithelial cells of renal proximal tubules, jejunum, bile duct, epididymis, seminal vesicles, choroid plexus, ciliary body, retinal pigment epithelium, bronchioles, and thyroid follicles; the canalicular regions of heptocytes; and the pancreatic acinar and ductile epithelial cells (5, 6). Early investigations showed that transpeptidase is associated with the particulate fraction of various tissue homogenates and these led to the inference that the enzyme is located either in cell plasma membranes or in microsomal membranes. In epithelial cells, such as those of the jejunum and renal proximal

tubule, which are characterized by the presence of numerous finger-like specializations of the plasma membrane (microvilli) on their lumenal surface (such cell surface is known as the brush border), the histochemical staining is consistent with location of the enzyme in or near the brush border. Subsequent subcellular fractionation studies, which yield membrane fractions enriched in microvilli are in accord with this conclusion (see (6) for references to the literature).

Ultrastructural studies utilizing a cytochemical technique have provided direct evidence that the major portion of the transpeptidase activity is associated with the microvillus membranes in the jejunum and kidney proximal tubules (15). No activity was seen on the basal-lateral membranes of these epithelial cells although low levels cannot be excluded because of the low sensitivity of this technique. Similarly, the poorly differentiated microvilli of the jejunal crypt cells exhibit little or no activity. Longer incubation of the tissue in the cytochemical medium reveals activity on the membranes of the endoplasmic reticulum and the Golgi. Since γ-glutamyl transpeptidase is a glycoprotein, the activity associated with the intracellular membranes may represent intermediates in its post-translational processing en route to its final destination in the plasma membranes. Recent studies demonstrate that in the rat epididymis, the transpeptidase activity is located in the membranes of the stereocilia, which are structurally analogous to the microvilli in other tissues (Kozak and Tate, unpublished). Evidence has also been obtained for plasma membrane localization of the enzyme in lymphoid cells (16). Furthermore, a combination of experiments involving solubilization of the enzyme with proteinases, use of impermeable substrates, immunocytochemical techniques utilizing antibodies conjugated to ferritin, and indirect immuno-precipitation using Fab antibodies, are in accord with location of transpeptidase on the outer surface of microvillus membranes and of lymphoid cell plasma membranes (15–18).

Catalytic properties

Mammalian γ-glutamyl transpeptidases exhibit rather similar catalytic properties and specificity. Thus, all of the enzymes thus far studied show a broad optical and steric specificity towards γ-glutamyl compounds; glutathione, a large number of its S-derivatives, and other γ-substituted glutamyl derivatives serve effectively as donor substrates (1, 6). The substrate most widely used in biochemical and clinical studies is L-γ-glutamyl-p-nitroanilide (19). Convenient spectrophotometric methods based on S-derivatives of glutathione are also available (20, 21). The fluorogenic substrate, L-γ-glutamyl-7-amino-4-methyl-coumarin, seems to provide a highly sensitive assay procedure (22).

Three separate subsites exhibiting characteristic preferences can be distinguished in the active center. Binding of L-γ-glutamyl, D-γ-glutamyl, and L-γ-(α-methyl)glutamyl compounds occurs at the γ-glutamyl binding subsite (23). The acceptor site, consisting of subsites for cysteinyl and glycine moieties, on the other hand, has restricted stereospecificity in that only L-amino acids and dipeptides in which both amino acids are of L-configuration serve as acceptors (20, 24). Kinetic and specificity studies indicate that the large variety of dipeptide acceptors bind to the Cys-Gly site and that amino acid acceptors interact with the cysteinyl subsite. The cysteinyl subsite prefers neutral amino acids such as the L-isomers of cystine, glutamine, methionine, alanine, and serine. Branched chain amino acids are relatively poor acceptors, whereas D-amino acids, L-proline, and α-substituted amino acids are inactive. The glycine subsite shown preference for glycine; other amino acid substitutions reduce the acceptor activity considerably. Thus, the best dipeptide acceptors include Gly-Gly, L-Met-Gly, L-Gln-Gly, L-Ala-Gly, L-Ser-Gly, etc. As indicated in reactions [1]–[3], the enzyme can degrade γ-glutamyl compounds by transpeptidation and hydrolysis. With L-γ-glutamyl compounds all three reactions occur in absence of an added acceptor. Separate determination of the hydrolytic and transpeptidase activities may be conveniently carried out with D-γ-glutamyl compounds (e.g., D-γ-glutamyl-p-nitroanilide (24, 25)) since the D-isomers do not serve as acceptors; such studies have been valuable in probing the mechanism of differential modulation of these two activities (see below). The hydrolytic reaction exhibits a broad optimum between pH 6 and 8, whereas optimum transpeptidation is seen between pH 8 and 9 (26–28). Thus, pH as well as the presence and concentration of an acceptor influence the relative rates of utilization of a γ-glutamyl substrate by hydrolysis and transpeptidation. The V_{max} for hydrolysis of glutathione in the absence of an added acceptor is about 10% of that for transpeptidation in presence of saturating concentrations (20 mM) of either L-methionine or L-alanine (6, 12). In the presence of 50 μM glutathione (a value approximating the normal plasma level of glutathione in the rat and mouse) and an amino acid mixture that closely approximates the amino acid composition of blood plasma, about 50% of the glutathione utilized participates in transpeptidation (29).

Kinetic studies are consistent with a ping-pong mechanism involving a γ-glutamyl-enzyme intermediate (20, 24):

Glutathione + enzyme ⇌ γ-glu-enzyme + Cys-Gly [4]

γ-Glu-enzyme + acceptor ⇌ γ-glu-acceptor + enzyme [5]

An activated γ-glutamyl intermediate is consistent with the observation that the enzyme catalyzes γ-glutamyl transfer to hydroxylamine (27, 30). The possibility that a covalent γ-glutamyl-enzyme intermediate is formed in the course of the transfer reactions receives strong support from the findings that the γ-glutamyl analogs, 6-diazo-5-oxo-L-norleucine (DON) and O-diazoacetyl-L-serine (L-azaserine) inactivate the enzyme by attaching covalently and stoichiometrically to the γ-glutamyl site (31, 32). Studies with DON-labeled enzyme indicate that the covalent attachment of the analog involves an O-ether linkage to a hydroxyl group located in the γ-glutamyl binding subsite (33). These results have led to the inference that an enzyme hydroxyl group also participates in the formation of the covalent γ-glutamyl-enzyme intermediate (Fig. 1).

Another aspect of the catalytic potential of the γ-glutamyl site was revealed during studies on the reversible dissociation of the enzyme. As discussed below, mammalian transpeptidases are dimeric enzymes consisting of a light subunit (M_r about 22 000) and a heavy subunit (M_r ranging between 46 000 and 65 000, depending upon the species). The γ-glutamyl binding site (as indicated by studies with the affinity labels DON and azaserine) is located on the light subunit. Treatment of the rat kidney enzyme (as well as other mammalian kidney transpeptidases) with dissociating agents such as

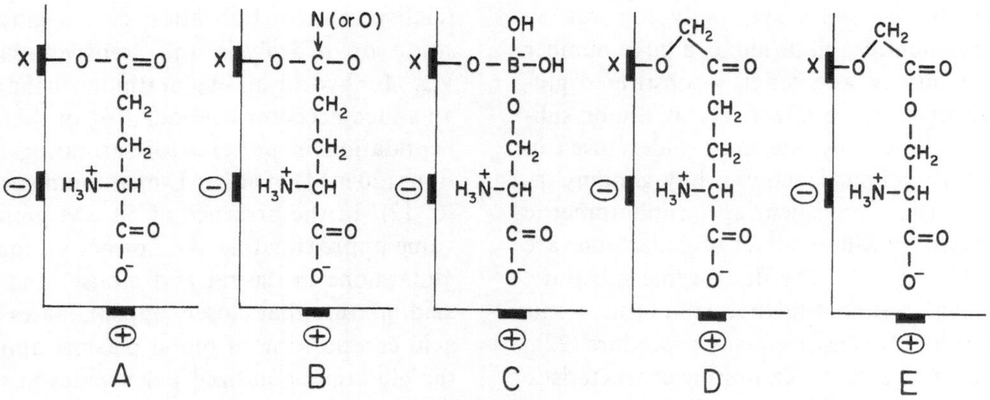

Fig. 1. Schematic representation of the active center of γ-glutamyl transpeptidase depicting the γ-glutamyl-enzyme intermediate (A), the expected tetrahedral transition state intermediate that would be formed during the transfer of the enzymebound γ-glutamyl moiety to the α-amino group of acceptor, or to water (B), the proposed enzyme-L-serine-borate complex (C), and the covalent derivatives obtained by treatment of the enzyme with the γ-glutamyl analogs 6-diazo-5-oxo-L-norleucine (D) and L-azaserine (E). The amino acid residue at the active center appears to be either a seryl or a threonyl residue (from 33).

urea and SDS at neutral pH values results inextensive proteolytic degradation of the heavy subunit (34). The proteinase activity, which is not evident with the native dimeric enzyme appears to be a catalytic function associated with the light subunit and involves the active center hydroxyl group at which γ-glutamylation of the enzyme also occurs during γ-glutamyl transfer reactions. Although the possible physiological significance of the proteinase activity remains to be elucidated, it should be noted that the hydrolysis and transfer reactions catalyzed by transpeptidase are analogous to those catalyzed by peptidases and proteinases of the serine and cysteine class, which also involve and acyl enzyme intermediate. It is interesting to note that several other polymeric proteins also contain subunits which exhibit proteinase activity upon separation from the native oligomer (35).

A significant activity which may be of physiological importance that is associated with γ-glutamyl transpeptidase has been illuminated by the recent finding that incubation of glutathione with the enzyme results in its rapid oxidation to glutathione disulfide (36–38). This apparent 'glutathione oxidase' activity of the enzyme has been ascribed to the transpeptidase-catalyzed production of cysteinyl-glycine. This dipeptide oxidizes rapidly and non-enzymatically to form cystinyl-*bis*-glycine. The oxidation of glutathione takes place by nonenzymatic transhydrogenation between glutathione and cystinyl-*bis*-glycine and between glu-

tathione and the mixed disulfide of Cys-Gly and glutathione (38) (Fig. 2). Other thiols such as cysteine can participate in similar nonenzymatic transhydrogenation reactions. Compounds such as cysteinyl-glycine and cysteine are rapidly converted to the respective disulfides in the presence of oxygen; glutathione, in contrast, reacts rather sluggishly with oxygen. Transpeptidase-mediated oxidation of glutathione may be significant in the extracellular metabolism of glutathione (37–40). Other sulfhydryl oxidases capable of oxidizing glutathione have been isolated. Thus, an iron-containing enzyme has been isolated from bovine milk membranes (41) and a flavoprotein has been

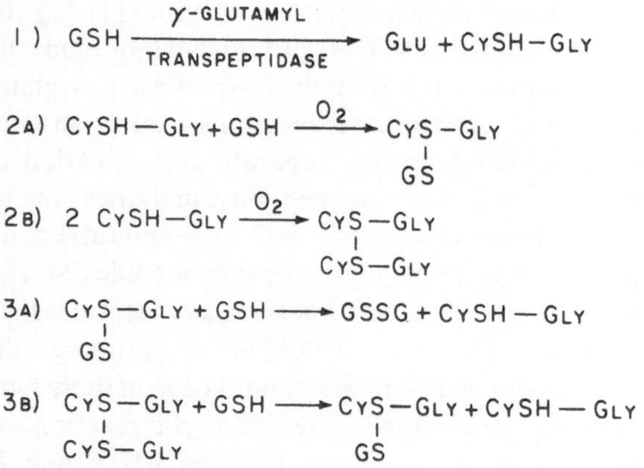

Fig. 2. Mechanism of γ-glutamyl transpeptidase-mediated conversion of glutathione (GSH) to glutathione disulfide (GSSG) (from 38).

purified from rat seminal vesicle secretion (42). Glutathione peroxidase, a widely distributed cytosolic enzyme, also catalyzes the oxidation of glutathione disulfide in the presence of H_2O_2 (43).

Inhibition

Both reversible and irreversible inhibitors of γ-glutamyl transpeptidase have been described and these have been used in studies on the function of the enzyme.

Reversible inhibitors

Revel and Ball made the interesting observation that L-serine in the presence of borate strongly inhibits transpeptidase (44), and later work showed that this combination inhibits transpeptidases from a variety of sources. Indeed, inhibition by L-serine plus borate is a valuable test for the enzyme. The serine-borate combination is particularly useful since its specificity can be tested by separately omitting either serine or borate; neither compound alone inhibits the enzyme. D-serine is also an effective inhibitor in the presence of borate. Studies on the mechanism of this inhibition indicate that serine and borate interact with the γ-glutamyl binding site. Thus, serine appears to occupy the active site region that accepts the α-amino and α-carboxyl groups of glutathione, and the borate anion forms a bridge-complex between the hydroxyl group of serine and an active site hydroxyl group (33). The tetrahedral borate complex thus serves as a transition-state analog (Fig. 1). The K_i values for L- and D-serine measured in the presence of 10 mM borate are, respectively, 20 and 170 μM (33).

γ-Glutamylhydrazones of α-keto acids are competitive inhibitors with respect to the γ-glutamyl donor; the K_i values for the γ-glutamylhydrazones of pyruvate and α-ketoglutarate are, about 400 μM (20). Particularly potent inhibitors are the γ-glutamylphenylhydrazides. L-γ-Glutamyl-(o-carboxy)-phenylhydrazide (L-OC) was isolated from the culture medium of a strain of *Penicillium oxalicum* and shown to be a strong competitive inhibitor with respect to the γ-glutamyl substrate ($K_i = 6 \mu$M) (45, 46). In an independent study, a number of γ-glutamyl-phenylhydrazide derivatives were synthesized and shown to inhibit transpep-

tidase (47). The most potent of these are the L- and D-isomers of γ-glutamyl (o-carboxy)phenylhydrazide (K_i values 8 and 23 μM, respectively). Interestingly, L-γ-glutamyl-(p-carboxy)phenylhydrazide is much less effective ($K_i = 800 \mu$M). L- and D-γ-glutamyl-(o-carboxy)phenylhydrazide have been used in in vivo studies. The phenylhydrazine derivatives, however, exhibit toxicity probably due to slow release of o-carboxypenylhydrazine, a potent convulsant. Other compounds that inhibit γ-glutamyl transpeptidase include sulfophthalein derivatives such as sulfobromophthalein and bromocresol green (48). The mechanism of inhibition by these compounds is not yet clear.

The dicarboxylic acid, maleate, exerts an unusual effect on transpeptidase (27, 49, 50). It reversibly stimulates the hydrolysis of glutathione and other γ-glutamyl compounds, but inhibits the formation of transpeptidation products. A large stimulatory effect is seen on the utilization of L-glutamine, which, is normally a relatively poor substrate that is converted to glutamate as well as to γ-glutamyl-glutamine. Maleate stimulates both these reactions but hydrolysis is increased to a greater extent relative to transpeptidation. These observations led to the finding that the so-called 'phosphate-independent glutaminase' of rat kidney is in fact a catalytic activity of γ-glutamyl transpeptidase (27, 49, 50). Maleate appears to bind to the Cys-Gly binding site of the enzyme accounting for the inhibition of the transfer of the γ-glutamyl moiety to acceptor amino acids and dipeptides (51). Recent studies have shown that hippurate (benzoylglycine), present in mammalian serum and urine, and several hippurate analogs affect transpeptidase in a manner similar to maleate and also appear to occupy the Cys-Gly site (52). Evidence has been obtained indicating that hippurate, commonly considered only as a detoxification product of benzoate, is formed in liver from benzoate originating from the degradative metabolism of phenylalanine (52). Normal concentrations of hippurate in serum are such that the activity of renal proximal tubule transpeptidase could be modulated by hippurate in the glomerular filtrate.

Irreversible inhibitors

Inactivation of transpeptidase by the glutamine antagonists, DON and L-azaserine, has been noted above. Recent studies have shown that the anti-tumor glutamine antagonist, L-(αS,5S)-α-amino-3-chloro-4,5-dihydro-5-isoxazole-acetic acid (AT-125), is also a very highly effective affinity label for the γ-glutamyl site of the enzyme (38, 53–55). Indeed, the rate of inactivation with AT-125 is about 20-fold greater than that seen with DON and the rates of inactivation by all three compounds are accelerated by maleate. In rat renal microvilli, transpeptidase appears to be the only protein labeled by AT-125 and this could serve as a useful in vitro experimental system to probe the function of the enzyme (56).

Phenylmethanesulfonyl fluoride (PMSF), a reagent that inactivates serine-type peptidases and proteinases, inactivates rat kidney transpeptidase slowly. The rate of inactivation is markedly accelerated by maleate (57). It seems likely that this reagent modifies the same active center hydroxyl group that is affinity-labeled by compounds such as DON and azaserine. Thus, the binding of PMSF and DON is mutually exclusive (Gardell and Tate, unpublished).

Both reversible and irreversible inhibitors of transpeptidase have been used in vivo to modulate glutathione metabolism. These studies have provided evidence that translocation out of the cell of intracellular glutathione is a normal and discrete step in the metabolism of glutathione via the γ-glutamyl cycle (7, 47, 54). Thus, inhibition of transpeptidase in animals prevents the normal extracellular breakdown of glutathione and, if the inhibition is extensive, glutathionuria results (Table 1). AT-125 is highly effective in this respect; its

administration to mice (2–5 mmol/kg) leads to massive glutathionuria in which the urinary concentration of glutathione is as high as 20–30 mM. The effectiveness of AT-125 is due to its very high affinity for the enzyme. All three glutamine antagonists, however, have the disadvantage of being non-specific; thus, they inhibit several glutamine amidotransferases and their high chemical reactivity might lead to nonspecific reaction with cellular nucleophiles. It is interesting to note that the competitive inhibitors, when administered to mice, also induce marked glutathionuria (Table 1).

Structural and topological studies

Since γ-glutamyl transpeptidase is bound to plasma membranes, the enzyme must be brought into a soluble form before attempting purification. Methods of solubilization that have been used include treatment of the particulate enzyme with detergents, organic solvents, and proteinases. The most highly purified preparations have been obtained from mammalian kidney. Table 2 summarizes some of the physical properties of proteinase-solubilized renal transpeptidases. Most of the work in our laboratory has been carried out with bromelain-solubilized rat kidney transpeptidase. Recently, a relatively rapid procedure in which papain is used for solubilization of the enzyme from renal microvilli has been developed (56). This method gives greater than 50% yields and the enzyme preparations obtained exhibit properties similar to those of the bromelain-solubilized enzyme. The method has also been used to purify the enzyme from rat jejunal and epididymal microvilli (Kozak and Tate, unpublished); these preparations exhibit properties that are similar to the kidney enzyme. The rat kidney enzyme has also been purified following solubilization with Triton X-100 (61). Both forms of the enzyme are composed of two non-identical glycopeptide subunits.

Purified rat kidney transpeptidase exhibits considerable heterogeneity on polyacrylamide gels and is separable by isoelectric focusing into twelve enzymatically active isozymes ranging in pI from 5 to 8 (58). The isoenzymes exhibit similar catalytic properties and their amino acid, hexose, and aminohexose compositions are similar; however, the sialic acid content varies from 14 to 61 nmol/mg of

Table 1.

Glutathionuria induced by inhibition of γ-glutamyl transpeptidase in mice	
Compound given (mmol kg^{-1})	Glutathionuria (mM)
None (control)	< 0.005
L-γ-Glu-(o-carboxy)phenylhydrazide (1.0)	3.6—5.6
D-γ-Glu-(o-carboxy)phenylhydrazide (2.5)	1.8–3.9
L-γ-Glu-(p-carboxy)phenylhydrazide (1.0)	0.09–1.5
6-Diazo-5-oxo-L-norleucine (DON) (2.0)	0.01–0.04
AT-125 (2.5)*	25–30

(From Griffith and Meister (47, 54))

* L-(αS, 5S)-α-amino-3-chloro-4,5-dihydro-isoxazoleacetic acid

protein. Neuraminidase treatment followed by iso-electric focusing indicates that the multiple forms are primarily due to different degrees of sialylation. Multiple forms, attributed to varying degrees of sialylation, have also been detected in adult, fetal, and regenerating rat liver (62), normal and neo-plastic rat mammary tissue (63), rat seminal vesicles and epididymis (64), and in purified human kidney enzyme (59).

The proteinase-solubilized rat kidney enzyme, $M_r = 68\,000$, consists of two subunits, $M_r = 46\,000$ and $22\,000$, respectively (58). As noted above, the light subunit contains the active site residue (an hydroxyl group), which is presumably involved in the formation of a covalent γ-glutamyl-enzyme intermediate (31, 33). Treatment of the enzyme with dissociating agents such as urea and SDS at neutral pH values results in extensive proteolytic degrada-tion of the large subunit due to unmasking of the proteinase activity of the light subunit (34). Intact subunits can, however, be isolated upon urea-treatment of the enzyme in 1 M acetic acid followed by gel filtration in the same medium (65). The denatured subunits are inactive and renaturation of individual subunits, by dialysis against pH 6.8 buffers containing no urea, does not restore ac-tivity. Mixing of the renatured subunits also fails to restore activity. The latter finding may be ascribed in part to the tendency of the denatured light subunit to form inactive polymers upon renatura-tion. Significant reconstitution of transpeptidase activity (up to 15% of the native enzyme) is achieved by prior mixing of denatured subunits followed by removal of urea by dialysis (65). The reconstituted active species can be further purified by gel filtra-tion; it has been shown to be similar to the native enzyme.

The proteinase-solubilized rat kidney transpep-tidase is soluble in aqueous solutions. In contrast, the Triton-solubilized enzyme is soluble only in presence of detergents, and can associate with unilamellar lecithin vesicles (61, 66). Treatment of the Triton-enzyme with papain yields a form which is identical in all respects to the papain-solubilized enzyme. The light subunits of papain- and Triton-solubilized enzymes exhibit identical molecular weights (61) and amino acid compositions (67). However, the heavy subunit of the latter is larger than that of the papain-enzyme by about 52 amino acid residues. The amino terminal residues of the

heavy and light subunits of the Triton-enzyme are methionine and threonine, respectively, whereas those of the papain-enzyme are glycine and threo-nine, respectively (67). On the basis of these data it has been suggested that the papain-sensitive amino terminal sequence of amino acids of the large subunit is responsible for association of transpep-tidase with the microvillus membranes (66, 67). The light subunit presumably does not interact directly with the lipid bilayer but is held by non-covalent interactions with the large subunit on the external surface of the membranes. A schematic model for the organization of the enzyme in the microvillus membranes is shown in Fig. 3. The exact mode of association of the enzyme with the microvillus membranes and conformation and extent of pene-

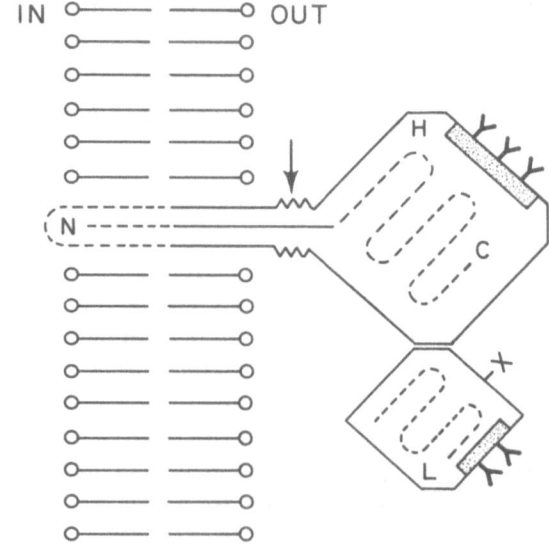

Fig. 3. Schematic representation of the topology of γ-glutamyl transpeptidase in microvillus membranes. H. and L, heavy and light subunits, respectively; X, active site hydroxyl group involved in γ-glutamyl-enzyme formation; shaded areas, glyco-sylated regions; the arrow indicates bonds cleaved by papain. Broken line near the amino terminal region of the anchor segment of H subunit indicates uncertainty regarding the extent of penetration of the anchor within the lipid bilayer. The bulk of the enzyme appears to be oriented towards the external (or lumenal) surface of microvilli. Similar membrane association has been proposed for other microvillus hydrolases (Kenny, A. G. & Booth, A. G., 1978. Essays in Biochem. 14: 1–44; Macnair, D. C. & Kenny, A. G., 1979. Biochem. J. 179: 379–395; Brunner, J., Hauser, H., Braun, H., Wilson, K. J., Wacker, H., O'Neill, B., and Semenza, G., 1979. J. Biol. Chem. 254: 1821–1828).

tration of the anchor requires further study.

Highly purified preparations of renal transpeptidase have also been obtained from other mammalian species (Table 2). These enzymes contain carbohydrate and are dimeric proteins. The light subunits have molecular weights of about 22 000. However, the enzymes fall into two groups with respect to the size of the heavy subunit: those with heavy subunits exhibiting M_r between 46–50 000 (rat and rabbit), and those with heavy subunits of M_r in excess of 60 000 (human, bovine, sheep, and hog). The γ-glutamyl binding site is located on the light subunit in all species tested. The mode of association of the enzyme with membranes, in species other than the rat, is not known.

Purified transpeptidase preparations have also been obtained from rat pancreas (68), jejunum and epididymis as noted above. These exhibit properties similar to those of the rat kidney enzyme. Apparently homogenous preparations have also been obtained from rat hepatomas (69) and human liver (70). Both proteins contain carbohydrate but their subunit structures are not yet known.

Function of γ-glutamyl transpeptidase

γ-Glutamyl transpeptidase catalyzes reactions in which there is transfer of the γ-glutamyl group of glutathione or of other γ-glutamyl compounds to acceptors (amino acids, dipeptides, glutathione), and hydrolysis of glutathione and other γ-glutamyl compounds (including glutamine) to yield glutamate. In both types of reactions, cysteinylglycine is formed, and this compound, which undergoes

rapid nonenzymatic oxidation, catalyzes the conversion of glutathione to glutathione disulfide ('glutathione oxidase'). Prior to the work of Hanes et al. (71, 72), who first showed that the enzyme can catalyze transpeptidation reactions, the enzyme was considered to be a glutathionase. Subsequently, largely because of studies stimulated by the γ-glutamyl cycle hypothesis, it has become apparent that transpeptidation is a physiologically significant function of the enzyme. According to this idea, γ-glutamyl transpeptidase catalyzes the formation of γ-glutamyl amino acids, which are translocated into the cell; free amino acids are released intracellularly. This hypothesis is consistent with the fact that γ-glutamyl transpeptidase is localized at anatomic sites at which there is substantial amino acid transport. There is evidence that the reactions of the γ-glutamyl cycle take place in vivo (1, 2), and that certain cells have a transport system for γ-glutamyl amino acids that is not shared by free amino acids (73).

A number of observations indicate the occurrence of in vivo transpeptidation; for example, γ-glutamyl amino acids are found in the urine (74, 75) and in various tissues (76–80). When isolated renal tubules were incubated with glutathione and glycine there was substantial formation of γ-glutamylglycine (81). Administration of glycylglycine (82) and of moderate doses of amino acids (83) to experimental animals leads to a marked decrease in the level of renal glutathione; this effect did not occur when the animals were also given an inhibitor of γ-glutamyl transpeptidase. Depletion of glutathione has also been observed in isolated renal cells suspended in media containing amino acids (84, 85), and in perfused kidneys when amino acids were present in the perfusate (84, 85); these effects were prevented by inhibition of transpeptidase.

It is notable that the V_{max} value for hydrolysis of glutathione in the absence of an added acceptor is about 10% of that for transpeptidation in the presence of saturating concentrations of amino acid acceptors (6). The rate of transpeptidation in the presence of 0.5 mM L-alanine and 50 μM L-methionine was found to be one-sixth of the rate of hydrolysis (28), and the K_m value for L-methionine was estimated to be 4.7 mM (86). Although these findings were considered as evidence for the conclusion that the sole function of the enzyme is to hydrolyze glutathione, such reasoning is not valid.

Tale 2. Proteinase-solubilized renal γglutamyl transpeptidases.

Source	M_r (X 10^{-3})	Subunit M_r[a] (X 10^{-3}) H	L	Carbohydrate	Reference
Rat	68	46	22	+	56, 58
Rabbit	71	48	23	+	34
Human	84	64	22	+	59
Bovine	83	63	20	+	34
Sheep	92	65	27	+	60
Hog	89	64	25	+	[b]

[a] H and L, heavy and light subunits, respectively.
[b] Tate, S. S. & Maack, M., unpublished.

Thus, the K_m values for the substrates of many enzymes are much higher than the physiological concentrations of the substrates (87). In fact, many of the glycolytic enzymes have K_m values that are 10–100 times the physiological substrate concentrations. Therefore, the finding that the K_m values for some amino acid acceptors of transpeptidase are higher than the plasma levels of these amino acids does not necessarily support the conclusion that transpeptidation involving these amino acids does not occur in vivo. Kinetic parameters are usually determined with very low concentrations of enzymes and it is doubtful that values obtained in this way can reliably predict in vivo activity of enzymes, especially in situations in which the concentration of the enzyme may be similar to that of the substrate concentrations (88). The in vivo concentration of γ-glutamyl transpeptidase is probably close to 0.1 mM in the renal brush-border, and is thus of about the same order of magnitude as many amino acid acceptor substrates.

Experiments which provide strong evidence that transpeptidation is a significant function of the enzyme were carried out by incubating catalytic amounts of the purified enzyme with 50 μM glutathione and a mixture of amino acids that closely approximates the amino acid composition of blood plasma; the relative extents of transpeptidation and hydrolysis were determined by quantitative measurement of the products formed (29). At pH 7.4, about 50% of the glutathione that was utilized participated in transpeptidation. Studies in which the formation of individual γ-glutamyl amino acids was determined showed that L-cystine and L-glutamine are the most active amino acid acceptors and also that other amino acids participate in transpeptidation. The extent to which glutathione is used for transpeptidation in vivo may increase under certain conditions. The level of plasma amino acids tends to increase postprandially; a 20–60% increase in total amino acid level would be expected to produce a significant increase in the fraction of glutathione used in transpeptidation. γ-Glutamyl transpeptidase is present on the external surface of certain cell membranes and is thus in close contact with amino acids and also with glutathione which is translocated across cell membranes. Thus, it would seem that γ-glutamyl amino acids must be continually produced. In certain locations, for example, the proximal renal tubule,

there is a very considerable uptake of water, and this may lead to relatively high local concentrations of amino acids at certain anatomic sites in the tubule.

The presence of substantial concentrations of amino acids at the membraneous sites at which γ-glutamyl transpeptidase is located suggests also that transpeptidation plays a role in the processing of glutathione conjugates. It is generally believed that transpeptidase catalyzes removal of the γ-glutamyl moiety of glutathione conjugates formed in the mercapturic acid pathway and in similar pathways of metabolism involving prostaglandins (89, 90), leukotrienes (91, 92), estrogens (93–97), and probably other compounds. Since this reaction presumably takes place on the surface of the cell membrane in the presence of amino acids, it is probable that it is facilitated by transpeptidation and thus coupled with the formation of γ-glutamyl amino acids. In vitro studies with purified transpeptidase preparations have shown that the enzyme acts effectively on a number of S-substituted glutathione conjugates, often more rapidly than it does on glutathione itself (see, for example (20)).

Although the data indicate that γ-glutamyl transpeptidase reactions in vivo, and that administered γ-glutamyl amino acids are transported into renal cells, direct evidence for the transport of γ-glutamyl amino acids formed in vivo by the action of transpeptidase is needed. Recent studies on azaserine toxicity in established cell lines suggest that azaserine may be transported into certain cells as γ-glutamyl azaserine. Thus, Perantoni et al (98) found that sensitivity to azaserine of several cell lines exhibited a positive correlation with γ-glutamyl transpeptidase activity. Earlier work had shown that azaserine-resistant cells are less efficient in concentrating azaserine than the more sensitive parental cells (99). Although human Wilms' tumor cells were found to be sensitive to azaserine, azaserine-resistant strains isolated from cultures of these cells had markedly reduced levels of transpeptidase. The findings suggest that transpeptidase is a significant determinant of cell sensitivity to azaserine toxicity and that sensitivity is a consequence of increased transport of azaserine, presumably an effect related to relatively high transpeptidase levels and the formation and transport of γ-glutamyl azaserine.

It would be expected that the physiological

function of transpeptidase would be illuminated by studies in which the activity of this enzyme is deficient or markedly inhibited. Thus far, two patients have been found who exhibit apparently generalized γ-glutamyl transpeptidase deficiency; these individuals were reported to have marked glutathionemia and glutathionuria (100, 101). Later studies on the urine of one of these patients showed that this patient also excretes substantial quantities of γ-glutamylcysteine and cysteine moieties (54). In these studies, the urine samples were treated with dithiothreitol and then with 2-vinylpyridine; subsequent chromatography revealed the presence of the 2-vinylpyridine derivatives of glutathione, γ-glutamylcysteine and cysteine. It is notable that in experiments in which mice were treated with γ-glutamyl transpeptidase inhibitors (L- and D-γ-glutamyl(o-carboxy)phenylhydrazide, AT-125), very high concentrations of glutathione, γ-glutamylcysteine and cysteine were also found in the urine (47, 54) (Table 1). These findings suggest that the physiological function of the transpeptidase is closely associated with the metabolism or transport (or both) of these sulfur-containing compounds. The appearance of urinary γ-glutamylcysteine might conveivably be explained if γ-glutamylcysteine formed intracellularly by γ-glutamylcysteine synthetase is translocated from cells to the blood plasma and thus to the glumerular filtrate. However, an intracellular origin of γ-glutamylcysteine seems unlikely because there are two highly active intracellular enzymes, i.e., glutathione synthetase and γ-glutamyl cyclotransferase, that are capable of utilizing this dipeptide, and the actions of these enzymes apparently maintain the intracellular concentration of γ-glutamylcysteine at a low level. It is notable that in the inborn error 5-oxoprolinuria in which there is a deficiency of glutathione synthetase, the excess γ-glutamylcysteine formed intracellularly is effectively converted to 5-oxoproline and little if any of this dipeptide is found extracellularly (102). Another possibility is that γ-glutamylcyst(e)ine might be formed from glutathione by the activity of a carboxypeptidase type enzyme. Although it is possible that some γ-glutamylcyst(e)ine is formed in this manner, an extensive series of experiments on a number of animal tissues has failed to reveal such an enzyme activity. Urinary γ-glutamylcyst(e)ine might be formed by still another pathway; thus, the residual

active transpeptidase present in both the patients with γ-glutamyl transpeptidase deficiency and in the experimental animals treated with inhibitors may be sufficient to catalyze the formation of γ-glutamylcystine from glutathione and cystine. It is notable that cystine is an exceptionally good acceptor substrate of the transpeptidase (25, 103). Thus, transpeptidation between glutathione and cystine may occur even in the presence of substantial transpeptidase deficiency or inhibition. Recent studies support this interpretation, and seem to explain the marked urinary excretion of cysteine and γ-glutamylcysteine moieties in patients with transpeptidase deficiency and in expermental animals treated with transpeptidase inhibitors. In these studies, mice were injected with glutathione and their urine was found to contain (after treatment with dithiothreitol and 2-vinylpyridine) the 2-vinylpyridine derivatives of glutathione, γ-glutamylcysteine, and cysteine (104). Studies in which the glutathione was labeled with ^{35}S, showed that the urinary γ-glutamylcysteine had a much lower specific radioactivity than the urinary glutathione; this finding does not support a pathway involving cleavage of the C-terminal glycine moiety of glutathione to form γ-glutamylcysteine. The data are consistent with the view that transpeptidase catalyzes a reaction between glutathione and cystine to form γ-glutamylcystine which is transported into the cell. In the presence of γ-glutamyl transpeptidase deficiency or of inhibition of this enzyme, it is evident that the formation of γ-glutamylcystine must be more rapid than its transport; it would therefore accumulate and appear in the urine. The findings suggest that the accumulation of glutathione which occurs in the presence of transpeptidase deficiency or inhibition, inhibits the transport of γ-glutamylcystine. This interpretation is consistent with recent studies which showed that glutathione inhibits the transport of γ-glutamyl amino acids (Bridges, unpublished).

In conclusion, the available data support the view that γ-glutamyl transpeptidase functions in transpeptidation leading to the formation of γ-glutamyl amino acids which are transported into cells. The enzyme also functions to remove the γ-glutamyl moiety of glutathione conjugates formed by reaction of glutathione with exogenous and endogenous compounds. The enzyme may also play a role in the extracellular metabolism of glutathione by promoting the conversion of glutathione to glutathione disulfide, which may be further metabolized to form cystine. A number of important questions remain to be answered, and additional data are required. The possibility that transpeptidase itself, or a closely associated protein in the membrane, functions in the transport of glutathione out of cells or of γ-glutamyl amino acids into cells needs to be investigated.

References

1. Meister, A. & Tate, S. S., 1976. Ann. Rev. Biochem. 45: 559–604.
2. Meister, A., 1981. In Current Topics of Cellular Regulation (Horecker, B. & Stadtman, E., eds.), vol. 18, 18: 21–57.
3. Meister, A., 1975. In Metabolism of Sulfur Compounds, Metabolic Pathways, 3rd edition (Greenberg, D. M., ed.), 7: 101–188, Academic Press.
4. Dakin, H. D. & Dudley, H. W., 1913. J. Biol. Chem. 15: 463–474.
5. Meister, A., Tate, S. S. & Ross, L. L., 1976. In The Enzymes of Biological Membranes (Martinosi, A., ed.), vol. 3, Plenum Press, New York, pp. 315–347.
6. Tate, S. S., 1980. In Enzymatic Basis of Detoxication (Jakoby, W. B., ed.), vol. 2, Academic Press, pp. 95–120.
7. Meister, A., Griffith, O. W., Novogrodsky, A. & Tate, S. S., 1980. Ciba Fdn. Symp. 72: 135–161.
8. Goldberg, D. M., 1980. Critical Reviews in Clinical Laboratory Sciences 12: 1–58.
9. Rosalki, S. B., 1975. Adv. Clin. Chem. 17: 53–107.
10. Cornell, J. S. & Meister, A., 1976. Proc. Natl. Acad. Sci. U.S.A. 73: 420–422.
11. Heinle, H., Wendel, A. & Schmidt, U., 1977. FEBS Lett. 73: 220–224.
12. Novogrodsky, A., Tate, S. S. & Meister, A., 1976. Proc. Natl. Acad. Sci. U.S.A. 73: 2414–2418.
13. Albert, Z., Orlowski, M. & Szewczuk, A., 1961. Nature (London) 191: 767–768.
14. Glenner, G. G., Folk, J. E. & McMillan, P. J., 1962. J. Histochem. Cytochem. 10: 481–489.
15. Marathe, G. V., Nash, B., Haschemeyer, R. H. & Tate, S. S., 1979. FEBS Lett. 107: 436–440.
16. Marathe, G. V., Damle, N. S., Haschemeyer, R H. & Tate, S. S., 1980. FEBS Lett. 115: 273–277.
17. Horiuchi, S., Inoue, M. & Morino, Y., 1978. Eur. J. Biochem. 87: 429–437.
18. Tsao, B. & Curthoys, N. P., 1980. J. Biol. Chem. 255: 7708–7711.
19. Orlowski, M. & Meister, A., 1963. Biochim. Biophys. Acta 73: 679–681.
20. Tate, S. S. & Meister, A., 1974. J. Biol. Chem. 249: 7593–7602.
21. Tate, S. S., 1975. FEBS Lett. 54: 319–322.
22. Smith, G. D., Ding, J. L. & Peters, T. J., 1979. Anal. Biochem. 100: 136–139.
23. Griffith, O. W. & Meister, A., 1977. Proc. Natl. Acad. Sci. U.S.A. 74: 3330–3334.
24. Thompson, G. A. & Meister, A., 1977. J. Biol. Chem. 252: 6792–6798.
25. Thompson, G. A. & Meister, A., 1976. Biochem. Biophys. Res. Commun. 71: 32–36.
26. Ball, E. G., Revel, J. P. & Cooper, O., 1956. J. Biol. Chem. 221: 895–908.
27. Tate, S. S. & Meister, A., 1974. Proc. Natl. Acad. Sci. U.S.A. 71: 3329–3333.
28. McIntyre, T. M. & Curthoys, N. P., 1979. J. Biol. Chem. 254: 6499–6504.
29. Allison, D. & Meister, A., 1981. J. Biol. Chem. 266: 2988–2992.
30. Orlowski, M. & Meister, A., 1965. J. Biol. Chem. 240: 338–347.
31. Tate, S. S. & Meister, A., 1977. Proc. Natl. Acad. Sci. U.S.A. 74: 931–935.
32. Inoue, M., Horiuchi, S. & Morino, Y., 1977. Eur. J. Biochem. 73: 335–342.
33. Tate, S. S. & Meister, A., 1978. Proc. Natl. Acad. Sci. U.S.A. 5: 4806–4809.
34. Gardell, S. J. & Tate, S. S., 1979, J. Biol. Chem. 254: 4942–4945.
35. Holzer, H. & Heinrich, P. C., 1980. Annu. Rev. Biochem. 49: 63–91.
36. Tate, S. S., Grau, E. M. & Meister, A., 1979. Proc. Natl. Acad. Sci. U.S.A. 76: 2715–2719.
37. Tate, S. S. & Orlando, J., 1979. J. Biol. Chem. 254: 5573–5575.
38. Griffith, O. W. & Tate, S. S., 1980. J. Biol. Chem. 255: 5011–5014.
39. Jones, D. P., Moldeus, P. & Orrenius, S., 1979. J. Biol. Chem. 254: 2787–2792.
40. Anderson, M. E., Bridges, R. J. & Meister, A., 1980. Biochim. Biophys. Res. Commun. 96: 848–853.
41. Janolino, V. G. & Swaisgood, H. E., 1975. J. Biol. Chem. 250: 2532–2538.
42. Ostrowski, M. C. & Kistler, W. S., 1980. Biochemistry 19: 2639–2645.
43. Flohé, L., Günzler, W. A. & Ladenstein, R., 1976. In Glutathione: Metabolism and Function (Arias, I. M. & Jakoby, W. B., editors), pp. 115–138, Raven Press, New York.
44. Revel, J. P. & Ball, E. G., 1959. J. Biol. Chem. 234: 577–582.
45. Kinoshita, T. & Minato, S., 1978. Bull. Chem. Soc. of Japan 51: 3282–3285.
46. Minato, S., 1979. Arch. Biochem. Biophys. 192: 235–240.
47. Griffith, O. W. & Meister, A., 1979. Proc. Natl. Acad. Sci. U.S.A. 76: 268–272.
48. Binkley, F., 1961. J. Biol. Chem. 236: 1075–1082.
49. Tate, S. S. & Meister, A., 1975. J. Biol. Chem. 250: 4619–4627.
50. Curthoys, N. P. & Kuhlenschmidt 1975. J. Biol. Chem. 250: 2099–2105.
51. Thompson, G. A. & Meister, A., 1979. J. Biol. Chem. 254: 2956–2960.
52. Thompson, G. A. & Meister, A., 1980. J. Biol. Chem. 255: 2109–2113.

53. Allen, L., Meck, R. & Yunis, A., 1980. Res. Commun. Chem. Pathol. Pharmacol. 27: 175–182.

54. Griffith, O. W. & Meister, A., 1980. Proc. Natl. Acad. Sci. U.S.A. 77: 3384–3387.

55. Gardell, S. J. & Tate, S. S., 1980. FEBS Lett. 122: 171–174.

56. Kozak, E. M. & Tate, S. S., 1980. FEBS Lett. 122: 175–178.

57. Inoue, M., Horiuchi, S. & Morino, Y., 1978, Biochem. Biophys. Res. Comm. 82: 1183–1188.

58. Tate, S. S. & Meister, A., 1976. Proc. Natl. Acad. Sci. U.S.A. 73: 2599–2603.

59. Tate, S. S. & Ross, M. E., 1977. J. Biol. Chem. 252: 6042–6045.

60. Zelazo, P. & Orlowski, M., 1976. Eur. J. Biochem. 61: 147–155.

61. Hughey, R. P. & Curthoys, N. P., 1976. J. Biol. Chem. 251: 7813–7870.

62. Köttgen, E., Reuter, W. & Gerok, W., 1978. Eur. J. Biochem. 82: 279–284.

63. Jaken, S. & Mason, M., 1978. Proc. Natl. Acad. Sci. U.S.A. 75: 1750–1753.

64. DeLap, L. W., Tate, S. S. & Meister, A., 1977. Life Sci. 20: 673–680.

65. Gardell, S. J. & Tate, S. S., 1981. J. Biol. Chem. 256: 4799–4804.

66. Hughey, R. P., Coyle, P. J. & Curthoys, N. P., 1979. J. Biol. Chem. 254: 1124–1128.

67. Tsuji, A., Matsuda, Y. & Katunuma, N., 1980. J. Biochem. (Tokyo) 87: 1567–1571.

68. Nash, B., 1980. Fed. Proc. 39: 1866.

69. Taniguchi, N., 1974. J. Biochem. (Tokyo) 75: 473–480.

70. Shaw, L. M., London, J. W. & Petersen, L. E., 1978, Clin. Chem. 24: 905–916.

71. Hanes, C. S., Hird, F. J. R. & Isherwood, F. A., 1950. Nature (Lond.) 166: 288–292.

72. Hanes, C. S., Hird, F. J. R. & Isherwood, F. A., 1952. Biochem. J. 51: 25–35.

73. Griffith, O. W., Bridges, R. J. & Meister, A., 1979. Proc. Natl. Acad. Sci. U.S.A. 76: 6319–6322.

74. Buchanan, D. L., Haley, E. E. & Markiw, R. T., 1962. Biochem. 1: 612–620.

75. Peck, H. & Pollitt, R. J., 1979. Clin. Chem. Acta 94: 237–240.

76. Kakimoto, Y., Nakajima, T., Kanazawa, A. Takesada, M. & Sano, I., 1964. Biochim. Biophys. Acta 93: 333–338.

77. Reichelt, K. L., 1970. J. Neurochem. 17: 19–25.

78. Versteeg, D. H. G. & Witter, A., 1970. J. Neurochem. 17: 41–52.

79. Kanazawa, A., Kakimoto, Y. Nakajima, T. & Sano, I., 1965. Biocheim. Biophys. Acta 111: 90–95.

80. Sano, I., 1970. Int. Rev. Neurobiol. 12: 235—263.

81. Wendel, A., Hahn, R. & Guder, W. G., 1976. Curr. Probl. Clin. Biochem. 6: 426–436.

82. Palekar, A. G., Tate, S. S. & Meister, A., 1975. Biochem. Biophys. Res. Commun. 62: 651–657.

83. Griffith, O. W., Bridges, R. J. & Meister, A., 1978. Proc. Natl. Acad. Sci. U.S.A. 75: 5405–5408.

84. Ormstad, K., Jones, D. P. & Orrenius, S., 1980. J. Biol. Chem. 255: 175–181.

85. Ormstad, K., Lastbom, T. & Orrenius, S., 1980. FEBS Lett. 112: 55–59.

86. Elce, J. S. & Broxmeyer, B., 1976. Biochem. J. 153: 223–232.

87. Fersht, A., 1977. Enzyme Structure and Mechanism, pp. 253–259, W. H. Freeman, San Francisco.

88. Srere, P. A., 1967. Science 158: 936–937.

89. Cagen, L. M., Fales, H. M. & Pisano, J. J., 1976. J. Biol. Chem. 251: 6500–6554.

90. Cagen, L. M. & Pisano, J. J., 1979. Biochim. Biophys. Acta 573: 547–551.

91. Örning, L., Hammarström, S. & Samuelsson, B., 1980. Proc. Natl. Acad. Sci. U.S.A. 77: 2014–2017.

92. Hammerstrom, S., Samuelsson, B., Clark, D. A., Groto, G., Marfat, A., Miowskowski, C. & Corey, E. J., 1980. Biochem. Biophys. Res. Commun. 92: 946–953.

93. Kuss, E., 1967. Hoppe-Seylers Z. Physiol. Chem. 348: 1707–1708.

94. Kuss, E., 1968. Hoppe-Seyler's Z. Physiol. Chem. 349: 1234–1236.

95. Kuss, E., 1969. Hoppe-Seyler's Z. Physiol. Chem. 350: 95–97.

96. Elce, J. S., 1970. Biochem. J. 116: 913–917.

97. Jellinck, P. H., Lewis, J. & Boston, F., 1967. Steroids 10: 329–346.

98. Perantoni, A., Berman, J. J. & Rice, J. M., 1979. Exp. Cell. Res. 122: 55–61.

99. Pine, E. K., 1958. J. Nat. Cancer Inst. 21: 973–984.

100. Schulman, J. D., Goodman, S. I., Mace, J. W., Patrick, A. D., Tietze, F. & Butler, E. J., 1975. Biochem. Biophys. Res. Commun. 65: 68–74.

101. Wright, E. C., Stern, J., Ersser, R. & Patrick, A. D., 1979. Journal of Inherited Metabolic Disease 2: 3–7.

102. Meister, A., 1977. In The Metabolic Basis of Inherited Disease (4th ed.), (Stanbury, J. B., Wyngaarden, J. B. & Frederickson, D. S., editors), pp. 328–336, McGraw-Hill.

103. Thompson, G. A. & Meister, A., 1976. Biochem. Biophys. Res. Commun. 71: 32–36.

104. Griffith, O. W., Bridges, R. J. & Meister, A., 1981. Proc. Natl. Acad. Sci. 78: 2777–2781.

Received April 27, 1981.

Dynamic utilization of GABA in substantia nigra: regulation by dopamine and GABA in the striatum, and its clinical and behavioral implications

K. Gale and M. Casu

Dept. of Pharmacology Georgetown University Schools of Medicine and Dentistry Washington, D.C., USA

Contents

Molecular and Cellular Biochemistry 39, 369–405 (1981). 0300-8177/81/0393-0369/$07.40.
© 1981, Martinus Nijhoff/Dr W. Junk Publishers, The Hague.

1. Introduction

The neural circuitry of the basal ganglia provides a challenging framework in which to consider the role and regulation of GABA-containing synapses. GABA-containing neurons and terminals are located throughout the various nuclei of the basal ganglia, including caudate and putamen (together referred to as 'striatum'), globus pallidus, and substantia nigra (SN). In fact, the concentration of GABA in the SN is the highest of all brain areas. In this system we can find an excellent example of a 'long-distance' GABAergic neural pathway projecting from the striatum to the SN, as well as a significant population of smaller GABAergic neurons intrinsic to the striatum (interneurons). Moreover, it is likely that the various GABA neurons in the basal ganglia are involved in circuits in which they mutually regulate each other's activity, as well as the activity of neurons containing other neurotransmitters. At the same time, these GABAergic neurons are subject to the control and influence of several pathways which converge on the striatum; in this context they may serve a significant integrating function.

Because of the complex neuronal circuitry in which the GABA neurons are embedded, a change in their functional activity can be elicited by a variety of drugs or lesions which do not affect the GABAergic neurons directly. Thus, a change in transmission at one synaptic junction may cause secondary changes to occur at subsequent synapses in the same neural circuit. These sequential trans-synaptic interactions are of particular importance in considering mechanisms of neural pathology and its pharmacological treatment. GABA-containing neurons in the basal ganglia are likely to be involved in the various pathological changes giving rise to movement disorders such as Huntington's chorea, neuroleptic-induced tardive dyskinesias and Parkinsonism. In some cases, such as Huntington's disease, GABA neurons themselves undergo degeneration (1, 2); in other cases such as Parkinsonism, changes in GABA neurons may be a secondary consequence of the degeneration of other neurons (i.e. dopamine neurons) (3, 4). In order to understand the ways in which a change in one element of a neural chain can alter the other linkages of that chain, we need to know more about the precise ways in which the various components of the circuit interact with each other. In this report, we will focus on a selected aspect of this complex circuitry: the relationship between nigrostriatal dopamine (DA) pathways and the GABAergic neurons of the striatum and SN. One aspect of this relationship, the influence of GABA on nigrostriatal DA function, has been actively investigated and repeatedly discussed in recent years; much less attention has been directed at the inverse aspect of this relationship, i.e. the influence of DA on striatal and nigral GABA function. Our emphasis will therefore be placed on the latter aspect, and we will consider experimental evidence demonstrating that changes in DA transmission can alter the activity of striatal and nigral GABA synapses.

1.1. Components of basal ganglia circuits

Before directing our attention specifically to the DA and GABA neurons of the nigrostriatal system, we need to appreciate the neuroanatomical and neurochemical context in which these neurons are situated. Almost every putative neurotransmitter and their respective receptors, can be found in one or another neural population in this system; the possibilities for interactions between these components is nearly infinite. The major 'receiving' end of the system, the striatum, collects information from widespread cortical projections, many of which contain glutamate (5, 6); these projections converge on cells, many of which also receive projections from intralaminar thalamic nuclei (centromedianum in particular) (7, 8). The latter two inputs are primarily excitatory on striatal interneurons; this may be counterbalanced by inhibitory

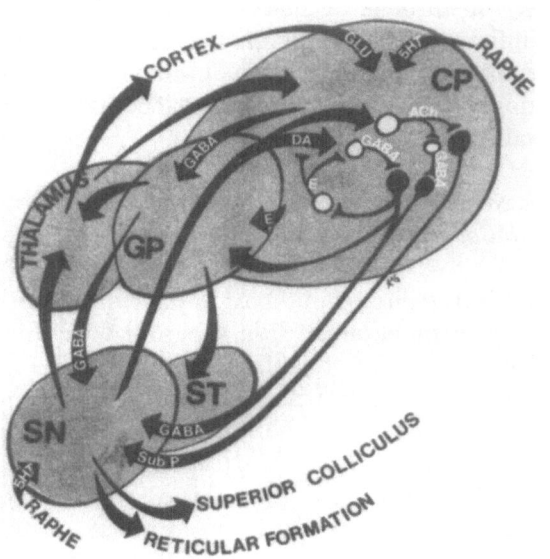

Fig. 1. Some circuits of the basal ganglia.

Ascending DA-containing fibers, arising from cell bodies in the zona compacta of SN, terminate in the caudate-putamen (striatum). These DA-containing terminals may form axo-dendritic synapses with striatal interneurons (cholinergic and GABAergic) as well as axo-axonic synapses with afferent projections from cortex (presumably glutamate-containing). The terminals of enkephalin-containing neurons in striatum may form axo-axonic synapses with DA terminals, and also may mutually interact with striatal GABA interneurons, forming a local 'feedback' circuit in the striatum. The various afferents to striatum (cortical, raphe, thalamic, nigral) converge on the striatal cholinergic and GABAergic interneurons which in turn act on striatonigral and striatopallidal pathways. Both GABA-containing and substance P-containing striatonigral pathways have been identified. The globus pallidus receives GABA projections from striatum and sends a GABA projection to SN.

Stimulation of DA receptors in striatum is associated with inhibition of striatal cholinergic and possibly GABAergic interneurons (these interneurons may be arranged in a series) and an increase in inhibitory transmission (presumably GABAergic) in SN. Conversely, reduction or blockade of striatal DA transmission is associated with an increase in excitatory transmission (substance P mediated?). The GABAergic terminals in SN may terminate directly on dendrites of DA neurons, and in addition may form synaptic connections with interneurons, terminals afferent to SN, and nigral efferent projections to thalamus, superior colliculus (tectum), and tegmental reticular formation.

afferent control from the nigrostriatal DA projections (9–12) and the serotonin-containing projections from the dorsal raphe nucleus (13–15). There is probably also a nigrostriatal pathway which is not DA-containing; the fibers of this pathway appear to exert an excitatory influence on striatal units (16–18). These neural pathways are illustrated schematically in Fig. 1.

Most of these afferent projections converge on the spines and dendrites of striatal interneurons (golgi type II neurons) many of which contain acetylcholine (19–21) or GABA (22–24). Recently, an additional population of striatal interneurons have been found to contain the opiate-like peptide, met-enkephalin (25–27). These striatal interneurons may be juxtaposed in any of several sequences and patterns which have yet to be established. Fig. 1 shows one such pattern; several others may exist. Some clues regarding the juxtaposition of the neural elements in striatum come from measurements of receptor-binding sites following lesions. Thus, receptors for met-enkephalin appear to be located on the striatal DA terminals, since lesions of the nigrostriatal DA neurons result in a significant decrease in these binding sites (27, 28). Receptor binding sites for DA agonists or antagonists have been found to decrease after destruction of 1) striatal interneurons and efferents (by kainic acid) and 2) corticostriatal afferents (by decortication) (29–32). Thus, DA may exert an influence on the presynaptic terminals of glutamate-containing afferents from cortex, as well as on the postsynaptic cholinergic and GABAergic striatal cells.

The afferent information coming into striatum may be amplified, filtered and reorganized as it proceeds through the network of synaptic switches and local circuits within the striatum. Once integrated, this information is funneled out of the striatum to each of two target regions: globus pallidus and SN. Pathways from striatum to SN include those containing GABA (33–36) and substance P (37–38), which appear to exert respectively inhibitory and excitatory influences on neurons in SN (39–42). The striatal projections to globus pallidus are primarily GABA-containing (43); there is also evidence for enkephalin-containing projections between these nuclei (44, 45). In addition to the projections from striatum, the globus pallidus receives projections from the subthalamic nucleus (7) which have not been characterized neurochem-

372

ically. Efferent projections of the globus pallidus include ventral anterior and ventrolateral thalamic nuclei, as well as SN (7). The pallidonigral pathway is primarily GABA-containing (33, 34).

Neurochemically, the SN is a 'hot-spot' of activity. This nucleus contains amongst the highest concentrations of GABA, substance P, serotonin and DA to be found in the brain. Almost all (>80%) of the GABA content of the SN is derived from terminals arising from cells located in forebrain structures including striatum and globus pallidus (46), while the entire substance P content of SN is associated with afferent terminals whose cells are located in the rostral striatum (37). Serotonin-containing projections arise from the median and/or dorsal raphe nuclei (47–50); it is possible that some serotonin terminals in SN are collaterals of projections to the striatum. In addition to the nigrostriatal projections, efferents from SN have been demonstrated to project to thalamus, superior colliculus, and the ponto-mesencephalic tegmentum (51–56). Nigrothalamic and nigrotectal projections include GABA-containing fibers (57–60). Indirect evidence suggests that the pars compacta cells of the SN which send projections to the mesencephalic central grey may be DA-containing (52); the neurochemical nature of the nigral projections to the pedunculopontine nucleus (53) is not presently known, but lesion studies have ruled out DA (52). The diagram in Fig. 1 summarizes these circuits.

The SN is generally described in terms of its two major subdivisions: pars compacta and pars reticulata. The pars compacta contains the majority of the cells giving rise to the nigrostriatal pathways, whereas cells in the more ventral reticulata region give rise to the thalamic, tectal and reticular projections. Although DA neurons are located primarily in pars compacta, their dendritic processes extend throughout the pars reticulata, where they may be contacted by GABAergic (61–63) and serotonergic (64) afferents. While most afferent terminals form synaptic contacts in the pars reticulata, many terminals have been found extending into the pars compacta region as well.

The nature of the neural connections within the SN have been under investigation for the past several years. As additional data are generated, the range of possible synaptic interactions in the SN continues to expand, making it increasingly diffi-

cult to specify the precise way in which nigral afferents and efferents interconnect. Not only can each of the various inputs to SN influence each of the various outputs, but the various afferent projections may be able to regulate one another via axo-axonic synapses. In addition, nigral efferents may have local effects on SN as a result of dendritic release of transmitter (as has been demonstrated for DA) or through recurrent collaterals. Since a significant portion of nigral afferents and efferents are GABA-containing, some of the synaptic interactions in which they participate will be discussed in detail in subsequent sections.

1.2. General considerations of the role of GABA in the basal ganglia

As is true throughout most of the brain, GABA neurons in the basal ganglia may be found synapsing upon each other, establishing serial inhibitory connections. The net result of this arrangement, 'disinhibition', is an important organizing feature of the central nervous system (see discussion of this in ref. 65). At the same time, this characteristic of GABAergic neurons makes experimental identification of their specific functions elusive, and makes the assignment of a unitary role for GABA, in a particular circuit, impossible. Augmentation of GABAergic transmission at one site may in turn depress GABAergic activity at another site in the same circuit. The functional role of GABA synapses must therefore be investigated and defined with respect to anatomical site. In this report, we will discuss evidence which suggests, in fact, that GABA synapses in striatum and SN play mutually counterposing roles and respond to changes in DA transmission in a reciprocal fashion.

Of the several ways in which the activity and functional changes in a neural circuit may be detected, we have chosen to concentrate on a neurochemical approach. Several aspects of pre- and post-synaptic GABA function can be assessed by the measurement of various neurochemical markers: 1) *Glutamic acid decarboxylase* (GAD), the enzyme responsible for GABA synthesis, is found in highest concentrations associated with GABA nerve terminals (66, 67) and its activity is sensitive to changes in the electrical activity of the neurons in which it is located (68–70). 2) *GABA levels* are a useful index for monitoring the effects of drugs which directly alter GABA synthesis or degradation. While measurement of GABA levels may indicate the amount of GABA available, it should be realized that in cases where a treatment does not directly influence GABA metabolism, levels may not reveal changes in the actual dynamic utilization of GABA. It is well known that drugs can influence turnover or utilization of a neurotransmitter without affecting steady-state levels (71). For example, if a treatment stimulates the synthesis of GABA and as a result more GABA is released into the synapse, an elevation of GABA might not be detected due to the rapid uptake and degradation of the GABA upon release. If, however, degradation of GABA is blocked, then GABA would be expected to accumulate at a rate proportional to the rate of synthesis. We have therefore included measurements of the rate of GABA accumulation after GABA transaminase inhibition in order to obtain an estimate of the synthesis and utilization of GABA in vivo. This type of approach has been used extensively for estimating the turnover rate of the monoamine neurotransmitters (72, 73). 3) *The density of receptor binding sites for GABA* has been demonstrated to increase (or 'upregulate') in response to the chronic loss of GABA innervation in SN (74, 75), and can therefore serve as an index of changes in the synaptic activity of GABA at specific loci. In addition, loss of specific binding sites for GABA after various lesions can provide information concerning the location of GABA receptors in a particular nucleus. In order to verify the functional significance of changes detected in GABA receptor binding measurements, we have also examined various behavioral responses to the direct stimulation of GABA receptors.

In the course of evaluating the synaptic role of GABA we must recognize that manipulations of GABA metabolism cannot be assumed to exert an exclusive effect on nerve-terminal related GABA, and conversely, changes in GABA content need not necessarily reflect alterations relevant to synaptic transmission. This is because GABA can be synthesized, taken up and degraded in cellular compartments other than GABAergic presynaptic terminals (e.g. neural perikarya, glial cells). The importance of discriminating between cellular compartments with respect to drug-induced changes in GABA levels or metabolism has been discussed at length elsewhere (76–79, see also

Iadarola and Gale, this volume), and will be considered here in the specific context of GABAergic nerve-terminals in SN. It will become evident that even large changes in GABA levels which are not associated with GABAergic nerve terminals, may have little or no direct impact on synaptic transmission. Thus, in addition to anatomical site, we will address ourselves to an evaluation of the cellular sites in which changes in GABA may occur.

With these considerations in mind, we will focus our attention on DA-GABA, GABA-GABA, and GABA-DA interactions in the striatum and SN. In this report, we are operating on the assumption that striatal neural activity, and hence the influence of striatal DA, is functionally expressed via relays in the globus pallidus and/or the SN. If the striatum is the heart of this system, the globus pallidus and SN are the sites where we can monitor its pressure and pulse. Although the experiments to be discussed will concentrate on the SN, it should be kept in mind that the pallidal outputs are probably equally important.

In the sections to follow, the interactions will be considered link-by-link, starting with the influence of DA on GABA in the striatum. Striatonigral GABA projections will lead us into the SN, where we can evaluate responses to manipulations of striatal DA and GABA. We will discuss the possibility that nigral GABA receptors mediate some of the behavioral changes which take place as a result of manipulations of striatal DA transmission; in the process we will consider the various influences that GABA can exert in SN.

2. Influence of dopamine neurons on GABAergic function in the striatum: effects of sustained reduction in dopaminergic transmission

2.1. Blockade of DA receptors or destruction of nigrostriatal DA neurons causes an increase in striatal GAD activity

The chronic blockade of DA receptors by drugs such as haloperidol and chlorpromazine, leads to an increase in GAD activity in the caudate-putamen without causing any significant change in steady-state levels of GABA in this nucleus (80, 81). As shown in Table 1, GAD values from the caudates of rats treated daily with haloperidol for

374

Table 1. Glutamic acid decarboxylase activity in rat striatum: increase after chronic haloperidol treatment and after 6-OHDA lesions of the nigrostriatal DA neurons.

| Treatment | Striatal GAD activity | |
	(μmol/mg prot/hr)	% control
Controls (saline injected)	.33 ± .02	
Haloperidol (1 mg/kg) (daily for 8 weeks)	.49 ± .04*	148%
6-OHDA lesion in medial forebrain bundle (4 weeks post. op.)	.56 ± .05*	160%
Sham lesion (saline)	.35 ± .03	

Values are the mean ± SEM from 8 animals.
* significantly different from control, p < .01.

Haloperidol treated rats were allowed three days drug-free before being killed. 6-OHDA (8 μg) was dissolved in 4 μl saline and infused over 10 min; sham lesioned rats received an equal volume of saline. GAD was measured as described by Sims and Pitts (180).

eight weeks, were more than 50% higher than the values from control rats. A similar increase in striatal GAD activity was obtained after destruction of nigrostriatal DA neurons (81–83). This destruction can be accomplished using the neurotoxin, 6-hydroxydopamine (6-OHDA), or by mechanical transection of the fibers; both lesioning procedures result in a marked (50–60%) increase in GAD activity measured in the striatum at four weeks post-operatively (Table 1).

The increase in striatal GAD activity found after either destruction of DA neurons or blockade of DA transmission suggests that striatal GABA synthesis and utilization may increase in the absence of regulation by nigrostriatal DA neurons. However, since the measurement of GAD activity in these experiments has been done in vitro, in the presence of a saturating concentration of exogenous cofactor (pyridoxal phosphate), these measurements do not necessarily reflect the synthetic activity of the enzyme in vivo (i.e. holoenzyme). In order to obtain an estimate of GABA synthesis in vivo, we examined the rate of accumulation of GABA in the caudate-putamen of rats treated with an inhibitor of GABA degradation.

2.2. Enhancement of striatal GABA turnover after loss of DA activity

For studies of GABA accumulation, we selected

an irreversible ('suicide') inhibitor of GABA transaminase, gamma-vinyl-GABA (GVG). This compound is one of the more specific agents of its class (84–86) and we, and others have previously documented its ability to elevate neuronal GABA (76, see also Iadarola and Gale, this volume). We chose to apply GVG directly into the caudate nucleus via the intracerebral microinjection route for two major reasons: 1) to examine the rate of GABA accumulation in a single brain nucleus without directly altering GABA levels in other regions with which the nucleus might be connected and 2) to avoid problems associated with absorption and distribution of the drug after peripheral administration. Our previous results with this method indicated that it is a reliable way of studying GABA synthesis and turnover in vivo (87).

After microinjection of GVG (20 μg) into the caudate-putamen, GABA-transaminase is maximally inhibited (<5% remaining) within 15 min and GABA levels increase in a linear fashion for at least 3 h (87). We examined the accumulation of GABA at 1.5 and 3 h after intracaudate GVG in rats which had received 6-OHDA lesions of the nigrostriatal

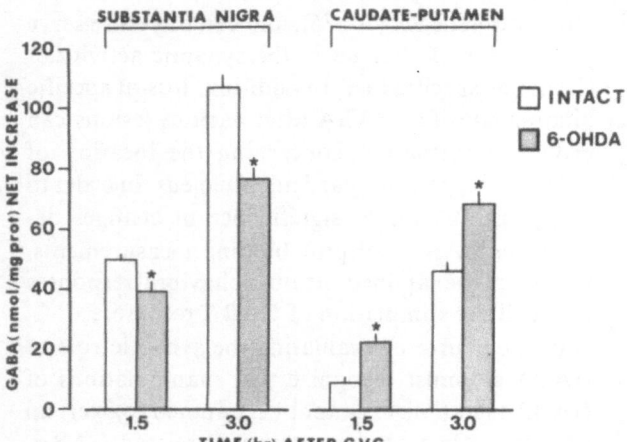

Fig. 2. GABA accumulation in substantia nigra and caudate-putamen in rats with unilateral 6-OHDA lesions.

GABA accumulation was measured after microinjection of GVG into SN (5 μg) or CP (20 μg), in separate groups of rats (n = 4–6 per group). Clear bars represent values obtained from controls; shaded bars represent values obtained from the lesioned hemisphere of rats which had been injected with 6-OHDA (8 μg/4 μl over 10 min) into the medial forebrain bundle four weeks previously. Basal GABA values (without GVG) were: SN: 101.3 ± 3 nmol/mg prot, CP: 22.1 ± 2 nmol/mg prot.

* Significantly different from respective control p < 0.05.

pathways four weeks before. The results, shown in Fig. 2, demonstrate that GABA accumulation is significantly greater in the DA-depleted caudates when compared to intact controls. The rate of accumulation, which can be derived from this data, is .40 nmol/mg prot/min in the caudates from the 6-OHDA lesioned hemispheres, as compared with .26 nmol/mg prot/min in controls. Since there was no difference between the groups with respect to steady-state levels of striatal GABA, it is likely that this difference in the in vivo rate of GABA accumulation reflects a difference in the turnover rate of GABA.

By studying the rate of incorporation of ^{13}C-glucose into GABA, Costa and co-workers have obtained an estimate of the turnover rate of GABA in several brain regions after acute and chronic blockade of DA receptors (71, 88, 89). These investigators found a marked enhancement of GABA turnover in the caudate-putamen after chronic, but not acute, treatment with haloperidol.

Thus, both in vitro measurements of GAD, as well as in vivo estimates of GABA turnover, suggest that the DA innervation of the striatum exerts an inhibitory influence on striatal GABA-ergic interneurons, and that sustained interference with DA function (by drugs or lesions) results in enhanced synthesis and utilization of GABA in the striatum.

3. Influence of striatal GABAergic transmission on GABA turnover in substantia nigra: evidence that GABA interneurons in striatum inhibit striato-nigral projections

It has been suggested (90) that the GABA neurons intrinsic to the striatum may be functionally linked to the GABAergic striatonigral projections. If the terminals of striatal GABA neurons exert an inhibitory influence on striato-nigral GABA neurons, we might expect that an increase in GABA transmission in striatum would reduce the turnover rate of GABA in the terminals in SN. To investigate this possibility, we examined the rate of GABA accumulation in SN after intra-nigral application of GVG (5 μg), as a function of various manipulations in the caudate.

We first examined the effect of enhancing GABA transmission in the caudate, on the rate of nigral

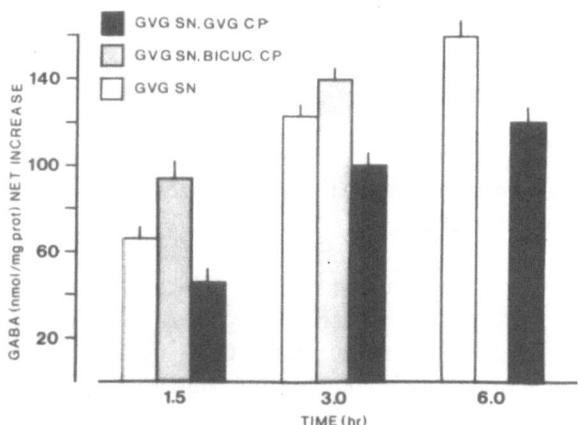

Fig. 3. GABA accumulation in substantia nigra (SN): effects of stimulation or blockade of GABA transmission in striatum (CP).

In all rats, GVG was microinjected into SN (5 μg) and the accumulation of GABA was subsequently measured (at times indicated on abscissa). Ten min after intranigral GVG, one of the following treatments was applied intrastriatally: Saline (controls, open bars), bicuculline methiodine (0.5 μg in 1.5 μl over 10 min, shaded bars), or GVG (20 μg in 2 μl over 10 min, black bars). The effect of bicuculline methiodide was not studied at 6 h after injection due to the short in vivo half life of this compound (<1 h). All experimental groups (shaded and black bars) were significantly different from controls, p < .05. Each value represents the mean ± S.E.M. of 4–7 rats.

GABA accumulation. To do this, we microinjected GVG into the caudate-putamen just prior to the intranigral application of GVG. At all time points examined intrastriatal GVG caused a depression in GABA accumulation in SN (Fig. 3).

Next, we examined the effect of striatal GABA receptor blockade on the rate of GABA accumulation in SN. Bicuculline methiodide, a specific GABA receptor antagonist, was microinjected into the caudate-putamen immediately following intranigral GVG; GABA accumulation in SN was measured at 1.5 and 3 h. At both times, nigral GABA accumulation was significantly enhanced by the intrastriatal bicuculline treatment (Fig. 3). Later time points were not examined in this experiment because of the short in vivo half-life of bicuculline methiodide (<1 h).

These results suggest that GABAergic transmission in the striatum exerts an inhibitory control on the striatonigral GABA projections; when this inhibition is blocked due to a reduction in striatal GABA receptor activity, the disinhibition of the striatonigral neurons is reflected in an enhanced rate of synthesis of GABA in the nigral nerve terminals.

4. The influence of nigrostriatal DA neurons on GABA transmission in SN: evidence for a disinhibitory role of DA

We have discussed evidence which suggests that striatal DA transmission may exert an inhibitory influence on intrinsic striatal GABA neurons. Evidence has also been presented which indicates that the striatal GABA neurons may inhibit the activity of the striatonigral GABA neurons. If we put these two linkages in tandem, we might expect that striatal DA transmission could cause *disinhibition* of striatonigral GABA projections. Or, in other words, the DA released in the striatum may be necessary for maintaining activity in the striatonigral GABA neurons.

4.1. Decreased GABA turnover in SN following interference with dopamine transmission

Evidence in support of the above hypothesis can be derived from several studies in which striatal DA

transmission has been disrupted. Chronic blockade of DA receptors by haloperidol results in a depression in the rate of GABA turnover in SN (71, 88). A similar change in nigral GABA turnover appears to take place after removal of the nigrostriatal DA pathways with 6-OHDA. The data presented in Fig. 2 demonstrate that the accumulation of GABA in the SN (after microinjection of GVG) was significantly reduced in rats which had been previously lesioned with 6-OHDA in the medial forebrain bundle. Steady-state levels of GABA were not significantly affected by the lesions (Fig. 2, legend), suggesting that the reduced accumulation of nigral GABA reflects a reduction in GABA turnover in this nucleus.

4.2. Increased GABA receptor binding sites in SN following chronic blockade of DA receptors

If the loss of striatal DA activity causes a concommitant loss of GABAergic transmission in SN, as suggested by the studies described above, then it might be expected that such a decrease in GABAergic presynaptic function in SN would be reflected in changes in nigral GABA receptors. It has been shown that the chronic removal of

Table 2. [^{3}H]GABA specific binding (femtomol/mg prot) in SN and in neostriatum after chronic treatment with antischizophrenic drugs.

Chronic treatment (mg/kg, s.c.) (8 weeks)	SN		Striatum	
		% of control		% of control
Control	382 ± 15		322 ± 13	
Haloperidol (0.7)	501 ± 32*	131	331 ± 18	103
Chlorpromazine (20)	521 ± 30*	136	348 ± 13	108
Clozapine (20)	360 ± 19	94	338 ± 15	105

Values represent the means of 15 rats (three separate experiments, five rats each) ± s.e.m. Rats were killed by decapitation and SN and striatum were dissected out as previously described (112) and placed on dry ice. For each SN determination, both SN (8 mg wet wt. tissue) from one rat were combined; this yielded enough protein (300–400 ug in the final membrane prep.) to run triplicate samples for binding. Tissue was prepared according to the method of Enna and Snyder (174); as described by Toffano et al. (175), this preparation results in the removal of a membrane-bound protein inhibitor of high-affinity GABA binding. Binding was measured at 0 °C in a Na$^+$-free medium in the presence of 30 nM [^{3}H]GABA; nonspecific binding was measured in the presence of 10^{-3} M cold GABA. The SN from groups of 3–4 rats were pooled to obtain values for Scatchard plots of high-affinity binding (10–90 nM [^{3}H]GABA). Under these conditions, linear regression analysis of the data indicated that the K_d values of haloperidol (42 ± 5 nM) and chlorpromazine (40 ± 5 nM) rats were not significantly different from controls (36 ± 4 nM). B_{max} values (pmol/mg prot) were: control, 1.19 ± .06; haloperidol, 1.61 ± .10*; chlorpromazine, 1.58 ± .12*.

* denotes values significantly different from controls, p < 0.05.

GABAergic projections to SN results in an increase in the number of GABA binding sites in SN (74, 75). We reasoned that a similar increase in nigral GABA binding might occur if a relative deficit of GABA transmission in SN were to be maintained by chronic blockade of DA receptors.

To test the above hypothesis, the specific binding of (³H)GABA to membrane preparations from nigral and striatal tissues were measured in rats which had been exposed to either acute or chronic treatment with DA receptor antagonists (91, 92). Three antischizophrenic drug treatments were studied: chlorpromazine, haloperidol and clozapine. The first two drugs represent classical neuroleptic compounds, while the third drug possesses an atypical biochemical and clinical profile. In particular, clozapine is relatively weak with respect to the production of extrapyramidal symptoms in animals and humans (96, 97).

Acute injections of chlorpromazine (20 mg/kg IP) haloperidol (0.7 mg/kg IP) or clozapine (20 mg/kg IP) were found to be without effect on specific GABA binding measured in SN and striatum of rats killed one hour after drug administration.

In the chronic experiments, rats were treated for eight weeks with daily subcutaneous injections of haloperidol (0.7 mg/kg), chlorpromazine (20 mg/kg) or clozapine (20 mg/kg). At the end of the eight-week period, five days elapsed without drug administration before the rats were killed for measurement of (³H)GABA binding. Table 2 shows the amount of specific (³H)GABA binding in the SN and striatum of chronically treated groups. When compared with values from control rats which received daily injections of vehicle, the values obtained from rats receiving either chronic chlorpromazine or haloperidol treatment were found to be significantly elevated. In the same rats in which this increase in specific (³H)GABA binding was found in SN, no change in specific (³H)GABA binding was obtained in striatum (Table 2). In contrast, clozapine treatment did not cause a significant change in GABA binding in SN. The SN from several chronically-treated rats were pooled for binding studies using a range of GABA concentrations (10–90 nM). Scatchard analysis revealed that the increased GABA binding in the SN of chlorpromazine and haloperidol-treated rats was due to an increase in B_{max} and not to a change in affinity (K_D) of the binding sites for GABA (see legend to Table 2).

Thus, chlorpromazine and haloperidol, while not acutely changing nigral binding sites for GABA, can, upon repeated administration cause an increase in the apparent number of these binding sites. Since GABA binding in striatum failed to change, the increase obtained in SN does not represent a general response of brain GABA receptors to these drugs and it is therefore unlikely that the changes observed could be due to a direct action of the drugs on GABA receptors. Instead the effects observed are probably related to the functional juxtaposition of specific neural pathways. As in the case of lesions of striatonigral GABAergic projections, the increase in nigral GABA binding after chronic drug treatment may represent a compensation for a decrease in the synaptic activity of nigral GABA. This possibility is consistent with the evidence that chronic treatment with haloperidol or chlorpromazine reduces the turnover of GABA in SN (71, 88).

The lack of effect of chronic clozapine treatment on GABA binding in SN is likely to be related to the unique pharmacology of this compound. It is possible that the DA receptors affected by clozapine may be functionally distinct from those affected by haloperidol and chlorprozamine (93, 94). In addition, clozapine's blockade of muscarinic cholinergic receptors (95) may interfere with this drug's ability to activate the striatal pathways required for suppressing GABAergic transmission in SN. Thus, acute clozapine treatment, unlike haloperidol or chlorpromazine, causes an increase in the turnover rate of GABA in SN (71, 88). The neurochemical effects of clozapine which distinguish this drug from the classical neuroleptics may in turn correlate with the low incidence of extrapyramidal side effects encountered with the use of this drug in man (96) and the inability of this drug to cause catalepsy in animals (97).

4.3. Functional supersensitivity of GABA receptors in SN after either blockade of DA receptors or lesions of nigrostriatal neurons: behavioral studies with intranigral muscimol

If the DA-antagonist-induced increase in nigral GABA receptor binding actually reflects a functional supersensitivity of nigral GABA receptors, responses to in vivo activation of these receptors should be enhanced. To determine if this was the case, we examined the behavioral response to intranigrally applied muscimol in rats which had been chronically treated with chlorpromazine.

The stereotyped behavioral response to bilateral intranigral application of the GABA-receptor agonist, muscimol, has been well described (98, 99). In a dose-dependent fashion, intranigral muscimol causes sniffing, repetitive vertical head movements, gnawing, and repetitive flexions and extensions of the forepaws. These behaviors resemble those elicited by systemic administration of DA agonists such as apomorphine or amphetamine. After the dose used in the present study (2.5 ng in 0.5 μl), control rats exhibited locomotor activity accompanied by sniffing, vertical head movements and occasional rearing against the cage walls. In contrast, rats which had been chronically treated with chlorpromazine showed a more intense behavioral response to intranigral muscimol: they exhibited gnawing, restricted vertical head movements close to the cage floor and repetitive flexing of the forelimbs accompanied by very brief periods of locomotor activity. The latter behavior patterns were similar to those observed in control rats with

doses of muscimol 2–3 times higher than that employed in this study. The comparison between the behavioral rating scores for the chlorpromazine-treated rats and control rats is shown in Table 3; the differences between the groups are significant at all time points evaluated.

If nigrostriatal DA function is in fact a critical factor in determining GABAergic synaptic activity in SN, then the 6-OHDA-induced degeneration of DA neurons should result in a supersensitivity of nigral GABA receptors, similar to what we observed with chronic chlorpromazine treatment. In animals in which the DA fibers of one hemisphere were destroyed by the unilateral injection of 6-OHDA into the medial forebrain bundle, we examined the response to the microinjection of muscimol into the SN of the lesioned hemisphere. Unlike the stereotyped behavior produced after bilateral intranigral application of muscimol, the behavior following unilateral intranigral muscimol injection consists of circling activity in a direction contraversive to the injected side; the rate of the circling behavior is dose-dependent (100, 101). As can be seen in Table 4, the rate of contralateral circling induced by muscimol (5 ng) was significantly greater in rats with 6-OHDA lesions than in

Table 3. Stereotypies induced by intranigral muscimol (bilateral) in rats treated chronically with chlorpromazine.

Chronic treatment (8 weeks)	Stereotypy score[1] after intranigral muscimol: 2.5 ng			
	time after injection			
	30 min	50 min	70 min	90 min
Saline (controls)	1.2 ± .4	2.2 ± .2	2.0 ± .2	1.2 ± .2
Chlorpromazine	3.0 ± .4	4.2 ± .3	4.2 ± .4	2.0 ± .3
% Chlorpromazine / Control	250	191	210	167

Chlorpromazine was administered (20 mg/kg daily) for eight weeks. Animals were tested five days after the cessation of chronic treatment. Muscimol was injected in a volume of 0.2 μl (saline) over 5 min.

[1] Stereotyped behavior was rated on a scale of 1–6 (1 = locomotor activity only, 2 = sniffing, rearing and locomotor activity, 3 = sniffing continuously, directed at ground or cage corners, 4 = sniffing and gnawing, with repetitive flexion-extension of forepaws, 5 = gnawing continuously, 6 = self-directed gnawing). Each value represents the mean ± S.E.M. of 5 rats; the same rats were observed at 20 min intervals over 90 min.

Table 4. Contralateral turning induced by intranigral muscimol (unilateral): effect of destruction of nigrostriatal dopamine neurons (6-OHDA lesions).

	Number of turns/minute (Intranigral muscimol: 5.0 ng)		
	time after injection		
	20 min	50 min	90 min
Controls	20 ± 1.5	25 ± 1.0	12 ± 1.5
Lesioned	27 ± 2.0*	32 ± 1.5*	25 ± 2.0*
% Lesioned / Controls	135	128	208

6-OHDA lesions were placed in the medial forebrain bundle (see Table 1) six weeks before behavioral testing. Muscimol was dissolved in saline and injected in a volume of 0.2 μl over 5 min.

Each value represents the mean ± S.E.M. obtained from eight rats. Complete turns/min for each rat were calculated at each time point by taking the average number of turns/min counted over a 3 min sampling period, during which the rat was placed on a large table top free of obstacles.

Note: Values obtained in 6-OHDA-lesioned rats tested six days after lesioning were similar to those shown above for rats tested at six weeks.

* Significantly different from controls p < .05.

control rats. This difference was evident throughout the duration of action of muscimol, but was especially pronounced at the time points during which the drug effect was submaximal.

Thus, it appears that either chronic systemic treatment with DA receptor antagonists, or 6-OHDA-induced destruction of DA neurons, results in an enhanced sensitivity of nigral GABA receptors to the GABA receptor agonist, muscimol. In view of the similarities between the behaviors induced by intranigral muscimol, and those behaviors produced by DA agonist agents, it is tempting to speculate that a supersensitivity of nigral GABA receptors may underly the enhanced responses to DA agonists observed after the long-term blockade of DA receptors or following 6-OHDA lesions of DA neurons. This would be consistent with the concept that the synaptic activity of DA in the striatum is expressed, in part, via enhanced GABA-ergic activity in SN.

5. Role of GABA in SN

5.1. Location of GABA receptors in SN

These are numerous neural elements in SN upon which GABA may act to directly influence neural excitability or transmitter release. One clue to this puzzle can be obtained from the measurement of GABA binding sites after lesions of various pathways afferent and/or efferent to the SN.

5.1.1. On nigrostriatal DA neurons

The first series of lesion experiments we performed were directed at the nigrostriatal DA neurons. In this study, we included a variety of lesions in an attempt to minimize any consistent source of non-specific damage which might result from one type of lesion. Thus, each of 74 rats received one of the following lesions: 1) 6-OHDA placed in the medial forebrain bundle (MFB) at the level of the lateral hypothalamus (28 rats); 2) 6-OHDA placed in the SN (14 rats); 3) 6-OHDA placed in the caudate-putamen (20 rats) or 4) electrolytic lesions of the MFB at the level of the lateral hypothalamus (12 rats). An additional group of 10 rats received sham lesions, in which saline was infused into the MFB. Postoperative survival time was 3–4 weeks before biochemical measurements were made.

A decrease in tyrosine hydroxylase (TH) activity in the caudate-putamen was taken as an index of the extent of destruction of DA neurons resulting from the lesions. Values of TH from the control (intact) caudates of the lesioned animals were not different from the values obtained from sham operated or unoperated control rats. Therefore, all lesioned values are expressed as a percentage of the respective control values obtained from the contralateral side. The extent of damage produced by the lesions ranged from very modest (25% loss) to virtually total (over 97% loss). Of the entire population of lesioned animals, 45% had greater than 85% destruction, 27% had 70–85% destruction, 10% had 55–70% destruction, 5% had 40–55% destruction, and 12% had 25–40% destruction. Although lesions in the MFB (electrolytic or 6-OHDA) resulted in a slightly higher incidence of maximal ($>90\%$) destruction, and rats with lesions in the caudate-putamen had a slightly higher incidence of subtotal (70–85%) destruction, nevertheless, the distributions obtained with each of the various types of lesions were remarkably similar. The natural variation in the effectiveness of the lesions allowed the (^{3}H)GABA binding measurements to be analyzed with respect to the amount of TH remaining.

No significant differences were found between the various lesion placements (MFB, SN, or caudate-putamen) with respect to effects on (^{3}H)GABA binding in SN, and therefore the data from these groups were combined for analysis as presented in Table 5. A significant decrease in binding was obtained in the group which had subtotal lesions (15–44% TH remaining), whereas no significant changes were apparent in rats with either maximal (less than 15% TH remaining) or minimal (over 45% TH remaining) damage. The relationship between (^{3}H)GABA binding in SN, and TH in caudate-putamen, expressed in terms of percent of control, is shown graphically in Fig. 4. A discontinuity in the relationship appears in the vicinity corresponding to 30% TH. A significant positive linear correlation was found ($r = +0.73$, $p < 0.05$) between striatal TH values in the 20–100% range and nigral GABA binding, with the line of best fit intercepting the ordinate at 69.4%. This would suggest that approximately 70% of nigral GABA binding is retained after complete loss of nigrostriatal DA neurons, or, conversely, that 30% of the GABA binding in SN is associated with DA neurons. However, when the values corresponding to 0–40% TH were analyzed, a significant *negative*

380

Table 5. Relationship between amount of striatal TH remaining after lesions and [³H]GABA binding in SN.

TH on lesioned (left) side (% of control side)	*Specific* [³H]GABA binding in SN (fmol/mg protein)		
	left	right	% Lesioned/Controls
(N) †			
0–14 (34)	403 ± 10	422 ± 7	95.5
15–44 (27)	306 ± 12*	408 ± 15	75.0¹
45–75 (13)	366 ± 25	397 ± 21	92.1
controls:			
sham (10)	418 ± 16	435 ± 15	96.0
unoperated controls	403 ± 8	410 ± 12	98.2

* Significantly different from contralateral (control) side p < .05.
¹ Significantly different from all other groups (p < .05) when analyzed by Duncan's new multiple range test.
† The distribution of TH loss was similar for each of the lesion techniques used (see text); therefore the various lesion placements were represented in similar proportions in each of the groupings for data analysis.

Tyrosine hydroxylase was assayed in homogenates (approximately 200 μg protein/assay tube) incubated at 37 °C for 30 min. in the presence of a saturating concentration of cofactor (DMPH₄) and tyrosine. Control mean value of TH was 5.2 + 0.4 nmol/mg prot/h. Specific GABA binding was measured in the presence of 30 nM [³H]GABA. Nonspecific [³H]GABA binding was measured in the presence of 10⁻³ M nonradioactive GABA and subtracted from the total [³H]GABA binding. In a separate group of 20 lesioned rats, membranes prepared from SN were pooled in order to assay the binding in the presence of several concentrations of [³H]GABA (15–90 nM). No significant differences were found between lesioned and control tissues with respect to K_D for GABA (control = 30 ± 4 nM; complete lesions = 36 ± 6 nM; partial lesions = 32 ± 5 nM).

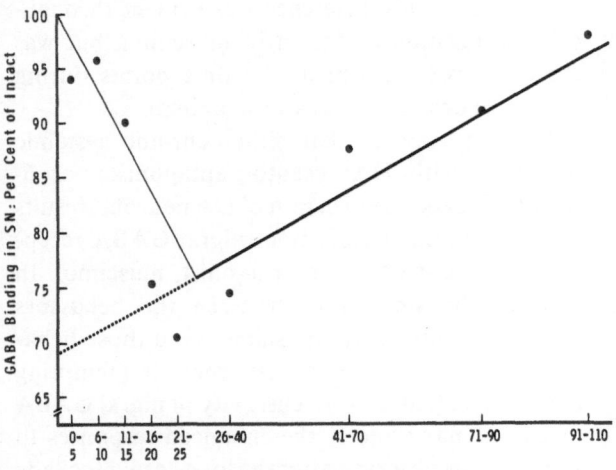

Fig. 4. Linear regression analysis of the relationship between loss of striatal tyrosine hydroxylase and nigral GABA binding after lesions of the nigrostriatal dopamine projection. Each point represents the mean value obtained from 6–10 rats.

linear correlation was found (r = – 0.77, p < 0.05) between striatal TH and nigral GABA binding, and it was evident that rats with the most complete loss of TH had (³H)GABA binding values in SN which were not significantly different from control values.

The biphasic relationship between the integrity of nigrostriatal DA neurons and the binding of (³H)GABA in SN, suggests that at least two different and apparently opposing processes are involved in determining the change in nigral GABA binding after DA neuron destruction. One process probably involves the loss of GABA binding sites associated with nigral DA neurons, and is observed with decreases in striatal TH down to 15% of control. The other process appears to involve a restoration of nigral GABA binding, under conditions in which DA neurons are almost completely destroyed. Changes in GABA binding associated with a population of nigral cells which are not dopaminergic could contribute to such an apparent 'restoration'. Thus, it may be postulated that a loss of GABA binding is associated with a loss of nigral DA neurons, and, in addition, an increase in nigral GABA binding, associated with non-DA cells, takes place under conditions of nearly total destruction of DA neurons.

The negative correlation between nigral GABA binding and TH values below 30% of control is understandable in the context of the pharmacological studies previously discussed (see Section 4.2.). When striatal DA transmission was interrupted pharmacologically, without actual destruction of DA neurons, the density of GABA binding sites in SN increased by 35%. A similar increase in nigral GABA binding probably occurs after 6-OHDA, lesions, as evidenced by the supersensitivity to intranigral muscimol (see Table 4). However, after 6-OHDA, the removal of the population of GABA receptors associated with DA neurons would result in a decreased baseline of (³H)GABA binding in SN; a 35% increase in the remaining population (70% of control) of nigral GABA bindings sites would therefore give a net value very close to that obtained in intact control tissue (135% × 70% = 95%).

Thus, when examining the relationship between the presence of nigrostriatal DA neurons and nigral GABA receptor binding, it is necessary to consider two distinct processes: 1) the direct physical association of GABA receptors with DA neurons in SN: Our study suggests that this can account for 25–30% of nigral GABA receptors, with the majority of the nigral GABA receptors located elsewhere; and 2) the indirect functional influence of DA transmission on nigral GABA receptors that are associated with non-DA neurons. Based on the data presented here, it may be postulated that the latter process becomes operative only when DA function is maximally compromised; this is perhaps because under such conditions compensatory mechanisms *within* the caudate (e.g. DA receptor supersensitivity) are not able to maintain sufficient output activity from the caudate to the SN.

5.1.2. On terminals of serotonin-containing afferents

From the above studies, it is evident that the majority of GABA binding sites in SN are located on neural elements which are not dopaminergic. These sites may be on efferent pars reticulata neurons, interneurons, or on the terminals of projections afferent to SN. To evaluate these possibilities, we examined changes in GABA receptor binding in SN after transections placed at various rostrocaudal levels.

After complete transection of pathways rostral to SN, no decrease in nigral GABA binding was obtained (75). In contrast, when transections were placed 2 mm caudal to SN, there was a 50% reduction in specific binding sites for GABA in SN (Table 6). Transections placed at the midcollicular level (3–4 mm caudal to SN) resulted in a 37% decrease in nigral GABA binding, but transections made even more caudally (in the rostral pons) failed to decrease GABA binding sites in SN (Table 6). The results suggest that a major portion of nigral GABA receptors are located on neurons which project between the SN and the caudal mesencephalon.

Since the 5HT projection to the SN represents a major source of afferent terminals deriving from the caudal mesencephalon, it was of interest to determine whether some of the nigral GABA binding sites might be associated with this projection. Lesions induced by 5,7-DHT in the SN caused a significant loss in GABA binding sites (28%) in SN; the loss of GABA binding in SN was directly correlated with the decrease in 5HT measured in the lesioned SN (Table 6, legend).

Several electrophysiological and anatomical studies suggest that the SN receives afferent projections from both the dorsal and median raphe nuclei (47–50, 102, 103). We therefore evaluated 5,7-DHT-induced lesions placed in the vicinity of the dorsal and median raphe nuclei, respectively, for

Table 6. Effect of various lesions on specific [³H]GABA binding in SN (see Fig. 5 for lesion placement).

Lesion	(n)	Specific [³H]GABA binding (fmol/mg prot)		
		Left[a]	Right	% Decrease
Control	(10)	440 ± 30	500 ± 42	
5,7 – DHT in				
SN[b]	(6)	352 ± 28*	488 ± 39	28%
Dorsal Raphe	(8)	448 ± 45	524 ± 40	
Median Raphe	(12)	334 ± 30*	445 ± 32	25%
Hemitransection				
Post. to SN	(8)	247 ± 20*†	515 ± 40	52%
Midcollicular	(8)	333 ± 38*	526 ± 45	37%
Postcollicular	(6)	452 ± 42	434 ± 20	
Sham injections	(6)	473 ± 35	496 ± 34	

* Significantly different from right (intact) side $p < .05$
† Significantly different from other lesioned groups $p < .05$
[a] Lesions were always placed on the left side
[b] Range of percent 5HT remaining on lesioned side: 16–25%
Note: rank order of samples with respect to decrease in 5HT was correlated with rank order with respect to decrease in specific GABA binding, which ranged from 25–35%; $r_s = 0.94$ $p < .05$.

382

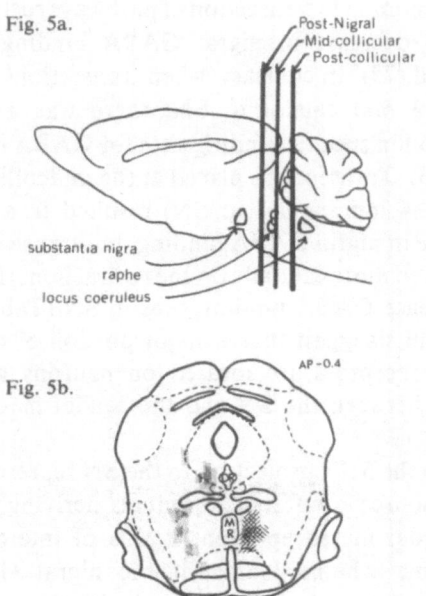

Fig. 5a.

Post-Nigral
Mid-collicular
Post-collicular

substantia nigra
raphe
locus coeruleus

Fig. 5b.

AP -0.4
M R

Fig. 5. Lesion placements for a) transections (sagittal view) and b) 5,7-DHT injections (coronal view).

a) Transections were made unilaterally by passing a blunt probe (see ref. 46 for description) several times in a medio-lateral direction between the midline and the lateral suture. The position of the transection was verified histologically in sagittal sections.

b) 5,7-DHT injections were made according to the procedure of Giambalvo and Snodgrass (137). In this procedure, injections of 5,7-DHT (28 μg/2 μl infused over 10 min) are made 1.0 mm lateral to the midline in order to achieve unilateral destruction. The lesion placements (based on location of cannula tip) effective for decreasing [³H]GABA binding in SN are indicated on the right side by hatch marks; ineffective placements are indicated on the left side by dotted areas. Stereotaxic coordinates are based on the atlas of Pellegrino and Cushman.

Effective placements were within 1 mm of the median raphe. These placements correspond to those which result in a 65–80% decrease in 5HT uptake in SN, cortex and hippocampus, restricted to the hemisphere ipsilateral to the injection. All animals were pretreated with desmethylimipramine (25 mg/kg) 30 min prior to surgery in order to minimize damage to catecholamine neurons.

effects on GABA binding in SN. The data (Table 6) indicated that whereas a significant decrease in nigral GABA binding sites resulted from median raphe lesions, no change in nigral GABA binding took place following dorsal raphe lesions. The placements of the 5,7-DHT lesions in the vicinity of the raphe nuclei were evaluated histologically; we used this information to generate a composite map of those regions in which 5,7-DHT placement

was effective (Fig. 5, right side), or ineffective (Fig. 5, left side) for causing decrease in GABA binding in SN. The resulting pattern suggests that 5,7-DHT injections placed within 1 mm of the median raphe are effective for decreasing GABA binding in SN.

These data suggest that one population of nigral GABA binding sites which decrease after transections caudal to SN are likely to be located on the afferent terminals of 5HT projections from the median raphe. It appears that this population accounts for 25% of the total nigral GABA binding sites. It is also possible that non-5HT pathways projecting between the raphe and SN (104) may account for some of the lesioned-induced decreases in SN GABA binding, since we cannot rule out a small amount of nonspecific damage in the vicinity of the 5,7-DHT injection site.

5.1.3. On non-dopaminergic descending efferents

Since hemitransections behind SN resulted in a significantly greater decrease in nigral GABA binding than could be obtained by 5,7-DHT lesions alone, it is possible that an additional 25% of the binding sites for GABA in SN may be located on descending nigral efferents which project into the caudal mesencephalon. Such a projection, although not extensively characterized, has been repeatedly demonstrated with anatomical tracing techniques (53—56) and appears to originate in SN pars reticulata. This pathway has been observed to terminate in the vicinity of the pedunculopontine nucleus of the pontomesencephalic tegmentum (53–56). The hemitransections that we placed just behind SN would have transected this pathway, and in addition may have damaged some of the projections from SN to superior colliculus. Our midcollicular lesions, which were less effective in decreasing GABA binding in SN were probably located too caudally to cause complete retrograde degeneration of this pathway (especially if this pathway branches into the nigrotectal projection as has been suggested in ref. 53).

In summary, we have provided evidence that receptor binding sites for GABA are located on neurons projecting between the SN and the caudal mesencephalon. While many of these sites are associated with afferent, probably 5HT-containing, terminals projecting from the median raphe to SN, other sites are likely to be located on efferent nigral descending projections.

5.2. Role of GABA for the activation of tyrosine hydroxylase (TH) in the nigrostriatal DA neurons

To examine the functional relationship between nigral GABA receptors and nigrostriatal DA activity, we have examined one index of nigrostriatal DA function: the affinity of striatal TH for the pteridine cofactor (105). When nigrostriatal DA neuronal activity is increased, either by direct electrical stimulation (106) or indirectly, in response to the blockade of DA receptors (107), an acceleration of the turnover rate of DA can be measured (108). Associated with these events is an increase in the apparent affinity of striatal TH for its pteridine cofactor; this allosteric activation of TH can be measured in vitro as a decrease in the Km of the enzyme for cofactor (109, 110). While the kinetics of striatal TH appears to be a useful indicator for enhanced function in nigrostriatal DA neurons, it is relatively insensitive to manipulations which depress the firing rate or metabolism of DA neurons below control values. Thus, there are few, if any, treatments which will cause a significant decrease

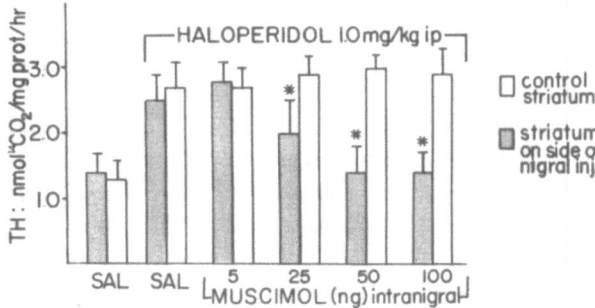

INTRANIGRAL MUSCIMOL: Attenuation (∗) of Haloperidol-Induced Activation of Striatal TH

Fig. 6. Intranigral muscimol: antagonism of the haloperidol-induced activation of striatal tyrosine hydroxylase (TH).

TH activity was measured in the right (open bars) and left (shaded bars) striatum of rats treated with saline (sal) or muscimol directly into the left substantia nigra via a chronically-implanted stainless-steel cannula. Muscimol was dissolved in saline and administered in a volume of 0.3 μl over 3 min. Ten min later, haloperidol (1.0 mg/kg), or its vehicle alone (.05% acetic acid, first pair of bars) was administered i.p. Animals were decapitated 40 min after intranigral injection. Assay for TH was done as previously described (109, 112) in the presence of a subsaturating amount of cofactor (.3 mM DMPH$_4$). Each value is the mean of eight rats. (Data from Gale and Guidotti, 113).

∗ p < .05 when compared with the contralateral (control) side.

(below control baseline) in the affinity of striatal TH for its cofactor. Therefore, in order to evaluate the inhibitory influence of GABAergic agents on DA neurons, we have selected a model in which striatal TH has been activated by systemic treatment with a DA receptor antagonist such as haloperidol. Against this background of TH activation (i.e. increased affinity for cofactor), it is possible to detect the actions of treatments which inhibit DA neuronal activity: these actions are manifest as a depression or reversal in the activation of striatal TH (105, 110, 112).

5.2.1. Blockade of striatal TH activation by direct stimulation of nigral GABA receptors

When GABA receptors in SN were stimulated by the local microinjection of muscimol, the haloperidol-induced activation of TH was blocked in the striatum ipsilateral to the muscimol treatment (113). In Fig. 6, Km values of striatal TH for pteridine cofactor are shown in the animals which received a unilateral intranigral injection of muscimol. The effect of muscimol could be reversed by intranigral injection of the GABA-receptor antagonist bicuculline methiodide (0.5 μg) which caused the reinstatement of striatal TH activation (112, 113). At the doses used, both muscimol and bicuculline were without effect on the Km of striatal TH for cofactor, when administered in the absence of haloperidol. These results suggest that nigral GABA receptors (most likely those located on the DA neurons) can exert an inhibitory action on nigrostriatal DA activity.

5.2.2. Blockade of striatal TH activation by elevation of nerve-terminal-associated nigral GABA

We have demonstrated that the direct stimulation of GABA receptors in SN can counteract the activating effect of haloperidol on striatal TH. Based on this, we were interested in determining whether the GABA produced by nerve terminals in SN could also be utilized to prevent the activation of the nigrostriatal DA neurons. Currently, several compounds are available which cause elevation of brain GABA after system administration; we selected 3 of these compounds each possessing a different mechanism of action, and a respectively distinct pharmacological profile. The compounds we investigated were: 1) amino-oxyacetic acid (AOAA), an agent that is thought to inhibit GABA-

384

transaminase (GABA-T) in vivo by interfering with the function of the pyridoxal phosphate cofactor (14, 115), 2) di-n-propylacetate (DPA, Depakene®, sodium valproate), which has been shown to inhibit GABA-T (116) and succinic semialdehyde dehydrogenase (117) competitively in vitro, but for which the in vivo mechanism of action remains controversial, and 3) gamma-vinyl-GABA (GVG), an analogue of the naturally occurring substrate for GABA-T, containing a latent reactive group which binds covalently to the enzyme's active site during catalytic conversion (84, 86).

These compounds have been demonstrated to have respectively different effects on GABA associated with the glial-perikarya compartment vs. that associated with nerve-terminal (see Iadarola and Gale, this volume). DPA appears to selectively increase GABA levels in synaptosomes (118) and causes regional increases in brain GABA which are in direct proportion to the respective GAD activity and basal GABA level of each area (79). Furthermore, in the SN, DPA was unable to significantly increase the GABA level under conditions in which the normally dense GABAergic innervation had been surgically removed (76). These data suggest that the increase in GABA after DPA is associated with the presence of nerve terminals.

In contrast, AOAA causes increases in brain GABA which, when analyzed on a regional basis, are not directly related to the density of GABAergic innervation (79). Moreover, this compound caused a net increase in GABA in the denervated SN which was nearly equivalent to that obtained in the intact SN (76). These results indicate that AOAA preferentially increases GABA in a compartment other than GABAergic nerve-terminals; this 'non-nerve-terminal' compartment is probably comprised mainly of GABAergic perikarya and glial cells.

Since GVG is an irreversible inhibitor of GABA-T, GABA levels are elevated for several days following a single injection of this agent. Analysis of the compartmental changes in GABA in the SN revealed that the portion of the GABA increase related to nerve-terminals varied a a function of time after GVG. While total GABA remained at a nearly constant level (several-fold over control) for several days after GVG, the proportion which was nerve-terminal dependent ranged from 0–50% between 12 and 60 h following i.p. treatment (77).

In view of the differences between these drugs

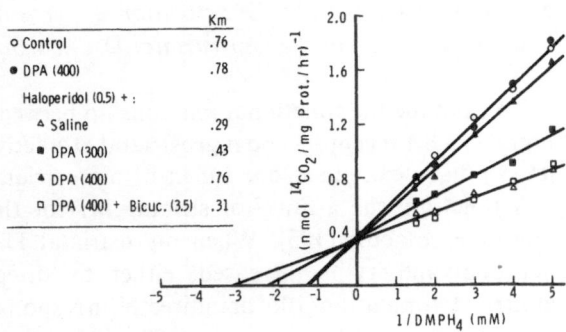

Fig. 7. Effect of DPA on the haloperidol-induced activation of striatal TH: reversal by bicuculline.

Double-reciprocal plot of the initial velocity of striatal TH against various concentrations of $DMPHA_4$ in the presence of 0.1 mM tyrosine. Time of administration of compounds before sacrifice was: haloperidol, 40 min; DPA, 30 min; and bicuculline (bicuc.), 15 min. Each point represents the mean obtained from ten rats. No seizure activity occurred in any of the animals which received the combined treatments. The S.E. was less than 10% of the mean.

with respect to their ability to influence nerve-terminal GABA in SN, we were interested in determining whether these differences would be related to the ability of the drugs to influence the functional activity of nigrostriatal DA neurons. We therefore assessed the ability of DPA, AOAA and GVG to antagonize the haloperidol-induced activation of striatal TH.

As shown in Fig. 7, DPA (400 mg/kg) completely prevented the haloperidol-induced decrease in the K_m of striatal TH for $DMPH_4$. A dose of 300 mg/kg was found to partially antagonize the action of haloperidol on striatal TH. DPA alone was without effect on the kinetic properties of striatal TH.

In order to determine whether GABA receptors were involved in the ability of DPA to reverse the haloperidol-induced activation of striatal TH, we treated rats with the GABA-receptor antagonist, bicuculline (3.5 mg/kg s.c.). As shown in Fig. 7, the antagonistic effect of DPA on the haloperidol-induced striatal TH-activation was completely reversed by bicuculline. Thus, it appears that in this situation, DPA is working via a GABA-receptor mediated mechanism.

The effect of DPA on nigral GABA was dose-dependent. A dose of 200 mg/kg of DPA did not produce a significant increase in GABA levels measured in SN. Doses of 300 mg/kg and 400

Table 7. Effect of AOAA on Km of striatal TH for DMPH$_4$ in rats treated with haloperidol. Drugs were administered intraperitoneally at the following times before decapitation: AOAA, 120 min; haloperidol, 40 min. Each value represents the mean ± S.E. of five animals.

Pretreatment	Dose (mg/kg)	Km of striatal TH for DMPH$_4$ (mM)		GABA in SN (nmol/mg prot)
		Saline	Haloperidol (.5 mg/kg)	
Saline		0.78 ± 0.05	0.28 ± 0.04*	102.1 ± 8.4
AOAA	(20)	0.76 ± 0.07	· 0.32 ± 0.05*	136.4 ± 8.5*
	(40)	0.80 ± 0.05	0.29 ± 0.02*	161.3 ± 9.8*
	(60)	0.76 ± 0.08	0.41 ± 0.04**	211.8 ± 13.4*

* p < .05 when compared with saline treated rats.

** p < .05 when compared with saline and haloperidol treated rats.

mg/kg of DPA, which were effective in attenuating the haloperidol-induced TH activation, significantly increased nigral GABA levels to 125 and 137% of control values. Based on our previous analysis of compartmental changes in GABA after DPA, these values would correspond to a 29 and 41% increase in nerve-terminal related GABA in SN. The results of the studies on striatal TH indicate that this increase in nerve-terminal GABA in SN can be utilized to influence the DA-containing nigral projections to striatum.

In contrast, AOAA only partially prevented the haloperidol-induced activation of striatal TH at a dose (60 mg/kg) that increased total GABA in SN by 100% over control (Table 7). With lower doses of AOAA, an increase in nigral GABA by as much as 60% over control was achieved without evidence of a functional impact on TH activity in nigrostriatal terminals: AOAA, at 20 and 40 mg/kg i.p. was without effect on the Km of striatal TH in the presence of haloperidol (Table 7). Doses of AOAA higher than 60 mg/kg could not be examined due to the toxicity of this agent at such doses.

The observation that an excessive increase in GABA was required for obtaining functional effects with AOAA, is consistent with the proposal that AOAA increases GABA to a large extent in compartments (GABA-containing neural perikarya and glial cells) which are not directly related to GABAergic neurotransmission (76, 119, 120). However, when changes specifically related to *nerve-terminal* GABA are evaluated (76, 77, 79), the estimated increase produced in this compartment by 60 mg/kg AOAA is, in fact, nearly equivalent to that produced by 300 mg/kg DPA

(approximately 30% over control). Thus, despite the differences in the mechanisms of action of these two compounds, it appears that when they are administered in doses which are equieffective with respect to elevating nerve-terminal GABA, their functional effects are quite similar.

The effect of GVG on the haloperidol-induced activation of striatal TH was studied over a time course of days, since we have previously determined

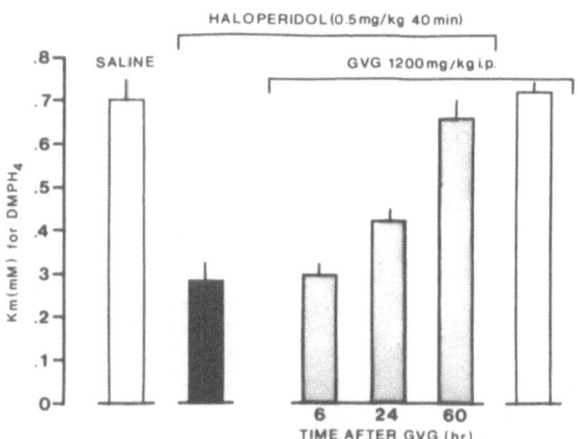

Fig. 8. Effect of gamma-vinyl GABA on the haloperidol-induced activation of striatal TH.

The Km of striatal TH for DMPH$_4$ was obtained from a Lineweaver-Burke analysis of TH activity obtained in the presence of five concentrations of DMPH$_4$ between .15 and .8 mM. Control rats did not receive haloperidol (clear bars); all other rats (black or shaded bars) received haloperidol (0.5 mg/kg i.p.) 40 min before decapitation. GVG (1200 mg/kg i.p.) was administered 6, 24 or 60 h prior to killing (as indicated in Fig.). Each value is the mean of 4–6 rats. The shaded bars corresponding to 24 and 60 h were significantly different from haloperidol alone (black bar), p < .05.

386

that a single intraperitoneal dose of GVG influences nerve-terminal GABA only after a delay of more than 12 h (77). Thus, the ability of GVG to prevent the haloperidol-induced decrease in the Km of striatal TH for DMPH$_4$, was evaluated at 6, 24 and 60 h following a single injection of GVG (1200 mg/kg i.p.). No effect on TH was seen at 6 h; at 24 h, the haloperidol-induced TH activation was partially antagonized, whereas 60 h after GVG, complete blockade of TH activation was obtained (Fig. 8). GVG alone did not affect the kinetic properties of striatal TH at any of the time points studied.

It is noteworthy that the GVG-induced increase in nigral GABA was maximal by 6 h after i.p. injection; despite this fact, no effect on striatal TH could be detected in our model. This observation is consistent with our finding that within the first 12 h after GVG treatment, no significant effect on the nerve-terminal-associated compartment of GABA could be detected (77). Moreover, the delayed functional effect of GVG on striatal TH is reminiscent of the time-course which we have observed in our studies of the anticonvulsant actions of GVG (77, see Iadarola and Gale, this volume): peak anticonvulsant actions, like the peak effect on striatal TH, were obtained at 60 h after a single i.p. injection of GVG.

To further analyze the impact of an elevation of nerve-terminal GABA in SN with respect to an influence of nigrostriatal DA neurons, we decided to restrict the drug-induced elevation of GABA to the vicinity of SN. As was previously done with muscimol, we applied GVG directly into one SN via a chronically implanted cannula. In these studies, we examined the effects of GVG within several hours of injection. This time course was chosen based on a compartmental analysis of the GABA elevation which took place following direct microinjection of GVG into the SN (see Iadarola and Gale, this volume). Since a significant portion of the GABA elevation was nerve-terminal-dependent at 3 and 6 h after direct microinjection, we selected these time points to evaluate the action of intranigral GVG on the haloperidol-induced activation of striatal TH. Fig. 9 shows that at 3 h after intranigral GVG (1 μg in 1 μl), there was a partial antagonism of the haloperidol-induced decrease in the Km of striatal TH for cofactor; by 6 h after GVG, the antagonism of the kinetic change in TH was complete. Intranigral GVG alone was without effect on the Km of striatal TH for cofactor.

Thus, although functional effects of GVG on the nigrostriatal system required a long latency to be manifest after systemic treatment, they emerged within a few hours after microinjection directly into SN. This was also true in our studies of the anticonvulsant action of GVG, in which seizure protection was obtained within hours after the intracerebral application of GVG (121, see Iadarola and Gale, this volume). The precise reason for the discrepancy between the latencies of action of systemic vs. intracerebrally-applied GVG is, at present, a matter of speculation. Nevertheless, it is clear that the functional effects on the nigrostriatal system (as well as anticonvulsant effects) are correlated with an elevation of GABA related to GABAergic nerve terminals. Moreover, the results obtained with the microinjection of GVG directly into SN add further support to the proposal that the GABA produced and released by GABAergic nerve-terminals in SN can exert an inhibitory influence on nigrostriatal DA function.

The ability of GABA agonists to depress metabolism and utilization of DA in nigrostriatal neurons has also been demonstrated using various indices of in vivo DA metabolism. Thus, DPA and muscimol were found effective in antagonizing the halo-

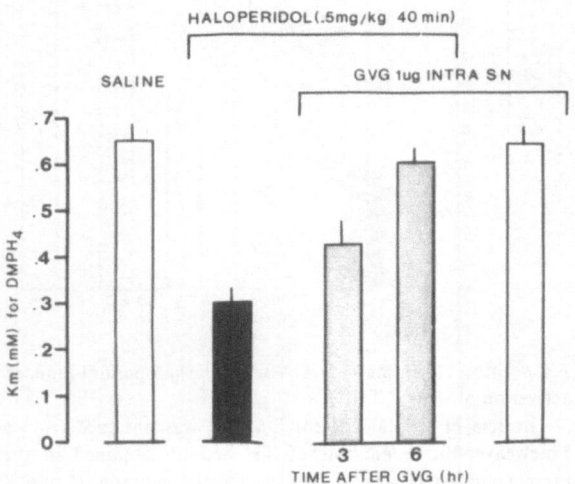

Fig. 9. Effect of intranigral GVG on the haloperidol-induced activation of striatal TH.

Experimental design was similar to that of Fig. 8 (see legend to Fig. 8) except that GVG (5 μg) was microinjected directly into SN, 3 or 6 h before killing rats (shaded bars).

Values represented by the shaded bars were significantly different from haloperidol alone (black bar), p < .05.

peridol-induced increase in striatal DOPA formation (122), and the GABA receptor agonists SL76002 and muscimol have been found to antagonize the neuroleptic-induced stimulation of DA utilization in striatum (123, 124 DA depletion following inhibition of DA synthesis was used as an index of DA utilization). In addition, systemic administration of muscimol and SL76002 (124), systemic or intranigral administration of gamma-acetylenic GABA (an irreversible GABA transaminase inhibitor) (125) and intranigral injection of muscimol (126) or gabaculline (an irreversible inhibitor of GABA-transaminase) (127) have been demonstrated to cause a depression in parameters associated with striatal DA utilization, including DA metabolite levels (125–127), DA release (124), DOPA formation (124), and the rate of DA depletion following inhibition of DA synthesis (124, 125). These data are consistent with our results on striatal TH and reinforce the notion that nigrostriatal DA neurons are sensitive to GABA-mediated inhibitory control.

5.2.3. Indirect influences of GABA on DA cells: dynamic role of GABA in SN

In contrast to the results just discussed, several studies have found that directly acting GABA receptor agonists can cause an apparent *stimulation* of metabolism and release of DA in striatum (128–131). Even in experiments in which muscimol was found to antagonize the stimulation of striatal DA metabolism induced by haloperidol, muscimol was able to cause a modest stimulation of DA metabolism by itself (122). Initially it seems paradoxical that activation of GABA receptors (presumably in SN) could both stimulate DA neurons and prevent their being stimulated by haloperidol. However, if we recognize that these two actions may be mediated by different mechanisms, the problem becomes more approachable.

Recent electrophysiological studies have demonstrated the ability of GABA agonists, as well as GABA itself, to cause stimulation of the activity of nigrostriatal DA neurons (132–134). This has been observed after systemic administration of low doses of muscimol (132–134) as well as after direct microiontophoretic application of muscimol or GABA into SN (133, 134). This excitatory effect of GABA on the nigrostriatal DA cells appears not to be exerted directly on the DA cells, but may be an indirect effect mediated by actions on other cellular elements in the pars reticulata of SN (133). Thus, GABA may cause the disinhibition of nigral DA cells under conditions in which selected GABAergic receptors in pars reticulata are activated. On the other hand, GABA and muscimol when applied directly onto DA neurons exerted a consistently inhibitory action (133, 134). It seems therefore, that the action of GABA on DA neurons in SN is highly dependent upon the population of receptors being occupied.

From this perspective, it is possible to view the influence of GABA in SN as highly dynamic and dependent upon the relative state of activity of the various nigral processes. Under conditions in which DA neurons are relatively inactive, it may be assumed that inhibitory influences (e.g. GABA, serotonin) on nigral DA neurons are predominating. In this situation it would be difficult to detect additional inhibition resulting from the activation of GABA receptors on DA neurons; instead the system would be prone to exhibiting disinhibitory responses to GABA. This would be true in most of the electrophysiological studies, as well as in many studies in which GABA agonists have been studied for actions on DA metabolism.

On the other hand, when DA neurons are relatively active, stimulation of nigral GABA receptors can provide the inhibitory influence necessary to counteract the excitatory drive on the DA neurons. In this case, the indirect disinhibitory actions of GABA would be relatively insignificant against the elevated baseline of DA activity, and the direct inhibitory influence of GABA on DA neurons is revealed. This would be true in cases in which DA neuronal firing rate and metabolism have been enhanced due to the presence of haloperidol. Thus, the mechanism by which GABA influences nigral DA neurons may depend upon the relative state of activity of the DA neurons; the resulting effects of GABA agonists must be interpreted within this context.

It is also important to consider whether directly-acting GABA-receptor agonists such as muscimol (or exogenous GABA) necessarily elicit the same responses as would be produced by the release of endogenous GABA from presynaptic terminals. The answer to this question is probably 'no', since directly-acting GABA receptor agonists act independently of the location and activity of presynaptic GABA terminals. In this context, it is interesting to note that excitatory influences on the firing rates and metabolism of nigrostriatal DA neurons have been observed with drugs which are primarily directly-acting GABA receptors agonists (122, 128–134), whereas inhibitory actions on DA metabolism are observed after drugs which elevate endogenous GABA (122, 124, 127); for example, muscimol and DPA were found to respectively increase and decrease striatal DOPA formation (122). Thus, while GABAergic transmission in SN appears to be capable of inhibiting DA neurons, we cannot assume that the system is normally (physiologically) capable of using GABA to *disinhibit* these neurons as well. While the excitatory influence which direct GABA receptor agonists have on DA neurons may be highly significant for the pharmacology of these agents, the physiological meaning of this phenomenon remains to be explored.

From the evidence discussed above, it is apparent that the nigrostriatal DA neurons are subject to control by GABAergic synapses in the SN. This link between GABA and DA in SN forms the final connection in what seems to be a closed loop between the nigra and striatum. As described earlier, the activity of striatal DA receptors influences striatonigral GABA function; the ability of nigral GABA receptors to influence nigrostriatal DA function completes a return trip through this neural loop (see Fig. 1).

5.3. Actions of GABA on non-dopaminergic nigral efferents

From a 'dopaminocentric' point of view, the most important way to get information out of SN is via the nigrostriatal DA neurons. It should be evident, however, that the flow of information in this system cannot merely proceed in endless circles; if it did, our attempts to relate this information to either normal or pathological behaviors would prove futile. We have documented the fact that the majority of nigral receptors for GABA are associated with non-DA neural pathways; it is likely that these pathways are at least as important as the DA efferents for transmitting the synaptic signals which have been integrated in SN.

Evidence that GABA can have functional effects on nigral neurons which are not dopaminergic derives from behavioral and electrophysiological studies of the actions of GABA and GABA agonists applied directly into SN.

The behavioral responses induced by the unilateral and bilateral activation of nigral GABA receptors in the rat (contralateral rotation and stereotypies, respectively) can still be obtained in animals in which DA receptors have been blocked by haloperidol (98, 100). Moreover, as we have already discussed (see section 4.3. above), the contralateral rotation induced by intranigral muscimol is not only maintained in rats with 6-OHDA-induced destruction of the nigrostriatal DA neurons, but exhibits an apparent supersensitivity. These observations indicate that nigrostriatal DA transmission is not essential for the expression of certain behavior patterns mediated by nigral GABA receptors.

Single units in the SN have been examined for their responses to the direct microiontophoretic application of GABA or GABA agonists, and it appears that the non-dopaminergic neurons of the zona reticulata are more sensitive to the inhibitory effects of GABA than are the DA cells of the zona compacta (133, 134). On this basis, it has been suggested that the non-dopaminergic neurons of the SN-zona reticulata may be more subject to GABAergic inhibitory regulation than are the nigral DA neurons (134).

Thus, it appears that by inhibiting non-DA nigral efferent projections, the activation of nigral GABA receptors can induce marked alterations in spontaneous behavior. Moreover, it is likely that the GABA receptors responsible for these effects normally are subject to activation by the striatonigral GABAergic projections. In support of this proposal are the findings that destruction of the striatonigral GABA projections results in an increase in nigral GABA receptor binding even when nigrostriatal DA neurons are concomitantly destroyed (74, 75); accompanying this increase in binding is an increase in the muscimol-induced behavioral (74, 75) and electrophysiological (135) effects on SN zona reticulata neurons. Thus, in the absence of normal inhibitory control by striatonigral afferents, GABA receptors located on the non-DA nigral efferents appear to become supersensitive.

In addition to DA and non-DA nigral efferents, the 5HT-containing afferent terminals in SN appear to contain GABA receptors (see section 5.1.2.

above). The functional role of these presynaptic GABA receptors is, at present, a matter of speculation, but it is possible that they may mediate the inhibitory action of GABA on nigral 5HT release in vivo (136). If these GABA receptors influence 5HT release in SN, then their impact on nigral output would depend upon the functional role of 5HT in SN. There is some electrophysiological and biochemical evidence for an inhibitory role of 5HT in SN (49, 50, 102, 103) and destruction of the median raphe has been found to cause an increase in DA turnover in nigrostriatal neurons (137). If GABA, released from terminals in SN, causes a reduction in 5HT release, then the net action of GABA in such a circuit would be disinhibitory (see hypothetical circuit in Fig. 10). It may be possible, for example, that some of the apparently disinhibitory effects of

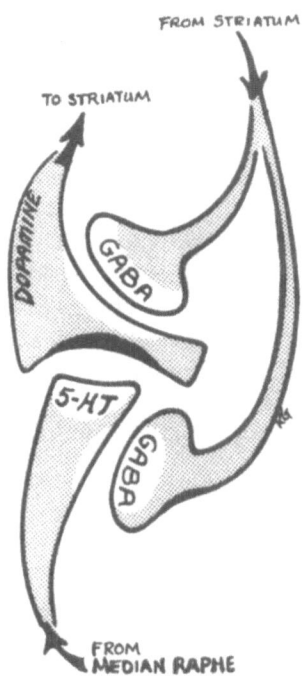

FROM STRIATUM

TO STRIATUM

DOPAMINE

GABA

5-HT

GABA

FROM MEDIAN RAPHE

Fig. 10. Hypothetical interaction between GABA, serotonin and DA neurons in SN.

Activation of GABA receptors, located on presynaptic serotonin terminals, may reduce or inhibit the release of serotonin. Serotonin can act on serotonin receptors located on DA neurons, causing inhibition of DA neuronal activity. A GABA agonist may inhibit DA neurons via a direct effect (on GABA receptors associated with DA neurons) and/or may disinhibit DA neurons via an indirect action mediated by serotonin. Conversely, a GABA receptor *antagonist,* could simultaneously block GABAergic inhibition and increase serotonergic inhibition on the DA neurons.

GABA and GABA agonists on nigral DA cells, as evidenced in studies of single unit activity in SN (133, 134), may be mediated by 5HT terminals.

The hypothetical circuit portrayed in Fig. 10 would also predict that, in certain circumstances, an increase in 5HT release could compensate for a reduction in GABAergic tone in SN. For example, we have previously reported that while the activation of nigrostriatal TH could be prevented by the stimulation of GABA receptors in SN, the blockade of nigral GABA receptors (e.g. by application of bicuculline) per se did not cause an activation of TH (112). Similarly, Waszczak et al. reported relatively slight effects of i.v. picrotoxin (a GABA antagonist) on the firing rate of nigral DA cells (134). If GABA exerts a tonic inhibitory effect on nigral DA neurons, it is difficult to explain why a blockade of GABA receptors would not release this inhibition. However, if 5HT terminals contain presynaptic receptors for GABA, this could account for why GABA receptor blockade might not necessarily stimulate nigral efferents: A GABA receptor antagonist would not only block the direct inhibitory influence of GABA on the nigral efferents, but at the same time would also reverse the inhibition of 5HT release (from 5HT terminals). In this context, the 5HT terminals in SN may serve a 'fail safe' function for the maintainance of inhibitory tone in SN. The significance of this interaction cannot be evaluated until the location of receptors for 5HT in SN is determined.

5.4. Nature of the non-dopaminergic nigral efferents

5.4.1. GABA-containing nigral efferents

As the scheme of the nigral neural circuity emerges, the next logical question concerns the nature of non-DA nigral efferents from zona reticulata. As described earlier (see Section 1.1.), these cells project to thalamus, superior colliculus, and reticular formation (51–56). Electrophysiological and anatomical evidence suggest that at least some of the nigrothalamic fibers and nigrotectal fibers may be collateral branches from the same nigral cells (138–141). These projections have been demonstrated to exert a predominantly inhibitory effect on cells in the superior colliculus and ventromedial or ventral lateral thalamus (139–143) and neurochemical evidence indicates that they are GABAergic (57–60). Less information exists with respect to the nigroreticular pathways, but anatomical tracing studies suggest that two pathways may exist: one projecting from the zona compacta to the central grey, and another projecting from the zona reticulata to the pedunculopontine nucleus of the mesencephalic tegmentum (53–56). The former projection may be DA-containing (52), while the latter projection has been suggested to be comprised of axonal branches of the nigrotectal neurons (53), and may be GABA-ergic (180).

Recently, it has been demonstrated that some of the efferent neurons of the zona reticulata give off axon collaterals within the SN (144). This raises the possibility that these neurons may control neural activity *within* the SN at the same time that they influence the various distant projection sites. If some of these collaterals are GABA-containing (which seems likely in view of the GABAergic nature of many of the nigral efferents), they may participate in local inhibitory (or disinhibitory) circuits.

5.4.2. GABA-GABA interactions in SN

From the results reviewed so far, it appears that GABAergic activity in SN can influence motor function via an interaction with non-DA nigral efferents, and that a portion of these efferents are likely to be GABA-containing. If such a GABA-GABA link is present in SN, it is possible that activation of GABA receptors in SN could influence the turnover of GABA in the nigral efferent neurons. We have obtained some preliminary

results which suggest that this may be the case. In animals into which muscimol (50 ng) was micro-injected into SN 10 min following GVG, we found that the initial rate of accumulation of GABA in SN was significantly less than that obtained in controls. To determine whether this depression in GABA accumulation was related to nigral afferents or efferents, we repeated these studies in rats in which we had eliminated the afferent GABAergic projections from the forebrain. In the GABA-denervated SN, muscimol was found to depress the GVG-induced accumulation of GABA; this reduction was of the same absolute value in the denervated and intact SN (Table 8). These data suggest, therefore, that the activation of nigral GABA receptors can inhibit the synthesis of GABA in cellular elements other than GABAergic afferent terminals. These elements may include the cell bodies of the GABAergic efferents and/or their local axon collaterals; it is also possible that GABAergic interneurons, if they exist in SN, could contribute to these changes.

5.4.3. Mediation of behavioral responses elicited by stimulation of nigral GABA receptors: importance of descending projections from SN

At this point it is pertinent to consider the relative importance of the various projections from SN zona reticulata with respect to the changes in motor function elicited by stimulation of nigral GABA receptors. The behavioral response which has received most attention in this context is the contra-

Table 8. Depression of GABA accumulation after intranigral application of muscimol in intact and denervated SN.

| Intranigral treatment | GABA (nmol/mg prot) | | Net decrease due to muscimol: | |
	Intact SN	Denervated SN	intact	denervated
Saline	99 ± 4	19 ± 2		
Muscimol (50 ng)	101 ± 5	18 ± 3	0	1
GVG (5 µg; 3h)				
+ Saline	202 ± 6	81 ± 4		
+ Muscimol (50 ng)	174 ± 8*	59 ± 4*	28	22

Values are means ± SEM from 4 animals
* Significantly different from GVG + Saline group $p < .05$

Muscimol was injected (0.2 µl over 5 min) 10 min following GVG (0.5 µl, over 10 min). Drugs were dissolved in saline. GABA was measured as previously described (179).

lateral asymmetry and rotational activity induced by unilateral stimulation of nigral GABA receptors (100, 101).

Kilpatrick et al. (59) studied the effects of lesions of the ventromedial nucleus of the thalamus on rotational behavior induced by intranigral muscimol application in rats. Unilateral lesions in the ventromedial thalamus produced either by electrocoagulation or by kainic acid injection were observed to attenuate the effect of muscimol (400 ng) placed in the ipsilateral SN. On the other hand, the local application of picrotoxin into this region of thalamus potentiated the response to intranigral muscimol, whereas elevation of thalamic GABA levels reduced the muscimol-induced rotation (59). Unilateral muscimol injections into the ventromedial thalamus produced a rotational response directed toward the side ipsilateral to the injection (59). These data suggest that a unilateral reduction in GABAergic transmission in the ventromedial thalamus can contribute to contralateral rotation; inhibition of the activity of nigrothalamic pathways which are presumably GABAergic (58–60, 143) represents one way of achieving such a reduction. Intranigral muscimol could therefore produce contralateral rotation by suppressing the activity of the nigrothalamic pathway, thereby disinhibiting thalamic neurons. Consistent with such a circuit is the observation that intranigral muscimol treatment increased the discharge rate of neurons in the parafascicular and ventromedial nuclei of the thalamus (60).

While thalamic projections may participate in the rotational response elicited by activation of nigral GABA receptors, these pathways do not appear to be *required* for the manifestation of this response to intranigral muscimol. This assertion is based on the observation that contraversive rotational activity was still obtained after intranigral muscimol treatment in rats in which all pathways rostral to SN were mechanically severed (46, 92, 145). The data, shown in Table 9, demonstrate that contralateral rotation induced by muscimol (50 ng) microinjected into the SN, was fully maintained even after complete cerebral hemitransections rostral to SN. Furthermore, equivalent responses to intranigral muscimol were obtained from microinjections into either hemisphere of the hemitransected rats. These data are in apparent contrast to those of Kilpatrick et al. (59) discussed above; although our transections severed the nigrothalamic pathways we found no attenuation of the behavioral response to intranigral muscimol. Several factors could account for this apparent discrepancy. Kilpatrick et al. employed very high doses of muscimol (almost an order of magnitude higher than the dose which we used and 100 times greater than the dose required for threshold effects); it is possible, that high doses may influence additional pathways or components of the circuitry not affected by lower doses. Another consideration is that our hemitransections destroyed the GABAergic afferents to SN, and as a result, may provoke a supersensitivity of nigral GABA receptors (75); it is possible that this could enhance (or reveal) an action of muscimol on those pathways (e.g. nigrotectal, nigroreticular) which are not damaged by our lesions. Finally, it is possible that lesions of the ventromedial thalamus indirectly alter corticofugal activity; a unilateral change in corticofugal activity could therefore account for the attenuation of muscimol-induced rotational behavior observed by Kilpatrick et al. (59). In contrast, our hemitransections would preclude the expression of any changes in forebrain activity.

Our hemitransection experiments indicate that descending nigral efferents are sufficient to main-

Table 9. Circling behavior (total turns in 3 min) in response to intranigral muscimol in rats with complete cerebral hemitransections rostral to SN.

| Hemisphere receiving microinjection | Intranigral injection | | | |
| | Saline | | Muscimol | |
	ipsi	contra	ipsi	contra
Hemitransected	4.0 ± .4	1.5 ± .2	0	55 ± 4
Intact	2.0 ± .2	5.0 ± .4	0	54 ± 3
Unlesioned controls	2.0 ± .3	3.0 ± .2	0	53 ± 3

All intranigral injections were made stereotaxically into SN in rats in which the transection was made seven days before. Values represent the mean number of total turns in a 3 min period for a group of 4–6 rats ± S.E.M. Ipsi = ipsilateral, Contra = contralateral (with respect to side of injection). Muscimol (0.2 nmol in 0.5 μl saline) was infused over 3 min; this dose was previously found to be maximally effective for producing circling behavior. The hemitransections, which were located 1–2 mm rostral to SN, completely severed all ascending and descending fibers connecting the midbrain and ipsilateral forebrain (46). Data is also shown for muscimol injections made into the SN in the intact hemisphere of hemitransected rats, and into the SN of rats which had not been lesioned.

tain expression of the rotational behavior following unilateral GABA receptor stimulation in SN. The pathways which are the most likely candidates for mediating this behavior would therefore be the nigroreticular and nigrotectal. At present, very little is known about the physiology of these pathways, but it is interesting that nigrotectal projections may impinge on the same neurons which receive afferents from neck muscles (146, 147).

6. Opposing actions of striatal and nigral GABA synapses

Having considered some of the functional effects in which GABAergic synapses participate in SN, we can return to the striatum in an attempt to assess the nature of the influence which striatal GABA neurons exert on the nigral outputs. The influence of striatal GABA interneurons on nigral activity is necessarily indirect, mediated by striatonigral and striatopallido-nigral pathways. At least one way in which striatal GABA interneurons may exert an influence in SN is by regulating the activity of the striatonigral GABA pathway; we have already discussed the ability of striatal GABA transmission to inhibit striatonigral GABA activity (see section 3). We might predict from this relationship that blockade of striatal GABA receptors could have an effect on nigral cells similar to that elicited by the stimulation of nigral GABA receptors.

6.1. Effect of intrastriatal GABA antagonists on nigrostriatal DA neurons

We selected the activation of nigrostriatal TH as a model system in which to test the above prediction. Since we have already demonstrated a clearcut inhibition of the activation of striatal TH by the intranigral application of GABA-agonists (see section 5.2.2.) we were interested in determining whether a similar effect could be obtained after intrastriatal application of GABA-antagonists. The compounds which we selected were: 1) the GABA receptor antagonist, bicuculline methiodide, and 2) an inhibitor of GABA synthesis, isoniazid; these compounds were microinjected directly into the head of the caudate-putamen (unilaterally) 10 min before the i.p. injection of haloperidol. The results

Table 10. Effect of intrastriatal microinjection of bicuculline or isoniazid on the haloperidol-induced activation of striatal tyrosine hydroxylase.

| Intrastriatal microinjection | Striatal TH: Km (mM) for DMPH$_4$ | |
	Control	Haloperidol (0.5 mg/kg i.p.)
Saline	0.75 ± 0.04	0.32 ± 0.05
Bicuculline (10 μg/1.5 μl)	0.73 ± 0.02	0.76 ± 0.06*
Isoniazid (140 μg/2 μl)	0.80 ± 0.06	0.71 ± 0.04*

* Significantly different from haloperidol-treated rats receiving saline microinjection. p < 0.01.

of this study, shown in Table 10, demonstrate the ability of both intrastriatal treatments to prevent the haloperidol-induced decrease in the Km of striatal TH for cofactor. On the other hand, as we might expect, these treatments do not prevent the activation of nigrostriatal TH when placed in the SN. The microinjections of isoniazid resulted in greater than a 50% reduction in GABA levels in the injected nucleus. These data are consistent with the proposal that striatonigral GABA projections are subject to inhibition by striatal GABA neurons. The blockade of striatal GABA receptors, or a reduction in striatal GABA levels, can withdraw this inhibition and allow release of GABA onto postsynaptic sites in the SN. Our examination of one of these sites, namely the nigrostriatal DA neurons, indicates that nigral GABA-ergic actions may, in fact, be augmented by a reduction in GABAergic tone in the striatum.

6.2. Opposing actions of striatal and nigral GABA on behavioral responses mediated by non-dopaminergic nigral efferents

In the study described above, behavioral manifestations which accompanied the unilateral injections are consistent with the concept of counterposing actions of GABAergic synapses in striatum and SN. The blockade of GABA receptors or the depletion of GABA content in SN was associated with ipsiversive rotational activity (Table 11), while similar manipulations in the striatum resulted in contraversive movements. On the other

Table 11. Circling behavior after intranigral isoniazid correlated with depletion of GABA in SN.

Time (min) after infusion of isoniazid, 1 µmol	GABA (nmol/mg prot.)			Turns in 3 min	
	Control side	Treated side	% treated/control	ipsi	contra
10	101 ± 8	92 ± 5	91	1	2
20	98 ± 6	70 ± 8	71	8	0
30	97 ± 5	40 ± 3	39	29	1

Isoniazid (1.0 µmol) dissolved in distilled H_2O was infused unilaterally into SN (1.0 µl over 5 min) via a stereotaxically-positioned stainless-steel cannula (28 g) while the rat was under ether anesthesia. Coordinates for injection were: AP + 2.6 mm, Lat 2.0 mm, DV −2.8 mm. Time after infusion of isoniazid was measured from the end of the injection period. Circling behavior was measured as the total number of complete (360°) turns made in each direction (defined with respect to side of injection) over a 3 min period during which the rat was placed on a large table top free of obstacles. Within 5 min after removal from the stereotaxic apparatus, all animals were awake and able to locomote. Rats were sacrificed immediately after the 3 min observation period. The data represent mean values obtained from six animals. S.E.M. for behavioral data was less than 10% of mean values.

hand, in experiments in which muscimol or GVG was applied to the striatum, rats exhibited asymmetrical postures and circling directed ipsiversively, in contrast to the contraversive rotation elicited by these agents in the SN. It is possible therefore that the manipulations of GABA activity in striatum are expressed, in part, through their opposing effects on GABA transmission in SN.

Table 12. Effects of DA or GABA agonists on spontaneous motor behavior: a disinhibitory zig-zag through the basal ganglia.

Nucleus	Transmitter system	Effect on motor behavior	
		Hyperactivity	Hypoactivity
Striatum	DA	X	
Striatum	GABA		X
SN	GABA	X	
Thalamus or superior colliculus	GABA		X

Hyperactivity includes bilateral manifestations such as stereotyped sniffing, chewing and gnawing, and unilateral manifestations such as contraversive circling.

Hypoactivity includes bilateral manifestations such as catalepsy, akinesia, decreased sensory responsiveness, and unilateral manifestations such as *ipsiversive* circling.

The 'X' designates the predominant nature of the response to local (e.g. intrastriatal, intranigral, etc.) application of DA or GABA agonist drugs (as indicated).

We have now collected what appears to be a series of GABA-GABA linkages: striatal GABA interneurons inhibit GABA projections to the SN, which in turn inhibit nigral efferents, some of which are GABAergic. This succession of inhibitory links means that the action of GABA on the final motor output of the system will alternate from facilitatory to inhibitory at each successive junction. The rotational behavior provides a very simple example of this sort of synaptic zigzag: the direction of this behavior after unilateral injection of GABA agonists is ipsiversive with striatal placements, contraversive with nigral placements, and ipsiversive with either thalamic or tectal placements (see Table 12). Moreover, bilateral activation of *striatal* GABA receptors can elicit both a reduction in motor activity and cataleptic responses, whereas the bilateral activation of *nigral* GABA receptors results in hyperactivity and stereotyped behaviors. Combined with our knowledge of the anatomical circuitry (22-24, 33-36, 43, 51-60) and some electrophysiological verification (35, 60, 139-143), these observations are consistent with a chain of disinhibitory synapses (see Fig. 11). Whether or not these sequences are related in a strictly linear fashion is less clear, since the absolute requirement for any single link in the expression of a particular function has yet to be demonstrated. We should also keep in

394

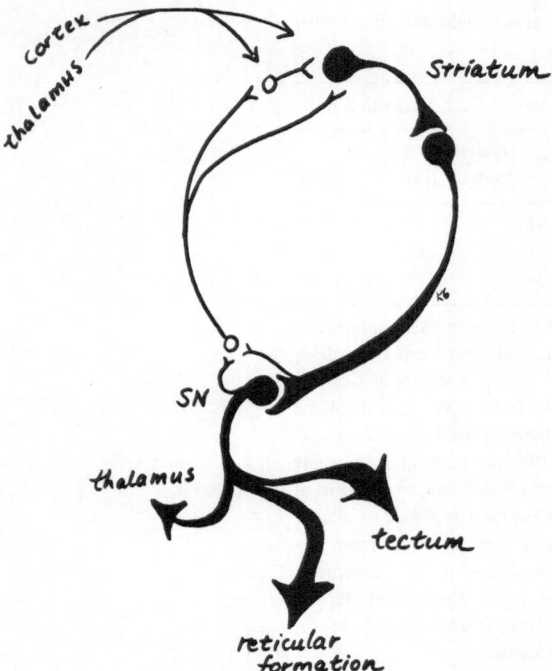

Fig. 11. Striatonigral outflow: Serial GABAergic links and regulation by DA.

Once neural information (coming from various cortical regions and thalamus) has been integrated in striatum, the striatonigral fibers provide a major outflow route for this information. Excitatory influences impinging on striatal GABAergic interneurons (from striatal afferents or intrinsic cholinergic neurons) increase the inhibitory action of these neurons on the striatonigral GABAergic projections; this in turn results in disinhibition of nigral efferents (to thalamus, reticular formation and tectum), many of which are GABAergic. These nigral efferents exert an important influence (possibly inhibitory) on motor activity and posture.

The information outflow through the nigral relay is monitored by DA neurons (and possibly by a non-DA nigrostriatal pathway as well), which can then regulate the information processing capacity of the striatum, either by modulating corticostriatal afferents or by inhibiting striatal interneurons, thereby causing disinhibition of striatonigral GABAergic activity.

GABAergic links are portrayed in heavy black in the figure.

mind that these circuits do not exist in isolation, but interdigitate and converge with a host of other circuits; these other circuits may exert actions which are regulatory, complementary, redundant or competitive with the synaptic functions that we have focused upon (see introductory section 1.1. for discussion of some of these circuits).

7. Serial GABA links and disinhibition in striato-nigral circuits: implications for the sites of action of GABAergic drugs

In order to evaluate or predict the impact which alterations in GABA transmission can have on neural processing in the striatum, SN and the nigral efferent projection areas, we need to gain some appreciation of the normal balance of GABAergic tone that exists between the various junctions. Each of the various GABAergic synaptic links that have been discussed have at one time or another been described as responsible for maintaining 'tonic inhibition'. Obviously, if the GABAergic neurons are connected in series it is not possible that they can all be simultaneously tonically active. Some sort of a reciprocal relationship must exist between these links with respect to their state of activity.

An indication of the degree of GABAergic tone at a particular site can be obtained by determining the relative sensitivity of the system to GABA agonists and antagonists at that site. If GABA is tonically active, then we might expect to see relatively slight effects of a GABA receptor agonist; under these conditions the *blockade* of GABA receptors should cause marked changes. These relationships would be reversed under conditions of little or no GABAergic tone; against this baseline, a GABA receptor agonist would have marked effects, whereas it might be difficult to measure a change produced by an antagonist. Although there has been very little systematic examination of these types of relationships in the basal ganglia, there are some observations that may be suggestive. We have examined the relative effects of local GABA receptor blockade and stimulation on the rate of accumulation of GABA within the striatum and the SN, respectively. These data are shown in Table 13, and it appears that in the striatum, bicuculline causes a marked increase in GABA accumulation whereas muscimol causes a relatively slight decrease. This may indicate that the GABA receptors which exert an inhibitory control over GABA synthesis in the striatum are normally tonically active; as a result, striatal GABA synthesis can be markedly enhanced by removing this source of inhibition. In contrast, the effect of muscimol in depressing *nigral* GABA synthesis is considerably more pronounced than the stimulatory effect of bicuculline (Table 13), suggesting that perhaps the GABAergic synaptic tone

Table 13. GVG-induced GABA accumulation in SN and CP: effects of stimulation or blockade of GABA receptors.

Brain region	Microinjection	GABA (nmol/mg prot)	Net changes: from control	from GVG + saline
SN	Saline	99.1 ± 2.9		
	GVG +			
	saline	158.7 ± 6.9	60	
	muscimol	138.2 ± 5.8*	39	−21
	bicuculline	150.5 ± 4.3	52	
CP	Saline	21.8 ± 0.6		
	GVG +			
	saline	68.2 ± 4.1	46	
	muscimol	54.7 ± 2.5*	33	−13
	bicuculline	96.0 ± 4.4*	74	+28

Muscimol (50 ng in SN; 500 ng in CP) or bicuculline (500 ng in SN; 10 μg in CP) were infused 10 min following GVG (5 μg in SN; 20 μg in CP). For measurement of GABA, rats with CP injections were killed at 3 h, rats with SN injections were killed at 1.5 h.

in SN is relatively low. The possibility that there is not a high degree of tonic GABAergic inhibition in SN is also suggested by observations from behavioral (49, 98, 148), neurochemical (112) and electrophysiological (134) studies in which nigral responses to GABA receptor stimulation were consistently more pronounced than were the nigral responses elicited by GABA receptor antagonism. Thus, we can adopt the following working hypothesis: Striatal GABA interneurons are tonically active and are, in part, responsible for keeping striatonigral GABAergic projections in a relatively inactive state. As a result, GABAergic efferents from SN would be expected to be tonically active; this has been suggested to be the case, for example, with the nigrothalamic projections (59, 60).

This dynamic relationship between GABAergic links in a neural circuit has significant implications for the pharmacology of GABA. The net effect which a GABA agonist will exert on specific features of motor function will depend critically on the brain regions which are most sensitive to the actions of the drug. This in turn will depend on the normal GABAergic tone (with respect to turnover, release and receptor activity) of the region and the mechanism of action of the drug (presynaptic vs.

postsynaptic, direct vs. indirect). An additional factor to be taken into account is the way in which the normal dynamic balances of the system are altered as a result of previous or concurrent treatment with other drugs, or as a result of pathology. Some of these considerations will be discussed below (Section 9) in the context of the clinical relevance of GABAergic agents.

8. DA – GABA interactions: synthesis and speculation

The chain of GABAergic links which starts in the striatum and relays through the nigral efferents, is subject to control by DA terminals in the striatum. As we have already discussed (see sections 2 & 4) DA terminals exert an inhibitory influence on the striatal GABA interneurons, and a disinhibitory influence on striatonigral GABA activity. From this point of view, the GABA-mediated synaptic activity in SN is downstream from the influence of DA neurons (see Fig. 1 and 11). It is likely therefore that many of the behavioral actions of DA stimulants are expressed via the release of GABA in SN. Consistent with this proposal is the observed similarity between the stereotyped behaviors induced by DA agonists and the behaviors induced by the bilateral activation of GABA receptors in SN. In addition, the behavioral responses to the unilateral stimulation of striatal DA receptors is qualitatively similar to the unilateral stimulation of nigral GABA receptors: both manipulations cause contraversive rotation. Furthermore, the blockade of nigral GABA receptors can attenuate the stereotyped behavior induced by the DA agonist, apomorphine (149) supporting the idea that some of the behavioral effects of DA stimulation may be dependent upon GABA transmission in SN.

Is it possible then, that chronic alterations of GABA transmission in SN could contribute to some of the behavioral changes observed after longterm treatment with DA antagonists? The answer is likely to be affirmative. It is well known, for example, that an enhanced behavioral response ('supersensitivity') to DA stimulants can be observed when animals are tested 5–10 days after cessation of chronic neuroleptic treatment (150, 151). We have demonstrated that chronic treatment with neuroleptic drugs results in an increased density of nigral GABA receptors (Table 2) and an enhanced behavioral response to stimulation of these receptors (Table 3). Thus, it is tempting to speculate that the enhanced response to DA agonists following chronic blockade of DA receptors is actually due to the fact that the nigral GABA receptors which mediate this response have become supersensitive.

A similar argument can be used to account for the contralateral turning induced by apomorphine in rats unilaterally lesioned with 6-OHDA (152, 153). Again, we have a situation in which GABA receptors show a supersensitive response, in the SN of the lesioned hemisphere. These receptors would therefore be more sensitive to GABA released into SN as an indirect result of striatal DA receptor stimulation; the rats would be expected to rotate contraversive to the supersensitive side.

An additional way in which DA receptor stimulation may influence nigral GABA activity is by a direct action in SN. There is evidence that DA-sensitive adenylate cyclase may be located on the terminals of GABAergic afferents to SN (154, 155) and it is possible that the activation of these receptors could enhance nigral GABA release. In this context, it is interesting that Kozlowski et al., could produce contralateral turning by injecting apomorphine directly into the SN of 6-OHDA lesioned rats and, moreover, that this turning was abolished by prior removal of the GABA afferents to SN (156). Thus, some of the behavioral actions of DA stimulants may be exerted via presynaptic receptors on GABAergic terminals in SN and this action may be revealed or exaggerated under conditions (e.g. 6-OHDA lesions) which induce receptor supersensitivity.

If an alteration in nigral GABA receptors can explain changes in behavioral responses to DA stimulants, what role do supersensitive DA receptors play? It has been assumed for several years that the enhanced behavioral responses to DA agonists (after DA receptor blockade or 6-OHDA lesions) is a direct result of DA receptor supersensitivity. The fact that unilateral 6-OHDA lesions or chronic neuroleptic treatment caused an increased in the binding of radiolabeled DA-antagonists was taken as strong evidence for DA-receptor supersensitivity. The binding studies and the behavioral studies were thereafter assumed to be reflections of the same phenomenon, and a causative relationship was inferred (152, 157). Recently, however, this relationship has been questioned, primarily on the basis that the respective time courses for the development of behavioral supersensitivity and the increase in ^{3}H-spiperone binding, are not coincident (158, 159). Moreover, marked behavioral supersensitivity to DA agonists has been reported under conditions in which no alteration of striatal DA receptors was detected (160).

Additional evidence in support of a critical role for GABA receptors in the development of supersensitive responses to DA agonists comes from chronic neuroleptic studies in which a GABA receptor agonist was administered concurrently. First, it should be noted that chronic administration of GABA agonists is unlikely to prevent the proliferation of striatal DA receptors (161); on the contrary, these agents have actually been observed to cause an *increase* in striatal DA receptors (162), probably an indirect result of depressing the activity of nigrostriatal neurons. Nevertheless, Lloyd (163) found that the behavioral supersensitivity to apomorphine, which is normally produced by chronic treatment with haloperidol, was significantly reduced in rats which had been treated chronically with a GABA agonist concurrently with the haloperidol treatment. This suggests that, by preventing the development of supersensitive GABA receptors, chronic GABA receptor stimulation may attenuate the development of behavioral supersensitivity to DA agonists.

At the same that information flows from the striatum to the SN and then to thalamus, colliculus and tegmentum, a certain amount of this information returns to the striatum via the nigrostriatal pathways. In this context, nigrostriatal DA neurons could be thought of as a feedback pathway: responsible for monitoring the relay activity passing through the SN, and accordingly adjusting the fine tuning in the striatum (see Fig. 1 and 11). The information which funnels into striatum from throughout the cortex must be integrated, condensed and inevitably channeled through pallidal or nigral outputs. Perhaps DA participates in this funnelling process by controlling the pattern and rate of information flow through the striatum, keeping this coordinated with the neural activity emanating from the SN.

9. Relevance to human disorders

Based on the evidence reviewed here and the foregoing discussion, some speculation concerning the role of GABA synapses in the therapy of basal ganglia disorders seems appropriate. Two types of disorders will be considered:
1) a drug-induced disorder, associated with chronic antischizophrenic drug therapy and
2) a degenerative disorder, Huntington's disease, involving loss of striatal neurons.

9.1. Chronic antischizophrenic drug treatment and the development of tardive dyskinesias

Based on the circuitry portrayed in Fig. 1 and 11, nigrostriatal DA neurons are responsible for adjusting the flow of information through striatum in order to keep pace with nigral (non-DA) efferent function. The blockade of striatal DA receptors by antischizophrenic drugs interrupts this feedback and causes a loss of GABAergic inhibitory activity in SN. At the same time, loss of DA inhibitory function in striatum probably allows cortical inputs to drive excitatory striatal outputs. The result is an increase in the ratio of excitatory (substance P?) to inhibitory (GABA) activity in the striatonigral pathway. When this situation is maintained by chronic drug treatment, nigral GABA receptors increase in response to the relative deficit in GABA activity.

By becoming more sensitive to GABA, the nigral cells would be less prone to disinhibition by the neuroleptic blockade of DA transmission. This adaptation could contribute to the development of tolerance to the cataleptogenic and Parkinson-like side effects of the classical antischizophrenic drugs.

With prolonged antischizophrenic drug treatment, the further development of supersensitivity to GABA in SN and, in addition, an enhanced sensitivity to DA, may combine to cause excessive inhibition of the non-DA nigral efferent pathways. Based on behavioral experiments in animals, excessive inhibition (e.g. GABAergic) in SN results in hyperactive and dyskinetic movement patterns. Thus, an increase in nigral GABA receptors may contribute to the tardive dyskinesias which develop with chronic neuroleptic treatment. Under these conditions, it is likely that DA continues to provide a stimulus for the release of GABA in SN, since

tardive dyskinesias can be suppressed by increasing the dose of DA antagonist. This is not an effective therapy, however, since the system continues to accomodate and the dyskinesias eventually re-emerge (164, 165).

If nigral GABA-receptor supersensitivity participates in the development of tardive dyskinesias, co-administration of a GABA receptor agonist with neuroleptic therapy might reduce the probability that these symptoms will emerge. Repeated administration of a GABA-receptor agonist can prevent the denervation-induced increase in GABA receptors in SN (75) and such treatment might similarly be able to counteract the influence of chronic neuroleptics on nigral GABA receptors. However, once dyskinesias have emerged, the stimulation of nigral GABA receptors (presumeably supersensitive) could actually worsen the severity of the abnormal movements by causing excessive inhibition of the non-DA nigral efferents.

The actions of an indirectly acting GABA agonist (e.g. a GABA-elevating agent, such as a GABA-T inhibitor) in an individual on chronic neuroleptic therapy might differ, in certain critical respects, from the actions of a GABA receptor agonist described above. The basis for the difference is the assumption that the GABA-elevating agent increases the amount of GABA available for release from the nerve-terminals; the liklihood that this GABA will interact with postsynaptic sites depends largely upon the activity of the presynaptic GABA terminal. Thus, elevation of GABA might be best utilized by the more active GABA synapses. This is in contrast to a directly-acting GABA receptor agonist that would act independently of presynaptic function; in fact, direct receptor agonists may actually have more pronounced effects at sites postsynaptic to a relatively *inactive* GABA terminal (e.g. at supersensitive receptors).

The following interactions might be postulated to take place in a situation in which a GABA-elevating agent is co-administered with a neuroleptic: Since the blockade of DA receptors results in a disinhibition of GABAergic striatal interneurons, a drug-induced GABA elevation would be utilized by these interneurons to further inhibit the striatonigral GABA projections. Thus, the combination of the GABA-elevating agent and neuroleptic might simply potentiate the short-term as well as long-term extrapyramidal effects of the neuroleptic. On the other hand, once nigral GABA receptors become supersensitive and tardive-dyskinesias emerge, treatment with a GABA-elevating agent might be useful in suppressing the symptoms of this disorder. In this case, one is interested in augmenting the function of the non-DA nigral efferents, some of which are GABAergic. A GABA-elevating agent could accomplish this by acting at two sites: 1) the striatum, to amplify the output of the GABA interneurons, and thus inhibit striatonigral fibers; and 2) the target areas of nigral GABAergic efferents (possibly tectum, thalamus or tegmentum), to amplify their inhibitory control on motor output. Unlike a direct GABA receptor agonist, a GABA-elevating agent would have relatively little impact on nigral GABA transmission because of the relative inactivity of these synapses in the presence of a neuroleptic. At least one clinical study with double-blind cross-over trials, has in fact demonstrated the effectiveness of DPA for suppressing dyskinetic movements associated with long-term neuroleptic treatment; this action of DPA was dependent upon the continued presence of the neuroleptic (166).

9.2. Huntington's disease

Of the various brain regions in which pathology can be found in Huntington's disease, the most striking is the striatum. There is marked loss of neural cells, striking decreases in the content of GABA and acetylcholine (1, 2) and a reduction in the density of muscarinic, DA and GABA binding sites (167–169). As a result of cell loss in the striatum, the nigral GABA and substance P levels are also decreased (170).

The pronounced decrease in GABA content in the basal ganglia of Huntington's disease brains has prompted interest in GABA agonist drugs as a possible therapeutic approach to this disorder. Due to the changes in neural circuitry associated with this disease, however, the action of GABA agonists may be mixed.

The most profound cells loss in the striatum is in the population of small neurons intrinsic to this nucleus. These would include the GABAergic interneurons, as well as the cholinergic cells. At the same time, DA concentrations are not significantly decreased, thus allowing a relative excess of inhibitory control on the few remaining GABA interneurons. As a result, the striatonigral GABA

pathways may be disinhibited. Although the striatal GABA efferents also undergo degeneration, the degree to which this occurs may not be as great as the degeneration associated with the small striatal interneurons (171, 172). Thus, despite some loss of the long striatonigral GABAergic neurons, it is nevertheless possible that the remaining nigral GABA afferents become overactive due to the loss of striatal regulation. This could result in excessive inhibition of non-DA nigral efferents. Moreover, the decrease in nigral substance P, a neurotransmitter candidate with excitatory actions on nigral neurons (37–42) could further enhance the net inhibitory impact of GABA on outputs from SN. Finally, some of the nigral reticulata cells themselves may be subject to pathological alteration. The net result of these imbalances would be a loss of activity in nigral efferents (possibly GABAergic) which normally exert inhibitory control on motor output.

Again, we have an example of a situation in which augmentation of GABAergic transmission could either exacerbate or suppress choreic symptoms depending on the major site of drug action. If, for arguments sake, we accept the hypothetical imbalances in activity proposed above, then augmentation of GABAergic function in the terminals of the nigral *efferent* projections would be therapeutic; increased GABAergic activity in *SN*, on the other hand, could be detrimental. While a GABA receptor agonist might not discriminate between these synapses, under certain circumstances a GABA-elevating agent might be able to preferentially enhance transmission at the 'therapeutic' site. This could be accomplished, for example by *combined* treatment with a DA receptor antagonist and a GABA-elevating agent. The DA receptor antagonist would indirectly cause the inhibition of striatonigral GABA activity, thereby reducing ongoing GABA transmission in SN. As a result, the nigral efferents will be disinhibited and, consequently, better able to utilize 'extra' GABA.

Administered alone, GABA agonist compounds have, in fact, met with relatively little success in the therapy of Huntington's disease (173). DA receptor antagonists are of significant, although very limited, value for controlling the choreic activity of these patients. Based on the analysis presented above, it would seem worthwhile to evaluate the effects of combined treatment with a GABA elevating agent and a DA antagonist. In 3 cases of Huntington's disease in which such a combination was tried (dipropylacetate and haloperidol) there was, in fact, marked clinical improvement when compared to haloperidol treatment alone (Dr. Stanley Cohan, personal communication). While the schemes described above are clearly speculative, they can serve as heuristic devices for generating novel approaches to pharmacological therapy.

10. Generalizations

This report has stressed the importance of GABA-containing neural sequences in the basal ganglia and the way in which they interact with DA, after both acute and chronic interventions. Although this is but one aspect of a dynamic system, the rich complexity of which we are only beginning to appreciate, the schemes presented in this report serve to illustrate certain features of these circuits which are of fundamental importance for preclinical neuropharmacology. These features may be summarized as follows:

1) As a consequence of the intricate functional relationships which exist between central neurotransmitter pathways, a chronic manipulation of one set of synapses will give rise to a series of transsynaptic changes. A cascade of adjustments could ensue, resulting in the reorganization of the original functional relationships. In situations in which the original relationships may have been pathological, their reorganization may be beneficial. Otherwise, such alterations may themselves be responsible for generating pathological patterns of activity. In the basal ganglia, the development of supersensitive GABA receptors in SN can occur as an indirect consequence of chronic DA receptor blockade. The subsequent response of the system to DA receptor stimulation may be altered as a result. Tardive-dyskinesias, which emerge after chronic neuroleptic therapy, may be a manifestation of this type of adjustment.

2) Patterns of activity and dynamic balances between components in a neural circuit are of much greater functional significance than the absolute quantity of a given component. Much in the same way that steady-state levels reveal little concerning neurotransmitter turnover, the numbers of neurons or their receptors tells us little of their functional activity. Thus, a partial loss of GABA neurons projecting to SN does not necessarily imply a loss of GABAergic function in SN; GABA receptor supersensitivity in SN, decreased striatal inhibition on striatonigral GABA projections) and reduction of the activity of transmitters with competing actions may all compensate (or even overcompensate) for the loss.

3) The level of ongoing activity at a particular synapse may be crucial for determining the impact of a drug on transmission at the synapse. Factors such as receptor occupancy and the rates of turnover and release of transmitter must be taken into account; in some circumstances these factors will influence the actions of direct receptor agonists and indirectly-acting agonists in opposite ways.

4) A drug which influences a particular transmitter system may simultaneously affect multiple neural projections which exert mutually opposing actions. This is particularly true for GABAergic systems which appear throughout the brain, often in sequential inhibitory links. The net drug effect will depend upon the respective activities of the various neural projections and the degree to which these have been altered by pathology or other drugs.

References

1. Perry, T. L., Hansen, S. & Kloster, M., 1973. Huntington's chorea. Deficiency of gamma-aminobutyric acid in brain. New Engl. J. Med. 288: 337–342.
2. McGeer, P. L. & McGeer, E. G., 1976. Enzymes associated with the metabolism of catecholamines, acetylcholine and GABA in human controls and patients with Parkinson's disease and Huntington's chorea. J. Neurochem. 26: 65–76.
3. McGeer, P. L., McGeer, E. G., Wada, J. A. & Jung, E., 1971. Effects of globus pallidus lesions and Parkinson's disease on brain glutamic acid decarboxylase. Brain Res. 32: 425–431.
4. Lloyd, K. G. & Hornykiewicz, O., 1973. L-Glutamic acid decarboxylase in Parkinson's disease: effect of l-dopa therapy. Nature, Lond. 243: 521–523.
5. McGeer, P. L., McGeer, E. G., Scherer, U. & Singh, K., 1977. A glutamatergic corticostriatal path? Brain Res. 128: 369–373.
6. Divac, I., Fonnum, F. & Storm-Mathisen, J., 1977. High affinity uptake of glutamate in terminals of corticostriatal axons. Nature, Lond. 266: 377–378.
7. Carpenter, M. B., 1976. Anatomical organization of the corpus striatum and related nuclei. In: The Basal Ganglia (M. D. Yahr, ed.) Raven Press, New York, pp. 1–35.

8. Hassler, R., 1978. Striatal control of locomotion, intentional actions and of integrating and perceptive activity. J. Neurol. Sci. 36: 187–224.

9. Ungerstedt, U., 1971. Stereotaxic mapping of the monoamine pathways in the rat brain. Acta Physiol. Scand., Suppl. 367: 1–48.

10. Lindvall, O. & Bjorklund, A., 1974. The organization of the ascending catecholamine neuron systems in the rat brain as revealed by the glyoxylic acid fluorescence method. Acta Physiol. Scand., Suppl. 412: 1–48.

11. Siggins, G. R., Hoffer, B. J., Bloom, F. E. & Ungerstedt, U., 1976. Cytochemical and electrophysiological studies of dopamine in the caudate nucleus. In: The Basal Ganglia (M. D. Yahr, ed.) Raven Press, New York, pp. 227–248.

12. Connor, J. D., 1970. Caudate nucleus neurones: correlation of the effects of substantia nigra stimulation with iontophoretic dopamine. J. Physiol., Lond. 208: 691–703.

13. Miller, J. J., Richardson, T. L., Fibiger, H. C. & McLennan, H., 1975. Anatomical and electrophysiological identification of a projection from the mesencephalic raphe to the caudate-putamen in the rat. Brain Res. 97: 133–138.

14. Samanin, R., Quattrone, A., Peri, G., Ladinsky, H. & Consolo, S., 1978. Evidence of an interaction between serotoninergic and cholinergic neurons in the corpus striatum and hippocampus of the rat brain. Brain Res 151. 73–82.

15. Olpe, H. R. & Koella, W. P., 1977. The response of striatal cells upon stimulation of the dorsal and medial raphe nuclei. Brain Res. 122: 357–360.

16. Ljungdahl, A., Hokfelt, T., Goldstein, M. & Park, D., 1975. Retrograde peroxidase tracing of neurons combined with transmitter histochemistry. Brain Res. 84: 313–319.

17. Fibiger, H. C., Pudritz, R. E., McGeer, P. L. & McGeer, E. G., 1972. Axonal transport in nigro-striatal and nigro-thalamic neurons: effects of medial forebrain bundle lesions and 6-hydroxydopamine. J. Neurochem. 19: 1697–1708.

18. Guyenet, P. G. & Aghajanian, G. K., 1978. Antidromic identification of dopaminergic and other output neurons of the rat substantia nigra. Brain Res. 150: 69–84.

19. Hattori, T., Singh, V. K., McGeer, E. G. & McGeer, P. L., 1976. Immunohistochemical localization of choline acetyltransferase containing neostriatal neurons and their relationship with dopaminergic synapses. Brain Res. 102: 164–173.

20. McGeer, P. L., McGeer, E. G., Fibiger, H. C. & Wickson, V., 1971. Neostriatal choline acetylase and cholinesterase following selective brain lesions. Brain Res. 35: 308–314.

21. McLennan, H. & York, D. H., 1966. Cholinergic mechanisms in the caudate nucleus. J. Physiol. 187: 163–175.

22. McGeer, P. L. & McGeer, E. G., 1975. Evidence for glutamic acid decarboxylase containing interneurons in the neostriatum. Brain Res. 91: 331–335.

23. Ribak, C. E., Vaughn, J. E. & Saito, K., 1978. Immunocytochemical localization of glutamic acid decarboxylase in neuronal somata following colchicine inhibition of axonal transport. Brain Res. 140: 315–332.

24. Ribak, C. E., Vaughn, J. E. & Roberts, E., 1979. The GABA neurons and their axon terminals in rat corpus striatum as demonstrated by GAD immunocytochemistry. J. Comp. Neurol. 187: 261–283.

25. Hong, J. S., Yang, H. Y. T. & Costa, E., 1977. On the location of methionine-enkephalin neurons in rat striatum. Neuropharm. 16: 451–453.

26. Schwarcz, R., Fuxe, K., Hokfelt, T., Terenius, L. & Goldstein, M., 1980. Effects of chronic striatal kainate lesions on some dopaminergic parameters and enkephalin immunoreactive neurons in the basal ganglia. J. Neurochem. 34: 772–778.

27. Pollard, H., Llorens, C., Schwartz, J. C., Gros, C. & Dray, F., 1978. Localization of opiate receptors and enkephalins in the rat striatum in relationship with the nigrostriatal dopaminergic system: Lesion studies. Brain Res. 151: 392–398.

28. Carenzi, A., Frigeni, V. & Della Bella, D., 1978. Synaptic localization of opiate receptors in rat striatum. Adv. Bioc. Psychopharm. 18: 265–270.

29. McGeer, E. G., Innanen, V. T. & McGeer, P. L., 1976. Evidence on the cellular localization of adenyl cyclase in the neostriatum. Brain Res. 118: 356–358.

30. Schwarcz, R., Creese, I., Coyle, J. T. & Snyder, S. H., 1978. Dopamine receptors localized on cerebral cortical afferents to rat corpus striatum. Nature, Lond. 271: 766–768.

31. Garau, L., Govoni, S., Stefanini, E., Trabucchi, M. & Spano, P. F., 1978. Dopamine receptors: pharmacological and anatomical evidence that two distinct dopamine receptor populations are present in rat striatum. Life Sci. 23: 1745–1750.

32. Creese, I., Usdin, T. & Snyder, S. H., 1979. Guanine nucleotides distinguish two dopamine receptors. Nature (Lond.) 278: 577–578.

33. Hattori, T., McGeer, P. L., Fibiger, H. C. & McGeer, E. G., 1973. On the source of GABA-containing terminals in the rat substantia nigra. Electron microscopic, autoradiographic and biochemical studies. Brain Res. 54: 103–114.

34. Ribak, C. E., Vaughn, J. E. & Roberts, E., 1980. GABAergic nerve terminals decrease in the substantia nigra following hemitransection of the striatonigral and pallidonigral pathways. Brain Res. 192: 413–420.

35. Precht, W. & Yoshida, M., 1971. Blockage of caudate-evoked inhibition of neurons in the substantia nigra by picrotoxin. Brain Res. 32: 229–233.

36. Minchin, M. C. W. & Fonnum, F., 1979. Metabolism of GABA and other amino acids in rat substantia nigra slices following lesions of the striatonigral pathway. J. Neurochem. 32: 203–209.

37. Kanazawa, I., Emson, P. C. & Cuello, A. C., 1977. Evidence for the existence of Substance P-containing fibers in striatonigral and pallidonigral pathways in rat brain. Brain Res. 119: 447–453.

38. Gale, K., Hong, J. S. & Guidotti, A., 1977. Presence of substance P and GABA in separate striatonigral neurons. Brain Res. 136: 371–375.

39. Davies, J. & Tongroach, P., 1979. Tetanus toxin and synaptic inhibition in the substantia nigra and striatum of the rat. J. Physiol. 290: 23–36.

40. Dray, A. & Straughn, D. W., 1978. Chemical transmission and the substantia nigra – some implications. In Chemical Communication Within the Nervous System and its Disturbance in Disease (A. Taylor & M. T. Jones, eds.) Pergamon Press, Oxford. pp. 65–82.

41. Walker, R. J., Kemp, J. A., Yajima, H., Kitagawa, K. & Woodruff, G. N., 1976. The action of substance P on mesencephalic reticular and substantia nigral neurones of the rat. Experientia 32: 214–215.

42. Davies, J. & Dray, A., 1976. Substance P in the substantia nigra. Brain Res. 107: 623–627.

43. Fonnum, F., Gottesfeld, Z. & Grofova, I., 1978. Distribution of glutamate decarboxylase, choline acetyltransferase and aromatic amino acid decarboxylase in the basal ganglia of normal and operated rats. Evidence for striato-pallidal, striatoentopeduncular and striatonigral GABA-ergic fibers. Brain Res. 143: 125–138.

44. Cuello, A. C. & Paxinos, G., 1978. Evidence for a long Leu-enkephalin striopallidal pathway in rat brain. Nature, Lond. 271: 178–180.

45. Cuello, A. C., 1978. Enkephalin and substance P containing neurons in the trigeminal and extrapyramidal systems. Adv. Bioc. Psychopharm. 18: 111–123.

46. Gale, K. & Iadarola, M. J., 1980. GABAergic denervation of rat substantia nigra: functional and pharmacological properties. Brain Res. 183: 217–223.

47. Bobillier, P., Seguin, S., Petitjean, F., Salvert, D., Touret, M. & Jouvet, M., 1976. The raphe nuclei of the cat brain stem: a topographic atlas of their efferent projections as revealed by autoradiography. Brain Res. 113: 449–486.

48. Palkovits, M., Saavedra, J. M., Jacobowitz, D. M., Kizer, J. S., Zaborszky, L. & Brownstein, M. J., 1977. Serotonergic innervation of the forebrain: effects of lesions on serotonin and tryptophan hydroxylase levels. Brain Res. 130: 121–134.

49. Dray, A., Davies, J., Oakley, N. R., Tongroach, P. & Vellucci, S., 1978. The dorsal and medial raphe projections to the substantia nigra in the rat: electrophysiological, biochemical and behavioral observations. Brain Res. 151: 431–442.

50. Dray, A., Gonye, T. J., Oakley, N. R. & Tanner, T., 1976. Evidence for the existence of a raphe projection to the substantia nigra in rat. Brain Res. 113: 45–57.

51. Graybiel, A. M., 1978. Organization in the nigrotectal connections: an experimental tracer study in the cat. Brain Res. 143: 339–348.

52. Hedreen, J. C., 1971. Separate demonstration of dopaminergic and non-dopaminergic projections of substantia nigra in the rat. Anat. Rec. 169: 338.

53. Beckstead, R. M., Domesick, V. B. & Nauta, W. J. H., 1979. Efferent connections of the substantia nigra and ventral tegmental area in the rat. Brain Res. 175: 191–217.

54. Jayaraman, A., Batton, R. R. & Carpenter, M. B., 1977. Nigrotectal projections in the monkey: an autoradiographic study. Brain Res. 135: 147–152.

55. Hopkins, D. A. & Niessen, L. W., 1976. Substantia nigra projections to the reticular formation, superior colliculus and central gray in the rat, cat and monkey. Neurosci. Lett. 2: 253–259.

56. Rinvik, E., Grofova, I. & Otterson, O. P., 1976. Demonstration of nigrotectal and nigroreticular projections in the cat by axonal transport of proteins. Brain Res. 112: 388–394.

57. Vincent, S. R., Hattori, T. & McGeer, E. G., 1978. The nigrotectal projection: a biochemical and ultrastructural characterization. Brain Res. 151: 159–164.

58. DiChiara, G., Porceddu, M. L., Morelli, M., Mulas, M. L. & Gessa, G. L., 1979. Evidence for a GABAergic projection from the substantia nigra to the ventromedial thalamus and to the superior colliculus of the rat. Brain Res. 176: 273–284.

59. Kilpatrick, I. C., Starr, M. S., Fletcher, A., James, T. A. & MacLeod, N. K., 1980. Evidence for a GABAergic nigro-thalamic pathway in the rat. I. Behavioral and Biochemical Studies. Exp. Brain Res. 40: 45–54.

60. MacLeod, N. K., James, T. A., Kilpatrick, I. C. & Starr, M. S., 1980. Evidence for a GABAergic nigrothalamic pathway in the rat. II. Electrophysiological studies. Exp. Brain Res. 40: 55–61.

61. Ribak, C. E., Vaughn, J. E., Saito, K., Barber, R. & Roberts, E., 1976. Immunocytochemical localization of glutamate decarboxylase in rat substantia nigra. Brain Res. 116: 287–298.

62. Hajdu, F., Hassler, R. & Bak, I. J., 1973. Electron microscopic study of the substantia nigra and the strianigral projection in the rat. Z. Zellforsch. Microsk. Anat. 146: 207–221.

63. McGeer, P. L., McGeer, E. G., Fibiger, H. C., Hattori, T., Singh, V. K. & Maler, L., 1974. Biochemical neuroanatomy of the basal ganglia. Adv. Behav. Biol. 10: 27–48.

64. Feltner, E. V., Meibach, R. C., Maayani, S. & Green, J. P., 1981. Radioautographic localization of ^{3}H-5-HT and ^{3}H-D-LSD binding sites on dopaminergic nigral-striatal neurons. Fed. Proc. 40: 265, Abst. #170.

65. Roberts, E., 1976. Disinhibition as an organizing principle in the nervous system: The role of the GABA system: Application to neurologic and psychiatric disorders. In: GABA in Nervous System Function. Raven Press, New York, pp. 515–540.

66. McLaughlin, B. J., Wood, J. G., Saito, K., Roberts, E. & Wu, J. Y., 1975. The fine structural localization of glutamate decarboxylase in developing axonal processes and presynaptic terminals of rodent cerebellum. Brain Res. 85: 355–371.

67. Fonnum, F., 1979. The localization of glutamate decarboxylase, choline acetyltransferase, and aromatic amino acid decarboxylase in mammalian and invertebrate nervous tissue. In: Metabolic Compartmentation and Neurotransmission (S. Berl, D. D. Clarke and D. Schneider, eds.) Plenum Press, N.Y. pp. 99–122.

68. Miller, L. P. & Walters, J. R., 1979. Effects of depolarization on cofactor regulation of glutamic acid decarboxylase in substantia nigra synaptosomes. J. Neurochem. 33: 533–539.

69. Gold, B. I. & Roth, R. H., 1979. Glutamate decarboxylase activity in striatal slices: characterization of the increase following depolarization. J. Neurochem. 32: 883–888.

70. Machiyama, Y., Balazs, R. & Richter, D., 1967. Effects of K$^+$-stimulation on GABA metabolism in brain slices in Vitro. J. Neurochem. 14: 591-594.

71. Mao, C. C. & Costa, E., 1978. Biochemical pharmacology of GABA transmission. In: Psychopharmacology: A Generation of Progress (M. A. Lipton, A. DiMascio & K. F. Killam, eds.), Raven Press, New York, pp. 307-318.

72. Neff, N. H. & Costa, E., 1968. Application of steady-state kinetics to the study of catecholamine turnover after monoamine oxidase inhibition or reserpine administration. J. Pharmacol. Exp. Therap. 160: 40-47.

73. Tozer, T. N., Neff, N. H. & Brodie, B. B., 1966. Application of steady state kinetics to the synthesis rate and turnover time of serotonin in the brain of normal and reserpine-treated rats. J. Pharmacol. Exp. 153: 177-182.

74. Waddington, J. L. & Cross, A. J., 1978. Denervation supersensitivity in the striatonigral GABA pathway. Nature, Lond. 276: 618-620.

75. Guidotti, A., Gale, K., Suria, A. & Toffano, G., 1979. Biochemical evidence for two classes of GABA receptors in rat brain. Brain Res. 172: 566-571.

76. Iadarola, M. J. & Gale, K., 1979. Dissociation between drug-induced increases in nerve terminal and non-nerve terminal pools of GABA in vivo. Eur. J. Pharmacol. 59: 125-129.

77. Gale, K. & Iadarola, M. J., 1980. Seizure protection and increased nerveterminal GABA: Delayed effects of GABA transaminase inhibition. Science (Wash. DC) 208: 288-291.

78. Iadarola, M. J. & Gale, K., 1980. GABA-elevating agents: Comparison of neurochemical and anticonvulsant effects in rats. In: Advances in Epileptology: XIth Epilepsy International Symposium (R. Canger, F. Angeleri & K. J. Penry, eds.), Raven Press, New York, pp. 449-455.

79. Iadarola, M. J. & Gale, K., 1980. Evaluation of increase in nerve terminal-dependent vs. nerve terminal-independent compartments of GABA in vivo. Brain Res. Bull. 5: suppl. 2, 13-19.

80. Lloyd, K. G., Shibuya, M., Davidson, L. & Hornykiewicz, O., 1977. Chronic neuroleptic therapy: Tolerance and GABA systems. Adv. Bioc. Psychopharm. 16: 409-415.

81. Gale, K. & Bernstein, H., 1981. Loss of neurochemical responses to acute and chronic haloperidol in the intact caudate-putamen of rats with unilateral lesions of nigro-striatal dopamine pathways. Soc. Neurosci. Abs. 274: 3.

82. Vincent, S. R., Nagy, J. I. & Fibiger, H. C., 1978. Increased striatal glutamate decarboxylase after lesions of the nigro-striatal pathway. Brain Res. 143: 168-173.

83. Casu, M. & Gale, K., 1981. Synthesis of GABA in caudate-putamen and substantia nigra in vivo: alterations induced by destruction of nigrostriatal dopamine neurons. Soc. Neurosci. Abst.

84. Schechter, P. J., Tranier, Y., Jung, M. J. & Bohlen, P., 1977. Audiogenic seizure protection by elevated brain GABA concentration in mice: effect of gamma-acetylenic GABA and gamma-vinyl GABA, two irreversible GABA-T inhibitors. Eur. J. Pharmac. 45: 319-328.

85. Loscher, W., 1980. A comparative study of the pharmacology of inhibitors of GABA-metabolism. Naunyn-Schmied. Arch. Pharmacol. 315: 119-128.

86. Lippert, B., Metcalf, B. W., Jung, M. J. & Casara, P., 1977. 4-Amino-hex-5-enoic acid, a selective catalytic inhibitor of 4-aminobutyric acid aminotransferase in mammalian brain. Eur. J. Biochem. 74: 441-445.

87. Casu, M. & Gale, K., 1981. Intracerebral injection of gamma-vinyl-GABA: Method for measuring rates of GABA synthesis in specific brain regions in vivo. Life Sci. 29: 681-688.

88. Mao, C. C., Cheney, D. L., Marco, E., Revuelta, A. & Costa, E., 1977. Turnover times of gamma-aminobutyric acid and acetylcholine in nucleus caudatus, nucleus accumbens, globus pallidus and substantia nigra: effects of repeated administration of haloperidol. Brain Res. 132: 375-379.

89. Marco, E., Mao, C. C., Cheney, D. L., Revuelta, A. & Costa, E., 1976. The effects of antipsychotics on the turnover rate of GABA and acetylcholine in rat brain nuclei, Nature, Lond. 264: 363-365.

90. Moroni, F., Peralta, E. & Costa, E., 1978. Turnover rates of GABA in striatal structures: Regulation and pharmacological implications. In: GABA-Neuro-transmitters (P. Krogsgaard-Larsen, J. Scheel-Kruger & H. Kofod, eds.), Munksgaard, Copenhagen, pp. 95-106.

91. Gale, K., 1980. Chronic blockade of dopamine receptors by antischizophrenic drugs enhances GABA binding in substantia nigra. Nature (Lond.) 283: 569-570.

92. Gale, K., 1980. Alteration of GABA receptors in rat substantia nigra after chronic treatment with antischizophrenic drugs. Brain Res. Bull. 5: Suppl. 2, 897-904.

93. Gale, K., 1980. Effects of chronic neuroleptic treatment on tyrosine hydroxylase in dopaminergic terminals: Comparisons between drugs and brain regions reveals different mechanisms of tolerance. In: Long-Term Effects of Neuroleptics, Pharmacological Basis and Clinical Implications (G. Racagni, F. Cattabeni, P. F. Spano & E. Costa, eds.), Raven ress, New York. pp. 23-29.

94. Hauser, D. & Closse, A., 1978. ^{3}H-Clozapine binding to rat brain membranes. Life Sci. 23: 557-562.

95. Miller, R. J. & Hiley, C. R., 1974. Anti-muscarinic properties of neuroleptics and drug-induced Parkinsonism. Nature 248: 596-597.

96. Gerlach, J., Koppelhus, P., Helweg, E. & Monrad, A., 1974. Clozapine and haloperidol in a single-blind cross-over trial: Therapeutic and biochemical aspects in the treatment of schizophrenia. Acta Psychiat. Scand. 50: 410-424.

97. Costall, B. & Naylor, R. J., 1975. Detection of the neuroleptic properties of clozapine, sulpiride and thioridazine. Psychopharmacology 43: 69-74.

98. Scheel-Kruger, J., Arnt, J. & Magelund, G., 1977. Behavioral stimulation induced by muscimol and other GABA agonists injected into the substantia nigra. Neurosci. Lett. 4: 351-356.

99. Scheel-Kruger, J., Arnt, J., Braestrup, C., Christensen, A. V. & Magelund, G., 1978. Development of new animal models for GABAergic actions using muscimol as a tool. In: GABA-Neurotransmitters (P. Krogsgaard-Larsen, J. Scheel-Kruger & H. Kofod, eds.), Munkgaard, Copenhagen, pp. 447-464.

100. Arnt, J. & Scheel-Kruger, J., 1979. GABAergic and glycinergic mechanisms within the substantia nigra: Pharmacological specificity of dopamine-independent contralateral turning behavior and interactions with other neurotransmitters. Psychopharm. 62: 267–277.

101. Oberlander, C., Dumont, C. & Boissier, J. R., 1977. Rotational behavior after unilateral intranigral injection of muscimol in rats. Eur. J. Pharmac. 43: 389–390.

102. Dray, A. & Straughan, D. W., 1976. Synaptic mechanisms in the substantia nigra. J. Pharm. Pharmacol. 28: 400–405.

103. Aghajanian, G. K. & Bunney, B. S., 1975. Dopaminergic and nondopaminergic neurons of the substantia nigra: differential responses to putative transmitters. In: Neuropsychopharmacology (J. R. Boissier, H. Hippius & D. Pichot, eds.), Excerpta Medica, Elsevier, Amsterdam, vol. 359: pp. 444–452.

104. Karabelas, A. B. & Purpura, D. P., 1979. Functional properties of dorsal raphe-substantia nigra projections in the cat. Soc. Neurosci., Abst. #238.

105. Guidotti, A., Gale, K., Hong, J. & Toffano, G., 1978. Models to study drug effects on the integrated function of GABAergic, peptidergic (substance P), and dopaminergic neurons. In: Interactions Between Putative Neurotransmitters in the Brain (S. Garattini, J. F. Pujol & S. Samanin, eds.), Raven Press, New York, pp. 217–229.

106. Roth, R. H., Walters, J. R., Murrin, L. C. & Morgenroth, V. H., 1975. In: Pre- and Postsynaptic Receptors (E. Usdin & W. E. Bunney, eds.), Masrcel-Dekker, New York, pp. 5–48.

107. Bunney, B. S., Walters, J. R., Roth, R. H. & Aghajanian, G. K., 1973. Dopaminergic neurons: Effect of antipsychotic drugs and amphetamine on single cell activity. J. Pharmacol. Exp. Therap. 185: 560–571.

108. Anden, N. E., Butcher, S. G., Corrodi, H., Fuxe, K. & Ungerstedt, U., 1970. Receptor activity and turnover of dopamine and noradrenaline after neuroleptics. Eur. J. Pharmacol. 11: 303–314.

109. Zivkovic, B., Guidotti, A., Revuelta, A. & Costa, E., 1975. Effects of thioridazine, clozapine, and other antipsychotics on the kinetic state of tyrosine hydroxylase on the turnover rate of dopamine in striatum and nucleus accumbens. J. Pharmac. Exp. Ther. 194: 37–46.

110. Zivkovic, B. & Guidotti, A., 1974. Changes of kinetic constant of striatal tyrosine hydroxylase elicited by neuroleptics that impair the function of dopamine receptors. Brain Res. 79: 505–509.

111. Zivkovic, B., Guidotti, A. & Costa, E., 1974. Effects of neuroleptics on striatal tyrosine hydroxylase: Changes in affinity for the pteridine cofactor. Mol. Pharm. 10: 727–735.

112. Gale, K., Costa, E., Toffano, G., Hong, J. S. & Guidotti, A., 1978. Evidence for a role of nigral gamma-aminobutyric acid and substance P in the haloperidol-induced activation of striatal tyrosine hydroxylase. J. Pharmac. Exp. Ther. 206: 29–37.

113. Gale, K. & Guidotti, A., 1976. GABA-mediated control of rat neostriatal tyrosine hydroxylase revealed by intranigral muscimol. Nature, Lond. 263: 691–693.

114. Tapia, R., 1975. Biochemical pharmacology of GABA in CNS. In: Handbook of Psychopharmacology, Plenum Press, New York, pp. 1–58.

115. Loscher, W. & Frey, H. H., 1978. Amino-oxyacetic acid: correlation between biochemical effects, anticonvulsant action and toxicity in mice. Biochem. Pharmacol. 27: 103–108.

116. Godin, Y., Heiner, L., Mark, J. & Mandel, P., 1969. Effects of di-n-propylacetate, an anticonvulsive compound, on GABA metabolism. J. Neurochem. 16: 869–873.

117. Sawaya, M. C. B., Horton, R. W. & Meldrum, B. S., 1975. Effects of anticonvulsant drugs on the cerebral enzymes metabolizing GABA. Epilepsia 16: 649–655.

118. Sarhan, S. & Seiler, N., 1979. Metabolic inhibitors and subcellular distribution of GABA. J. Neurosci. Res. 4: 399–421.

119. Waniewski, R. A. & Suria, A., 1977. Alterations in gamma-aminobutyric acid content in the rat superior cervical ganglion and pineal gland. Life Sci. 21: 1129–1142.

120. Wood, J. D., Kurylo, E. & Newstead, J. D., 1978. Aminooxyacetic acid induced changes in gamma-aminobutyrate metabolism at the subcellular level. Canadian J. Biochem. 56: 667–672.

121. Gale, K. & Iadarola, M. J., 1980. Drug-induced elevation of GABA after intracerebral microinjection: Site of anticonvulsant action. Eur. J. Pharmacol. 68: 233–235.

122. Walters, J. R., Lakoski, J. M., Eng, N. & Waszczak, B. L., 1978. Effect of muscimol, AOAA and Na valproate on the activity of dopamine neurons and dopamine synthesis. In: GABA-Neurotransmitters, Alfred Benzon Symposium, ed. by P. Krogsgaard-Larsen, J. Scheel-Kruger and H. Kofod, pp. 119–133, Munksgaard, Copenhagen, 1978.

123. Scheel-Kruger, J., Arnt, J., Braestrup, C., Christensen, A. V. & Magelund, G., 1978. Development of new animal models for GABAergic actions using muscimol as a tool. In: GABA-Neutrotransmitters, Alfred Benzon Symposium, ed. by P. Krogsgaard-Larsen, J. Scheel-Kruger and H. Kofod, pp. 447–464, Munksgaard, Copenhagen.

124. Bartholini, G., Scatton, B., Zivkovic, B. & Lloyd, K. G., 1978. On the mode of action of SL 76002, a new GABA receptor agonist. In: GABA Neurotransmitters (P. Krogsgaard-Larsen, J. Scheel-Kruger & H. Kofod, eds.). Munkgaard, Copenhagen pp. 326–329.

125. Palfreyman, M. G., Huot, S., Lippert, B. & Schechter, P. J., 1978. GABA-Dopamine interactions: Studies using a new enzyme-activated irreversible inhibitor of GABA transaminase, gamma-acetylenic-GABA. In: GABA Neurotransmitters (P. Krogsgaard-Larsen, J. Scheel-Kruger & H. Kofod, eds.), Munksgaard, Copenhagen, pp. 432–446.

126. Waldmeier, P. C., personal communication.

127. Matsui, Y. & Kamioka, T., 1978. The effects of elevating gamma-amino butyrate content in substantia nigra on the behavior of rats. Eur. J. Pharmacol. 50: 243–251.

128. Biggio, G., Casu, M., Corda, M. G., Vernaleone, F. & Gessa, G. L., 1977. Effect of muscimol, a GABA mimetic agent, on dopamine metabolism in the mouse brain, Life Sci. 21: 525–532.

129. Carlsson, A., Biswas, B. & Lindquist, M., 1977. Influence of GABA and GABA-like drugs on monoaminergic mechanisms. Adv. Bioc. Psychopharm. 16: 471–475.

130. Cheramy, A., Nieoullon, A. & Glowinski, J., 1978. GABAergic processes involved in the control of dopamine release from nigrostriatal dopaminergic neurons in the cat. Eur. J. Pharmacol. 48: 281–295.

404

131. Martin, G. E. & Haubrich, D. R., 1978. Striatal dopamine release and contraversive rotation elicited by intranigrally applied muscimol. Nature 275: 230–231.

132. MacNeil, D., Gower, M. & Szymanska, I., 1978. Response of dopamine neurons in substantia nigra to muscimol. Brain Res. 154: 401–403.

133. Grace, A. A. & Bunney, B. S., 1979. Paradoxical GABA excitation of nigral dopaminergic cells: indirect mediation through reticulata inhibitory neurons. Eur. J. Pharmacol. 59: 211–218.

134. Waszczak, B., Eng, N. & Walters, J. R., 1980. Effects of muscimol and picrotoxin on single unit activity of substantia nigra neurons. Brain Research 188: 185–197.

135. Waszczak, B. L. & Walters, J. R., 1980. Do substantia nigra pars reticulata neurons become supersensitive to GABAergic drugs after striatal kainic acid lesions? Poster presentation at 10th Annual Mtg. of Soc. Neurosci. Cincinnati, Ohio.

136. Soubrie, P., Montastruc, J. L., Bourgoin, S., Reisine, T., Artaud, F. & Glowinski, J., 1981. In vivo evidence for GABAergic control of serotonin release in the cat substantia nigra. Eur. J. Pharmacol. 69: 483–488.

137. Giambalvo, C. T. & Snodgrass, S. R., 1978. Biochemical and behavioral effects of serotonin neurotoxins on the nigrostriatal dopamine system: Comparison of injection sites. Brain Research 152: 555–566.

138. Bentivoglio, M., Van der Kooy, D., Kuypers, H. G. J. M., 1979. The organization of the efferent projections of the substantia nigra of the rat. A retrograde fluorescent double labelling study. Brain Res. 174: 1–17.

139. Anderson, M. & Yoshida, M., 1977. Electrophysiological evidence for branching nigral projections to the thalamus and superior colliculus. Brain Res. 137: 361–364.

140. Deniau, J. M., Hammond, C., Riszk, A. & Feger, J., 1978. Electrophysiological properties of identified output neurons in the rat substantia nigra (pars compacta and pars reticulata): Evidence for the existence of branched neurons. Exp. Brain Res. 32: 409–422.

141. Guyenet, P. G. & Aghajanian, G. K., 1978. Antidromic identification of dopaminergic and other output neurones of the rat substantia nigra. Brain Res. 150: 69–84.

142. Yoshida, M. & Omata, S., 1979. Blocking by picrotoxin of nigra-evoked inhibition of neurons of ventromedial nucleus of the thalamus. Experientia 35: 794.

143. Ueki, A., Uno, M., Anderson, M. & Yoshida, M., 1977. Monosynaptic inhibition of thalamic neurons produced by stimulation of the substantia nigra. Experientia 33: 1480–1482.

144. Karabelas, A. B. & Purpura, D. P., 1980. Axon collaterals of substantia nigra pars reticulata neurons. Soc. Neurosci. Abst. #124.7.

145. Gale, K., 1979. GABA receptors in rat substantia nigra: changes in response to lesions and chronic drug treatment. Soc. Neurosci. Abstr. No. 231.

146. Motamedi, F. & York, D. H., 1978. A descending pathway involving nigral-induced head turning movements. Soc. Neurosci. Abstract #142.

147. York, D. H. & Faber, J. E., 1977. An electrophysiological study of nigrotectal relationships: a possible role in turning behavior. Brain Research 130: 383–386.

148. Arnt, J., Scheel-Kruger, J., Magelund, G. & Krogsgaard-Larsen, P., 1979. Muscimol and related GABA receptor agonists: the potency of GABAergic drugs in vivo determined after intranigral injection. J. Pharm. Pharmacol. 31: 306–313.

149. DeMontis, G. M., Olianas, M. C., Serra, G., Tagliamonte, A. & Scheel-Kruger, J., 1979. Evidence that a nigral GABAergic-cholinergic balance controls posture. Eur. J. Pharmacol. 53: 181–190.

150. Klawans, H. L. & Rubovits, R., 1972. An experimental model of tardive dyskinesia. J. Neural Transm. 33: 235–246.

151. Tarsy, D. & Baldessarini, R. J., 1974. Behavioral supersensitivity to apomorphine following chronic treatment with drugs which interfere with the synaptic function of the catecholamines. Neuropharm. 13: 927–940.

152. Creese, I., Burt, D. R. & Snyder, S. H., 1977. Dopamine receptor binding enhancement accompanies lesion-induced behavioral supersensitivity. Science 197: 596–598.

153. Ungerstedt, U., 1971. Postsynaptic supersensitivity after 6-hydroxydopamine induced degeneration of the nigrostriatal dopamine system in the rat brain. Acta Physiol. Scand. 82: Suppl. 367: 69–93.

154. Gale, K., Guidotti, A. & Costa, E., 1977. Dopamine-sensitive adenylate cyclase: Location in substantia nigra. Science 195: 503–505.

155. Premont, J., Thierry, A. M., Tassin, J. P., Glowinski, J., Blanc, G. & Bockaert, J., 1976. FEBS Letters 68: 99–104.

156. Kozlowski, M. R., Sawyer, S. & Marshall, J. F., 1980. Behavioral effects and supersensitivity following nigral dopamine receptor stimulation. Nature, Lond. 287: 52–54.

157. List, S. & Seeman, P., 1980. Neuroleptic/Dopamine receptors: Elevation and reversal. Adv. Bioc. Psychopharmacol. 24: 95–101.

158. Neve, K., personal communication.

159. Staunton, D. A., Wolfe, B. B., Groves, P. M. & Molinoff, P. B., 1981. Dopamine receptor changes following destruction of the nigrostriatal pathway: Lack of a relationship to rotational behavior. Brain Research 211: 315–327.

160. Mailman, R. B., Kilts, C. D., Beamont, K. & Breese, G. R., 1981. 'Supersensitivity' of dopamine systems: Comparisons between haloperidol withdrawal, intracisternal, and unilateral 6-hydroxydopamine treatments. Fed. Proc. 40: 291.

161. Bartholini, G., Scatton, B. & Zivkovic, B., 1980. Effect of the new gamma-aminobutyric acid agonist SL 76002 on striatal acetylcholine: Relation to neuroleptic-induced extrapyramidal alterations. Adv. Bioc. Psychopharm. 24: 207–213.

162. Ferkany, J. W., Strong, R. & Enna, S. J., 1980. Dopamine receptor supersensitivity in the corpus striatum following chronic elevation of brain gamma-aminobutyric acid. J. Neurochem.

163. Lloyd, K. G. & Worms, P., 1980. Sustained gamma-aminobutyric acid receptor stimulation and chronic neuroleptic effects. Adv. Bioc. Psychopharm. 24: 253–258.

164. Baldessarini, R. J. & Tarsy, D., 1978. Tardive dyskinesia. In: Psychopharmacology: A Generation of Progress (M. A. Lipton, A. DiMascio & K. F. Killam, eds.), Raven Press, N.Y. pp. 993–1004.

165. Marsden, C. D., Tarsy, D. & Baldessarini, R. J., 1975. Spontaneous and drug-induced movement disorders in psychiatric patients. In: Psychiatric Aspects of Neurologic Disease (D. F. Benson & D. Blumers, eds.), Grune and Stratton, N.Y. pp. 219–265.

166. Nair, N. P. V., Lal, S., Schwartz, G. & Thavundayil, J. X., 1980. Effect of sodium valproate and baclofen in tardive dyskinesia: clinical and neuroendocrine studies. Adv. Bioc. Psychopharm. 24: 437–441.

167. Hiley, C. R. & Bird, E. D., 1974. Decreased muscarinic receptor concentration in postmortem brain in Huntington's chorea. Brain Res. 80: 355–358.

168. Reisine, T. D., Fields, J. Z., Stern, L. Z., Johnson, P. C., Bird, E. D. & Yamamura, H. I., 1977. Alterations in dopaminergic receptors in Huntington's disease. Life Sci. 21: 1123–1128.

169. Enna, S. J., Bennet, J. P., Bylund, D. B., Bird, E. D., Iversen, L. L. & Snyder, S. H., 1976. Alterations of brain neurotransmitter receptor binding in Huntington's chorea. Brain Res. 116: 531–537.

170. Kanazawa, I., Bird, E., O'Connell, R. & Powell, D., 1977. Evidence for decrease in substance P content of substantia nigra in Huntington's chorea. Brain Res. 120: 387–392.

171. Lange, H., Thorner, G., Hopf, A. & Schroder, K. F., 1976. Morphometric studies of the neuropathological changes in choreatic diseases. J. Neurol. Sci. 28: 401–425.

172. Dom, R., Baro, F. & Brucher, J. M., 1973. A cytometric study of the putamen in different types of Huntington's chorea. Adv. Neurol. 1: 369–385.

174. Enna, S. J. & Snyder, S. H., 1977. Influence of ions, enzymes and detergents on gamma-aminobutyric acid receptor binding in synaptic membranes of rat brain. Molec. Pharmac. 13: 442–453.

175. Toffano, G., Guidotti, A. & Costa, E., 1978. Purification of an endogenous protein inhibitor for the high binding affinity of gamma-aminobutyric acid to synaptic membranes of rat brain. Proc. Nat. Acad. Sci., U.S.A. 75: 4024–4028.

176. Gale, K., 1981. Relationship between the presence of dopaminergic neurons and GABA receptors in substantia nigra: Effects of lesions. Brain Res. 210: 401–406.

177. Casu, M. & Gale, K., 1981. Effects of gamma-vinyl-GABA on dopamine neurons: Relationship between elevation of GABA in nerve terminals and change in tyrosine hydroxylase activity. Fed. Proc. 40: 290.

178. Gale, K. & Bernstein, H., 1980. Development of supersensitive GABA receptors in substantia nigra after either chronic blockade of dopamine receptors or destruction of nigrostriatal dopamine neurons. Soc. Neurosci. Abst. #124.9.

179. Casu, M. & Gale, K., 1981. Differential effects of GABA-elevating agents on the neuroleptic-induced activation of striatal tyrosine hydroxylase: Evidence that di-n-propylacetate augments GABAergic neurotransmission. J. Pharm. Exp. Therap. 217: 177–180.

180. Childs, J. A. & Gale, K., 1981. Neurochemical characterization of the nigrotegmental projections in the rat. Soc. Neurosci. Abst. 64: 21.